Handbook of Psychiatry

Handbook of Psychiatry

Editor: Fernando Hogan

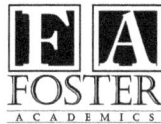

FOSTER ACADEMICS

www.fosteracademics.com

www.fosteracademics.com

F A
FOSTER
ACADEMICS

Cataloging-in-Publication Data

Handbook of psychiatry / edited by Fernando Hogan.
    p. cm.
Includes bibliographical references and index.
ISBN 978-1-63242-783-0
1. Psychiatry. 2. Psychology, Pathological. 3. Mental health. 4. Medicine and psychology.
I. Hogan, Fernando.
RC456 .H36 2019
616.89--dc23

Foster Academics,
118-35 Queens Blvd., Suite 400,
Forest Hills, NY 11375, USA

ISBN 978-1-63242-783-0 (Hardback)

Contents

Preface

The world is advancing at a fast pace like never before. Therefore, the need is to keep up with the latest developments. This book was an idea that came to fruition when the specialists in the area realized the need to coordinate together and document essential themes in the subject. That's when I was requested to be the editor. Editing this book has been an honour as it brings together diverse authors researching on different streams of the field. The book collates essential materials contributed by veterans in the area which can be utilized by students and researchers alike.

Psychiatry is a branch of medicine concerned with the diagnosis, prevention and treatment of mental disorders. The assessment of a patient's condition usually begins with a case history and mental status examination. In order to obtain the case history of the patient, the psychiatrist asks the patient several questions. The answers to those questions aid the psychiatrist in the diagnosis and treatment process. A mental status examination is meant to assess a patient's mental state at a fixed point of time, by observing his appearance, attitude, speech, mood, behaviour and thought process. It is very useful in assessing a person's suicidal thoughts. This book unfolds the innovative aspects of psychiatry which will be crucial for the progress of this field in the future. It studies, analyzes and upholds the pillars of psychiatry and its utmost significance in modern times. Students, researchers, experts and all associated with psychiatry will benefit alike from this book.

Each chapter is a sole-standing publication that reflects each author's interpretation. Thus, the book displays a multi-facetted picture of our current understanding of application, resources and aspects of the field. I would like to thank the contributors of this book and my family for their endless support.

Editor

The relationship between dispositional empathy, psychological distress, and posttraumatic stress responses among Japanese uniformed disaster workers

Masanori Nagamine[1]* (iD), Jun Shigemura[2], Toshimichi Fujiwara[3], Fumiko Waki[3], Masaaki Tanichi[2], Taku Saito[2], Hiroyuki Toda[2], Aihide Yoshino[2] and Kunio Shimizu[1]

Abstract

Background: Disaster workers suffer from psychological distress not only through the direct experience of traumatic situations but also through the indirect process of aiding disaster victims. This distress, called secondary traumatic stress, is linked to dispositional empathy, which is the tendency for individuals to imagine and experience the feelings and experiences of others. However, the association between secondary traumatic stress and dispositional empathy remains understudied.

Methods: To examine the relationship between dispositional empathy and mental health among disaster workers, we collected data from 227 Japan Ground Self-Defense Force personnel who engaged in international disaster relief activities in the Philippines following Typhoon Yolanda in 2013. The Impact of Event Scale-Revised and the Kessler Psychological Distress Scale were used to evaluate posttraumatic stress responses (PTSR) and general psychological distress (GPD), respectively. Dispositional empathy was evaluated through the Interpersonal Reactivity Index, which consists of four subscales: Perspective Taking, Fantasy, Empathic Concern, and Personal Distress. Hierarchial linear regression analyses were performed to identify the variables related to PTSR and GPD.

Results: High PTSR was significantly associated with high *Fantasy* (identification tendency, $\beta = 0.21$, $p < .01$), high *Personal Distress* (the self-oriented emotional disposition of empathy, $\beta = 0.18$, $p < .05$), and no experience of disaster relief activities ($\beta = 0.15$, $p < .05$). High GPD was associated with high *Personal Distress* ($\beta = 0.28$, $p < .001$), marital status (married, $\beta = 0.22$, $p < .01$), being female ($\beta = 0.18$, $p < .01$), medical unit ($\beta = 0.18$, $p < .05$), and no experience of disaster relief activities ($\beta = 0.13$, $p < .05$).

Conclusions: Among Japanese uniformed disaster workers, high PTSR was associated with two subtypes of dispositional empathy: the self-oriented emotional disposition of empathy and high identification tendency, whereas high GPD was associated with high identification tendency. Educational interventions that aim to mitigate these tendencies might be able to relieve the psychological distress of disaster workers.

Keywords: Disaster workers, Empathy, Interpersonal reactivity index, Identification, Secondary traumatic stress, Posttraumatic stress response, Psychological distress

* Correspondence: nagaminemasanori@gmail.com
[1]Division of Behavioral Science, National Defense Medical College Research Institute, 3-2 Namiki, Tokorozawa, Saitama 359-8513, Japan
Full list of author information is available at the end of the article

Background

On November 8, 2013, Typhoon Yolanda struck the Philippines and caused large-scale damage: 6300 individuals were killed, 28,688 were injured, and 1062 were missing [1]. The Japanese government responded to a humanitarian assistance request from the Filipino government and sent Japan Self-Defense Forces' personnel to the affected area. Disaster relief activities consisted of medical assistance, epidemic prevention, and transport of relief supplies [2], which continued until December 18, 2013.

Disasters result in mental health distress not only among survivors but also among disaster workers [3, 4]. These individuals have the burden of rescuing lives in disaster-stricken sites fraught with life-threatening danger. In addition to such direct traumatic stresses, disaster workers can also experience indirect psychological effects of aiding disaster victims, which is defined as secondary traumatic stress [5]. These psychological effects can result in various reactions, including depression and anxiety disorder, in addition to stress-related disorders, such as acute and post-traumatic stress disorder [6]. According to a recent meta-analysis, the pooled prevalence of posttraumatic stress disorder among rescue workers was 10% [7], indicating the magnitude of their work-related traumatic experience on worker's mental health. Countermeasures for work-related traumatic stress are crucial for disaster workers to prevent adverse mental health outcomes. Coping strategies to mitigate such impacts include sufficient training prior to missions [8–10], awareness of and pride in one's duties [11, 12], and humor [8, 13, 14]. Minimization of excessive empathy and identification with victims is also recommended to prevent traumatic stress [8, 15–17], which is supported by two empirical studies [15, 17].

Empathy is a multi-dimensional concept with emotional and cognitive components [18]. Davis defined empathy as the "reactions of one individual to the observed experiences of another" and developed the Interpersonal Reactivity Index (IRI), which is a multi-dimensional scale of empathic traits [19]. The IRI consists of four subscales: Perspective Taking (PT; the tendency to spontaneously adopt the psychological point of view of others), Fantasy (FS; the respondents' tendencies to transpose themselves imaginatively into the feelings and actions of fictitious characters in books, movies, and plays), Empathic Concern (EC; "other-oriented" feelings of sympathy and concern for unfortunate others), and Personal Distress (PD; "self-oriented" feelings of personal anxiety and unease in tense interpersonal settings). Although the construct of self-oriented negative feeling (e.g., PD) is not included in the narrowly defined empathy [20], IRI provides multifaceted information on aspects of dispositional empathy and thus, is one of the most widely used measures to evaluate empathy [21].

As to the relationships between empathy and secondary traumatic stress, Figley reported that individuals who have a great capacity to feel and express empathy tend to be more vulnerable to the traumatic stress in his studies of healthcare workers [22]. Klimecki and Singer suggest that the consequence of empathy take on two paths; one is an "other-oriented," or compassion that results in prosocial motivation or positive feelings, and the other is a "self-oriented" personal distress that results in withdrawal or the experience of negative feelings [23]. In disaster workers, the latter path might explain their development of posttraumatic stress responses. However, to the best of our knowledge, the relationship between the empathy and secondary traumatic stress has yet to be fully investigated. To expand the theoretical and professional knowledge regarding secondary traumatic stress in the field of traumatic stress, we examined the relationships between dispositional empathy (measured with the IRI) and mental health (posttraumatic stress and psychological distress) among Japan Ground Self-Defense Force (JGSDF) personnel who were deployed on a humanitarian mission in response to the disaster of Typhoon Yolanda in 2013.

Methods

Participants and procedure

This survey was conducted as part of the mandatory occupational health management of all JGSDF personnel who were engaged in the humanitarian mission after Typhoon Yolanda ($N = 283$). The self-report survey was administered immediately after they returned home using registered (i.e., non-anonymous) forms. Of all the personnel, only 227 participated and provided written consent (response rate: 80.2%).

Psychological evaluation

We assessed two outcome measures—posttraumatic stress responses (PTSR) and general psychological distress (GPD)—using the Japanese versions of the Impact of Events Scale-Revised (IES-R) [24] and the Kessler Psychological Distress Scale (K10) [25], respectively. The IES-R is a 22-item self-administered questionnaire (score range: 0–88) that is used to evaluate three domains of PTSR—intrusion, avoidance, and hyperarousal—following a traumatic event [26]. The K10 is a 10-item self-administered questionnaire (score range: 10–50) that was developed by Kessler [27] and is widely used as a tool for evaluating GPD. The originally reported Cronbach's alpha for internal consistency was 0.91 for the K10 [28] and 0.92 to 0.95 for the IES-R [24]. In this study, Cronbach's alphas of 0.91 for the IES-R and 0.89 for the K10 were obtained.

Dispositional empathy was evaluated using the IRI [19]. The IRI is a 28-item self-report measure answered on a 5-point Likert scale. It consists of four subscales (PT, FS, EC, and PD), and each subscale contains seven different items (score ranges from 0 to 28). A previous paper reported Cronbach's alphas of 0.65 for PT, 0.76 for FS, 0.77 for EC, and 0.76 for PD [29]. In this study we obtained Cronbach's alphas of 0.63 for PT, 0.62 for FS, 0.57 for EC, and 0.65 for PD.

In addition to these psychological measures, the following information was collected based on the previous report by Berger and colleagues [7]: age, sex, marital status, rank, unit (e.g., medical, airlift, others), previous disaster relief experience, exposure to human bodies during relief efforts, and previous psychiatric treatment history.

Statistical analyses

First, Pearson correlation analyses were performed to explore the correlation between dispositional empathy and PTSR or GPD. Second, analysis of variance was used for the univariate analyses of each personal attribute. Finally, hierarchical linear regression analyses were conducted to investigate factors related to PTSR and GPD. In Step 1, personal attributes including age, sex, marital status, previous deployment experience, psychiatric treatment history were entered as covariates. In Step 2, work-related factors such as rank, unit (e.g., medical or airlift), and exposure to bodies were added as covariates. In Step 3, dispositional empathy evaluated using the four subscales of the IRI (PT, FS, EC, and PD) that were entered as predictor variables.

We used a significance level of $p < .05$. IBM SPSS Statistics for Windows version 22 was used for the statistical tests [30].

Results

Personal attributes and the results of the univariate analyses

The average age of the participants was 35.59 ± 7.99 years (mean $\pm SD$). As Table 1 demonstrates, those with no previous disaster relief experience scored significantly higher on both PTSR and GPD than those with previous disaster relief experience. In addition, women, officers, and individuals assigned to medical units showed significantly higher scores on GPD than did men, those who were Enlisted/Private, and individuals assigned to "others" units, respectively.

Psychological measures and correlation analyses

Table 2 presents the summary statistics for the psychological measures and the results of the Pearson correlation analyses between the measures. IES-R was significantly correlated with two IRI subscales: FS ($r = .28$, $p < .001$) and PD ($r = .25$, $p < .001$). K10 showed a significant correlation with three IRI subscales: PD ($r = .35$, $p < .001$), FS ($r = .23$, $p < .001$), and EC ($r = .18$, $p < .01$). There were significant correlations between the IRI subscales, except for PT and PD.

Table 1 Personal attributes and the results of the univariate analyses

	N	%	PTSR Mean	SD	GPD Mean	SD
Sex						
Male	214	94.3	4.6	6.7	12.7	3.6
Female	13	5.7	7.7	6.3	17.2***	8.0
Marital status						
Single	81	35.7	4.0	5.9	12.4	3.5
Married	146	64.3	5.2	7.1	13.2	4.4
Rank						
Enlisted/Private	143	63.0	4.3	5.8	12.3	3.1
Officer	84	37.0	5.6	7.9	13.9**	5.3
Unit						
Medical	53	23.3	5.9	7.1	14.1ᵃ	5.3
Airlift	97	42.7	4.8	7.5	13.0	3.8
Others	77	33.9	3.9	5.3	12.0	3.2
Disaster relief experience						
Yes	193	85.0	4.3	6.1	12.6	3.9
No	34	15.0	7.5*	8.9	14.9**	4.6
Exposure to bodies						
No	216	95.2	4.8	6.8	12.9	4.1
Yes	11	4.8	3.5	4.4	13.5	4.6
Psychiatric treatment history						
No	219	98.2	4.8	6.7	12.9	4.1
Yes	4	1.8	8.5	7.2	11.0	2.0

$N = 227$. *PTSR* Posttraumatic stress response evaluated by the Impact of Event Scale-Revised, *GPD* General psychological distress evaluated by the Kessler Psychological Distress Scale, *SD* standard deviation
ᵃIndividuals who were assigned to medical units showed significantly higher scores than others ($p < .05$, multiple comparisons with the Bonferroni correction)
*$p < .05$, **$p < .01$, ***$p < .001$

Hierarchical linear regression analyses

The results of the hierarchical linear regression analyses for high PTSR and GPD are shown in Table 3. It is reported that any variance inflation factor (VIF) exceeds 10 and tolerance value lower than 0.10 indicates a potential problem of multicollinearity [31]. In this study, variance inflation factor (VIF) ranged from 1.007 to 1.621 and tolerance ranged from 0.617 to 0.993 throughout the hierarchical linear regression analyses, no multicollinearity was observed. Regarding the correlates of PTSR, significant associations were observed for two IRI subscales: FS ($\beta = 0.21$, SE $= 0.11$, $p < .01$) and PD ($\beta = 0.18$, SE $= 0.13$, $p < .05$). Having no experience of disaster relief was also significantly associated with high PTSR ($\beta = 0.15$, SE $= 1.3$, $p < .05$). For the correlates of high GPD status, significant relations were shown for PD ($\beta = 0.28$, SE $= 0.07$, $p < .001$), marital status (married, $\beta = 0.22$, SE $= 0.61$, $p < .01$), being female ($\beta = 0.18$, SE $= 1.15$, $p < .01$), medical unit ($\beta = 0.18$, SE $= 0.68$, $p < .05$), and no disaster relief experience ($\beta = 0.13$, SE $= 0.73$, $p < .05$). Therefore, the

Table 2 Results of the psychological measures and Pearson correlation analyses

	IES-R	K10	IRI_PT	IRI_FS	IRI_EC	IRI_PD	Mean	SD	Median	Range	Cronbach's alpha
IES-R	–	.59***	.07	.28***	.05	.25***	4.77	6.70	2	0–40	0.91
K10		–	.13	.23***	.18**	.35***	12.91	4.09	11	10–39	0.89
IRI_PT			–	.14*	.43***	.04	15.90	4.09	16	5–28	0.63
IRI_FS				–	.22**	.39***	9.67	4.28	9	0–22	0.62
IRI_EC					–	.28***	16.89	3.59	17	8–28	0.57
IRI_PD						–	10.31	3.88	10	2–22	0.65

Note. $N = 227$. IES-R Impact of Event Scale-Revised, K10 Kessler Psychological Distress Scale, IRI Interpersonal Reactivity Index, PT Perspective Taking, FS Fantasy, EC Empathic Concern, PD Personal Distress, SD standard deviation
$^*p < .05$, $^{**}p < .01$, $^{***}p < .001$

two IRI subscales, FS and PD, showed the largest standardized coefficient β in the multiple linear regression models for PTSR and GPD, respectively.

Discussion

We examined the associations between dispositional empathy and the mental health status (PTSR and GPD) of JGSDF personnel who were engaged in the international disaster relief activity after Typhoon Yolanda in 2013. High PTSR was significantly related to both high FS and PD. High GPD was significantly related to high PD. To our knowledge, this is the first paper to report a link between psychological distress or posttraumatic stress and dispositional empathy among disaster workers using quantitative empathy measures.

Table 3 Results of the hierarchical multiple linear regression analysis

	PTSR Hierarchial Models Standardized Coefficient β			GPD Hierarchial Models Standardized Coefficient β		
	Step 1	Step 2	Step 3	Step 1	Step 2	Step 3
Personal Attributes						
Age	0.02	0.02	0.02	−0.05	−0.05	−0.04
Sex[a]	0.11	0.11	0.07	0.26***	0.23**	0.18**
Marital status[b]	0.11	0.12	0.13	0.19**	0.18*	0.22**
Disaster relief experience[c]	−0.18**	−0.17*	−0.15*	−0.19**	−0.17*	−0.13*
Psychiatric treatment history[c]	0.09	0.09	0.1	−0.05	−0.05	−0.06
Work-related factors						
Rank[d]		0.03	0.01		0.09	0.04
Medical unit[c]		0.09	0.1		0.18*	0.18*
Airlift unit[c]		0.10	0.06		0.16*	0.12
Exposure to bodies[c]		−0.06	−0.03		0.03	0.06
Dispositional Empathy						
IRI_PT			0.05			0.04
IRI_FS			0.21**			0.08
IRI_EC			−0.11			0.03
IRI_PD			0.18*			0.28***
Statistics						
R^2	0.057	0.071	0.164	0.13	0.166	0.271
ΔR^2		0.014	0.093		0.036	0.106
F	2.635*	1.815	3.150***	6.475***	4.696***	5.984***

$N = 227$. PTSR Posttraumatic stress response evaluated by the Impact of Events Scale-Revised, GPD General psychological distress evaluated by the Kessler Psychological Distress Scale, IRI Interpersonal Reactivity Index, PT Perspective Taking, FS Fantasy, EC Empathic Concern, PD Personal Distress
[a]Dummy variable was created (male = 0, female = 1). [b]Dummy variable was created (single = 0, married = 1). [c]Dummy variables were created (no = 0, yes = 1).
[d]Dummy variables were created (enlisted/private = 0, officer = 1)
$^*p < .05$, $^{**}p < .01$, $^{***}p < .001$

PD reflects emotional dispositional empathy and represents "self-oriented" feelings of personal anxiety and unease in tense interpersonal settings. Previous research that targeted clinical physicians reported that PD was closely related to secondary traumatic stress [32]. Cognitive neuroscience studies have outlined control mechanisms that regulate whether someone's empathic reactions are self- or other-oriented, indicating the importance of being aware of the distinction between experiences of the self and others [33, 34]. Our study suggests that individuals with high PD—who have a poor ability to distinguish between self- and other-oriented empathic reactions—are prone to suffering from psychological distress when faced with persons experiencing adversity.

FS, which is the tendency to transpose oneself imaginatively into the feelings and actions of fictitious characters, was also extracted as a significant factor related to high PTSR in this study. Ursano and colleagues have shown the importance of "identification with disaster victims" as a mechanism through which relief workers experience secondary trauma [17]. Cetin and colleagues also reported results that support this finding [15] and warned against excessive identification with disaster victims. Considering the conceptual similarity between FS, which is a type of dispositional empathy, and "identification with disaster victims," our results also support these previous findings.

Previous disaster relief-related literature suggests the importance of maintaining professional distance and avoiding excessive empathy and identification with victims [8, 15, 17, 35]. A similar trend has been observed in the field of clinical medicine; "detached concern"—a purely cognitive understanding of patients' emotions, while establishing emotional distance to maintain objectivity and limit exposure to negative emotions—has been traditionally recommended for physicians [36]. Given that those with high FS or PD are prone to suffering from psychological distress when faced with distressed individuals, it is likely that maintaining professional or emotional distance, such as "detached concern," is especially helpful for such emergency relief workers in order to minimize their psychological distress. However, this does not necessarily suggest that a complete absence of empathy is appropriate. Empathy is multifaceted; "other-oriented" empathy provide individuals with a variety of positive effects such as compassion satisfaction [37] and positive clinical outcomes [38]. One study targeted at physicians reported that compassion satisfaction was strongly associated with EC and PT, while compassion fatigue was more closely related to PD [32]. Therefore, an educational intervention that could reinforce other-oriented empathic reactions while inhibiting self-oriented empathic reactions might be effective for mitigating the psychological distress of emergency relief workers. It will be crucial to examine the

effectiveness of such educational interventions through in-depth follow-up studies. These programs may specifically target workers with high PD or FS in order to prevent their posttraumatic mental health difficulties.

In this study, those with no disaster relief experience were identified as being at risk for both high PTSR and GPD, and women, married individuals, and medical unit were identified as being at risk for high GPD. Previous studies that focused on body handlers also reported that women and inexperienced workers had higher levels of distress than men and experienced workers [39]. Our results are consistent with this previous report. As for marital status, the previous literature has reported that unmarried individuals are more prone to suffer from psychological distress than those who are married [40]. Although our study demonstrated the opposite result, we theorize that being married could be not only protective but also risk factor depending on the marital relationship or family situation. For example, for the married personnel who have not built a good marital relationship, the existence of spouse could work as a concern rather than a social support when they are suddenly assigned for disaster relief work. Such background might induce inconsistent outcomes. Since medical staff were more likely to suffer from direct or indirect traumatic stress in such a major disaster, it was reasonable that being a member of medical unit was identified as the risk factor for high GPD.

Limitations

Our findings should be interpreted within the context of some limitations. First, our study participants were limited to JGSDF personnel and they did not include other defense services; therefore, our results do not represent all JGSDF personnel engaged in disaster relief activities in the Philippines. Second, this study employed a registered (non-anonymous) questionnaire, which has been reported to cause participants to conceal their symptoms, as compared to an anonymous questionnaire [41]. Furthermore, the Japanese sociocultural background strongly stigmatizes the expression of emotional suffering [42]. Thus, there is a strong possibility that participants' psychological effects were underreported in this study. Third, our cross-sectional study design limits the causal association between the dependent and the independent variables. Finally, this study did not examine other factors that might confound our findings (e.g., pre-deployment mental health status, personal characteristics for coping with stress, previous traumatic experiences, numbers of years of disaster relief experience, compassion satisfaction, and major life event experience). Further studies that include such information are needed to more rigorously identify the psychological effects of these factors for disaster workers.

Conclusions

Despite some limitations, we demonstrated that PD and FS, which are subscales of the IRI, are related to psychological distress among disaster workers. Situations that increase the risk of secondary trauma are not limited to disaster relief activities but also include humanitarian aid, such as medical and welfare activities. More precise and better understanding of the relationship between dispositional empathy and psychological distress is needed to design better educational interventions to protect the mental health of people who engage in such activities.

Abbreviations

EC: Empathic Concern; FS: Fantasy; GPD: General psychological distress; IES-R: Impact of Events Scale-Revised; IRI: Interpersonal Reactivity Index; JGSDF: Japan Ground Self-Defense Force; K10: Kessler Psychological Distress Scale; PD: Personal Distress; PT: Perspective Taking; PTSR: Posttraumatic stress response

Acknowledgements

We wish to thank all the participants and medical staff of the JGSDF who supported our research. The authors would also like to thank Dr. Yumi Suzuki of the International College of Arts and Sciences, Fukuoka Women's University, Fukuoka, Japan, for use of the Japanese version of the IRI. The views expressed in this article are those of the authors and do not reflect the position or policy of the National Defense Medical College or the Japan Ministry of Defense.

Funding

This work was supported by the Japanese Society for the Promotion of Science KAKENHI Grant number 26461779.

Authors' contributions

MN conceived and designed the study, and developed it in discussion with JS, MT, TS, HT, AY, and KS. MN, TF, and FW were involved in the acquisition and analysis of the data, and all authors participated in the interpretation of the data. MN wrote the first draft of the article and all authors contributed to critically revising the paper. Finally, all authors read and approved the final manuscript.

Consent for publication

Not applicable.

Competing interests

The authors declare that they have no competing interests.

Author details

^{1}Division of Behavioral Science, National Defense Medical College Research Institute, 3-2 Namiki, Tokorozawa, Saitama 359-8513, Japan. ^{2}Department of Psychiatry, School of Medicine, National Defense Medical College, 3-2 Namiki, Tokorozawa, Saitama, Japan. ^{3}Japan Ground Self-Defense Force Medical School, 1-2-24, Ikejiri, Setagaya-ku, Tokyo, Japan.

References

1. National Disaster Risk Reduction and Management Council. Final report re: effects of typhoon "Yolanda" (Haiyan). In: NDRRMC update; 2013. http://ndrrmc.gov.ph/attachments/article/1329/FINAL_REPORT_re_Effects_of_Typhoon_YOLANDA_(HAIYAN)_06-09NOV2013.pdf. Accessed 24 Apr 2018.
2. Cabinet Office of Japan. International contributions of Japan self-defense forces. In: We are Tomodachi; 2014. http://www.japan.go.jp/tomodachi/2014/spring-summer2014/international_contributions_of_apan.html. Accessed 24 Apr 2018.
3. Norris FH, Friedman MJ, Watson PJ, Byrne CM, Diaz E, Kaniasty K. 60,000 disaster victims speak: part I. an empirical review of the empirical literature, 1981–2001. Psychiatry. 2002;65:207–39.
4. Perrin MA, DiGrande L, Wheeler K, Thorpe L, Farfel M, Brackbill R. Differences in PTSD prevalence and associated risk factors among world trade center disaster rescue and recovery workers. Am J Psychiatry. 2007;164:1385–94.
5. Figley CR. Compassion fatigue as secondary traumatic stress disorder. In: Figley CR, editor. Compassion fatigue: coping with secondary traumatic stress disorder in those who treat the traumatized. New York: Routledge; 1995. p. 1–20.
6. Benedek DM, Fullerton C, Ursano RJ. First responders: mental health consequences of natural and human-made disasters for public health and public safety workers. Annu Rev Public Health. 2007;28:55–68.
7. Berger W, Coutinho ES, Figueira I, Marques-Portella C, Luz MP, Neylan TC, et al. Rescuers at risk: a systematic review and meta-regression analysis of the worldwide current prevalence and correlates of PTSD in rescue workers. Soc Psychiatry Psychiatr Epidemiol. 2012;47:1001–11. https://doi.org/10.1007/s00127-011-0408-2.
8. Fullerton CS, McCarroll JE, Ursano RJ, Wright KM. Psychological responses of rescue workers: fire fighters and trauma. Am J Orthop. 1992;62:371–8.
9. Guo YJ, Chen CH, Lu ML, Tan HK, Lee HW, Wang TN. Posttraumatic stress disorder among professional and non-professional rescuers involved in an earthquake in Taiwan. Psychiatry Res. 2004;127:35–41. https://doi.org/10.1016/j.psychres.2004.03.009.
10. Marmar CR, Weiss DS, Metzler TJ, Ronfeldt HM, Foreman C. Stress responses of emergency services personnel to the Loma Prieta earthquake interstate 880 freeway collapse and control traumatic incidents. J Trauma Stress. 1996; 9:63–85.
11. Leffler CT, Dembert ML. Posttraumatic stress symptoms among U.S. navy divers recovering TWA flight 800. J Nerv Ment Dis. 1998;186:574–7.
12. Ursano RJ, McCarroll JE. Exposure to traumatic death: the nature of the stressor. In: Ursano RJ, McCaughey BG, Fullerton CS, editors. Individual and community responses to trauma and disaster: the structure of human chaos. Cambridge: Cambridge University Press; 1994. p. 46–71.
13. Alexander DA, Wells A. Reactions of police officers to body-handling after a major disaster. A before-and-after comparison. Br J Psychiatry. 1991;159:547–55.
14. Jones DR. Secondary disaster victims: the emotional effects of recovering and identifying human remains. Am J Psychiatry. 1985;142:303–7.
15. Cetin M, Kose S, Ebrinc S, Yigit S, Elhai JD, Basoglu C. Identification and posttraumatic stress disorder symptoms in rescue workers in the Marmara, Turkey, earthquake. J Trauma Stress. 2005;18:485–9. https://doi.org/10.1002/jts.20056.
16. Regehr C, Goldberg G, Hughes J. Exposure to human tragedy, empathy, and trauma in ambulance paramedics. Am J Orthop. 2002;72:505–13.
17. Ursano RJ, Fullerton CS, Vance K, Kao TC. Posttraumatic stress disorder and identification in disaster workers. Am J Psychiatry. 1999;156:353–9. https://doi.org/10.1176/ajp.156.3.353.
18. Decety J, Svetlova M. Putting together phylogenetic and ontogenetic perspectives on empathy. Dev Cogn Neurosci. 2012;2:1–24. https://doi.org/10.1016/j.dcn.2011.05.003.
19. Davis MH. Measuring individual differences in empathy: evidence for a multidimensional approach. J Pers Soc Psychol. 1983;44:113–26. https://doi.org/10.1037/0022-3514.44.1.113.
20. Batson CD, Fultz J, Schoenrade PA. Distress and empathy: two qualitatively distinct vicarious emotions with different motivational consequences. J Pers. 1987;55:19–39.
21. Stepien KA, Baernstein A. Educating for empathy. A review. J Gen Intern Med. 2006;21:524–30.

22. Figley CR. Compassion fatigue: Psychotherapists' chronic lack of self care. J Clin Psychol. 2002;58:1433–41. https://doi.org/10.1002/jclp.10090.

23. Klimecki O, Singer T. Empathic distress fatigue rather than compassion fatigue? Integrating findings from empathy research in psychology and social neuroscience. In: Oakley B, Knafo A, Madhavan G, Wilson D, editors. Pathological altruism. New York: Oxford University press; 2012. p. 368–83.

24. Asukai N, Kato H, Kawamura N, Kim Y, Yamamoto K, Kishimoto J, et al. Reliability and validity of the Japanese-language version of the impact of event scale-revised (IES-R-J): four studies of different traumatic events. J Nerv Ment Dis. 2002;190:175–82.

25. Furukawa TA, Kawakami N, Saitoh M, Ono Y, Nakane Y, Nakamura Y, et al. The performance of the Japanese version of the K6 and K10 in the world mental health survey Japan. Int J Methods Psychiatr Res. 2008;17:152–8. https://doi.org/10.1002/mpr.257.

26. Weiss DS, Marmar CR. The impact of event scale-revised. In: Wilson JP, Keane TM, editors. Assessing psychological trauma and PTSD. New York: The Guilford Press; 1997. p. 339–411.

27. Kessler RC, Andrews G, Colpe LJ, Hiripi E, Mroczek DK, Normand SL, et al. Short screening scales to monitor population prevalences and trends in non-specific psychological distress. Psychol Med. 2002;32:959–76.

28. Sakurai K, Nishi A, Kondo K, Yanagida K, Kawakami N. Screening performance of K6/K10 and other screening instruments for mood and anxiety disorders in Japan. Psychiatry Clin Neurosci. 2011;65:434–41.

29. Himichi T, Osanai H, Goto T, Fujita H, Kawamura Y, Davis MH, et al. Development of a Japanese version of the interpersonal reactivity index. Shinrigaku Kenkyu. 2017;88:61–71.

30. Corp IBM. SPSS statistics for windows version 22.0.0. Armonk: IBM Corp; 2013.

31. Hair JF, Black WC, Babin BJ, Anderson RE. Multivariate data analysis. 7th ed. Upper Saddle River: Pearson Prentice Hall; 2010.

32. Gleichgerrcht E, Decety J. Empathy in clinical practice: how individual dispositions, gender, and experience moderate empathic concern, burnout, and emotional distress in physicians. PLoS One. 2013;8:e61526. https://doi.org/10.1371/journal.pone.0061526.

33. Decety J, Jackson PL. The functional architecture of human empathy. Behav Cogn Neurosci Rev. 2004;3:71–100. https://doi.org/10.1177/1534582304267187.

34. Decety J, Lamm C. Human empathy through the lens of social neuroscience. Sci World J. 2006;6:1146–63. https://doi.org/10.1100/tsw.2006.221.

35. Pross C. Burnout, vicarious traumatization and its prevention. Torture. 2006;16:1–9.

36. Fox R, Lief H. Training for "detached concern" in medical students. In: Lief HI, Lief VF, Lief NR, editors. The psychological basis of medical practice. New York: Harper & Row; 1963. p. 12–35.

37. Sodeke-Gregson EA, Holttum S, Billings J. Compassion satisfaction, burnout, and secondary traumatic stress in UK therapists who work with adult trauma clients. Eur J Psychotraumatol. 2013;4. https://doi.org/10.3402/ejpt.v4i0.21869.

38. Derksen F, Bensing J, Lagro-Janssen A. Effectiveness of empathy in general practice: a systematic review. Br J Gen Pract. 2013;63:e76–84.

39. McCarroll JE, Ursano RJ, Fullerton CS, Lundy A. Traumatic stress of a wartime mortuary: anticipation of exposure to mass death. J Nerv Ment Dis. 1993;181:545–51. https://doi.org/10.1097/00005053-199309000-00003.

40. Fullerton CS, Ursano RJ, Wang L. Acute stress disorder, posttraumatic stress disorder, and depression in disaster or rescue workers. Am J Psychiatry. 2004;161:1370–6.

41. McLay RN, Deal WE, Murphy JA, Center KB, Kolkow TT, Grieger TA. On-the-record screenings versus anonymous surveys in reporting PTSD. Am J Psychiatry. 2008;165:775–6. https://doi.org/10.1176/appi.ajp.2008.07121960.

42. Goto T, Wilson JP. A review of the history of traumatic stress studies in Japan: from traumatic neurosis to PTSD. Trauma Violence Abuse. 2003;4:195–209 doi: July 1, 2003. https://doi.org/10.1177/1524838003004003001.

2

Hospital utilization rates following antipsychotic dose reductions: implications for tardive dyskinesia

Stanley N. Caroff[1]* ⓘ, Fan Mu[2], Rajeev Ayyagari[2], Traci Schilling[3], Victor Abler[3] and Benjamin Carroll[3]

Abstract

Background: Data are limited on the benefits and risks of dose reduction in managing side effects associated with antipsychotic treatment. As an example, antipsychotic dose reduction has been recommended in the management of tardive dyskinesia (TD), yet the benefits of lowering doses are not well studied. However, stable maintenance treatment is essential to prevent deterioration and relapse in schizophrenia.

Methods: A retrospective cohort study was conducted to analyze the healthcare burden of antipsychotic dose reduction in patients with schizophrenia. Medical claims from six US states spanning a six-year period were analyzed for ≥10% or ≥30% antipsychotic dose reductions compared with those from patients receiving a stable dose. Outcomes measured were inpatient admissions and emergency room (ER) visits for schizophrenia, all psychiatric disorders, and all causes, and TD claims.

Results: A total of 19,556 patients were identified with ≥10% dose reduction and 15,239 patients with ≥30% dose reduction. Following a ≥ 10% dose reduction, the risk of an all-cause inpatient admission increased (hazard ratio [HR] 1.17; 95% confidence interval [CI] 1.11, 1.23; $P < 0.001$), and the risk of an all-cause ER visit increased (HR 1.09; 95% CI 1.05, 1.14; $P < 0.001$) compared with controls. Patients with a ≥ 10% dose reduction had an increased risk of admission or ER visit for schizophrenia (HR 1.27; 95% CI 1.19, 1.36; $P < 0.001$) and for all psychiatric disorders (HR 1.16; 95% CI 1.10, 1.23; $P < 0.001$) compared with controls. A dose reduction of ≥30% also led to an increased risk of admission for all causes (HR 1.23; 95% CI 1.17, 1.31; $P < 0.001$), and for admission or ER visit for schizophrenia (HR 1.31; 95% CI 1.21, 1.41; $P < 0.001$) or for all psychiatric disorders (HR 1.21; 95% CI 1.14, 1.29; $P < 0.001$) compared with controls. Dose reductions had no significant effect on claims for TD.

Conclusion: Patients with antipsychotic dose reductions showed significant increases in both all-cause and mental health–related hospitalizations, suggesting that antipsychotic dose reductions may lead to increased overall healthcare burden in some schizophrenia patients. This highlights the need for alternative strategies for the management of side effects, including TD, in schizophrenia patients that allow for maintaining effective antipsychotic treatment.

Keywords: Tardive dyskinesia; antipsychotic medication, Schizophrenia, Relapse, Healthcare burden

---

* Correspondence: caroffs@pennmedicine.upenn.edu
[1]Department of Psychiatry, Corporal Michael J. Crescenz VA Medical Center and the Perelman School of Medicine at the University of Pennsylvania, 3900 Woodland Avenue, Philadelphia, PA 19104, USA
Full list of author information is available at the end of the article

Background

Antipsychotic medication is the mainstay of treatment for schizophrenia [1]. Agreement on the therapeutic doses of antipsychotics has been controversial; doses are determined empirically based on assessment of efficacy and tolerability for individual patients [1]. When side effects emerge, management options include discontinuation of the current antipsychotic, switching to a different drug, or lowering the dose [2–4].

For example, tardive dyskinesia (TD), which occurs in up to 30% of patients receiving antipsychotics, is a serious side effect of antipsychotics for which dose reduction has been proposed [2–4]. However, controlled evidence on the effect of dose reduction for the management of TD remains limited. [5]. Although novel drugs for treatment of TD are now available, management begins with consideration of antipsychotic prescribing decisions. In non-psychotic patients with TD, antipsychotic drug discontinuation may be considered and drugs may be tapered off if clinically appropriate [6]. Early diagnosis and drug cessation may facilitate remission, but evidence is limited on whether or how often TD resolves, and how long it takes to do so, after discontinuation of antipsychotics [7, 8]. In psychotic patients, maintenance antipsychotic treatment is essential to prevent deterioration and relapse [9]. Approximately 50% of patients taking antipsychotics are being treated for schizophrenia [10], which has a relapse rate of 53% within 9 months after antipsychotic discontinuation [11]. Antipsychotic discontinuation, which is associated with increased risk of violence, incarceration, hospitalization, increased healthcare resource utilization, and interruption of rehabilitation efforts, may be impractical in most patients with schizophrenia [12, 13].

Although some published evidence supports increasing doses or switching to other antipsychotics to suppress TD symptoms [14–16], these changes may raise concerns about increasing acute extrapyramidal symptoms, limiting chances of TD reversibility, and possibly destabilizing psychiatric status. Dose reduction has also been recommended in past reviews of treatment options [5, 6, 17]. However, published meta-analyses have concluded that available data are insufficient to either support or refute treatment of TD by antipsychotic dose reduction [5, 18]. Furthermore, published studies of dose-reduction strategies to minimize the risk of developing extrapyramidal symptoms including TD, involving dose reductions of 50% or more, have been inconsistent but generally reported significant risks of psychotic exacerbation and relapse [9, 19–23].

To further address the risks of dose reduction as a recommended treatment intervention for side effects of antipsychotic treatment, including TD, we conducted a retrospective cohort study to analyze the healthcare burden in terms of utilization of hospital-based resources resulting from ≥10% and ≥30% reductions in antipsychotic doses for patients with schizophrenia.

Methods

Study objective and data sources

A large retrospective cohort study using electronic medical records was conducted to compare the risk of all-cause and mental health–related inpatient admissions and emergency room (ER) visits for schizophrenia patients who were treated with a stable dose versus those who experienced a dose reduction of an oral antipsychotic monotherapy.

Medicaid data was extracted from six US states (Iowa, Kansas, Mississippi, Missouri, New Jersey, and Wisconsin). These states were chosen based on the availability of data for the analysis. Each state has its own policies regarding use and sharing of their data, and these six states had agreements in place allowing this analysis to be performed compiling and using Medicaid data from each state. All states for which data were available were included. Data representing the most recent six years from each state were analyzed, the dates of which varied by state. The overall study period ranged from 2008 to 2017 for all medical records. The Medicaid records contained complete medical claims, including diagnosis, procedures, paid amounts, pharmaceutical claims, enrollment history, and patient demographics.

Patient selection

Patients for the analysis met the following inclusion criteria: 18 years or older as of the index date; at least one diagnosis of schizophrenia in the most recent 6 years of data for each state; at least two fills of an oral antipsychotic after the first schizophrenia diagnosis; at least one antipsychotic monotherapy period that was ≥90 days with a stable dose; and a baseline period of at least 6 months of continuous enrollment prior to the index date.

Exclusion criteria included: patients receiving long-acting injectable antipsychotics; patients receiving more than one antipsychotic concurrently during the study period; and patients from New Jersey who turned 65 after 2012, as these patients were eligible for both Medicare and Medicaid, potentially preventing complete capture of drug claim information via the Medicaid database.

"Cases" were defined as patients with a stable-dose monotherapy period of ≥90 days who then experienced a dose reduction, defined as a reduction ≥10% from the stable dose. The date of the initial dose reduction was defined as the index date for cases. Controls were defined as patients with a stable-dose monotherapy period that lasted for ≥91 days without a dose reduction greater than 10%. The first prescription fill after the first 90-day stable-dose period was defined as the index date for controls. If a patient had multiple potential index dates that met all of the inclusion criteria, the index date used for the purposes of the study was randomly selected from the eligible potential index dates. A randomly chosen potential index date was used rather than the first such index date to avoid biasing the analysis towards earlier stages of the disease.

Cases and controls were matched 1:1 based on age, gender, state, healthcare plan type (health maintenance organization [HMO] vs fee-for-service [FFS]), index treatment (first- vs second-generation antipsychotic), and index year. All patients were followed for 2 years after the index date or until they were removed from the analysis due to either the earliest event of dose escalation (disqualification from dose-reduction analysis) or the end of eligibility (defined as any change outside of the original inclusion criteria, including medication switch, additional medication added, dose escalation, or occurrence of an outcome event). Mean duration of the follow-up period was also reported. Additional subgroup analyses were performed on the subset of cases experiencing a dose reduction of ≥30% together with matched controls.

The following patient characteristics were assessed for cases and controls during the baseline period or on the index date: characteristics (age, gender, state, and healthcare plan type); index year; index treatment; psychiatric comorbidity profile; Charlson Comorbidity Index (CCI) score, including individual comorbidities; psychotherapy; psychiatric medication; and observed disease duration, defined as the first observed schizophrenia diagnosis date prior to the index date.

Outcome measurements

Patients were assessed for all-cause inpatient admission and ER visits as well as healthcare utilization related to an inpatient admission or ER visit for either schizophrenia or another psychiatric diagnosis. Schizophrenia inpatient admissions or ER visits were identified using the International Classification of Diseases, 9th revision (ICD-9) code 295.xx and ICD-10 codes F20.x and F25.x. Psychiatric inpatient admissions or ER visits were identified by ICD-9 or ICD-10 codes for schizophrenia-spectrum and other psychotic disorders, substance-related and addictive disorders, depressive disorders, bipolar and related disorders, trauma- and stressor-induced disorders, anxiety disorders, sleep-wake disorders, and personality disorders (Additional file 1: Table S1). Patients were also assessed for TD diagnosis, corresponding to ICD-9 code 333.85 (subacute dyskinesia due to drugs) or ICD-10 code G24.01 (drug-induced subacute dyskinesia).

Statistical analysis

Descriptive statistics (mean, standard deviation, percentage) were used to describe patient demographics between case and control cohorts. Patient characteristics between cohorts were evaluated using Wilcoxon signed-rank tests for continuous variables and McNemar's tests for dichotomous variables. For comparison of study outcomes (all-cause inpatient admission or ER visit, schizophrenia-related inpatient admission or ER visit, psychiatric-related inpatient admission or ER visit), Kaplan−Meier analyses with log-rank test were used. Multivariable Cox proportional hazard models were used to compare outcomes between cases and controls, adjusting for 19 covariates, including additional patient characteristics such as age (continuous), disease duration, CCI score, psychiatric comorbidity profile, psychotherapy use, and psychiatric medication use.

Results

Baseline characteristics

A total of 185,267 patients were diagnosed with schizophrenia during the study period, and 19,556 case patients meeting the final inclusion criteria were matched 1:1 with control patients for the ≥10% dose-reduction analyses (Fig. 1). The resulting distribution of age, gender, state, and healthcare plan type were nearly identical between cases and controls. In both cohorts, the mean age was ~ 45.3 years and 52% were male, and ~ 44% and 18% of patients subscribed to FFS and HMO insurance plans (Table 1). Differences between the cohorts include the mean observed disease duration, which was 27 months for case patients and 20 months for control patients. In addition, the mean duration of follow-up time was 4.5 months for case patients and 8.0 months for control patients (Table 1). The demographics for the ≥30% dose-reduction cohorts are shown in Additional file 1: Table S2.

The distribution of index drug class was also identical between the case and control cohorts (Table 1). Eighty-eight percent of patients were using second-generation antipsychotics, with ~ 12% using first-generation antipsychotics. Cases had lower rates of psychiatric comorbidities and substance use disorders than controls, with the exception of personality disorders. In addition, the CCI score was also similar between cases and controls except for AIDS/HIV, dementia, and peripheral vascular disease. The number of TD claims reported for patients in both cohorts was extremely low, representing approximately 0.2–0.3% of the patient population.

Dosing patterns

Table 2 shows the mean dose distribution between the case and control cohorts for the ten most commonly prescribed antipsychotic medications. Mean doses were higher in the case cohort versus the control cohort for all of the top ten medications.

The mean and distribution of the percent reduction among cases for each of the top ten antipsychotics are shown in Table 3. Patients on all ten antipsychotic medications had

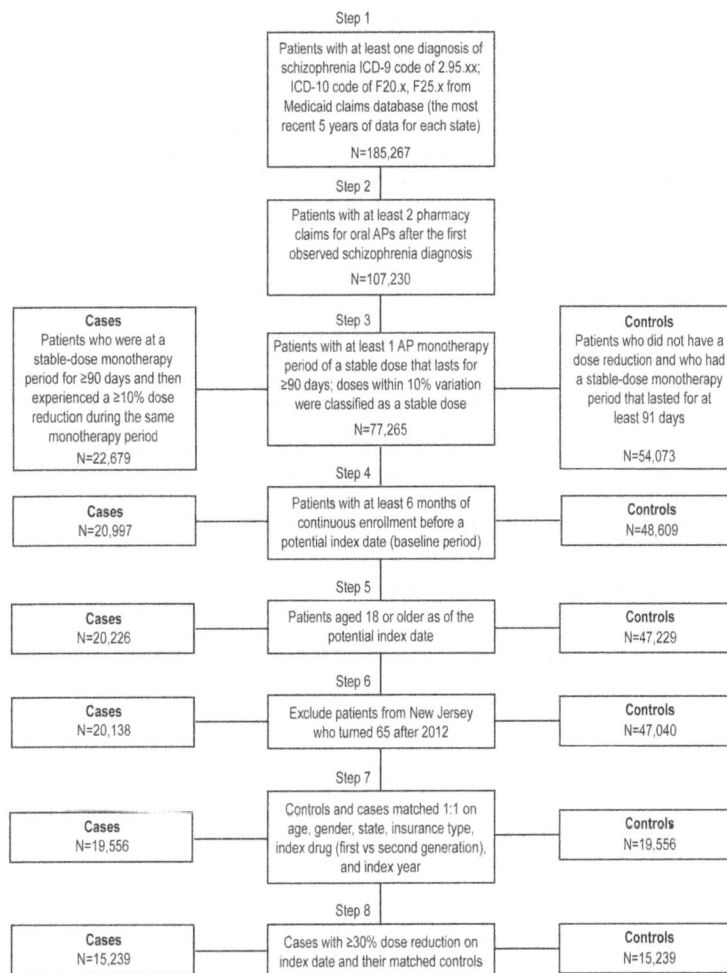

Fig. 1 Patient Selection Flow Diagram. Patients were selected for case and control cohorts from a Medicaid claims database representing six US states and the most recent 6 years of data as detailed in Methods. AP, antipsychotic; ICD, International Classification of Diseases

similar dose reductions throughout; mean dose reductions ranged from 45.3% (ziprasidone) to 57.3% (paliperidone) (Table 3). For most antipsychotics, 25% of patients had a dose reduction of ~ 33% or less, and approximately half of patients had a dose reduction of 50% or less (Table 3).

All-cause hospital utilization

Patients in the case and control cohorts were evaluated for all-cause healthcare utilization by assessing the likelihood of experiencing either an inpatient admission or an ER visit. For all-cause inpatient admissions, cases with a ≥ 10% dose reduction had a first-year event rate of 34.2%, compared with a 30.9% event rate for the control group, an absolute difference of 3.3% (Fig. 2a). Dose-reduction cases were more likely to have an inpatient admission compared with controls, and this increased likelihood persisted after adjusting for differences in baseline characteristics (Table 4).

Cases with a ≥ 30% dose reduction showed a slightly higher rate of all-cause inpatient admission compared

with the ≥10% dose-reduction cases. The difference in first-year event rate between cases and controls was 4.9% (35.4% cases vs 30.5% controls) (Fig. 2b). Dose-reduction cases again showed an increased likelihood for inpatient admission compared with controls, which remained increased after adjusting for additional patient characteristics (Table 4).

For ER visits, cases with a ≥ 10% dose reduction had a first-year event rate difference of 1.4% (43.9% cases vs 42.5% controls) (Fig. 3a), whereas cases with a ≥ 30% dose reduction had a first-year event rate of difference of 3.4% (46.3% cases vs 42.9% controls) (Fig. 3b). Cases with ≥10% and ≥ 30% dose reductions were more likely to have an all-cause ER visit than controls, and this increased likelihood remained after adjusting for baseline patient characteristics (Table 4).

Mental health–related hospital utilization

Patients in the case and control cohorts were also evaluated for mental health–related healthcare utilization by

Table 1 Baseline demographics of ≥10% dose-reduction case and control cohorts

Characteristic	Case N = 19,556	Control N = 19,556	P Value
Demographics			
Age	45.3 ± 13.8	45.3 ± 13.8	0.86
Schizophrenia duration (months)	27.0 ± 17.9	20.1 ± 17.5	< 0.001
Male	10,075 (51.5%)	10,075 (51.5%)	–
Duration of follow-up (months)	4.5 ± 8.1	8.0 ± 11.7	< 0.001
Insurance type			
FFS	8562 (43.8%)	8562 (43.8%)	–
HMO	3603 (18.4%)	3603 (18.4%)	–
Mixed	7391 (37.8%)	7391 (37.8%)	–
State			
Iowa	1024 (5.2%)	1024 (5.2%)	–
Kansas	1294 (6.6%)	1294 (6.6%)	–
Mississippi	1761 (9.0%)	1761 (9.0%)	–
Missouri	7765 (39.7%)	7765 (39.7%)	–
New Jersey	5578 (28.5%)	5578 (28.5%)	–
Wisconsin	2134 (10.9%)	2134 (10.9%)	–
Index characteristics			
Index drug class			
First generation	2384 (12.2%)	2384 (12.2%)	–
Second generation	17,172 (87.8%)	17,172 (87.8%)	–
Index year			
2008	480 (2.5%)	480 (2.5%)	–
2009	1388 (7.1%)	1388 (7.1%)	–
2010	1799 (9.2%)	1799 (9.2%)	–
2011	2516 (12.9%)	2516 (12.9%)	–
2012	3280 (16.8%)	3280 (16.8%)	–
2013	3378 (17.3%)	3378 (17.3%)	–
2014	2196 (11.2%)	2196 (11.2%)	–
2015	2223 (11.4%)	2223 (11.4%)	–
2016	1910 (9.8%)	1910 (9.8%)	–
2017	376 (1.9%)	376 (1.9%)	
Comorbidity profile			
Substance-related and addictive disorders	4638 (23.7%)	4879 (25.0%)	< 0.01
Anxiety disorders	2973 (15.2%)	3264 (16.7%)	< 0.001
Bipolar and related disorders	4452 (22.8%)	4672 (23.9%)	< 0.01
Depressive disorders	4942 (25.3%)	5472 (28.0%)	< 0.001
Personality disorders	809 (4.1%)	757 (3.9%)	0.19
Schizophrenia-spectrum disorders (excluding schizophrenia)	2426 (12.4%)	2699 (13.8%)	< 0.001
Sleep–wake disorders	1516 (7.8%)	1565 (8.0%)	0.36
Tardive dyskinesia	37 (0.2%)	51 (0.3%)	0.17
Trauma- and stressor-related disorders	1312 (6.7%)	1446 (7.4%)	< 0.01
CCI	0.6 ± 1.2	0.6 ± 1.2	0.29
AIDS/HIV	238 (1.2%)	288 (1.5%)	< 0.05

Table 1 Baseline demographics of ≥10% dose-reduction case and control cohorts *(Continued)*

Characteristic	Case N = 19,556	Control N = 19,556	P Value
Cancer	391 (2.0%)	399 (2.0%)	0.80
Cerebrovascular disease	765 (3.9%)	717 (3.7%)	0.21
Congestive heart failure	759 (3.9%)	722 (3.7%)	0.33
Chronic pulmonary disease	3901 (20.0%)	3836 (19.6%)	0.41
Dementia	512 (2.6%)	430 (2.2%)	< 0.01
Diabetes with chronic complication	791 (4.0%)	751 (3.8%)	0.30
Diabetes without chronic complication	3201 (16.4%)	3066 (15.7%)	0.06
Hemiplegia or paraplegia	220 (1.1%)	188 (1.0%)	0.12
Mild liver disease	800 (4.1%)	834 (4.3%)	0.40
Metastatic solid tumor	60 (0.3%)	50 (0.3%)	0.39
Myocardial infarction	189 (1.0%)	197 (1.0%)	0.72
Moderate or severe liver disease	68 (0.4%)	59 (0.3%)	0.48
Peptic ulcer disease	112 (0.6%)	111 (0.6%)	1.00
Peripheral vascular disease	883 (4.5%)	784 (4.0%)	< 0.05
Renal disease	559 (2.9%)	544 (2.8%)	0.67
Rheumatic disease	198 (1.0%)	221 (1.1%)	0.27
Psychotherapy			
Psychotherapy in crisis	36 (0.2%)	41 (0.2%)	0.65
Psychotherapy non-crisis	2587 (13.2%)	2791 (14.3%)	< 0.01
Psychoanalysis	0 (0%)	2 (0.01%)	0.48
Additional psychiatric medications			
ADHD medication	523 (2.7%)	513 (2.6%)	0.77
Anticholinergic	3998 (20.4%)	3465 (17.7%)	< 0.001
Antidepressant	9176 (46.9%)	9214 (47.1%)	0.63
Anxiety medication	4961 (25.4%)	4964 (25.4%)	0.98
Mood stabilizer	5980 (30.6%)	5388 (27.6%)	< 0.001
Sedative	1946 (10.0%)	2112 (10.8%)	< 0.01

Error represents standard deviation
ADHD attention-deficit/hyperactivity disorder; *AIDS* acquired immunodeficiency syndrome; *CCI* Charlson Comorbidity Index; *FFS* fee-for-service; *HIV* human immunodeficiency virus; *HMO* health maintenance organization

Table 2 Dose distribution for ten most frequently used antipsychotics during stable-dose period among case and control cohorts

Drug	Case (N, %)	Case Stable Dose (mg), Mean ± SD	Control (N, %)	Control Stable Dose (mg), Mean ± SD
Risperidone	4564 (23.3)	7 ± 7	4135 (21.1)	5 ± 6
Quetiapine	3871 (19.8)	463 ± 278	3226 (16.5)	331 ± 254
Olanzapine	2558 (13.1)	22 ± 13	2422 (12.4)	17 ± 12
Aripiprazole	1838 (9.4)	29 ± 47	2712 (13.9)	22 ± 38
Paliperidone	1180 (6.0)	70 ± 68	1704 (8.7)	56 ± 63
Haloperidol	1472 (7.5)	31 ± 30	1396 (7.1)	22 ± 19
Ziprasidone	1185 (6.1)	147 ± 61	1026 (5.2)	125 ± 55
Clozapine	1251 (6.4)	407 ± 180	683 (3.5)	405 ± 190
Lurasidone	467 (2.4)	93 ± 42	820 (4.2)	68 ± 35
Fluphenazine	301 (1.5)	20 ± 13	277 (1.4)	15 ± 11

SD standard deviation

Table 3 Dose reductions for patient percentiles for the ten most frequently used antipsychotic drugs

Drug	N	Mean	10th Percentile	25th Percentile	50th Percentile	75th Percentile	90th Percentile
Risperidone	4564	48.6%	25.0%	33.3%	50.0%	66.7%	83.3%
Quetiapine	3871	48.3%	25.0%	33.3%	50.0%	66.7%	80.0%
Olanzapine	2558	46.0%	25.0%	30.0%	50.0%	60.0%	75.0%
Aripiprazole	1838	47.4%	25.0%	33.3%	50.0%	60.0%	75.0%
Paliperidone	1180	57.3%	25.0%	33.3%	50.0%	90.0%	96.3%
Haloperidol	1472	54.9%	25.0%	34.3%	50.0%	75.0%	90.0%
Ziprasidone	1185	45.3%	25.0%	33.3%	50.0%	52.0%	75.0%
Clozapine	1251	47.3%	16.7%	23.1%	40.0%	75.0%	88.2%
Lurasidone	467	46.9%	25.0%	33.3%	50.0%	50.0%	75.0%
Fluphenazine	301	45.7%	25.0%	33.3%	50.0%	50.0%	70.0%

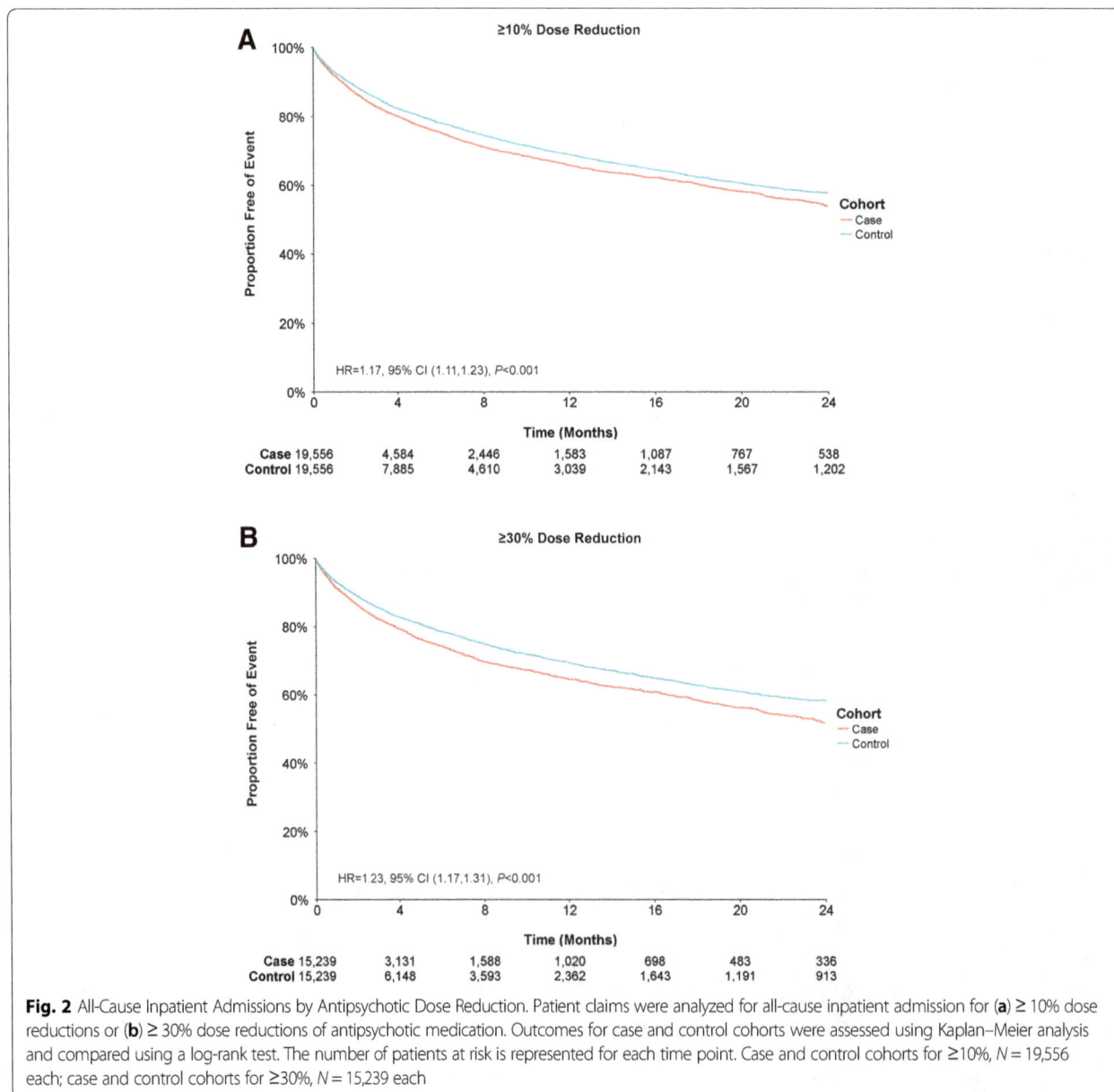

A ≥10% Dose Reduction

HR=1.17, 95% CI (1.11,1.23), *P*<0.001

Case 19,556	4,584	2,446	1,583	1,087	767	538
Control 19,556	7,885	4,610	3,039	2,143	1,567	1,202

B ≥30% Dose Reduction

HR=1.23, 95% CI (1.17,1.31), *P*<0.001

Case 15,239	3,131	1,588	1,020	698	483	336
Control 15,239	6,148	3,593	2,362	1,643	1,191	913

Fig. 2 All-Cause Inpatient Admissions by Antipsychotic Dose Reduction. Patient claims were analyzed for all-cause inpatient admission for (**a**) ≥ 10% dose reductions or (**b**) ≥ 30% dose reductions of antipsychotic medication. Outcomes for case and control cohorts were assessed using Kaplan–Meier analysis and compared using a log-rank test. The number of patients at risk is represented for each time point. Case and control cohorts for ≥10%, *N* = 19,556 each; case and control cohorts for ≥30%, *N* = 15,239 each

Table 4 Multivariate cox regression analysis for comparison of outcome measures between case and control cohorts

Outcome	Dose Reduction	HR	95% CI	P Value
Inpatient admission	≥10%	1.17	1.11, 1.23	< 0.001
Inpatient admission	≥30%	1.23	1.17, 1.31	< 0.001
ER visit	≥10%	1.09	1.05, 1.14	< 0.001
ER visit	≥30%	1.14	1.08, 1.19	< 0.001
Schizophrenia admission or ER visit*	≥10%	1.27	1.19, 1.36	< 0.001
Schizophrenia admission or ER visit*	≥30%	1.31	1.21, 1.41	< 0.001
Psychiatric admission or ER visit*	≥10%	1.16	1.10, 1.23	< 0.001
Psychiatric admission or ER visit*	≥30%	1.21	1.14, 1.29	< 0.001
TD claim	≥10%	1.39	0.80, 2.41	0.24
TD claim	≥30%	1.60	0.86, 3.00	0.14

*See Additional file 1: Table S1 for ICD-9 and ICD-10 diagnostic codes
CI confidence interval; *ER* emergency room; *HR* hazard ratio; *ICD* International Classification of Diseases

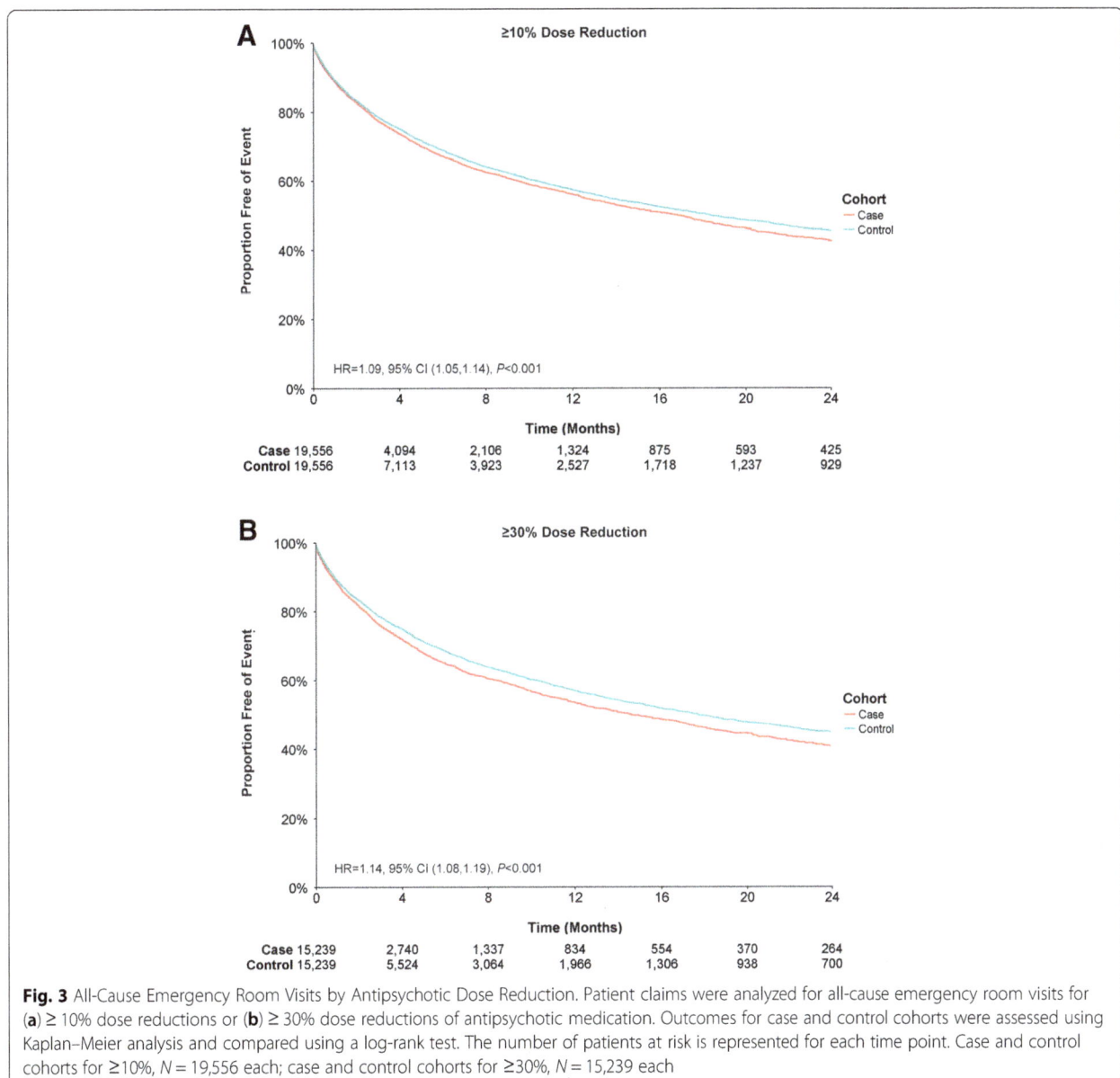

Fig. 3 All-Cause Emergency Room Visits by Antipsychotic Dose Reduction. Patient claims were analyzed for all-cause emergency room visits for (**a**) ≥ 10% dose reductions or (**b**) ≥ 30% dose reductions of antipsychotic medication. Outcomes for case and control cohorts were assessed using Kaplan–Meier analysis and compared using a log-rank test. The number of patients at risk is represented for each time point. Case and control cohorts for ≥10%, *N* = 19,556 each; case and control cohorts for ≥30%, *N* = 15,239 each

assessing the likelihood of experiencing an inpatient admission or ER visit for either a schizophrenia or psychiatric diagnosis (Additional file 1: Table S1). For schizophrenia, cases with a ≥ 10% dose reduction had a first-year event rate of 22.1%, compared with a 17.5% event rate for the control group, an absolute difference of 4.6% (Fig. 4a), and were more likely to have an inpatient admission or ER visit for schizophrenia than their control counterparts. After adjusting for differences in baseline characteristics, patients with a dose reduction of ≥10% were still more likely to have an inpatient admission or ER visit for schizophrenia than their counterparts with no dose reduction (Table 4). Cases with a ≥ 30% dose reduction showed a slightly higher rate of

schizophrenia admissions or ER visits than the ≥10% dose-reduction cases; the difference in first-year event rate between cases and controls was 5.5% (22.8% cases vs 17.3% controls) (Fig. 4b). These cases showed an increased likelihood for inpatient admission or ER visit for schizophrenia, which persisted after adjusting for additional patient characteristics (Table 4).

For psychiatric diagnoses, cases with a ≥ 10% or ≥ 30% dose reduction had a first-year event rate difference of 2.5% (27.7% cases vs 25.2% controls) and 3.8% (29.0% cases vs 25.2% controls) respectively (Fig. 5a, b). Cases with ≥10% and ≥ 30% dose reductions were more likely to have an inpatient admission or ER visit for psychiatric diagnoses than controls;

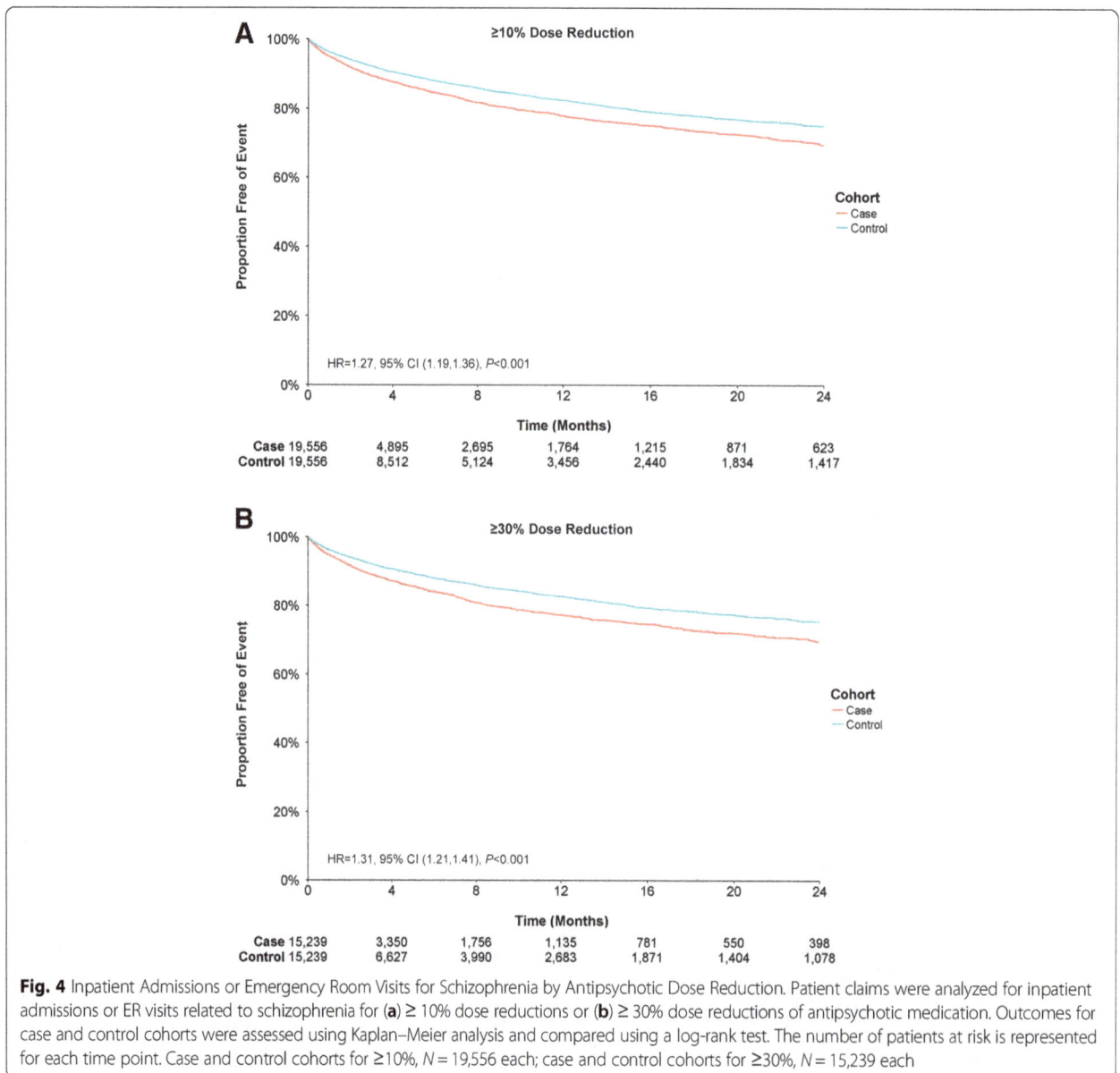

Fig. 4 Inpatient Admissions or Emergency Room Visits for Schizophrenia by Antipsychotic Dose Reduction. Patient claims were analyzed for inpatient admissions or ER visits related to schizophrenia for (**a**) ≥ 10% dose reductions or (**b**) ≥ 30% dose reductions of antipsychotic medication. Outcomes for case and control cohorts were assessed using Kaplan–Meier analysis and compared using a log-rank test. The number of patients at risk is represented for each time point. Case and control cohorts for ≥10%, N = 19,556 each; case and control cohorts for ≥30%, N = 15,239 each

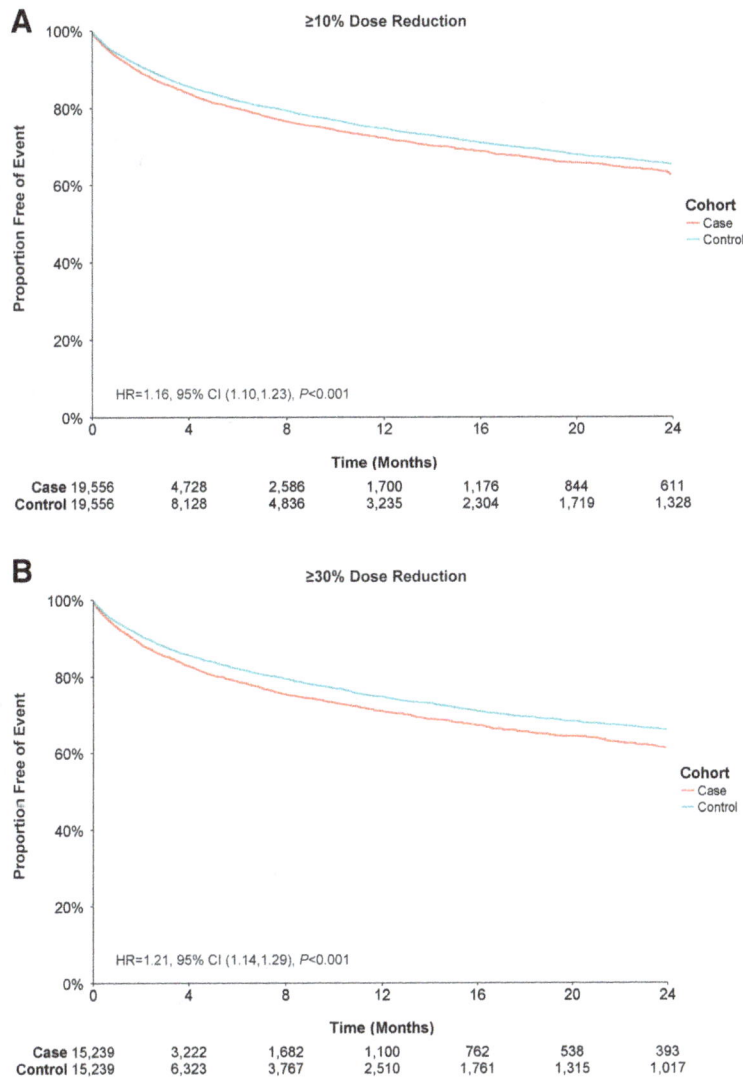

Fig. 5 Inpatient Admissions or Emergency Room Visits for Psychiatric-Related Diagnosis by Antipsychotic Dose Reduction. Patient claims were analyzed for inpatient admissions or ER visits related to psychiatric diagnoses for (**a**) ≥ 10% dose reductions or (**b**) ≥ 30% dose reductions of antipsychotic medication. Outcomes for case and control cohorts were assessed using Kaplan–Meier analysis and compared using a log-rank test. The number of patients at risk is represented for each time point. Case and control cohorts for ≥10%, $N = 19,556$ each; case and control cohorts for ≥30%, $N = 15,239$ each

when adjusted for baseline characteristics, this likelihood remained increased (Table 4).

TD claims

Although analysis of TD claims was limited by the small sample size of TD claims, we assessed the existing claims for the emergence of any trends. Data from all patients in both cohorts, with and without TD at baseline, were analyzed with respect to the risk of a TD diagnosis during the study period. Cases with a ≥ 10% dose reduction did not show a lower risk of having a TD claim than controls (first-year event rate of 0.21% cases vs 0.24% controls; HR: 1.39, 95% CI 0.80, 2.41, $P = 0.24$). Patients with a ≥ 30% dose reduction also showed similar

results (first-year event rate of 0.23% cases vs 0.22% controls; HR: 1.60, 95% CI 0.86, 3.00, $P = 0.14$). Both comparisons represented a non-significant difference in risk of having a TD claim after adjusting for baseline characteristics (Table 4).

Dose-reduction groups were also analyzed with respect to new cases of TD diagnosis during the study period compared with controls. To determine the risk of a new TD diagnosis, patients with TD at baseline were excluded (cases, $n = 37$; controls, $n = 51$). The resulting cases with a dose reduction did not have lower risk of having a TD claim compared with controls in the ≥10% group (first-year event rate of 0.16% cases vs 0.16% controls; HR: 1.66, 95% CI 0.87, 3.18, $P = 0.12$) and in the

≥30% group (first-year event rate of 0.18% cases vs 0.14% controls; HR: 1.84, 95% CI 0.89, 3.83, $P = 0.10$) after adjusting for baseline characteristics.

In addition, among patients with a TD claim during the baseline period, the percentages of patients having at least one additional TD claim during the first year of the study period were comparable between the dose-reduction cohort and the control cohort in both the ≥10% (21/37 [57%] vs 28/51 [55%], $P = 0.33$) and the ≥30% dose-reduction analyses (17/30 [57%] vs 21/40 [53%]; $P = 0.46$).

Discussion

Patients with antipsychotic dose reductions showed significant increases in both all-cause and mental health–related admissions and ER visits. Absolute percentage differences in first-year hospital event rates were small (1–6%), but were statistically significant given the large sample size. The clinical meaningfulness of the observed differences should be considered by healthcare decision makers, because even a 1% difference in event rates reflected an additional 196 patients using hospital services during the study period. In addition, the shorter duration of follow-up observed for cases compared with controls suggests that dose reduction not only may increase the risk of hospital utilization, but also may result in shorter periods of treatment stability.

Hospital re-admissions for schizophrenia may be an indicator of an adverse outcome or failure of antipsychotic treatment after dose reductions. The chronic nature and severity of schizophrenia contribute to its large overall healthcare burden; direct healthcare costs for schizophrenia were estimated at 38 billion US dollars in 2013 [24]. Inpatient admissions represent one of the largest portions of the healthcare burden for schizophrenia, estimated in one study as 60–70% of direct costs [25]. The cost for schizophrenia patients who relapse is estimated to be two to five times higher than that for non-relapsed patients [26].

However, antipsychotic dose reduction in patients with schizophrenia may be necessary and appropriate for a variety of reasons; for example, patients in the dose-reduction cohort had higher mean doses to start with, as well as more cases of diabetes, which may have prompted reductions of antipsychotic doses. Although dose reduction has also been recommended to manage TD in previous practice guidelines for patients with schizophrenia who require maintenance antipsychotic treatment [5, 6], our results suggest that even relatively modest reductions in antipsychotic dosing, regardless of the rationale, may have significant adverse effects on outcomes for some patients. Therefore, prescribing decisions on maintenance antipsychotic treatment for preventing or treating TD should be carefully considered on an individualized basis for each patient. Apart from antipsychotic prescribing decisions, other measures, e.g., discontinuation or modification of anticholinergic drugs or

treatment with vesicular monoamine transporter-2 inhibitors, may be considered in the management of TD.

The current study also attempted to evaluate antipsychotic dose reduction with respect to the diagnosis of TD and found no significant difference between stable dosing and dose reduction groups in either the number of new claims for TD during the study period based solely on the ICD-9 code of 333.85 and the ICD-10 code of G24.01 or in the persistence of a TD diagnosis following dose reduction. However, the duration of follow-up was significantly shorter in the dose-reduction group, and there were too few claims for TD in the databases compared with an expected prevalence of up to 30% in some previous studies [27]. This severely limits any interpretation of the relationship between dose reduction and the treatment of TD that was present at baseline, as well as the risk of new cases of TD developing in the total patient population. We suspect that TD is vastly underreported in claims databases [28], possibly due to complacency or a lack of clinical awareness, screening, approved treatments, standardization of the diagnosis or clarity regarding ICD codes. This study therefore highlights the need to document TD in a more systematic fashion. In addition, further study is needed to evaluate whether antipsychotic dose reduction is an effective treatment strategy for established cases of TD.

Strengths of the current study include the use of large patient cohorts with a 2-year follow-up period. In addition, claims data were analyzed from multiple states, with closely matched case and control groups. Study limitations include the possibility that the dose-reduction group had more hospitalizations because it represented a more-severe or chronically ill population compared with controls as suggested by the slightly longer duration of underlying schizophrenia among the case patients, the higher mean doses of antipsychotics they received, and the higher number of patients receiving clozapine at baseline. However, patients with more-severe disease would have been less likely to have doses reduced by prescribers and qualify as cases. In addition, more-severely ill patients were excluded from the analysis if they received multiple antipsychotics during the study period, had recent increases in doses (dose-reduction group), or were receiving long-acting injectable antipsychotics, all reflective of more-resistant disease. Comorbid psychiatric diagnoses that contribute to severity and hospitalizations, especially substance use, were actually more common among controls and may have biased results against our findings, resulting in worse outcomes among controls. Finally, outcome measures were controlled for numerous covariates in the Cox model that may reflect severity of illness, including psychiatric, substance use and medical co-morbidities, illness duration, and concomitant medication use. Nonadherence to treatment is another major contributor to relapse and hospitalization that may have affected differences in outcomes. However, enrollment criteria screened against including recognized nonadherent patients; patients were excluded if they received long-acting injectable antipsychotics or if they had fewer than 90 days of stable prescription monotherapy with antipsychotics prior to the index study date. Even if the dose reduction group showed greater rates of hospitalization because of nonadherence after the index date, that would still be clinically meaningful evidence suggesting untoward treatment effects of dose reduction. The high attrition during the 2 years of the study and the difference in attrition rates between cohorts were due to the cohort definitions, the differences in outcomes, and possibly nonadherence. Specifically, patients in the dose-reduction and control groups were censored at any change in antipsychotic use outside of the original inclusion criteria or after occurrence of an outcome event. The attrition and censoring of patients were accounted for in the Kaplan–Meier analyses and in the Cox models, which are statistical tools designed to handle censored or truncated time-to-event data [29]. Finally, given the retrospective nature of this claims-based study, we could not confirm the reasons for antipsychotic dose reductions and whether dose reduction affected outcomes positively in relation to other clinical domains.

Conclusion

Results from this study show statistically significant differences in hospital utilization event rates, and suggest that dose reductions of antipsychotics may destabilize psychiatric status and lead to increased hospitalization rates in some patients with schizophrenia, resulting in damaging effects on recovery and adding to overall healthcare costs. Dose reductions had no effect on claims for TD, but this finding was confounded by the limited duration of follow-up and underreporting of the diagnosis. Therefore, decisions on dose reduction of antipsychotics in schizophrenia patients who require maintenance antipsychotic treatment, whether to prevent or reduce TD symptoms or for other reasons, should be carefully considered on an individualized basis. These results may highlight the need for alternative management strategies apart from dose reduction to reduce distressing side effects that would allow physicians to maintain effective maintenance treatment for patients with schizophrenia.

Additional file

Additional file 1: Table S1. Diagnostic Codes for Schizophrenia and Psychiatric Relapse. Listing of ICD-9 and ICD-10 codes for disorders identified as causes for hospitalization and ER visits. **Table S2.** Baseline Demographics of ≥30% Dose-Reduction Case and Control Cohorts. Comparison of baseline demographic data between cases undergoing ≥30% dose reduction of antipsychotics versus controls on stable doses. (DOCX 25 kb)

Abbreviation
ADHD: Attention-deficit/hyperactivity disorder; AIDS: Acquired immunodeficiency syndrome; CCI: Charlson Comorbidity Index; CI: Confidence interval; ER: Emergency room; FFS: Fee-for-service; HIV: Human immunodeficiency virus; HMO: Health maintenance organization; HR: Hazard ratio; ICD: International Classification of Diseases; TD: Tardive dyskinesia

Acknowledgments
We thank the personnel involved with this study, and Michael Howell, PhD (Chameleon Communications International with funding from Teva Pharmaceutical Industries) for editorial assistance in the preparation of this manuscript.

Funding
This study was funded by Teva Pharmaceuticals. The sponsor was involved only in providing funding for aspects of the research and presentations of the manuscript. The design of the study, and collection, analysis, and interpretation of data, and writing of the manuscript was conducted solely by the authors, as specified below, including those affiliated with the study sponsor.

Authors' contributions
SNC design and conceptualization of the study, significant content-related direction, data acquisition and analysis, contribution to the writing of the draft, and feedback on all relevant materials throughout the development of the manuscript. FM design and conceptualization of the study, significant content-related direction, data acquisition and analysis, contribution to the writing of the draft, and feedback on all relevant materials throughout the development of the manuscript. RA design and conceptualization of the study, significant content-related direction, data acquisition and analysis, contribution to the writing of the draft, and feedback on all relevant materials throughout the development of the manuscript. TS design and conceptualization of the study, significant content-related direction, data acquisition and analysis, contribution to the writing of the draft, and feedback on all relevant materials throughout the development of the manuscript. VA design and conceptualization of the study, significant content-related direction, data acquisition and analysis, contribution to the writing of the draft, and feedback on all relevant materials throughout the development of the manuscript. BC design and conceptualization of the study, significant content-related direction, data acquisition and analysis, contribution to the writing of the draft, and feedback on all relevant materials throughout the development of the manuscript. All authors read and approved the final manuscript.

Consent for publication
Not applicable.

Competing interests
SNC: Consultant for Teva Pharmaceutical Industries and Neurocrine Biosciences Inc., research grant from Neurocrine Biosciences Inc.; FM, TS, VA, BC: Employee of Teva Pharmaceutical Industries; RA: Employee of Analysis Group

Author details
[1]Department of Psychiatry, Corporal Michael J. Crescenz VA Medical Center and the Perelman School of Medicine at the University of Pennsylvania, 3900 Woodland Avenue, Philadelphia, PA 19104, USA. [2]Analysis Group, 111 Huntington Ave, Boston, MA 02199, USA. [3]Teva Pharmaceutical Industries, 41 Moores Rd, Frazer, Malvern, PA 19355, USA.

References

1. Lehman AF, Lieberman JA, Dixon LB, McGlashan TH, Miller AL, Perkins DO, et al. Practice guidelines: practice guideline for the treatment of patients with schizophrenia (second edition). Am J Psychiatry. 2004;161(2 Suppl):1–56.

2. Aquino CC, Lang AE. Tardive dyskinesia syndromes: current concepts. Parkinsonism Relat Disord. 2014;20(Suppl 1):S113–S7.

3. Caroff SN, Campbell EC. Drug-induced extrapyramidal syndromes: Implications for contemporary practice. Psychiatr Clin North Am. 2016;39:391–411.

4. Waln O, Jankovic J. An update on tardive dyskinesia: from phenomenology to treatment. Tremor Other Hyperkinet Mov (N Y). 2013:3.

5. Bhidayasiri R, Fahn S, Weiner WJ, Gronseth GS, Sullivan KL, Zesiewicz TA. Evidence-based guideline: treatment of tardive syndromes: report of the guideline development Subcommittee of the American Academy of neurology. Neurology. 2013;81:463–9.

6. American Psychiatric Association. Tardive dyskinesia: a task force report of the American Psychiatric Association. American Psychiatric Association, Washington, DC, 1992.

7. Glazer WM, Moore DC, Schooler NR, Brenner LM, Morgenstern H. Tardive dyskinesia. A discontinuation study. Arch Gen Psychiatry. 1984;41:623–7.

8. Zutshi D, Cloud LJ, Factor SA. Tardive syndromes are rarely reversible after discontinuing dopamine receptor blocking agents: experience from a university-based movement disorder clinic. Tremor Other Hyperkinet Mov (N Y). 2014;4:266.

9. Schooler NR. Maintenance medication for schizophrenia: strategies for dose reduction. Schizophr Bull. 1991;17:311–24.

10. Dhir A, Schilling T, Abler V, Potluri R, Carroll B. estimation of epidemiology of tardive dyskinesia incidence and prevalence in the United States. The American Academy of Neurology annual meeting; April 22–28, 2017; Boston, MA.

11. Gilbert PL, Harris M, McAdams L, Jeste DV. Neuroleptic withdrawal in schizophrenic patients: a review of the literature. Arch Gen Psychiatry. 1995; 52:173–88.

12. Sariah AE, Outwater AH, Malima KI. Risk and protective factors for relapse among individuals with schizophrenia: a qualitative study in Dar Es Salaam, Tanzania. BMC Psychiatry. 2014;14:240.

13. Pigott TA, Carson WH, Saha AR, Torbeyns AF, Stock EG, Ingenito GG, Apriprazole Study Group. Aripiprazole for the prevention of relapse in stabilized patients with chronic schizophrenia: a placebo-controlled 26-week study. J Clin Psychiatry. 2003;64:1048–56.

14. Brar JS, Parepally H, Chalasani L, Gopalani A, Appel N, Chengappa KN. The impact of olanzapine on tardive dyskinetic symptoms in a state hospital population. Ann Clin Psychiatry. 2008;20:139–44.

15. Caroff SN, Davis VG, Miller DD, Davis SM, Rosenheck RA, McEvoy JP, et al. Treatment outcomes of patients with tardive dyskinesia and chronic schizophrenia. J Clin Psychiatry. 2011;72:295–303.

16. Mentzel CL, Bakker PR, van Os J, Drukker M, Matroos GE, Hoek HW, Tijssen MA, van Harten PN. Effect of antipsychotic type and dose changes on tardive dyskinesia and parkinsonism severity in patients with a serious mental illness: the curacao extrapyramidal syndromes study XII. J Clin Psychiatry. 2017;78:e279–ee85.

17. Kane JM, Woerner M, Sarantakos S, Kinon B, Lieberman J. Do low dose neuroleptics prevent or ameliorate tardive dyskinesia? In: Casey D, Gardos G, editors. Tardive Dyskinesia and Neuroleptics: From Dogma to Reason. Washington, D.C.: American Psychiatric Press, Inc. p. 100–7.

18. Soares KV, McGrath JJ. The treatment of tardive dyskinesia--a systematic review and meta-analysis. Schizophr Res. 1999;39:1–16 discussion 7–8.

19. Tarsy D, Baldessarini RJ. Epidemiology of tardive dyskinesia: is risk declining with modern antipsychotics? Mov Disord. 2006;21:589–98.

20. Davis JM, Matalon L, Watanabe MD, Blake L, Metalon L. Depot antipsychotic drugs. Place in therapy Drugs. 1994;47:741–73.

21. Wang CY, Xiang YT, Cai ZJ, Weng XY, Bo QJ, Zhao JP, et al. Risperidone maintenance treatment in schizophrenia: a randomized, controlled trial. Am J Psychiatry. 2010;167:676–85.

22. Cookson IB. The effects of a 50% reduction of cis(z)-flupenthixol decanoate in chronic schizophrenic patients maintained on a high dose regime. Int Clin Psychopharmacol. 1987;2:141–9.

23. Kane JM, Rifkin A, Woerner M, Reardon G, Sarantakos S, Schiebel D, Ramos-Lorenzi J. Low-dose neuroleptic treatment of outpatient schizophrenics. I. Preliminary results for relapse rates. Arch Gen Psychiatry. 1983;40:893–6.

24. Cloutier M, Aigbogun MS, Guerin A, et al. The economic burden of schizophrenia in the United States in 2013. J Clin Psychiatry. 2016;77:764–71.

25. Svarstad BL, Shireman TI, Sweeney JK. Using drug claims data to assess the relationship of medication adherence with hospitalization and costs. Psychiatr Serv. 2001;52:805–11.

26. Ascher-Svanum H, Zhu B, Faries DE, Salkever D, Slade EP, Peng X, Conley RR. The cost of relapse and the predictors of relapse in the treatment of schizophrenia. BMC Psychiatry. 2010;10:2.

27. Carbon M, Hsieh CH, Kane JM, Correll CU. Tardive dyskinesia prevalence in the period of second-generation antipsychotic use: a meta-analysis. J Clin Psychiatry. 2017;78:e264–e78.

28. Cortese L, Jog M, McAuley TJ, Kotteda V, Costa G. Assessing and monitoring antipsychotic-induced movement disorders in hospitalized patients: a cautionary study. Can J Psychiatr. 2004;49:31–6.

29. Kleinbaum D, Klein M. Survival analysis: a self-learning text. 3rd ed. New York, NY: Springer; 2012.

3

The moderating roles of bedtime activities and anxiety/depression in the relationship between attention-deficit/hyperactivity disorder symptoms and sleep problems in children

Lian Tong[1][*][†], Yan Ye[2][†] and Qiong Yan[1]

Abstract

Background: Children with attention-deficit/hyperactivity disorder (ADHD) often experience sleep problems, but the comorbidity mechanism has not been sufficiently studied. This study aimed to determine the comorbidity of ADHD symptoms and sleep problems as well as the moderating effects of bedtime activities and depression/anxiety symptoms on the relationship between ADHD symptoms and sleep problems.

Methods: We recruited 934 primary students from third to fifth grade and their parents by stratified random sampling from three primary schools in Shanghai, China. This study used parent-reported versions of the ADHD Rating Scale-IV, Children's Sleep Habits Questionnaire, and Achenbach Child Behavior Checklist. We used hierarchical linear regression analysis to clarify the moderating effects of bedtime activities and depression/anxiety symptoms.

Results: We found that children with more ADHD symptoms had shorter sleep durations and more sleep problems on weekdays. Screen time before bedtime strengthened the relationship between ADHD symptoms and sleep-disordered breathing. Children with more screen time were more likely to have sleep onset delay, while those with less screen time had more sleep onset problems with increasing ADHD symptoms. The high bedtime eating group experienced more night waking with increasing ADHD symptoms compared with the low bedtime eating group. Anxiety/depression exacerbated total sleep problems and further interacted with ADHD symptoms to predict sleep length and sleep duration problems.

Conclusions: Bedtime activities and emotional problems had important moderating effects on the relationship between ADHD symptoms and sleep problems. These findings indicate that appropriate bedtime management and emotional management may reduce sleep problems and improve sleep duration for children with ADHD symptoms.

Keywords: ADHD, Sleep problems, Bedtime activities, Anxiety/depression

* Correspondence: ltong@fudan.edu.cn
†Lian Tong and Yan Ye contributed equally to this work.
[1]Department of Maternal, China and Adolescent Health, School of Public Health, Fudan University/Key laboratory Public Health Safety, Chinese Ministry of Education, P.O. Box 244, 138 Yixueyuan Road, Shanghai 200032, China
Full list of author information is available at the end of the article

Background

Attention-deficit/hyperactivity disorder (ADHD) is a common neurodevelopmental disorder among children, characterized by hyperactivity, inattention, and impulsivity. It affects 5–10% of school-age children worldwide [1–3]. ADHD is commonly associated with a number of other behavioral and emotional disorders, such as conduct disorder, anxiety disorder, depression disorder [4, 5], and sleep problems, one of the most common comorbidities [6]. Children with ADHD symptoms are more likely to report sleep problems such as prolonged sleep onset latency, difficulty falling asleep, bedtime resistance problems, sleep-disordered breathing, restless leg movements during sleep, night awakenings, and difficulties with morning awakening [7, 8]. As many as 55–74% of children with ADHD are affected by sleep disturbances [9]. A population-based study with a sample of 9486 adolescents found that ADHD symptoms were linked to shorter sleep duration, longer sleep latency, longer nocturnal wake time, and sleep deficiency [10].

The underlying mechanism of comorbid ADHD and sleep problems is complicated. A biopsychosocial and contextual model of sleep suggests that biological factors, psychosocial factors (i.e., mental health, family, and peer factors), and contextual factors (i.e., electronic media use, homework, and extracurricular activities) contribute to the association of ADHD symptoms and sleep problems [8]. The present study narrowly focuses on mental health problems of anxiety/depression and bedtime activities including screen time and diet behaviors. Evidence from epidemiological and clinical studies has suggested that lifestyle behaviors, such as screen time, diet, and physical activity, are closely correlated with both ADHD symptoms and sleep problems [11]. One study found that children with ADHD symptoms were almost twice as likely to have unhealthy behaviors compared with typically developing children. For example, children with ADHD symptoms spent more time watching TV, playing video games, and using computers and consumed more sugar and artificially sweetened juice than their counterparts [12]. A meta-analysis of 45 empirical studies has suggested that there is a significant relationship between ADHD symptoms and media use [13].

As is well known, for typical children and adolescents worldwide, exposure to the Internet, computers, video gaming, and caffeine is related to various sleep problems [14]. Longitudinal research also has shown a link between electronic media use and sleep problems [15]. The mechanisms beneath this phenomenon may be explained by a model [16]. According to this model, electronic media use may replace children's sleep time, or may deteriorate sleep quality through increased psychophysiological arousal leading by the contents of the

media or through too much light exposure. However, little is known about how increased screen time is related to sleep problems in children with ADHD. A recent study found that playing games significantly reduced the average sleep hours of boys with ADHD, although no such relationship was found among typically developing boys [17]. Another study found that the use of an electronic device for 1 hour before bedtime did not influence the relationship between ADHD symptoms and sleep problems in teenagers [10]. Thus, a clear conclusion cannot be drawn from the inconsistent findings of previous studies. There has been particularly little research on the effects of screen exposure before bedtime in children with ADHD.

In addition, increased screen time is associated with unhealthy eating habits, including lower vegetable consumption, higher consumption of unhealthy snacks and drinks, higher consumption of fast food, and higher overall caloric intake [18]. As screen activities such as watching TV, playing video games, and using mobile phones have become predominant bedtime activities for children [19], this has led to more night eating. Our recent study indicated that children with ADHD have more screen time, and more eating behaviors co-occur with screen time than children without ADHD symptoms [20]. A clinical study showed that treatment with an elimination diet reduced sleep complaints and physical problems in children diagnosed with ADHD [21]. This finding suggests that food consumption may be related to sleep problems in children with ADHD. However, it remains unknown whether bedtime eating contributes to sleep problems in the context of ADHD.

Beyond lifestyle-related behaviors, the combination of ADHD and emotional problems in children leads to more sleep problems. Studies have indicated that more than 50% of children with ADHD suffer from anxiety/depression problems that contribute to specific sleep problems [22, 23]. Youth with comorbid ADHD and anxiety were found to have the longest sleep onset delay, shortest sleep duration, and greatest daytime sleepiness in comparison to typically developing youth and youth with ADHD alone [24]. A clinical study found that children with ADHD comorbid with anxiety/depression showed more total sleep problems, difficulty falling asleep, restlessness during sleep, waking during the night, nightmares, walking or talking during sleep, waking too early, and sleeping less than typical children [25]. A large population-based study suggested that ADHD symptoms and anxiety/depression symptoms independently contribute to delayed sleep phase syndrome in adolescents [26]. However, it is still unknown whether ADHD and anxiety/depression contribute to sleep problems in children separately or via an interactive effect between these factors.

The first purpose of this study is to explore the relationship between screen time and eating behaviors before bedtime with sleep problems, particularly the interaction between ADHD and bedtime activities. The second purpose of this study is to clarify the moderating role of anxiety/depression in the relationship between ADHD symptoms and sleep problems.

Methods

Participants

We recruited 934 primary students, ages 9 to 12 years old (mean = 10.5, $SD = 1.1$), and their parents by stratified random sampling of three primary schools (third grade to fifth grade) in Shanghai, China. The sample covered different socioeconomic strata in China. Parents in School A had the highest socioeconomic status (SES; e.g., high educational attainment, high household income, and young parents), and parents in School C had the lowest SES. Of the students, 501 (53.8%) were boys and 430 (46.2%) were girls.

Measures

Both a student self-report questionnaire and a parent-completed questionnaire were used in this study. The two questionnaires were matched by student identification (ID). The specific assessment instruments used in this study were as follows:

ADHD symptoms

ADHD symptoms were assessed by the parent-reported version of the ADHD Rating Scale-IV (ADHDRS-IV) [27]. The ADHDRS-IV is an 18-item ADHD assessment scale, and it consisted of two subscales, inattention and hyperactivity-impulsivity, each containing nine items. For example, the following items were used to assess hyperactivity and impulsivity symptoms: 1) Fidgets with hands or feet or squirms in seat, 2) Is "on the go" or acts as if "driven by a motor", 3) Runs about or climbs excessively in situations in which it is inappropriate; The items, like "Fails to give close attention to details or makes careless mistakes in schoolwork", "Loses things necessary for tasks or activities", and "Is easily distracted" were used to evaluate inattention symptoms. Each item mapped onto one of the 18 DSM-IV (Diagnostic and Statistical Manual of Mental Disorders-IV) symptoms of ADHD. Parents were required to rate the frequency of each of the ADHD symptoms occurred over the past 6 months on a five-point Likert scale with 0 for never or rarely, 1 for sometimes, 2 for often, and 3 for very often. The sum of all the scores on the 18 items results in a total score. The reliability and validity of the home version of the ADHDRS-IV had been verified in a sample of Chinese children ages 6–17 years old [28]. Cronbach's alpha of the ADHDRS-IV for the present

sample was 0.92. A cutoff of 26 points was used to define children with or without clinically significant ADHD symptoms [28].

Sleep problems and sleep length

Parents completed the Children's Sleep Habits Questionnaire (CSHQ) to report their children's sleep problems [29]. The CSHQ contains 45 (only 33 items for scoring) items in eight subscales. There are bedtime resistance (six items, e.g., goes to bed at same time), sleep onset delay (one item, falls asleep in 20 min), sleep duration (three items, e.g. sleep the right amount), sleep anxiety (four items, e.g. afraid of sleeping alone), night waking (three items, e.g. awakes more than once), parasomnias (seven items, e.g. talks during sleep), sleep-disordered breathing (three items, e.g. snores loudly), and daytime sleepiness (eight items, e.g. seems tired).

Parents were required to rate the frequency of certain sleep-related behaviors that occurred in the previous week. A response of "usually" (given a score of 3) indicated that the behavior had occurred between five and seven times, "sometimes" (scored 2) meant it had happened two to four times, and "rarely" (scored 1) meant that the behavior was observed once at most. The reliability and validity of the instrument had been verified in a sample of Chinese primary school students [30]. The Cronbach's alpha coefficient in the current sample was 0.75, which was similar to other studies [22, 23]. Parents were required to report the time their children fell asleep and woke up on weekdays and weekends. Sleep length was calculated by the investigators.

Bedtime activities

Diet behaviors Children were asked to rate the frequency of their consumption of snacks, soft drinks, tea, and coffee before bedtime in a typical week on a five-point Likert scale ranging from 0 (never) to 4 (seven times a week).

Screen time Children were asked to rate how frequently they used a smart phone or computer (including an or any electronic music player, tablet, or other device) or watched TV before bedtime in a typical week using a five-point Likert scale ranging from 0 (never) to 4 (seven times a week).

Anxiety/depression symptoms

Parents filled out the subscale of the Achenbach Child Behavior Checklist (CBCL, the version fit for children ages 6–18 years old) to evaluate children's anxiety/depression symptoms. The subscale of anxiety/depression included 17 items, for example, fears he / she might think or do something bad; Feels or complains that no one loves him / her. Parents were required to rate the frequency of each anxiety/depression symptom over the past 6 months on a three-point Likert scale (0 = not true, 1 = sometimes true, and 2 = often true). The reliability and validity of the instrument had been verified among Chinese children and teenagers [31]. The Cronbach' s alpha coefficient in the current sample was 0.87.

Data analysis

We conducted statistical analyses with SPSS version 20.0. The cutoff point of 26 was used to define children with or without ADHD. A chi-squared test was used to examine the differences in categorical variables of demographic information between the ADHD symptomatic and non-symptomatic groups, while a t-test was used for continuous variables (i.e., age). The Wilcoxon rank-sum test was used to clarify the differences in sleep length, sleep problems, bedtime activities, and anxiety/depression between two ADHD groups. Additionally, we used hierarchical regression analyses to examine the predictors of sleep length and sleep problems and the interactive effect of moderators. Both moderators and independent variables were centralized by a Z-score to avoid potential multicollinearity among the variables in the regression equation [32]. The moderating effects of bedtime screen time and diet and anxiety/depression are shown in Figs. 1, 2, 3, 4, 5 and 6.

Results

Table 1 presents the demographics of the participants. Of the 934 children, 82 (10.3%) belonged to the ADHD symptomatic group, and more boys (14.5%) were symptomatic than girls (6.1%; $\chi^2 = 14.456$, $P < 0.01$). The proportion of ADHD children did not differ by grades ($\chi^2 = 2.187$, $P > 0.1$). The mean age of the ADHD symptomatic group was 10.3 years, slightly younger than the ADHD non-symptomatic group (10.6; $t = 2.691$, $P < 0.01$). No significant differences in parents' education level (father: $\chi^2 = 3.172$, $P > 0.1$; mother: $\chi^2 = 1.634$, $P > 0.1$) and annual household income ($\chi^2 = 2.187$, $P > 0.1$) were found between the ADHD symptomatic and non-symptomatic groups, which means the proportion of non-symptomatic and symptomatic children was similar across parents' education levels and across household incomes.

We found that children's average sleep time was 9.3 h on weekdays, significantly less than the average 10.1 h on weekends ($t = -18.152$, $P < 0.001$; Table 2). However, there was no difference in sleep hours between the ADHD symptomatic group and non-symptomatic group. The ADHD symptomatic group had more sleep problems in general. Compared with the non-symptomatic group, the symptomatic group had more bedtime resistance problems ($U = 14,984.5$, $P < 0.001$), sleep onset delay ($U = 24,284.5$, $P < 0.05$), sleep duration problems ($U = 17,729.0$, $P < 0.001$), sleep anxiety problems ($U = 20,815.0$, $P < 0.05$), night waking problems($U = 20,552.5$, $P < 0.0001$), parasomnias problems ($U = 17,845.0$, $P < 0.0001$), sleep-disordered breath problems ($U = 20,407.0$, $P < 0.0001$), and daytime sleepiness problems ($U = 17,546.0$, $P < 0.0001$) (Table 2). In addition, children in the ADHD symptomatic group had more screen time ($U = 22,595.0$, $P < 0.05$) and consumed more snacks, soft

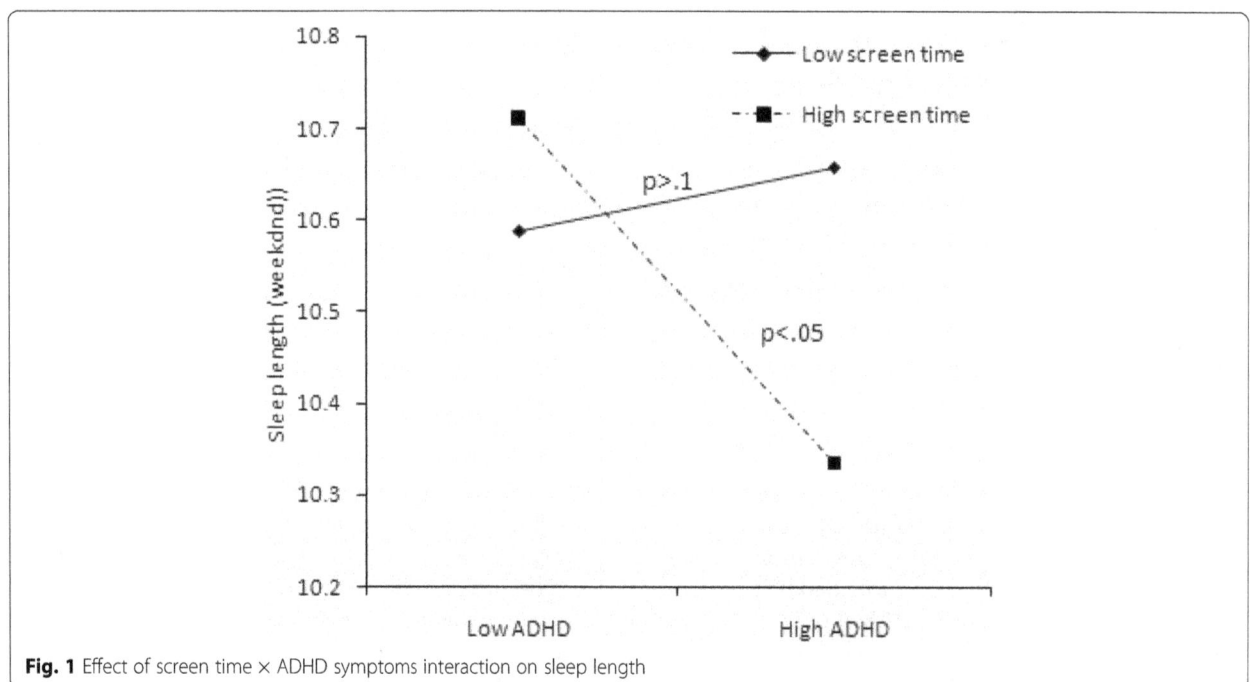

Fig. 1 Effect of screen time × ADHD symptoms interaction on sleep length

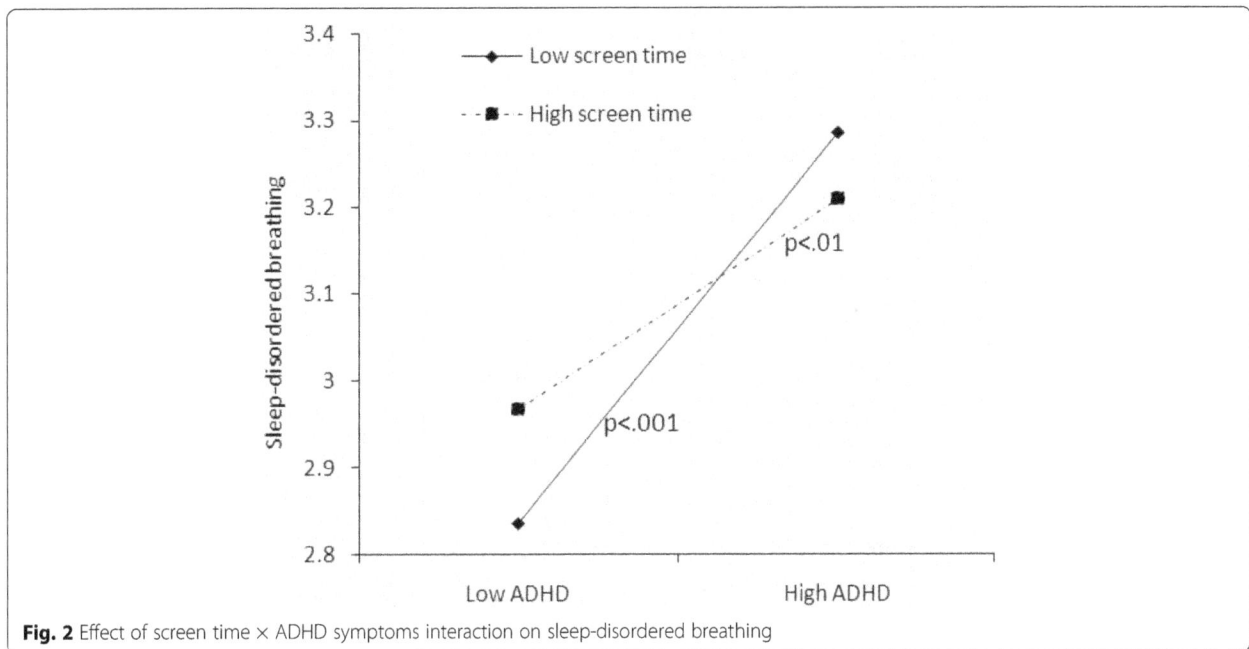

Fig. 2 Effect of screen time × ADHD symptoms interaction on sleep-disordered breathing

drinks, tea, and coffee before bedtime than children without ADHD symptoms ($U = 22,705.0$, $P = 0.071$). Furthermore, children in the ADHD symptomatic group had more anxiety/depression symptoms than those in the non-symptomatic group ($U = 13,516.0$, $P < 0.001$).

The results of correlation analysis were presented in Table 3. After controlling for children's gender and age and parents' education and annual household income, ADHD symptoms were significantly correlated with sleep problems ($r = .48$, $p < .001$), sleep length on weekday ($r = -.11$, $p < .05$), diet behavior ($r = .14$, $p < .01$), and anxiety/depression problems ($r = .24$, $p < .001$). It was found that sleep problems were associated with diet behavior ($r = .12$, $p < .01$), and anxiety/depression problems ($r = .69$, $p < .001$), and only marginally associated with sleep length on weekday($r = -.10$, $p = .02$) and screen activities ($r = .08$, $p = .08$).

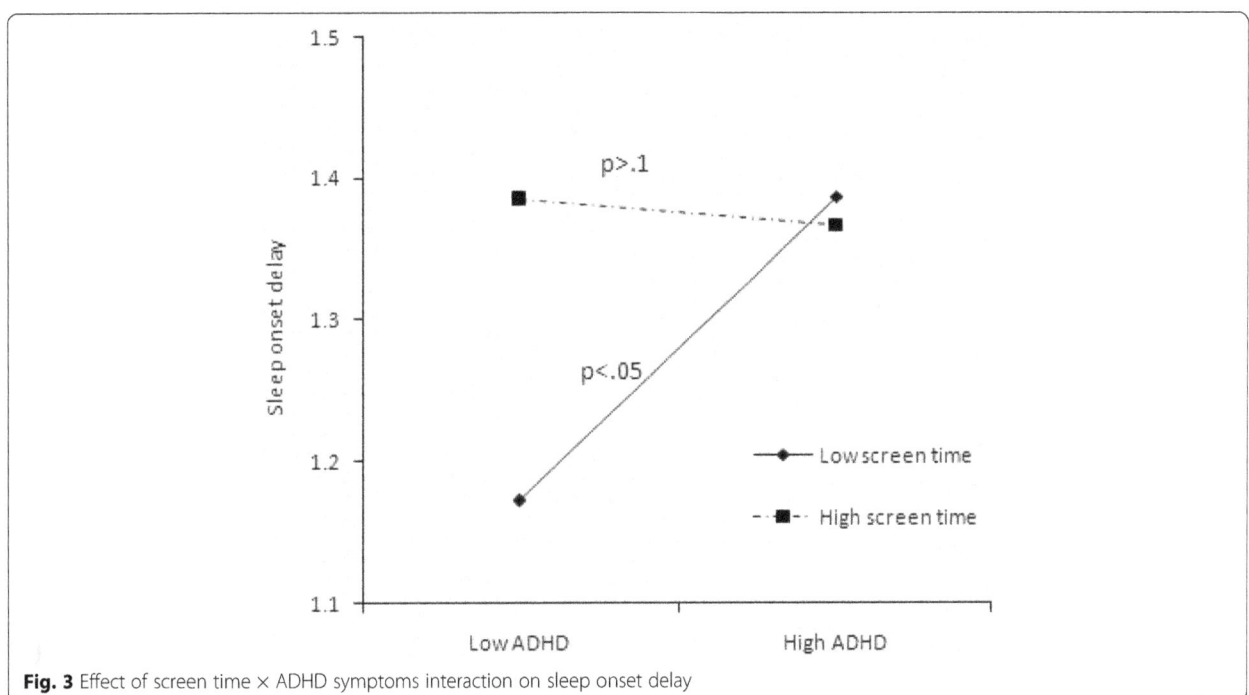

Fig. 3 Effect of screen time × ADHD symptoms interaction on sleep onset delay

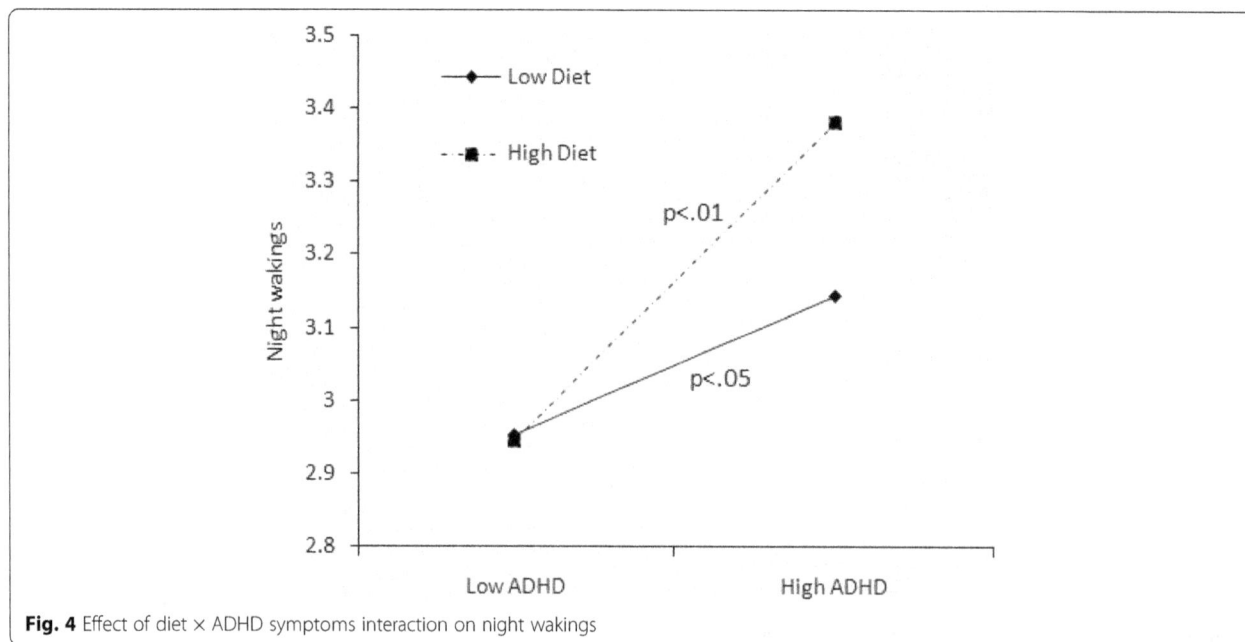

Fig. 4 Effect of diet × ADHD symptoms interaction on night wakings

We used hierarchical linear regression analysis to examine the predictors of ADHD, bedtime activities, anxiety/depression, and each sleep problem. The main findings are shown in Table 4. In Model 2, after controlling for children's gender and age and parents' education and annual household income, ADHD symptoms significantly predicted children's sleep length on weekdays ($B = -0.107$, $P < 0.001$), total sleep problems ($B = 2.792$, $P < 0.001$), bedtime resistance problems ($B = 0.625$, $P < 0.001$), sleep duration problems ($B = 0.325$, $P < 0.001$), sleep anxiety problems ($B = 0.314$, $P < 0.001$), night waking problems($B = 0.164$, $P < 0.001$), parasomnias problems

($B = 0.361$, $P < 0.001$), sleep-disordered breathing problems ($B = 0.170$, $P < 0.001$), and daytime sleepiness problems($B = 0.779$, $P < 0.001$). Anxiety/depression was another important factor associated with weekend sleep time ($B = 0.195$, $P < 0.01$) and total sleep problems ($B = 1.413$, $P < 0.001$).

In Model 3, when the interaction effect with ADHD was taken into consideration, bedtime activities more strongly predicted sleep length and sleep problems (see Table 4). We found that the interaction between screen time and ADHD predicted sleep duration on weekends ($B = -0.111$, $P < 0.05$), sleep onset delay ($B = -0.058$, $P < 0.05$),

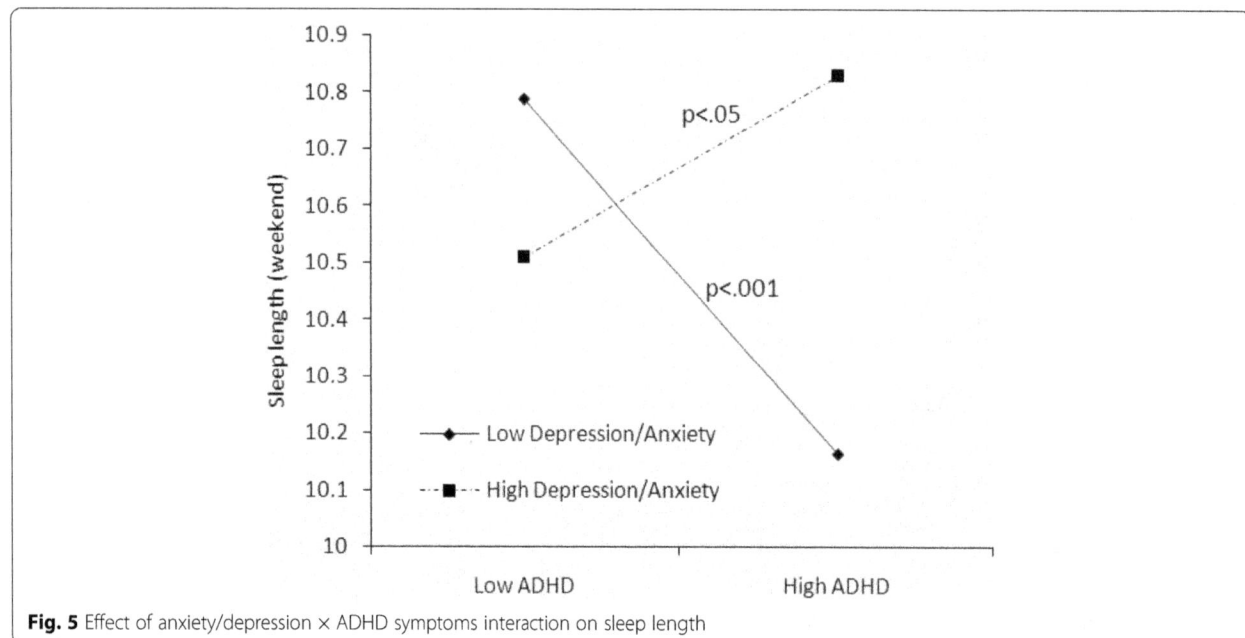

Fig. 5 Effect of anxiety/depression × ADHD symptoms interaction on sleep length

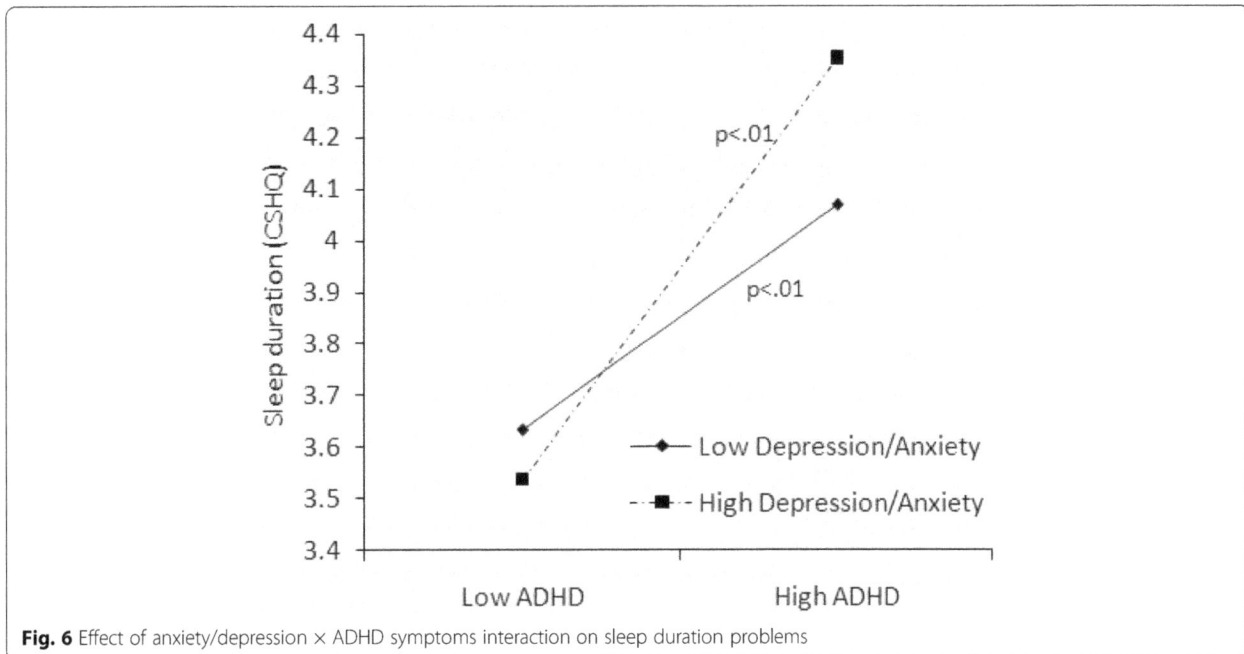

Fig. 6 Effect of anxiety/depression × ADHD symptoms interaction on sleep duration problems

and sleep-disordered breathing ($B = -0.052$, $P = 0.057$). These interactive effects are presented in Figs. 1–4. For children with low screen time before bedtime, sleep length decreased with increasing ADHD symptoms (Fig. 1). For children with low as well as with high screen time before bedtime, sleep disorder breathing problems increased with increasing ADHD symptoms (Fig. 2). For children with low screen time before bedtime, sleep onset delay exacerbated with increasing ADHD symptoms (Fig. 3). Additionally, eating before bedtime was associated with longer sleep length on weekdays ($B = 0.070$, $P < 0.05$) and more night waking problems ($B = 0.076$, $P < 0.1$). Furthermore, eating before bedtime played a moderating role in the relationship between ADHD and night waking ($B = 0.061$, $P < 0.1$). For children with low as well as with high screen time before bedtime, night waking problems increased with increasing ADHD symptoms (Fig. 4).

Taking emotional problems into account, anxiety/depression exacerbated total sleep problems ($B = 1.413$, $P < 0.001$), particularly sleep anxiety ($B = 0.285$, $P < 0.001$), parasomnias ($B = 0.305$, $P < 0.001$), and daytime sleepiness ($B = 0.488$ $P < 0.001$). In Model 2, we found that more anxiety/depression symptoms predicted longer sleep duration on weekends ($B = 0.195$, $P < 0.01$). Furthermore, in Model 3, the interaction of anxiety/depression and ADHD predicted longer sleep periods on weekends ($B = 0.236$, $P < 0.001$) as well as sleep duration problems ($B = 0.095$, $P = 0.08$). The interaction effects illustrated in Fig. 5 show that for children with low Depression/Anxiety scores, sleep duration on weekends decreased with increasing ADHD symptoms while for children with high Depression/Anxiety scores, sleep duration rather increased with increasing ADHD symptoms.

For children with low as well as with high Depression/Anxiety scores, sleep duration problems increased with increasing ADHD symptoms (Fig. 6). Additionally, the mother's educational attainment independently contributed to children's sleep problems in general ($B = -0.902$, $P < 0.05$) and was related to sleep onset delay ($B = -0.088$, $P < 0.05$), sleep duration problems ($B = -0.157$, $P < 0.1$), and night waking ($B = -0.160$, $P < 0.05$), as well as parasomnias ($B = -0.231$, $P < 0.05$).

Discussion

Children with ADHD often experience sleep problems [33], and this association was supported by the present study. We found that children with more ADHD symptoms had more bedtime resistance problems, sleep onset delay, sleep duration problems, sleep anxiety, night waking problems, parasomnias, sleep-disordered breath, and daytime sleepiness problems. Other findings of the present study offered new evidence for interpreting the potential mechanisms. For example, we found that children with ADHD symptoms had more unhealthy bedtime activities, including more screen time and eating. These behaviors associated with sleep problems independently in addition to moderating the relationship between ADHD symptoms and sleep problems.

Specifically, children with more ADHD symptoms and screen time before bedtime tended to have shorter sleep times on weekends. A previous study also suggested that high exposure to games and TV decreased sleep hours among boys diagnosed with ADHD [17]. This may be

Table 1 Characteristics of study populations with and without ADHD symptoms

	Total % (n)	ADHD Non-Symptomatic % (n)	Symptomatic % (n)	χ^2
Gender				
Male	53.8 (501)	85.5 (428)	14.5 (73)	14.456***
Female	46.2 (430)	93.9 (404)	6.1 (26)	
Grade				
Three	36.6 (342)	87.3 (299)	12.7 (43)	2.187
Four	30.0 (280)	90.6 (253)	9.4 (27)	
Five	33.4 (312)	90.8 (283)	9.2 (29)	
Father's education level				
Primary school and below	3.7 (28)	89.3 (25)	10.7 (3)	3.172
Junior high school	37.4 (286)	88.1 (252)	11.9 (34)	
Senior high school	26.8 (205)	89.8 (184)	10.2 (21)	
College	29.5 (226)	92.5 (209)	7.5 (17)	
Graduate	2.6 (20)	85.0 (17)	15.0 (3)	
Mother's education level				
Primary school and below	11.9 (91)	87.9 (80)	12.1 (11)	1.634
Junior high school	35.8 (273)	88.6 (242)	11.4 (31)	
Senior high school	24.0 (183)	90.2 (165)	9.8 (18)	
College	27.7 (211)	91.0 (192)	9.0 (19)	
Graduate	0.7 (5)	100 (5)	0	
Annual household income (USD)				
≤ 3000	6.9 (50)	88.0 (44)	12.0 (6)	1.080
3000–6000	11.8 (86)	88.4 (76)	11.6 (10)	
6000–9000	19.5 (142)	88.7 (126)	11.3 (16)	
9000–12,000	14.4 (105)	91.4 (96)	8.6 (9)	
12,000–15,000	17.5 (127)	89.8 (114)	10.2 (13)	
≥ 15,000	29.8 (217)	90.8 (197)	9.2 (20)	
Total	100.0 (934)	91.2 (852)	8.8 (82)	

***$P < 0.01$

because parents allow their children to use electronics before bedtime for longer periods on weekends than on weekdays, so as to reduce unexpected behaviors for children with ADHD. Additionally, we found bedtime screen activities to be a strong moderating factor for the relationship between ADHD symptoms and sleep-disordered breathing problems. Children with high ADHD symptoms showed more sleep-disordered breathing problems than those with low ADHD symptoms; moreover, both low screen time and high screen time significantly strengthened this association. This suggests that even a short period of exposure to screen activities before bedtime may make children with ADHD symptoms more hyperactive and impulsive [16, 34], which may lead to more breathing problems and snoring [35].

With regard to the problem of sleep onset delay, neither ADHD symptoms nor screen time associated with sleep onset delay independently; however, the interaction of the two factors significantly affected sleep onset delay. Regardless of ADHD symptoms, children with high screen time always experienced longer sleep onset delay, while the children with low screen time experienced more sleep onset delay with increasing ADHD symptoms. This suggests that children with ADHD symptoms should avoid screen activities before bedtime, because even a short screen time may excite them and make it hard for them to fall asleep. This explanation is supported by the fact that violent or age-inappropriate content, the fast pace of entertainment media, and higher overall screen time can lead to ADHD-related behaviors (e.g., intense arousal, poor self-control) [13].

Table 2 The differences in sleep status, bedtime activities, and anxiety/depression between the two groups

	ADHD		U
	Non-Symptomatic $\bar{x}$ (SD)	Symptomatic $\bar{x}$ (SD)	
Sleep length			
Weekdays	9.3 (0.6)	9.3 (0.7)	25,424.0
Weekends	10.1 (0.9)	10.3 (2.8)	26,846.0
Sleep problems (total score)	46.3 (6.7)	52.9 (6.9)	9237.0***
Bedtime resistance	8.2 (2.2)	9.6 (2.6)	14,984.5***
Sleep onset delay	1.4 (0.6)	1.6 (0.7)	24,284.5*
Sleep duration	4.4 (1.4)	5.3 (1.5)	17,729.0***
Sleep anxiety	5.4 (1.8)	6.1 (1.9)	20,815.0*
Night waking	3.5 (0.8)	4.1 (1.2)	20,552.5***
Parasomnias	8.4 (1.4)	9.3 (1.9)	17,845.0***
Sleep-disordered breath	3.3 (0.6)	3.8 (1.2)	20,407.0***
Daytime sleepiness	11.8 (2.8)	13.1 (2.7)	17,546.0***
Bedtime activities			
Screen activities	5.3 (2.2)	6.0 (2.9)	22,595.0*
Diet	4.7 (1.9)	5.4 (2.9)	22,705.0$^+$
Anxiety/depression	2.7 (2.9)	5.9 (4.1)	13,516.0***

$^+P < 0.1$, *$P < 0.05$, ***$P < 0.0001$

Moreover, we found that bedtime diet moderated the relationship between ADHD symptoms and sleep problems. More bedtime eating behaviors were associated with more night waking problems with increasing ADHD symptoms. As of now, the mechanism of the relationship between bedtime diet and ADHD symptoms is unclear. Children with ADHD often have eating disorders, which may increase the risk of night eating behaviors. Our previous study also demonstrated that children with ADHD symptoms showed more frequent bedtime eating behaviors than non-ADHD children [19]. Another study showed that young adults with night eating syndrome were significantly more likely to have histories of ADHD, depression, and eating disorders [36]. These studies showed that hypersensitivity to food may play an

Table 3 Correlations among the study variables

Main variables	1	2	3	4	5	6
1. ADHD symptoms	1					
2. Sleep problems	.48***					
3. Sleep length (weekday)	−.11*	−.10$^+$				
4. Sleep length (weekend)	.01	.06	.21***			
5. Bedtime activities (screen)	.05	.08$^+$	.02	−.02		
6. Bedtime activities (diet)	.14**	.12*	.04	−.02	.55***	
7. Anxiety/depression	.24***	.69***	−.08$^+$	0	.05	.08$^+$

$^+P < 0.1$, *$P < 0.05$, **$P < 0.001$, ***$P < 0.0001$

etiologic role in sleep complaints in children with ADHD and suggest a relationship between diet and sleep problems in children with ADHD. However, previous studies of night eating syndrome have been conducted in clinical samples. Our study findings add to the literature suggesting that bedtime eating may associate with sleep problems in general school-age children.

An interesting finding of the current study was that emotional problems (i.e., anxiety/depression) played a moderating role in the relationship between ADHD symptoms and sleep problems. Children with more ADHD symptoms and high levels of anxiety/depression had longer sleep durations on weekends, but poorer sleep quality (wake up more during the night). The finding is consistent with a recent study, which found that that children combined ADHD and anxiety/depression had shorter sleep durations and more sleep problems than their counterparts [37]. It also suggests that children with ADHD may have different sleep patterns on weekdays and weekends. Especially for school-age children in China, the strict school schedule on weekdays is a great challenge for children with mental health problems, and to compensate, they sleep longer on weekends. As shown in the present study, children with ADHD and emotional problems experienced more sleep problems, so they were likely tired on weekdays and slept longer on weekends to compensate. Furthermore, the parent-reported sleep times for children may be biased, because the time the child goes to bed may not equal the time the child falls asleep, especially for children with emotional problems. It has been suggested that anxiety/depression symptoms may increase nighttime fears related to personal safety, separation, loss, pressures, and so on, leading these children to stay awake in bed or even lose sleep at night [23].

Additionally, a mother's higher level of education appears to be a protective factor for some sleep problems, including sleep onset delay, sleep duration, night waking, and parasomnias. Some previous studies showed that parental education and SES were associated with sleep hours and sleep problems. For example, one study found that higher parental education was associated with longer sleep time in their children [38]. Children in low-SES families have more sleep problems than children in high-SES families [39, 40]. The mother is generally the primary caregiver in both Western countries and Asian countries [41] and therefore tends to have a greater impact on the child. Mothers with higher education know more about healthy sleep habit and are more likely to provide their children regular bedtimes and bedtime routines [42]. One evidence-based survey reported that parental control of night activities could considerably improve children's sleep quality [43].

Table 4 Hierarchical linear regression analysis

	Model 1[a]	Model 2[b]	Model 3[c]
	Beta	Beta	Beta
Sleep length(weekend)			
Child's gender	.134	.088	.086
Child's age	−.074	−.079	−.065
Father's education	−.118	−.119	−.116
Mother's education	−.110	−.107	−.121
Annual household income	−.012	−.007	−.007
ADHD		−.080	−.076
Screen behaviors in bedtime (Screen)		−.038	−.050
Diet behaviors in bedtime		.003	.044
Anxiety/Depression		.195**	.097
Screen × ADHD			−.111*
Diet × ADHD			−.027
Anxiety/Depression × ADHD			.236***
$R^2(F)$	.029 (3.7**)	.047 (3.4***)	.094 (5.3***)
Sleep problems (total)			
Child's gender	−.029	1.260	1.267*
Child's age	−.358	.096	.102
Father's education	−.127	.108	.113
Mother's education	−.902*	−.530	−.531
Annual household income	−.301	−.354*	−.353*
ADHD		2.792***	2.811***
Screen behaviors in bedtime		.504	.545+
Diet behaviors in bedtime		.087	.037
Anxiety/Depression		1.413***	1.437***
Screen × ADHD			−.272
Diet × ADHD			.165
Anxiety/Depression × ADHD			−.060
$R^2(F)$	.034(3.649***)	.292(23.820***)	.293(17.874***)
Sleep onset delay			
Child's gender	.029	.057	.062
Child's age	.021	.026	.031
Father's education	.061	−.060	−.061
Mother's education	−.088*	−.076*	−.075*
Annual household income	.009	.010	.010
ADHD		.039	.049
Screen behaviors in bedtime		.038	.048
Diet behaviors in		.001	.005

Table 4 Hierarchical linear regression analysis *(Continued)*

	Model 1[a]	Model 2[b]	Model 3[c]
	Beta	Beta	Beta
bedtime			
Anxiety/Depression		.025	−.025
Screen × ADHD			.058*
Diet × ADHD			.0
Anxiety/Depression × ADHD			−.002
$R^2(F)$	.044(5.6***)	.054(3.9***)	.064(3.5***)
Sleep duration			
Child's gender	.050	.192	.188
Child's age	.051	.097+	.100+
Father's education	−.054	−.026	−.025
Mother's education	−.157+	−.140+	−.145+
Annual household income	−.083*	−.086*	−.085*
ADHD		.325***	.313***
Screen behaviors in bedtime		.020	.002
Diet behaviors in bedtime		.031	.046
Anxiety/Depression		.087	.046
Screen × ADHD			.033
Diet × ADHD			−.021
Anxiety/Depression × ADHD			.095+
$R^2(F)$	.041 (5.0***)	.102 (7.4***)	.107 (5.8***)
Night wakings			
Child's gender	.039	.108	.103
Child's age	.045	.075*	.077*
Father's education	−.043	−.027	−.029
Mother's education	−.160**	−.152**	−.152**
Annual household income	.018	.019	.021
ADHD		.164***	.157***
Screen behaviors in bedtime		−.025	−.018
Diet behaviors in bedtime		.076+	.057
Anxiety/Depression		.065	.050
Screen × ADHD			−.043
Diet × ADHD			.061+
Anxiety/Depression × ADHD			.049
$R^2(F)$	.046 (5.7***)	.098 (7.2***)	.107 (5.9***)
Sleep-disordered breathing			
Child's gender	−.133*	−.061	−.061
Child's age	.010	.035	.036

Table 4 Hierarchical linear regression analysis *(Continued)*

	Model 1[a] Beta	Model 2[b] Beta	Model 3[c] Beta
Father's education	−.021	−.009	−.010
Mother's education	−.018	−.011	−.009
Annual household income	.010	.009	.010
ADHD		.170***	.173***
Screen behaviors in bedtime		.003	.014
Diet behaviors in bedtime		.025	.014
Anxiety/Depression		−.009	−.008
Screen × ADHD			−.052+
Diet × ADHD			.036
Anxiety/Depression × ADHD			.006
$R^2(F)$	.012 (1.5)	.067 (4.8***)	.074 (3.9***)

+p < .1, *p < .05, **p < .001, ***p < .01
[a]Model 1: Gender, age, father's education, mother's education, Annual household income. These variables were adjusted in model 2–3;
[b]Model 2: Variables of ADHD, Screen behavior (Screen), Diet before sleep (Diet), Anxiety/Depression were added;
[c]Model 3: Interactive terms of Screen × ADHD, Diet × ADHD, Anxiety/Depression× ADHD were added

Limitations

Some limitations of this study should be mentioned. First, the study design was a cross-sectional design, limiting our ability to draw causal inferences. For example, it is impossible to clarify whether media use causes sleep onset difficulties or whether children with ADHD who have trouble falling asleep turn to electronics as a way to cope with their sleep onset problems. Second, the sleep hours and sleep problems were assessed by parent-reported rating scales rather than measured by devices, so the data may have been imprecise. Child report of sleep problems was not collected - this is particularly important for aspects of sleep that parents may not observe such as night wakings and parasomnias. Third, this study used a questionnaire and not an interview-based assessment to assess ADHD symptoms. Forth, the data on medication was not collected, so the role of medication in these relationships is unknown. Therefore, more research is needed to determine the causal effects of bedtime activities on sleep problems in children with ADHD.

Conclusions

Bedtime activities and emotional problems had important moderating effects on the relationship between ADHD and sleep problems. Bedtime management—including consistent parent-set bedtimes, a clear structure surrounding house rules, and bedtime behavior management—could reduce sleep problems for children with ADHD. Moreover, paying attention to children's emotional status and strengthening their emotion management could potentially improve sleep quality as well.

Abbreviations
ADHD: Attention Deficit Hyperactivity Disorder;; ADHDRS-IV: ADHD Rating scale-IV;; CBCL: Achenbach Child Behavior Checklist; CSHQ: Children's Sleep Habits Questionnaire; DSM-IV: Diagnostic and Statistical Manual of Mental Disorders-IV;; SES: Social-economic Status

Acknowledgements
The authors appreciated all the participated families.

Funding
The study was funded by Award from Shanghai Municipal Health Bureau (Grant No. 15GWZK0402) for the publication fee; the National Natural Science Foundation of China (Grant No. 81402693) and Shanghai Pujiang Program (Grant No. 14PJC012) supported the study design, data collection and analysis. Shanghai Municipal People's Government Decision-making Consultation Research Project Education Policy Special (Grant No. 2018-Z-R12) supported the writing and editing of this manuscript.

Authors' contributions
LT designed the study, supervises the data collection, and revised the manuscript. YY analyzed the data and wrote the manuscript. LT and QY collected the data. All authors read and approved the final manuscript.

Consent for publication
Not applicable.

Competing interests
The authors declare that they have no competing interests.

Author details
[1]Department of Maternal, China and Adolescent Health, School of Public Health, Fudan University/Key laboratory Public Health Safety, Chinese Ministry of Education, P.O. Box 244, 138 Yixueyuan Road, Shanghai 200032, China. [2]Department of Behavior and Psychology Science, Zhejiang University, Hangzhou, China.

References
1. Willcutt EG. The prevalence of DSM-IV attention-deficit/hyperactivity disorder: a Meta-analytic review. Neurotherapeutics. 2012;9(3):490–9.
2. Polanczyk G, et al. The worldwide prevalence of ADHD: a systematic review and metaregression analysis. Am J Psychiatr. 2007;164(6):942–8.
3. Tong L, Shi H, Zang J. Prevalence of ADHD in children of China:a systematic review and meta analysis. Chin J Public Health. 2013;29(9):1279–83.

4.   Dulcan M. Practice parameters for the assessment and treatment of children, adolescents, and adults with attention-deficit/hyperactivity disorder. J Am Acad Child Adolesc Psychiatry. 1997;36(10, Supplement):85S–121S.

5.   Mulraney M, et al. The bidirectional relationship between sleep problems and internalizing and externalizing problems in children with ADHD: a prospective cohort study. Sleep Med. 2016;17:45–51.

6.   Jensen CM, Steinhausen H-C. Comorbid mental disorders in children and adolescents with attention-deficit/hyperactivity disorder in a large nationwide study. ADHD Attention Deficit and Hyperactivity Disorders. 2015;7(1):27–38.

7.   Cortese S, et al. Sleep in children with attention-deficit/hyperactivity disorder: meta-analysis of subjective and objective studies. J Am Acad Child Adolesc Psychiatry. 2009;48(9):894–908.

8.   Becker SP, Langberg JM, Byars KC. Advancing a biopsychosocial and contextual model of sleep in adolescence: a review and introduction to the special issue. Journal of Youth and Adolescence. 2015;44(2):239–70.

9.   Lycett K, et al. Behavioral sleep problems and internalizing and externalizing comorbidities in children with attention-deficit/hyperactivity disorder. European Child & Adolescent Psychiatry. 2015;24(1):31–40.

10. Hysing M, et al. Association between sleep problems and symptoms of attention deficit hyperactivity disorder in adolescence: results from a large population-based study. Behav Sleep Med. 2016;14(5):550–64.

11. Billows M, et al. Family disorganization, sleep hygiene, and adolescent sleep disturbance. J Clin Child Adolesc Psychol. 2009;38(5):745–52.

12. Holton KF, Nigg JT. The Association of Lifestyle Factors and ADHD in children. J Atten Disord. 2017. https://www.ncbi.nlm.nih.gov/pmc/articles/PMC5205565/pdf/nihms835190.pdf.

13. Nikkelen SW, et al. Media use and ADHD-related behaviors in children and adolescents: a meta-analysis. Dev Psychol. 2014;50(9):2228.

14. Bartel KA, Gradisar M, Williamson P. Protective and risk factors for adolescent sleep: a meta-analytic review. Sleep Med Rev. 2015;21:72–85.

15. Maume DJ. Social ties and adolescent sleep disruption. J Health Soc Behav. 2013;54(4):498–515.

16. Cain N, Gradisar M. Electronic media use and sleep in school-aged children and adolescents: a review. Sleep Med. 2010;11(8):735–42.

17. Engelhardt CR, Mazurek MO, Sohl K. Media use and sleep among boys with autism spectrum disorder, ADHD, or typical development. Pediatrics. 2013;132(6):1081–9.

18. Pearson N, Biddle SJH. Sedentary behavior and dietary intake in children, adolescents, and adults: a systematic review. Am J Prev Med. 2011;41(2):178–88.

19. Foley LS, et al. Presleep activities and time of sleep onset in children. Pediatrics. 2013;131(2):276–82.

20. Tong L, Xiong X, Tan H. Attention-deficit/hyperactivity disorder and lifestyle-related behaviors in children. PLoS One. 2016;11(9):e0163434.

21. Pelsser LM, et al. Effects of food on physical and sleep complaints in children with ADHD: a randomised controlled pilot study. Eur J Pediatr. 2010;169(9):1129–38.

22. Leirbakk MJ, Clench-Aas J, Raanaas RK. ADHD with co-occurring depression/anxiety in children: the relationship with somatic complaints and parental socio-economic position. J Psychol Abnorm. 2015;4(1);702–8.

23. Lovato N, Gradisar M. A meta-analysis and model of the relationship between sleep and depression in adolescents: recommendations for future research and clinical practice. Sleep Med Rev. 2014;18(6):521–9.

24. Moreau V, Rouleau N, Morin CM. Sleep of children with attention deficit hyperactivity disorder: actigraphic and parental reports. Behav Sleep Med. 2013;12(1):69.

25. Mayes SD, et al. ADHD subtypes and comorbid anxiety, depression, and oppositional-defiant disorder: differences in sleep problems. J Pediatr Psychol. 2009;34(3):328–37.

26. Sivertsen B, et al. Mental health problems in adolescents with delayed sleep phase: results from a large population-based study in Norway. J Sleep Res. 2015;24(1):11–8.

27. DuPaul GJ, et al. Parent ratings of attention-deficit/hyperactivity disorder symptoms: factor structure and normative data. J Psychopathol Behav Assess. 1998;20(1):83–102.

28. Su YE, et al. Parent ratings of ADHD symptoms in Chinese urban schoolchildren: assessment with the Chinese ADHD rating scale–IV: home version. J Atten Disord. 2012;9. https://doi.org/10.1177/1087054712461177.

29. Owens JA, Spirito A, McGuinn M. The Children's sleep habits questionnaire (CSHQ): psychometric properties of a survey instrument for school-aged children. Sleep-New York. 2000;23(8):1043–52.

30. Sheng-hui L, et al. Development and psychometric properties of the Chinese version of Children's sleep habits questionnaire. Chinese Journal of Pediatrics. 2007;45(3):176–80.

31. Su L-Y, Li X. The norms of Achenbach child behavior checklist in Hunan Province. Chinese Journal of Clinical Psychology. 1996;12(2):67–9.

32. Frazier PA, Tix AP, Barron KE. Testing moderator and mediator effects in counseling psychology research. J Couns Psychol. 2004;51(1):115.

33. Lycett K, et al. A prospective study of sleep problems in children with ADHD. Sleep Med. 2014;15(11):1354–61.

34. Alexandru G, et al. Epidemiological aspects of self-reported sleep onset latency in Japanese junior high school children. J Sleep Res. 2006;15(3):266–75.

35. Beebe W. Neurobehavioral morbidity associated with disordered breathing during sleep in children: a comprehensive review. Sleep-New York Then Westchester. 2006;29(9):1115.

36. Runfola CD, et al. Prevalence and clinical significance of night eating syndrome in university students. J Adolesc Health. 2014;55(1):41–8.

37. Moreau V, Rouleau N, Morin CM. Sleep of children with attention deficit hyperactivity disorder: Actigraphic and parental reports. Behav Sleep Med. 2014;12(1):69–83.

38. Adam EK, Snell EK, Pendry P. Sleep timing and quantity in ecological and family context: a nationally representative time-diary study. J Fam Psychol. 2007;21(1):4–19.

39. Owens JA, Spirito A, Mcguinn M. The Children's sleep habits questionnaire (CSHQ): psychometric properties of a survey instrument for school-aged children. Sleep. 2000;23(8):1043–51.

40. Stamatakis KA, Kaplan GA, Roberts RE. Short sleep duration across income, education, and race/ethnic groups: population prevalence and growing disparities during 34 years of follow-up. Ann Epidemiol. 2008;17(12):948–55.

41. Shek DT. Differences between fathers and mothers in the treatment of, and relationship with, their teenage children: perceptions of Chinese adolescents. Adolescence. 2000;35(137):135–46.

42. Hale L, et al. Social and demographic predictors of preschoolers' bedtime routines. J Dev Behav Pediatr. 2009;30(5):394–402.

43. Pieters D, et al. Effects of pre-sleep media use on sleep/wake patterns and daytime functioning among adolescents: the moderating role of parental control. Behav Sleep Med. 2014;12(6):427–43.

4

Effects of long-term methylphenidate use on growth and blood pressure: results of the German Health Interview and Examination Survey for Children and Adolescents (KiGGS)

Suzanne McCarthy[1]* [ID], Antje Neubert[2], Kenneth K. C. Man[3,4,5], Tobias Banaschewski[6], Jan Buitelaar[7], Sara Carucci[8], David Coghill[9,10,11], Marina Danckaerts[12,13], Bruno Falissard[14], Peter Garas[15], Alexander Häge[6], Chris Hollis[16], Sarah Inglis[17], Hanna Kovshoff[18], Elizabeth Liddle[16,19], Konstantin Mechler[6], Peter Nagy[15], Eric Rosenthal[20], Robert Schlack[21], Edmund Sonuga-Barke[22,23], Alessandro Zuddas[8] and Ian C. K. Wong[3,24]

Abstract

Background: Concerns have been raised over the safety of methylphenidate (MPH), with regard to adverse effects on growth and blood pressure. Our study investigates whether, and to what extent, methylphenidate use in boys with ADHD is associated with having low body mass index (BMI), having low height, and increased systolic and diastolic blood pressure.

Methods: Data used for this study stem from the German KiGGS dataset. Three different groups of boys aged 6–15 years were included in the analysis: ADHD patients who used MPH for less than 12 months; ADHD patients who used MPH for 12 months or more; and ADHD patients without current MPH treatment. Each of these three groups was compared to a non-ADHD control group regarding low weight (BMI $\leq$ 3rd percentile), low height ($\leq$3rd percentile) and raised systolic and diastolic blood pressure. For growth outcomes, boys were categorized according to age (< 11 years/$\geq$11 years, to account for pubertal maturation). Multivariable logistic regression was conducted to test for associations.

Results: 4244 boys were included in the study; MPH < 12 months: $n = 65$ ($n = 36 < 11$ years), MPH $\geq$ 12 months: $n = 53$ ($n = 22 < 11$ years), ADHD controls: $n = 320$ ($n = 132 < 11$ years), non-ADHD controls: $n = 3806$ ($n = 2003 < 11$ years). Pre-pubertal boys with MPH use less than 12 months and pubertal/postpubertal boys with MPH use of 12 months or greater were significantly more likely to have a BMI $\leq$ 3rd percentile compared to non-ADHD controls. Boys from the ADHD control group were significantly less likely to have a raised systolic blood pressure compared to non-ADHD controls. Beyond that, no significant between group differences were observed for any other growth and BP parameter.

Conclusion: The analyses of the KiGGS dataset showed that MPH use in boys with ADHD is associated with low BMI. However, this effect was only observed in certain groups. Furthermore, our analysis was unable to confirm that MPH use is also associated with low height ($\leq$3rd percentile) and changes in blood pressure.

Keywords: ADHD, Methylphenidate, Safety, Growth, BMI, Blood pressure

* Correspondence: s.mccarthy@ucc.ie
[1]School of Pharmacy, University College Cork, Cork, Ireland
Full list of author information is available at the end of the article

Background

Attention deficit hyperactivity disorder (ADHD) is characterized by pervasive and impairing hyperactivity, inattention and impulsiveness [1]. The worldwide prevalence of ADHD among school-aged children and adolescents is around 5% [2, 3]. Methylphenidate (MPH), the most commonly prescribed psychopharmacological treatment of ADHD in Europe, is effective at improving ADHD symptoms [4]. However, there have been reports in the literature concerning the effect of MPH on growth [5] and adverse cardiovascular outcomes [6].

Height and weight

Effects on growth are usually reported as minor at the group level, but there is wide variability with some children unaffected [7–9] and others reporting moderate growth suppression [10–12]. Longitudinal studies suggest an overall height stunting of approximately 1 cm/year during the first three years of treatment which can be clinically relevant. These effects appear to attenuate over time and terminal adult height is not necessarily reduced [5, 13]. A Cochrane review published in 2015 examined the literature on the beneficial and harmful effects of methylphenidate on children and adolescents with ADHD [14]. With respect to the effect of methylphenidate on weight, five trials including 805 participants reported that children taking methylphenidate weighed significantly less than controls and six trials (859 participants) reported a decrease in weight among children taking methylphenidate. Children were also more likely to have a lower body mass index (BMI) based on the findings from one study with 215 participants [14]. However, disentangling these effects from growth deficits that may be associated with ADHD itself is challenging [5, 10, 15–17].

Cardiovascular outcomes

A number of studies have investigated cardiovascular events (e.g. stroke, myocardial infarction, ventricular arrhythmia, sudden death) and cardiovascular effects (e.g. changes in BP and heart rate) associated with MPH.

Dalsgaard et al. [18] conducted a prospective longitudinal cohort study in Denmark ($n = 714{,}258$) to determine the risk of cardiovascular events among stimulant users. They reported a stimulant-related increase in risk for cardiovascular events (adjusted Hazard Ratio = 1.83 (1.10–3.04)) that persisted after restricting the analysis to only children with ADHD ($n = 8300$) (adjusted Hazard Ratio = 2.20 (2.15–2.24)).

A pooled analysis of three large data sets (19–21) including more than 1.8 million patients (ages 2–24 years [19], 25–64 years [20], 3–17 years [21]) reported no association between methylphenidate, amphetamine (AMP) and atomoxetine and sudden death or stroke

(adjusted Odds Ratio = 0.93 (0.731.17)) [22]. However, in the study by Cooper et al. [19], it was reported that while there was no evidence of an association of serious cardiovascular events with ADHD drug use identified (adjusted Hazard Ratio = 0.70 (0.31–1.85)), "the upper limit of the 95% confidence interval indicated that a doubling of the risk could not be ruled out. However, the absolute magnitude of such an increased risk would be low". A population-based, retrospective cohort study, conducted by Winterstein et al. [23], reported no significant association between central nervous stimulants and cardiovascular events (stroke, acute myocardial infarction and sudden cardiac death as a primary composite endpoint and the previous events plus ventricular arrhythmia as a secondary composite endpoint (adjusted Odds Ratio = 0.62 (0.27–1.44) and 0.74 (0.38–1.46) for the primary and secondary endpoints respectively [23]).

In terms of cardiovascular effects, stimulant medication can cause small increases in heart rate and BP. On average, heart rate increases of 1–2 beats per minute are reported at the group level, although larger increases can occur in some individuals. Average increases in systolic and diastolic BP range between 1 and 4 mmHg and 1 and 2 mmHg respectively [24]. Few studies report categorical hypertension data (defined as BP beyond the 95th centile) although anecdotally and from case reports, it is reported that MPH can cause a rise in BP above the 95th centile in some individuals [25].

The Committee for Medicinal Products for Human Use at the European Medicines Agency concluded in January 2009 that the overall benefits of MPH outweigh the risks; at the same time they highlighted the need for more data on the long-term effects of MPH on children and young adults as many of the trials conducted to date had focused only on short-term effects [26].

The aim of this study was to examine associations between MPH use in ADHD, body mass index (BMI) and height and BP in boys. Data from the German Health and Examination Survey for Children and Adolescents (KiGGS), a population-based German representative sample, were analyzed to evaluate the hypothesis that boys with ADHD and current MPH use show higher percentages of having low BMI, having low height, and of increased systolic blood pressure (SBP) and diastolic blood pressure (DBP) compared to controls.

Methods
Data source

Data for the present study stem from the KiGGS database. KiGGS was conducted by the Robert Koch Institute, Berlin, Germany, between May 2003 and May 2006. A two-stage sampling strategy was utilised: in the first stage, a representative sample of 167 German municipalities was identified. In the second stage, random samples of children and adolescents aged between 0 and 17, and stratified by sex and age, were then selected from these municipalities through local population registries. The resulting sample included 17,461 children and adolescents (8985 boys, 8656 girls). Detailed information on the KiGGS dataset and the sampling strategy have been reported elsewhere [27, 28].

Sample selection

Individuals were classified as having ADHD if a parent reported that a diagnosis of ADHD had been made by a physician or psychologist [29]. Current ADHD-medication use (defined as use of medication within the seven days prior to interview) was documented using a standardized computer-assisted personal drug use interview which was conducted with the participants and their parents by a study physician [29]. The study design ensured that the study subjects were not interviewed during school holidays to exclude discontinuity of ADHD medication due to school breaks [30]. Duration of current medication use was categorized as either: less than 12 months or 12 months and longer. Patients with a record of current AMP use were excluded from the analyses in line with this study's aim to focus on methylphenidate exclusively. Information on past use of medication was not recorded in the database. Patients who did not have a value recorded for a particular outcome variable (BMI, height, systolic blood pressure (SBP) and diastolic blood pressure (DBP)) were excluded from that specific variable analysis.

Four groups of individuals were identified for inclusion in the study: two groups who were taking MPH (< 12 months and ≥ 12 months), an ADHD group not currently taking MPH and a non-ADHD control group. Matching of controls to the medicated cohort was not undertaken. Preliminary analyses revealed that there were low numbers of females and older adolescents amongst the ADHD groups generally and the MPH groups specifically and so the study was restricted to males aged between 6 and 15 years inclusive.

Outcome variables/ assessments

BMI, height: Body weight was measured in underwear to the nearest 0.1 kg with a calibrated scale (SECA, Birmingham, UK). Body height was measured by trained staff according to a standardized protocol to the nearest 0.1 cm using portable devices (standing height with Harpenden stadiometer for ages 2–17; Holtain Ltd., Crymych, UK). Measurement procedures were subject to internal and external quality control measures [31]. BMI was calculated as the ratio of weight (kg) to height (m) squared [31].

BP: Two readings of SBP and DBP were obtained using an automated oscillometric device (Datascope Accutorr Plus) at 2-min intervals after a non-strenuous part of the examination and an additional 5-min rest. The measurements were taken using the right arm, in the sitting position with the elbow at the level of the right atrium, using 1 of 4 cuff sizes which had to cover at least two-thirds of the upper arm length (from the axilla to the ante-cubital fossa). The mean of the two measurements was used for analysis [32]. The KiGGS dataset included a variable *cardiac disease* (code ca07); this variable, based on parents' reports, was recorded in the dataset as 'yes', 'no' or 'don't know'.

Outcome references
BMI and height

German reference data for BMI and height were obtained [31, 33]. The main focus of the data analyses was the percentage of boys with low BMI, defined as BMI <3rd percentile and the percentage of boys with a height ≤ 3rd percentile [34]. Analyses were conducted on the cohort as a whole (from 6 to 15 years) as well as according to two age categories, defined as 6–10 years and 11–15 years. By splitting the sample according to age, we use a simplified method that allows us to separate prepubertal children from peri and pubertal boys in the analyses, thus amplifying the power to detect an impact of MPH on growth.

BP

For the analysis of SBP and DBP, guidelines from the European Society of Hypertension [35] were used since these guidelines did not exclude overweight children unlike German reference data. (32).

Definition and classification of hypertension was as follows [35]:

Class	SBP / DBP percentile
Normal	<90th
High-normal	≥90th to < 95th ≥120/80 even if below 90th percentile in adolescents
Stage 1 hypertension	95th percentile to the 99th percentile plus 5 mmHg
Stage 2 hypertension	>99th percentile plus 5 mmHg

Both high-normal BP (≥90th to <95th percentile) and hypertension (Stage 1 (95th percentile to the 99th percentile plus 5 mmHg) or Stage 2 hypertension (>99th percentile plus 5 mmHg)) were collapsed to form "Raised SBP" and "Raised DBP" categories for the purposes of the regression analyses.

Statistical methods

For each outcome variable, mean and standard deviations (sd) was calculated. Odds Ratios (OR) and 95% Confidence Intervals (95% CI) were derived from logistic regression analyses. Each of the three ADHD groups was compared to a non-ADHD control group regarding weight (BMI ≤ 3rd percentile), height (≤3rd percentile) and raised SBP and DBP.

For the outcomes BMI and height, boys were categorized according to age (< 11 years/≥11 years, to account for pubertal maturation). The relationship between blood pressure and MPH use was examined using logistic regression adjusting for age, BMI and cardiac disease. Sensitivity analysis was conducted removing patients who had a cardiac disease code of yes or don't know.

A p-value of < 0.05 was considered significant for all analyses.

Results

i)   Sample characteristics:

A total of 4244 boys were included in the study: n = 65 in MPH < 12 months, n = 53 in MPH ≥ 12 months, n = 320 ADHD controls, and n = 3806 non-ADHD controls; 2193 (51.7%) boys of the total sample were 6–10 years old, 2051 boys (48.3%) were aged 11–15 years. For details see Table 1.

Body mass index

BMI data were available for 4229 boys (99.65%). Data of the group of boys aged 6–10 years (n = 2185) and those aged 11–15 years (n = 2044) were analyzed separately. The focus of the analyses was the percentage of boys who had low BMI, defined as BMI ≤ 3rd percentile. In the group of boys aged 6–10 years, those with MPH use of less than 12 months were significantly more likely to have a BMI ≤ 3rd percentile compared to the non-ADHD control group (OR 4.52 (95% CI, 1.54–13.28), p = 0.006). Whereas in the subsample of boys aged 11–15 years, those with MPH use ≥12 months were significantly more likely to have a BMI ≤ 3rd percentile compared to the non-ADHD control group (OR 3.59 (1.06–12.22), p = 0.040). Moreover, when compared to the non-ADHD control group no significant differences

with regard to low weight were observed for the other groups (see Table 2).

Height

Height data were available for 4242 boys (99.95%). In accordance with the analysis of the BMI data we distinguished between boys aged 6–10 years and 11–15 years. In both age-groups, no significant differences between the MPH and ADHD control groups and the non-ADHD control group were observed with regard to the percentage of boys with a height ≤ 3rd percentile (see Table 3).

Blood pressure

Blood pressure data were available for 4238 boys (99.86%). Mean SBP and mean DBP were similar across the different groups. Stage 2 hypertension based on SBP and/or DBP was generally very rare and was not observed in boys currently taking MPH. However, stage 1 hypertension based on SBP and/or DBP could be observed most frequently in those taking MPH ≥ 12 months (for details see Table 4). The percentage of boys in the ADHD control group with raised SBP was statistically significantly lower than in the non-ADHD control group (OR 0.65 (95% CI 0.46–0.92), p = 0.016). Moreover, no statistically significant differences between the MPH groups and ADHD control groups and the non-ADHD control group with regard to raised SBP nor to raised DBP could be found (See Table 5). These findings persisted after removal of such patients with a cardiac disease code of *yes* or *don't know*.

Discussion

This study investigated naturalistic data from a cohort of children collected within a large nation-wide survey in Germany. The aim of this study was to explore growth and cardiovascular outcomes across different patient groups, in particular to evaluate the hypothesis that boys with ADHD and current MPH use show a higher percentage of having low BMI, having low height, and increased systolic and diastolic BP compared to controls.

Height and BMI

Our analysis was unable to confirm our hypotheses that MPH use is also associated with low height (height ≤ 3rd percentile).

Table 1 Number (%) of boys in each study cohort

	MPH < 12 months	MPH ≥ 12 months	ADHD control	Non-ADHD control	Total (n)
Boys 6–10 years (n / %)	36 (0.85)	22 (0.52)	132 (3.11)	2003 (47.20)	2193
Boys 11–15 years (n / %)	29 (0.68)	31 (0.73)	188 (4.43)	1803 (42.48)	2051
Total (n / %)	65 (1.53)	53 (1.25)	320 (7.54)	3806 (89.68)	4244

Table 2 BMI data for 4229 boys

BMI ≤ 3rd percentile, n (%)	MPH < 12 months (n = 65)	MPH ≥ 12 months (n = 53)	ADHD control (n = 317)	Non-ADHD control (n = 3794)
Boys 6–15 years (n = 4229)				
Yes	5 (7.69)	4 (7.55)	11 (3.47)	108 (2.85)
No	60 (92.31)	49 (92.45)	306 (96.53)	3686 (97.15)
OR (95% CI), p-value	2.84 (1.12–7.22) 0.028	2.79 (0.99–7.89) 0.053	1.23 (0.65–2.31) 0.523	Reference
Boys 6–10 years (n = 2185)				
Yes	4 (11.11)	1 (4.55)	3 (2.29)	56 (2.81)
No	32 (88.89)	21 (95.45)	128 (97.71)	1940 (97.19)
OR (95% CI), p-value	4.52 (1.54–13.28), 0.006	1.83 (0.24–14.04), 0.561	0.84 (0.26–2.71), 0.766	Reference
Boys 11–15 years (n = 2044)				
Yes	1 (3.45)	3 (9.68)	8 (4.30)	52 (2.89)
No	28 (96.55)	28 (90.32)	178 (95.70)	1746 (97.11)
OR (95% CI), p-value	1.20 (0.16–8.98), 0.860	3.59 (1.06–12.22) 0.040	1.51 (0.71–3.23), 0.289	Reference

Several studies in children with ADHD have investigated associations between ADHD medication and height. Hanć and colleagues reported that the height of drug-naïve boys with ADHD was not significantly different from the norm [17]. Zhang and colleagues examined the impact of long-term treatment of MPH on height and weight of school age children with ADHD and reported a small but significant deceleration of height velocity, the magnitude of which was related to the duration of treatment [36].

Our analyses of the KiGGS dataset overall showed that MPH use in boys with ADHD was associated with low BMI. This effect was observed in the younger boys aged 6–10 years with MPH use of less than 12 months (OR: 4.52, 95% CI: 1.54–13.28, $p = 0.006$). There was a trend towards an effect in the boys aged 11–15 years with MPH use ≥12 months (OR: 3.59, 95% CI: 1.06–12.22, $p = 0.04$). Boys aged 6–10 years with MPH use ≥12 months and boys 11–15 years with MPH use less than 12 months did not significantly differ from the non-ADHD control group in that respect. Several considerations might help to interpret these findings:

A *fast* weight lost within a short amount of time (weeks or months) can raise concerns and lead to discontinuation of medication (in particular in younger children). This could explain why low BMI was more often in boys 6–10 years of age with MPH use of less than 12 months compared to controls, but not in the group with an MPH use ≥12 months (as this sample was reduced by the number of those who had to discontinue due to earlier weight loss).

However, we found the opposite effect in pubertal/post-pubertal boys. This might be due to a higher proportion of *slow* weight loss resulting in low BMI after more than one year of treatment. One reason for this might be a less severe post-pubertal effect of MPH on

Table 3 Height data for 4242 boys

Height ≤ 3rd percentile, n (%)	MPH < 12 months (n = 65)	MPH ≥ 12 months (n = 53)	ADHD control (n = 319)	Non-ADHD control (n = 3805)
Boys 6–15 years (n = 4242)				
Yes	2 (3.08)	3 (5.66)	11 (3.45)	104 (2.73)
No	63 (96.92)	50 (94.34)	308 (96.55)	3701 (97.27)
OR (95% CI), p-value	1.13 (0.27–4.68) 0.866	2.10 (0.64–6.85) 0.219	1.25 (0.67–2.36) 0.483	Reference
Boys 6–10 years (n = 2191)				
Yes	2 (5.56)	2 (9.09)	3 (2.29)	53 (2.65)
No	34 (94.44)	20 (90.91)	128 (97.71)	1949 (97.35)
OR (95% CI), p-value	2.22 (0.52–9.53), 0.282	3.94 (0.88–17.62), 0.073	0.88 (0.27–2.86), 0.830	Reference
Boys 11–15 years (n = 2051)				
Yes	0 (0.00)	1 (3.23)	8 (4.26)	51 (2.83)
No	29 (100.00)	30 (96.77)	180 (95.74)	1752 (97.17)
OR (95% CI), p-value	-	1.19 (0.16–8.95), 0.863	1.55 (0.72–3.32), 0.260	Reference

Table 4 Blood Pressure data for 4238 boys

	MPH < 12 months (n = 65)	MPH ≥ 12 months (n = 53)	ADHD control (n = 318)	Non-ADHD control (n = 3802)
i) Mean SBP (SD) / mmHg	107.71 (9.43)	107.23 (9.48)	107.71 (10.75)	108.61 (11.02)
ii) SBP Category				
Normal, n (%)	53 (81.54)	45 (84.91)	273 (85.85)	3142 (82.64)
Normal-high, n (%)	8 (12.31)	3 (5.66)	27 (8.49)	328 (8.63)
Stage 1 hypertension, n (%)	4 (6.15)	5 (9.43)	17 (5.35)	308 (8.10)
Stage 2 hypertension, n (%)	0 (0.00)	0 (0.00)	1 (0.31)	24 (0.63)
iii) Mean DBP (SD) / mmHg	64.65 (5.75)	67.19 (7.38)	64.86 (7.51)	65.31 (7.44)
iv) DBP Category				
Normal, n (%)	62 (95.38)	46 (86.79)	292 (91.82)	3494 (91.90)
Normal-high, n (%)	3 (4.62)	3 (5.66)	21 (6.60)	197 (5.18)
Stage 1 hypertension, n (%)	0 (0.00)	4 (7.55)	5 (1.57)	100 (2.63)
Stage 2 hypertension, n (%)	0 (0.00)	0 (0.00)	0 (0.00)	11 (0.29)

weight either due to metabolic reasons or due to a better way of coping with reduced appetite in this age group (eating larger meals in the later evening). These findings should be interpreted with caution due to the small numbers and wide confidence intervals and further research is required to verify these considerations.

The relationships between ADHD, methylphenidate use and growth appear to be complex. Some evidence suggests that there is a significant association between ADHD per se and obesity/overweight among patients, however this relationship is not consistent across studies [37]. Schwartz and colleagues used longitudinal health record data to examine associations between ADHD diagnosis and stimulant use on BMI trajectories throughout childhood and adolescence [15]. Their findings suggested that ADHD during childhood not treated with stimulants was associated with higher childhood BMIs whereas BMI was reduced in those

Table 5 Multivariable logistic regression for SBP and DBP, adjusting for age, bmi and cardiac disease (n = 4225)

	OR (95% CI)	Std Err	P-value
Normal SBP (base outcome)			
Raised SBP			
MPH < 12 months	1.09 (0.56–2.12)	0.37	0.796
MPH ≥12 months	0.91 (0.41–1.99)	0.36	0.807
ADHD Control	0.65 (0.46–0.92)	0.12	0.016*
Non-ADHD Control	Reference		
Normal DBP (base outcome)			
Raised DBP			
MPH < 12 months	0.55 (0.17–1.77)	0.32	0.315
MPH ≥12 months	1.80 (0.80–4.06)	0.75	0.159
ADHD Control	0.88 (0.57–1.35)	0.19	0.554
Non-ADHD Control	Reference		

* significant

whose ADHD was treated with stimulants but for this group there was a rebound later in adolescence to levels above those for children without stimulant use or without a history of ADHD [15]. Taking into account findings for both parameters (height and BMI) our data suggests that MPH may have more of an effect on weight than on height, a finding also highlighted by previous studies [10, 38].

Cardiovascular outcomes

Our analyses of the KiGGS dataset were unable to confirm the hypotheses that MPH use in boys with ADHD is associated with increased systolic and/or diastolic BP (≥90th percentile).

A review of the cardiovascular effects associated with MPH published in 2014 reported that changes in BP across the eight included studies (n = 970) ranged from − 4.3 to + 21.2 mmHg for mean SBP, and − 4.7 to + 4.0 mmHg for mean DBP. When duration of treatment was examined, the authors concluded that short-term use (≤6 months) of MPH was associated with small increases in BP that were not statistically significant whereas the data for MPH ≥ 6 months' duration provided "a more mixed picture …with some decreases in SBP and DBP… reported. However, it should be noted that these longer-term results were not corrected for age" [39].

Clinicians need to be cognisant however of the effects that even small changes in BP can have. Meta-analytic data from adult studies at ages 40–69 years estimate that each difference of 20 mmHg in usual SBP or 10 mmHg in DBP is associated with a two-fold increase in the rate of death from ischaemic heart disease and other vascular causes and more than a two-fold increase in the death rate from stroke [40]. In children, the exact level and duration of elevated BP that causes target organ damage are not established. However, there is increasing evidence that even very small elevations in BP can have long-term adverse effects on vascular structure and function [41].

Limitations

There are a number of limitations which should be considered in the current study. This study is cross-sectional in nature and thus inferences of causality cannot be made. For example, confounding factors (e.g. genes) may influence the likelihood of being treated via symptom severity and also influence body weight. Follow-up data were not available which would be particularly important for assessment of growth trajectories in children. However, analyses of growth outcomes were conducted stratified by age (< 11 years and ≥ 11 years) to account for the correlation between height velocity, growth spurts and pubertal maturation. The ADHD control group consists of children with an ADHD diagnosis but no current use of MPH. However, data were not available as to whether these children were stimulant-naïve or had prior exposure to MPH. The data were not gathered for the primary purpose of investigating the current research question and such secondary analyses cannot gather additional data on prior exposure to MPH; it is acknowledged that this potential contamination effect may attenuate differences among the groups. Information on dosing of MPH was not complete for all patients and, therefore, could not be included in the analyses. Identifying the ADHD cohort within the KiGGS sample was done by parent report of an ADHD diagnosis that had been made by a physician or psychologist. Due to the large number of children included and the wide range of competing physical, psychological and social health indicators which comprised the dataset, a full psychiatric diagnostic interview was not possible. However, other studies which have examined prevalence of ADHD in the KiGGS cohort have obtained a rate of 4.8% which is well in line with other population-based estimates [42]. The numbers of children within the two MPH groups were low and thus this may have contributed to a lack of precision around the estimates reported and the potential for Type II errors should be considered. Selection bias may be an issue within the MPH ≥ 12 months group insofar as individuals in whom adverse effects emerge may be less likely to persist with MPH treatment in the long-term. Finally, although the original study sample was assessed over ten years ago and the total number of children and adolescents in Germany decreased since then (as in many Western countries), we do not feel that this impacts on the findings of the current study.

Conclusion and implications for practice

When looking at the balance between risks and benefits of MPH treatment for ADHD, it needs to be considered that ADHD itself is associated with a broad range of psychosocial impairments such as; school failure, parental and family conflict, social rejection by peers, low self-esteem, higher risk for delinquent behaviour, smoking and substance use disorders. Adverse outcomes continue into adolescence and adulthood to include academic and vocational underachievement, reduced occupational functioning, emotional dysregulation, anxiety, depression, unemployment and suicide attempts, higher rates of traffic accidents, unwanted pregnancies, preterm mortality [43].

Secondly, findings from national registry studies indicate that the use of medication, particularly stimulants, reduces the risk of accidents and trauma-related emergency department admissions and might have protective effects on substance abuse, suicidality and delinquent behaviour [44–46].

We have used cross-sectional data from a German national representative sample to identify adverse growth and cardiovascular outcomes associated with MPH. Effects on BMI were observed among the MPH cohorts; clinicians should discuss with all patients and their parents the potential effects on growth and balance these effects with the outcomes of not treating ADHD symptoms. Particular attention should be paid to those patients in the lower growth percentiles. Serious concerns about growth warrant referral to a paediatric endocrinologist or growth expert [24]. This study is also one of the first to present categorical data on hypertension in patients taking MPH. While these data did not highlight significant differences overall between MPH cohorts and controls with respect to raised BP, the data do not preclude clinically significant BP increases in single cases, and so it is recommended to check BP and pulse prior to initiating MPH treatment and to monitor regularly throughout treatment. Sustained elevated BP before or during MPH treatment requires assessment and treatment. Further details on the management of adverse effects of medication for ADHD are presented by Graham and colleagues [24], Cortese and colleagues [47] and the 2018 NICE Clinical Guideline [NG87] [4].

Abbreviations

ADHD: Attention deficit hyperactivity disorder; AMP: Amphetamine; BMI: Body Mass Index; BP: Blood Pressure; DBP: Diastolic Blood Pressure; KiGGS: The German Health and Examination Survey for Children and Adolescents; MPH: Methylphenidate; OR: Odds Ratio; SBP: Systolic Blood Pressure; SD: Standard Deviation

Funding

This study was conducted as part of the European Commission 7th Framework Programme for research; Attention Deficit/hyperactivity Drugs Use Chronic Effects (ADDUCE; www.adhd-adduce.org/page/view/2/Home).

Authors' contributions

ESB: Contributed to interpretation of data, drafting of the manuscript, final approval of the manuscript. TB: Contributed to conception and design, data analysis, interpretation of data, drafting of the manuscript, final approval of the manuscript. JB: Contributed to interpretation of data, interpretation of data, drafting of the manuscript, final approval of the manuscript. SC: Contributed to interpretation of data, interpretation of data, drafting of the manuscript, final approval of the manuscript. DC: Contributed to interpretation of data, interpretation of data, drafting of the manuscript, final approval of the manuscript. MD: Contributed to interpretation of data, interpretation of data, drafting of the manuscript, final approval of the manuscript. BF: Contributed to conception and design, data analysis and interpretation, interpretation of data, drafting of the manuscript, final approval of the manuscript. PG: Contributed to interpretation of data, interpretation of data, drafting of the manuscript, final approval of the manuscript. CH: Contributed to interpretation of data, interpretation of data, drafting of the manuscript, final approval of the manuscript. SI: Contributed to interpretation of data, interpretation of data, drafting of the manuscript, final approval of the manuscript. HK: Contributed to interpretation of data, interpretation of data, drafting of the manuscript, final approval of the manuscript. EL: Contributed to interpretation of data, interpretation of data, drafting of the manuscript, final approval of the manuscript. K KC M: Contributed to data analysis and interpretation, interpretation of data, drafting of the manuscript, final approval of the manuscript. KM: Contributed to interpretation of data, interpretation of data, drafting of the manuscript, final approval of the manuscript. SM: Contributed to conception and design, data analysis and interpretation, interpretation of data, drafting of the manuscript, final approval of the manuscript. AN: Contributed to conception and design, data acquisition, data analysis, interpretation of data, interpretation of data, drafting of the manuscript, final approval of the manuscript. PN: Contributed to interpretation of data, interpretation of data, drafting of the manuscript, final approval of the manuscript. ER: Contributed to interpretation of data, interpretation of data, drafting of the manuscript, final approval of the manuscript. RS: Contributed to data acquisition, interpretation of data, interpretation of data, drafting of the manuscript, final approval of the manuscript. AH: Contributed to interpretation of data, interpretation of data, drafting of the manuscript, final approval of the manuscript. AZ: Contributed to interpretation of data, interpretation of data, drafting of the manuscript, final approval of the manuscript. ICKW: Contributed to conception and design, interpretation of data, interpretation of data, drafting of the manuscript, final approval of the manuscript. All authors read and approved the final manuscript.

Consent for publication

Not applicable.

Competing interests

ESB: Financial.
Speaker fees, consultancy, research funding and conference support from Shire Pharma. Speaker fees from American University of Beirut, Janssen Cilag, Consultancy from Neurotech solutions, Copenhagen University and Berhanderling, Skolerne, KU Leuven. Book royalties from OUP and Jessica Kingsley. Financial support received from Arrhus Univeristy and Ghent University for visiting Professorship. Grants awarded from MRC, ESRC, Wellcome Trust, Solent NHS Trust, European Union, Child Health Research Foundation New Zealand, NIHR, Nuffield Foundation, Fonds Wetenschappelijk Onderzoek-Vlaanderen (FWO), MQ – Transforming Mental health. Editor-in-Chief JCPP – supported by a buy-out of time to University of Southampton and personal Honorarium.
Non-financial.
Member of the European ADHD Guidelines Group.
TB: Dr. Banaschewski served in an advisory or consultancy role for Actelion, Hexal Pharma, Lilly, Medice, Novartis, Oxford outcomes, PCM scientific, Shire and Viforpharma. He received conference support or speaker's fee by Medice, Novartis and Shire. He is/has been involved in clinical trials conducted by Shire & Viforpharma. He received royalties from Hogrefe,

Kohlhammer, CIP Medien, Oxford University Press. The present work is unrelated to the above grants and relationships.
JB: Jan K Buitelaar has been in the past 3 years a consultant to / member of advisory board of /.
and/or speaker for Janssen Cilag BV, Eli Lilly, Lundbeck, Shire, Roche, Medice, Novartis,
and Servier. He has received research support from Roche and Vifor. He is not an employee.
of any of these companies, and not a stock shareholder of any of these companies. He has no.
other financial or material support, including expert testimony, patents, royalties.
SC: During the last three years collaboration within projects from the European Union (7th Framework Program) and collaboration as sub-investigator in sponsored clinical trials by Shire Pharmaceutical Company. Travel support from Shire Pharmaceutical Company.
DC: Prof. Coghill reports grants from European Commission, during the conduct of the study; grants and personal fees from Shire, personal fees from Eli Lilly, grants from Vifor, personal fees from Novartis, personal fees from Oxford University Press, other than the EC grants these are all outside the submitted work.
MD: MD is a member of the European ADHD Guideline Group (EAGG) and holds grants from the European Union FP7 programme.
BF: The author declares that they have no conflict of interest.
PG: The author declares that they have no conflict of interest.
CH: Grants from European Union FP7 programme, H2020, National Institute of Health Research (NIHR) and Medical Research Council (MRC) during the conduct of the study; CH is a member of the European ADHD Guideline Group (EAGG) and NICE ADHD Guideline Committee.
SI: The author declares that they have no conflict of interest.
HK: The author declares that they have no conflict of interest.
EL: The author declares that they have no conflict of interest.
K KC M: The author declares that they have no conflict of interest.
KM: The author declares that they have no conflict of interest.
SM: Dr. McCarthy has received speaker's fee, travel support and research support from Shire.
AN: The author declares that they have no conflict of interest.
PN: The author declares that they have no conflict of interest.
ER: The author declares that they have no conflict of interest.
RS: The author declares that they have no conflict of interest.
AH: A. Häge received speakers' fees, was on advisory boards or has been involved in clinical trials by Shire, Janssen-Cilag, Otsuka, Lundbeck and Servier.
AZ: Dr. Zuddas served in an advisory or consultancy role for Angelini, Lundbeck, Otsuka, EduPharma, Shire and Viforpharma. He received conference support or speaker's fee by Angelini and EduPharma. He is/has been involved in clinical trials conducted by Roche, Lundbeck, Shire & Viforpharma. He received royalties from Oxford University Press and Giunti OS. The present work is unrelated to the above grants and relationships.
ICKW: Prof. Wong reports grants from European Union FP7 programme, during the conduct of the study; grants from Shire, grants from Janssen-Cilag, grants from Eli-Lily, grants from Pfizer, outside the submitted work; and Prof Wong was a member of the National Institute for Health and Clinical Ex-cellence (NICE) ADHD Guideline Group and the British Association for Psy-chopharmacology ADHD guideline group and acted as an advisor to Shire.

Author details

[1]School of Pharmacy, University College Cork, Cork, Ireland. [2]Department of Paediatrics and Adolescents Medicine, University Hospital Erlangen, Erlangen, Germany. [3]Centre for Paediatric Pharmacy Research, Research Department of Practice and Policy, UCL School of Pharmacy, London, UK. [4]Department of Paediatrics and Adolescent Medicine, Li Ka Shing Faculty of Medicine, The University of Hong Kong, Hong Kong, Hong Kong. [5]Department of Medical Informatics, Erasmus University Medical Center, Rotterdam, Netherlands. [6]Department of Child & Adolescent Psychiatry and Psychotherapy, Medical Faculty Mannheim, Central Institute of Mental Health, University of Heidelberg, Mannheim, Germany. [7]Department of Cognitive Neuroscience,

Donders Institute for Brain, Cognition and Behavior, Radboud University Medical Centre, & Karakter Child and Adolescent Psychiatry University Centre, Nijmegen, The Netherlands. [8]Child and Adolescent Neuropsychiatry Unit, Department of Biomedical Science, University of Cagliari & "A. Cao" Pediatric Hospital, Brotzu Hospital Trust, Cagliari, Italy. [9]Departments of Paediatrics and Psychiatry, Faculty of Medicine, Dentistry and Health Sciences, University of Melbourne, Melbourne, Australia. [10]Murdoch Children's Research Institute, Melbourne, Australia. [11]Division of Neuroscience, School of Medicine, University of Dundee, Dundee, UK. [12]Department of Child and Adolescent Psychiatry, University Psychiatric Center, Leuven, KU, Belgium. [13]Department of Neurosciences, University Psychiatric Center, Leuven, KU, Belgium. [14]University Paris-Sud, Univ. Paris-Descartes, AP-HP, INSERM U1178, Paris, France. [15]Vadaskert Child and Adolescent Psychiatric Hospital, Budapest, Hungary. [16]Division of Psychiatry and Applied Psychology, Institute of Mental Health, School of Medicine, University of Nottingham, Nottingham, UK. [17]Tayside Clinical Trials Unit, University of Dundee, Dundee, UK. [18]Department of Psychology, University of Southampton, Southampton, UK. [19]Institute of Mental Health, Nottingham, UK. [20]Department of Paediatric Cardiology, Evelina Children's Hospital, St Thomas' Hospital, London, UK. [21]Unit of Mental Health Department of Epidemiology and Health Reporting, Robert Koch Institute, Berlin, Germany. [22]Department of Child and Adolescent Psychiatry, Institute of Psychiatry, King's College London, London, UK. [23]Department of Experimental Clinical & Health Psychology, Ghent University, Ghent, Belgium. [24]Centre for Safe Medication Practice and Research, Department of Pharmacology and Pharmacy, Li Ka Shing Faculty of Medicine, The University of Hong Kong, Hong Kong, Hong Kong.

References

1. American Psychiatric Association. Diagnostic and statistical manual of mental disorders. Fifth ed. Arlington: Americal Psychiatric Publishing; 2013.
2. Polanczyk G, de Lima MS, Horta BL, Biederman J, Rohde LA. The worldwide prevalence of ADHD: a systematic review and metaregression analysis. Am J Psychiatry. 2007;164(6):942–8.
3. Polanczyk GV, Willcutt EG, Salum GA, Kieling C, Rohde LA. ADHD prevalence estimates across three decades: an updated systematic review and meta-regression analysis. Int J Epidemiol. 2014;43(2):434–42.
4. National Institute for Health and Clinical Excellence. Attention deficit hyperactivity disorder: diagnosis and management. NICE Clinical Guideline 87 2018. Available from https://www.nice.org.uk/guidance/ng87/resources/attention-deficit-hyperactivity-disorder-diagnosis-andmanagement-pdf-1837699732933. Accessed 23 Sept 2018.
5. Faraone SV, Biederman J, Morley CP, Spencer TJ. Effect of stimulants on height and weight: a review of the literature. J Am Acad Child Adolesc Psychiatry. 2008;47(9):994–1009.
6. Nissen SE. ADHD drugs and cardiovascular risk. N Engl J Med. 2006;354(14): 1445–8.
7. Biederman J, Spencer TJ, Monuteaux MC, Faraone SV. A naturalistic 10-year prospective study of height and weight in children with attention-deficit hyperactivity disorder grown up: sex and treatment effects. J Pediatr. 2010; 157(4):635–40, 40 e1.
8. Harstad EB, Weaver AL, Katusic SK, Colligan RC, Kumar S, Chan E, et al. ADHD, stimulant treatment, and growth: a longitudinal study. Pediatrics. 2014;134(4):e935–44.
9. Spencer TJ, Faraone SV, Biederman J, Lerner M, Cooper KM, Zimmerman B, et al. Does prolonged therapy with a long-acting stimulant suppress growth in children with ADHD? J Am Acad Child Adolesc Psychiatry. 2006;45(5):527–37.
10. Swanson JM, Elliott GR, Greenhill LL, Wigal T, Arnold LE, Vitiello B, et al. Effects of stimulant medication on growth rates across 3 years in the MTA follow-up. J Am Acad Child Adolesc Psychiatry. 2007;46(8):1015–27.
11. Charach A, Figueroa M, Chen S, Ickowicz A, Schachar R. Stimulant treatment over 5 years: effects on growth. J Am Acad Child Adolesc Psychiatry. 2006; 45(4):415–21.
12. Poulton AS, Melzer E, Tait PR, Garnett SP, Cowell CT, Baur LA, et al. Growth and pubertal development of adolescent boys on stimulant medication for attention deficit hyperactivity disorder. Med J Aust. 2013;198(1):29–32.
13. Peyre H, Hoertel N, Cortese S, Acquaviva E, Limosin F, Delorme R. Long-term effects of ADHD medication on adult height: results from the NESARC. J Clin Psychiatry. 2013;74(11):1123–4.
14. Storebo OJ, Krogh HB, Ramstad E, Moreira-Maia CR, Holmskov M, Skoog M, et al. Methylphenidate for attention-deficit/hyperactivity disorder in children and adolescents: Cochrane systematic review with meta-analyses and trial sequential analyses of randomised clinical trials. BMJ. 2015;351:h5203.
15. Schwartz BS, Bailey-Davis L, Bandeen-Roche K, Pollak J, Hirsch AG, Nau C, et al. Attention deficit disorder, stimulant use, and childhood body mass index trajectory. Pediatrics. 2014;133(4):668–76.
16. Cortese S, Vincenzi B. Obesity and ADHD: clinical and neurobiological implications. Curr Top Behav Neurosci. 2012;9:199–218.
17. Hanc T, Cieslik J, Wolanczyk T, Gajdzik M. Assessment of growth in pharmacological treatment-naive polish boys with attention-deficit/hyperactivity disorder. J Child Adolesc Psychopharmacol. 2012;22(4):300–6.
18. Dalsgaard S, Kvist AP, Leckman JF, Nielsen HS, Simonsen M. Cardiovascular safety of stimulants in children with attention-deficit/hyperactivity disorder: a nationwide prospective cohort study. J Child Adolesc Psychopharmacol. 2014;24(6):302–10.
19. Cooper WO, Habel LA, Sox CM, Chan KA, Arbogast PG, Cheetham TC, et al. ADHD drugs and serious cardiovascular events in children and young adults. N Engl J Med. 2011;365(20):1896–904.
20. Habel LA, Cooper WO, Sox CM, Chan KA, Fireman BH, Arbogast PG, et al. ADHD medications and risk of serious cardiovascular events in young and middle-aged adults. JAMA. 2011;306(24):2673–83.
21. Schelleman H, Bilker WB, Strom BL, Kimmel SE, Newcomb C, Guevara JP, et al. Cardiovascular events and death in children exposed and unexposed to ADHD agents. Pediatrics. 2011;127(6):1102–10.
22. Mazza M, D'Ascenzo F, Davico C, Biondi-Zoccai B, Fratie G, Romagnolig E, et al. Drugs for attention deficit-hyperactivity disorder do not increase the mid-term risk of sudden death in children: a meta-analysis of observational studies. Int J Cardiol. 2013;168(4):4320–1. https://doi.org/10.1016/j.ijcard.2013.04.169. Epub May 11.
23. Winterstein AG, Gerhard T, Kubilis P, Saidi A, Linden S, Crystal S, et al. Cardiovascular safety of central nervous system stimulants in children and adolescents: population based cohort study. BMJ. 2012;345:e4627.
24. Graham J, Banaschewski T, Buitelaar J, Coghill D, Danckaerts M, Dittmann RW, et al. European guidelines on managing adverse effects of medication for ADHD. Eur Child Adolesc Psychiatry. 2011;20(1):17–37.
25. Hamilton RM, Rosenthal E, Hulpke-Wette M, Graham JG, Sergeant J, European network of hyperkinetic D. Cardiovascular considerations of attention deficit hyperactivity disorder medications: a report of the European network on hyperactivity disorders work group, European attention deficit hyperactivity disorder guidelines group on attention deficit hyperactivity disorder drug safety meeting. Cardiol Young. 2012;22(1):63–70.
26. European Medicines Agency. EMEA 2010 Priorities for Drug Safety Research. Long-term effects in children and in young adults of methylphenidate in the treatment of attention deficit hyperactivity disorder (ADHD). Available from http://www.ema.europa.eu/docs/en_GB/document_library/Other/2010/03/WC500076318.pdf. Accessed 10/11/2015.
27. Huss M, Holling H, Kurth BM, Schlack R. How often are German children and adolescents diagnosed with ADHD? Prevalence based on the judgment of health care professionals: results of the German health and examination survey (KiGGS). Eur Child Adolesc Psychiatry. 2008;17(Suppl 1):52–8.
28. Kurth BM, Kamtsiuris P, Holling H, Schlaud M, Dolle R, Ellert U, et al. The challenge of comprehensively mapping children's health in a nation-wide health survey: design of the German KiGGS-study. BMC Public Health. 2008;8:196.
29. Knopf H, Holling H, Huss M, Schlack R. Prevalence, determinants and spectrum of attention-deficit hyperactivity disorder (ADHD) medication of children and adolescents in Germany: results of the German Health Interview and Examination Survey (KiGGS). BMJ Open. 2012;2:e000477. https://doi.org/10.1136/bmjopen-2011-000477.
30. Holling H, Kamtsiuris P, Lange M, Thierfelder W, Thamm M, Schlack R. The German health interview and examination survey for children and adolescents (KiGGS): study management and conduct of fieldwork. Bundesgesundheitsblatt Gesundheitsforschung Gesundheitsschutz. 2007;50(5–6):557–66.
31. Rosario AS, Kurth BM, Stolzenberg H, Ellert U, Neuhauser H. Body mass index percentiles for children and adolescents in Germany based on a nationally representative sample (KiGGS 2003-2006). Eur J Clin Nutr. 2010; 64(4):341–9.

32. Neuhauser HK, Thamm M, Ellert U, Hense HW, Rosario AS. Blood pressure percentiles by age and height from nonoverweight children and adolescents in Germany. Pediatrics. 2011;127(4):e978–88.

33. Rosario AS, Schienkiewitz A, Neuhauser H. German height references for children aged 0 to under 18 years compared to WHO and CDC growth charts. Ann Hum Biol. 2011;38(2):121–30.

34. Nützenadel W. Failure to thrive in childhood. Dtsch Ärztebl Int. 2011; 108(38):642–9.

35. Lurbe E, Cifkova R, Cruickshank JK, Dillon MJ, Ferreira I, Invitti C, et al. Management of high blood pressure in children and adolescents: recommendations of the European Society of Hypertension. J Hypertens. 2009;27(9):1719–42.

36. Zhang H, Du M, Zhuang S. Impact of long-term treatment of methylphenidate on height and weight of school age children with ADHD. Neuropediatrics. 2010;41(2):55–9.

37. Cortese S, Castellanos FX. The relationship between ADHD and obesity: implications for therapy. Expert Rev Neurother. 2014;14(5):473–9.

38. Faraone SV, Giefer EE. Long-term effects of methylphenidate transdermal delivery system treatment of ADHD on growth. J Am Acad Child Adolesc Psychiatry. 2007;46(9):1138–47.

39. Awudu GA, Besag FM. Cardiovascular effects of methylphenidate, amphetamines and atomoxetine in the treatment of attention-deficit hyperactivity disorder: an update. Drug Saf. 2014;37(9):661–76.

40. Lewington S, Clarke R, Qizilbash N, Peto R, Collins R, Prospective Studies C. Age-specific relevance of usual blood pressure to vascular mortality: a meta-analysis of individual data for one million adults in 61 prospective studies. Lancet. 2002;360(9349):1903–13.

41. The Fourth Report on the Diagnosis. Evaluation, and treatment of high blood pressure in children and adolescents. Pediatrics. 2004; 114(Supplement 2):555–76.

42. Schlack R, Holling H, Kurth BM, Huss M. The prevalence of attention-deficit/ hyperactivity disorder (ADHD) among children and adolescents in Germany. Initial results from the German health interview and examination survey for children and adolescents (KiGGS). Bundesgesundheitsblatt Gesundheitsforschung Gesundheitsschutz. 2007;50(5–6):827–35.

43. Faraone SV, Asherson P, Banaschewski T, Biederman J, Buitelaar JK, Ramos-Quiroga JA, et al. Attention-deficit/hyperactivity disorder. Nat Rev Dis Primers. 2015;1:15020.

44. Chang Z, Lichtenstein P, Halldner L, D'Onofrio B, Serlachius E, Fazel S, et al. Stimulant ADHD medication and risk for substance abuse. J Child Psychol Psychiatry. 2014;55(8):878–85.

45. Lichtenstein P, Halldner L, Zetterqvist J, Sjolander A, Serlachius E, Fazel S, et al. Medication for attention deficit-hyperactivity disorder and criminality. N Engl J Med. 2012;367(21):2006–14.

46. Man KK, Chan EW, Coghill D, Douglas I, Ip P, Leung LP, et al. Methylphenidate and the risk of trauma. Pediatrics. 2015;135(1):40–8.

47. Cortese S, Holtmann M, Banaschewski T, Buitelaar J, Coghill D, Danckaerts M, et al. Practitioner review: current best practice in the management of adverse events during treatment with ADHD medications in children and adolescents. J Child Psychol Psychiatry. 2013;54(3):227–46.

5

The Erlangen test of activities of daily living in persons with mild dementia or mild cognitive impairment (ETAM) – an extended validation

Stephanie Book[1]*[iD], Katharina Luttenberger[1], Mark Stemmler[2], Sebastian Meyer[3] and Elmar Graessel[1]

Abstract

Background: The ability to perform activities of daily living (ADLs) is a central marker in the diagnosis and progression of the dementia syndrome. ADLs can be identified as basic ADLs (BADLs), which are fairly easy to perform, or instrumental ADLs (IADLs), which involve more complex activities. Presently, the only performance-based assessment of IADL capabilities in persons with cognitive impairment is the Erlangen Test of Activities of Daily Living in Persons with Mild Dementia or Mild Cognitive Impairment (ETAM). The aim of the present study was to revalidate the ETAM in persons with mild cognitive impairment (MCI) or mild dementia and to analyze its application to persons with moderate dementia.

Methods: We used baseline data from a cluster randomized controlled trial involving a sample of 443 users of 34 day-care centers in Germany. We analyzed groups of persons with MCI, mild dementia, and moderate dementia, categorized on the basis of the Mini-Mental State Examination (MMSE) and the Montreal Cognitive Assessment (MoCA). An item analysis was performed, and new discriminant validities were calculated. We computed a confirmatory factor analysis (CFA) to examine the postulated theoretical model of the ETAM with all six items loading on a single IADL factor. This was the first time that the ETAM's sensitivity to change was analyzed after a time period of 6 months.

Results: The overall sample scored on average 17.3 points (SD = 7.2) on the ETAM (range: 0–30 points). Persons with MCI scored on average 23.2 points, persons with mild dementia scored 18.4 points, and persons with moderate dementia scored 12.9 points, $p < .001$ (ANOVA). The item analysis yielded good difficulty indices and discrimination powers. The CFA indicated a good fit between the model and the observed data. After 6 months, both the ETAM score at baseline and the change in MMSE score (t0-t1) were significant predictors of the ETAM score at t1.

Conclusions: The ETAM is a valid and reliable instrument for assessing IADL capabilities in persons with MCI or mild dementia. It is sensitive to changes in cognitive abilities. The test parameters confirm its application to persons with moderate dementia.

Keywords: Activities of daily living, Cognitive impairment, Dementia, Performance test, Validation

* Correspondence: stephanie.book@uk-erlangen.de
[1]Center for Health Services Research in Medicine, Department of Psychiatry and Psychotherapy, Friedrich-Alexander Universität Erlangen-Nürnberg, Schwabachanlage 6, 91054 Erlangen, Germany
Full list of author information is available at the end of the article

Background

The mastery of everyday practical capacities is essential for the elderly to maintain their independence. Lawton and Brody [1] defined a set of everyday activities for the elderly, so-called activities of daily living (ADLs). They differentiated between basic ADLs (BADLs), which refer to self-maintenance skills such as feeding, dressing, and toileting, and instrumental ADLs (IADLs), which cover more complex behaviors of domestic functioning and enable independent living. IADLs include food/meal preparation, financial administration, housekeeping, laundry, use of the telephone, responsibility for one's own medication, mode of transportation, and shopping.

With an aging population, the number of people with dementia has dramatically increased in recent decades, and dementia has become a public health challenge [2]. Alzheimer's disease is the most common form of dementia and begins years before the onset of clinical symptoms. Its pathology can be described on a continuum that ranges from a preclinical stage (changes in biomarkers) to a prodromal stage with minor cognitive symptoms/mild cognitive impairment, to a symptomatic stage that includes dementia [3, 4]. At different stages of the disease, different assessments are needed. While a patient is in the preclinical stage, an assessment of biomarkers is most important, whereas functional assessments become more important in the prodromal and symptomatic stages [5]. IADLs can be used for a functional assessment as early as in the prodromal stage because it has been shown that impairments in IADLs are associated with the diagnosis and development of dementia [6–10] and, more important, deficits in BADLs and IADLs seem to occur at different stages of the dementing process [10, 11]. Whereas BADLs have been found to be more strongly correlated with motor functioning and coordination [12] and thus are more likely to remain preserved until the later stages of the disease, IADLs have been found to be more sensitive to the earlier stages of cognitive decline as these activities are more complex and require greater neuropsychological organization [11]. Even more, IADL impairments have been shown to predict the progression to dementia and can be used to help distinguish between dementia and early forms of cognitive decline, such as mild cognitive impairment (MCI) [6, 13]. MCI refers to a state that is defined by the presence of the first cognitive impairments that do not yet constitute dementia [14] but have a high probability of progressing to dementia [15]. Persons with MCI can experience subtle changes in everyday functional competence [8]. There is scientific evidence showing that IADLs can be impaired in MCI [8, 16–18]. In addition, in a systematic review, Jekel et al. [17] reported that patients with MCI and IADL deficits seem to have a higher risk of developing dementia than patients with MCI without IADL deficits, again stressing the importance of IADLs.

Because there is ample evidence that the ability to perform IADLs plays a crucial role in identifying the development of the dementia syndrome, there is a need for assessment tools that have been specifically designed and validated for patients with the first signs of impairments in IADLs (i.e. persons with MCI or mild dementia). As one study showed that several informant-based IADL questionnaires were limited in their quality [19], it remains important to identify an optimal way to measure IADLs. A promising approach is the use of performance tests as these tests provide standardized and more objective results [17]. To move in this conceptual direction, the Erlangen Test for Activities of Daily Living (E-ADL) [20] was developed in 2009 and can be characterized by its excellent economy. In contrast to other performance tests, it requires only about 10 min to be performed and does not require any tasks to be done outside the test room. The E-ADL was designed to assess BADL capabilities and can be used with persons with moderate or severe dementia [21]. Because it is too easy for persons with less severe dementia, there is a need for a performance test that has been validated for persons with mild dementia or even MCI. For this reason, the Erlangen Test of Activities of Daily Living in Persons with Mild Dementia or Mild Cognitive Impairment (ETAM) was developed as a performance-based tool for the assessment of IADLs [22]. The ETAM addresses some of the disadvantages of existing performance tests for ADL capabilities as some of these are very time-consuming (from 45 min, Functional Living Skills Assessment [FLSA] [23], up to 1.5 h, Direct Assessment of Functional Abilities [DAFA] [24]), cover only a limited range of relevant domains of IADLs, or include culture-specific items (e.g. "calling directory assistance" or "refilling a prescription" in the Revised Direct Assessment of Functional Status [DAFS-R] [25]). Above all, the ETAM can be used with persons with MCI [22]. In a first validation study of 107 study participants, including participants with normal cognition, persons with MCI, and persons with mild dementia, the ETAM was shown to be a feasible performance-based assessment tool with good psychometric parameters [22]. In this first study, the final structure of the ETAM was developed, and the items were reduced from ten to six items on the basis of an exploratory factor analysis and other criteria.

However, because this study was only cross-sectional, there is currently no longitudinal data on the ETAM's sensitivity to change. This is essential because sensitivity to change or responsiveness is an essential aspect of validity. It provides important information about the ETAM's ability to measure change over time, and consequently, it determines whether the ETAM can be used in intervention studies. At this time, there are currently no performance tests for assessing IADLs in persons with MCI that can be used in intervention studies. Thus, one aim of the present study was to analyze the ETAM's sensitivity to change. In addition, we wanted to investigate whether the original target group of persons with MCI or mild dementia could also be extended to include persons with moderate dementia. This would extend the application of the ETAM enormously because dementia is a progressive disease. Other aims of the present study involve other test construction criteria. The exploratory factor analysis in the validation study supported a one-factor structure for the ETAM. In the current study, we conducted a confirmatory factor analysis and investigated whether this structure could be supported. This was important to do in order to determine whether actual data were consistent with the hypothesis that the ETAM consists of a single IADL factor. Other test construction criteria included analyzing discriminant validity with additional instruments and determining criterion-related validity.

Methods

Design

The data for the extended validation were obtained from the two-arm cluster randomized controlled trial "DeTaMAKS project" (ISRCTN16412551) to evaluate a six-month-long multimodal non-pharmacological therapy (MAKS therapy) in day-care centers in Germany with day-care-center users and their caregivers. The study protocol was published previously [26]. For the current study, we included baseline data (t0) from all day-care-center users and follow-up data after six months (t1) for the control group that received no study-specific treatment (Fig. 1). The MAKS intervention is a multimodal nonpharmacological therapy for older adults with mild to moderate dementia and has been shown to be an effective treatment for dementia [27]. Because of the influence of the MAKS therapy on the ETAM scores [28], all analyses with t1 data were computed only on data from the control group, which did not receive any special therapy during that time. Cross-sectional analyses from the first measurement point (t0) were computed on data from all participants (the later control and the later intervention groups).

All procedures were approved by the Friedrich-Alexander-Universität Erlangen-Nürnberg Ethics Committee (Re.-No. 170_14 B).

Recruitment

All users of the 34 day-care centers throughout Germany and their caregivers were included in the screening process. All dyads (consisting of a day-care center user and caregiver) that fulfilled the criteria for inclusion were informed about the study and asked to take part in the project. Exclusion criteria for the day-care-center users were: blindness, deafness, lacking a caregiver, lacking the ability to communicate, more than one stroke, severe depression, schizophrenia, an addictive disorder, concrete plans for institutionalization, and attendance at the day-care center of less than once a week. The day-care centers' documentation contained all medical diagnoses and doctors' prescriptions known to the informal caregivers. Inclusion criteria were informed consent and an MMSE score of 10 or higher. For persons with an MMSE score of 24 or higher, we required them to also have an MoCA score of 22 or lower. Recruitment strategies are described in detail in [26].

Instruments

Tool under investigation

Erlangen Test of Activities of Daily Living in Persons with Mild Dementia or Mild Cognitive Impairment (ETAM) [22] The ETAM is a feasible (19 min on average), reliable, and valid performance test for IADL capabilities in persons with MCI or mild dementia. Thus, it can be administered to investigate the capacity to accomplish complex activities of daily living relevant to older adults living alone. The development of the ETAM was theoretically driven by the International Classification of Functioning, Disability, and Health (ICF), which was published by the World Health Organization (WHO) in 2001 [29]. The ICF is a classification of health and health-related domains including a list of "Body Functions," "Body Structures," "Activity and Participation," and "Environmental Factors." Activity can be described as the "execution of a task or action by an individual" (p. 123) and Participation can be described as "involvement in a life situation" (p. 123). The domain "Activity and Participation" consists of nine main categories, five of which are particularly relevant for the independent living of persons with dementia [30]: Communication, Mobility, Self-Care, Domestic Life, and Major Life Areas, especially Economic Life. These main categories are represented by six items in the ETAM (one 6-point item for each main category with the exception of two 3-point items for the main category Domestic Life). The total possible score is 30 points with higher values indicating greater competence in the mastery of IADLs. In a first validation study [22], Cronbach's alpha was .71, and the inter-rater reliability was .97.

Control tools

Mini-Mental State Examination (MMSE) [31] The MMSE is the most frequently used short screening instrument for dementia [32]. It assesses five areas of cognitive function: orientation, registration, attention and calculation, recall, and language. Designed to be a short (5–10 min) pencil-and-paper test that is easy to administer, it is based

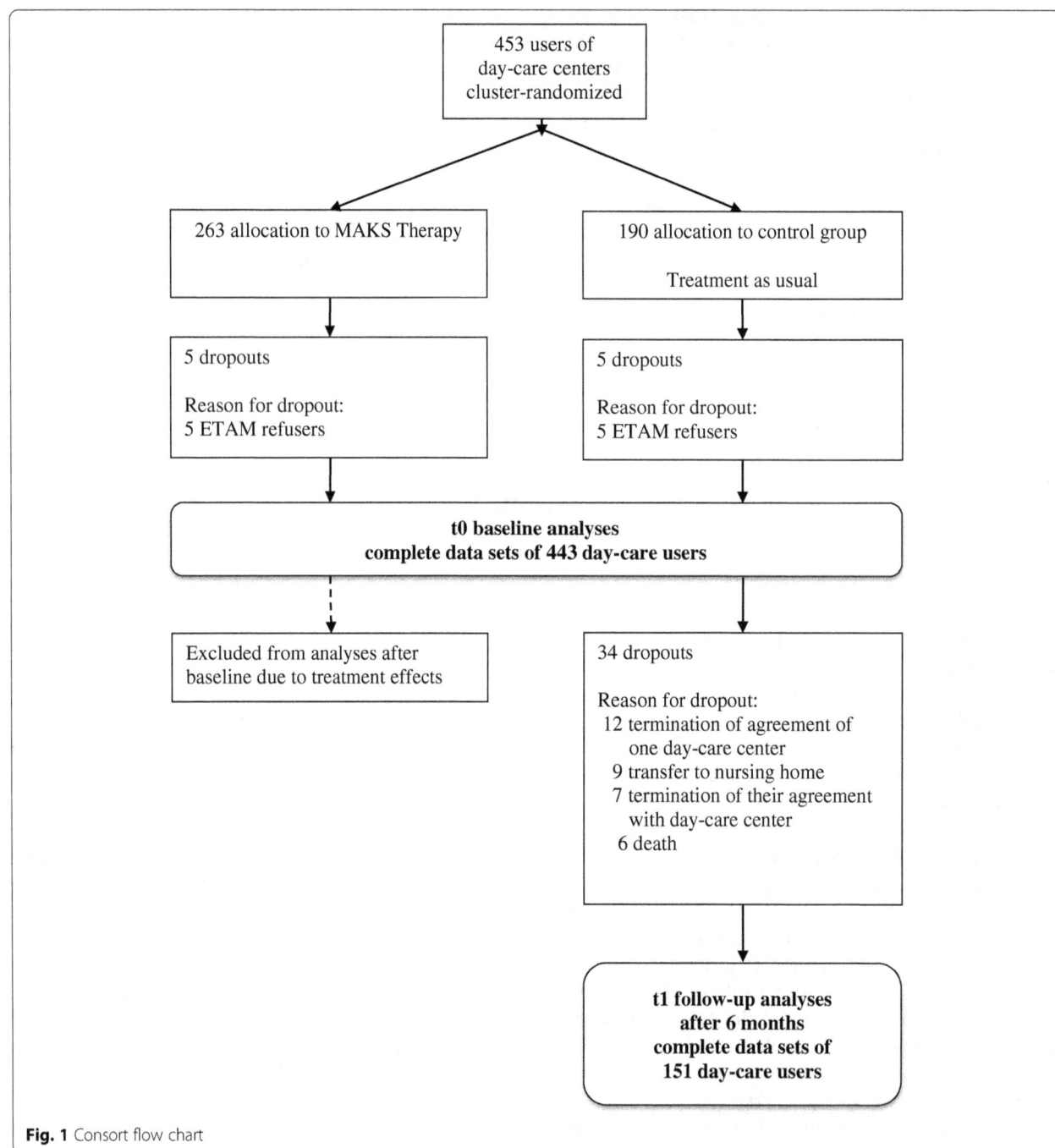

Fig. 1 Consort flow chart

on a total possible score of 30 points, with higher values indicating greater performance capacity. Scores ≥24 points are considered to be indicative of "normal" cognition (not associated with dementia), whereas scores below this can be indicative of mild dementia (18–23 points), moderate dementia (10–17 points), or severe dementia (0–9 points) [33].

Montreal Cognitive Assessment (MoCA) [34] The MoCA is a measure that is used to screen for MCI. It

consists of more difficult items than the MMSE and is thus able to better detect MCI [34–37]. Scores range from 0 to 30 points, with higher scores indicating better cognitive performance. A score of 22 or lower indicates cognitive impairment [35].

EuroQol five dimensions questionnaire (EQ-5D) [38] The EQ-5D is a cognitively simple, brief instrument providing a simple description of a person's generic health status. It consists of five items covering Mobility,

Self-Care, Usual Activities, Pain/Discomfort, and Anxiety/Depression. Each item is rated on a 5-point scale indicating the level of severity with higher scores reflecting more complaints.

Nurses' Observation Scale for Geriatric Patients (NOSGER) [39] The NOSGER is an observer rating scale covering the impairments that are found most frequently in geriatric patients. It consists of six subscales (Mood, Disturbing Behavior, Social Behavior, Memory, ADLs, and IADLs) that contain five items each. We included the Social Behavior subscale in the present study. Each item is rated on a scale that ranges from 1 (always) to 5 (never) with higher scores indicating less impairment.

Other measures

Each participant's age, gender, nursing care needs, and other sociodemographic data were provided by their caregivers or nurses at the day-care center. In Germany, nursing care needs are determined on the basis of a three-level scale to establish eligibility for nursing care benefits. Three care levels describe the extent to which the patient is eligible to receive assistance from long-term care insurance ranging from mild care (level 1) to moderate care (level 2) to a great need for care (level 3).

Classification of the level of cognitive impairment (MCI, mild or moderate dementia)

In order to differentiate between day-care-center users with MCI, mild dementia, or moderate dementia, we administered a combination of the MMSE and the MoCA at baseline. The MoCA was administered when the MMSE values ranged from 24 to 30 points, as the MMSE is widely regarded as not being sensitive enough to be able to detect MCI in the range of non-dementia cases [33, 34, 40]. Freitas [35] suggested using a cut-off score of 22 points to discriminate between normal cognition and MCI for the MoCA. To differentiate between mild and moderate dementia, we used the MMSE values and the recommendations by Tombaugh et al. [33]. We considered scores between 18 and 23 points to be indicative of mild dementia and scores between 10 and 17 points to be indicative of moderate dementia. With this procedure, we defined the level of cognitive impairment in a psychometric way.

Data recording

The MMSE, MoCA, ETAM, and anamnestic data were recorded by staff at the day-care centers who had attended training sessions. The EQ-5D and the NOSGER subscale Social Behavior were completed via computer-assisted telephone interviews (CATIs) with the caregivers. All of the persons involved in data recording were thoroughly trained in the use of each instrument.

Data quality management

In order to ensure the validity of the data, the data sources (tests, CATIs, day-care centers) are subjected to a random internal audit. To obtain evidence of the inter-rater reliability of the ETAM test and the CATI, 5% of the baseline data were collected with the participation of a second person who was there to observe. For additional information, please see [28].

Sample

For the purpose of this study, our analyses were based on 443 day-care-center users with baseline data. The proportion of women in the sample was 61.4%, and the mean age was 81.7 years (SD = 7.7). All analyses except for one were based on these 443 day-care-center users and their baseline data (Table 1). Only for the analysis of sensitivity to change did we use the baseline and follow-up data of 151 control-group participants (because of treatment effects, we excluded the intervention group, see Fig. 1).

Statistical analysis
Reliability and item analysis

In order to determine the test construction characteristics of the ETAM, measures of reliability were computed

Table 1 Sample characteristics

Characteristics	$N = 443$
Age, M (SD)	81.7 (7.7)
Women, n (%)	272 (61.4%)
Education, n (%)	
Not completed	24 (5.4%)
9 years	317 (71.6%)
10 years	51 (11.5%)
13 years	23 (5.2%)
More than 13 years	28 (6.3%)
Care level	
No care level	71 (16%)
Level 1	232 (52.4%)
Level 2	136 (30.7%)
Level 3	4 (0.9%)
MMSE score, M (SD)	19.4 (4.7)
Cognitive Impairment according to MMSE/MoCA	
MCI (MMSE 24–30 and MoCA ≤22)	91 (20.5%)
Mild dementia (MMSE 18–23)	186 (42.0%)
Moderate dementia (MMSE 10–17)	166 (37.5%)
ETAM score at baseline, M (SD)	17.3 (7.2)

MMSE mini-mental status examination, *ETAM* Erlangen test of activities of daily living in persons with mild dementia or mild cognitive impairment and an item analysis was conducted. Means and standard deviations were calculated at the item level and for the ETAM total score. Cronbach's α was computed as a measure of internal consistency, and values higher than 0.7 were considered acceptable [41]. The difficulty index and discrimination power were calculated at the item level. As the ETAM items use a multilevel (4- or 7-step) response format, the difficulty index was calculated as the ratio of the subjects' squared points to the number of subjects times the squared item maximum ($\frac{\sum_{i=1}^{n} x_i^2}{n \cdot x_{max}^2}$) [42]. The item difficulty index ranges from 0 (most difficult item) to 1 (easiest item). Item difficulties in the range of .2 to .8 are preferred [43]. Discrimination power was calculated as the corrected item-total correlation. A discrimination power of .3 to .5 should be rated as moderate, whereas a discrimination power > .5 should be rated as high [43].

In order to assess the extent to which the ETAM could discriminate between different levels of severity of cognitive impairment, we computed a one-way ANOVA with the total ETAM score as the dependent variable and the severity of cognitive impairment (MCI, mild dementia, moderate dementia) as the independent variable. For a post hoc analysis, we computed a Games-Howell test because the groups did not have equal variances. Cohen's d was used to examine the magnitude of the differences in ETAM scores between the subgroups (MCI, mild dementia, moderate dementia).

Confirmatory factor analysis

A confirmatory factor analysis was computed to determine whether the six ETAM items fit the proposed one-factor model as found when the exploratory factor analysis was conducted in the first validation study [22]. The asymptotic distribution free (ADF) method of estimation was chosen because the ETAM items were not normally distributed.

To evaluate the model, we used the adjusted chi-square test statistic in conjunction with other fit indices as recommended by Brown [44]. Schreiber et al. [45] recommended the ratio of χ^2 to df ≤ 2, a root mean square error of approximation (RMSEA) < .06, a comparative fit index (CFI) $\geq$ .95, and a Tucker-Lewis index (TLI) $\geq$ .96.

Validity

Discriminant validity To test for discriminant validity, the ETAM score at baseline was correlated with several scales or items that measured different constructs (Spearman Rank Sum Correlation) at baseline. The MMSE was used to measure cognition, the Social Behavior scale of the NOSGER was used to measure social

behavior, and the five items of the EQ-5D were used to measure specific topics that are relevant for health status: Mobility, Self-Care, Usual Activities, Pain/Discomfort, and Anxiety/Depression. We hypothesized that the correlation between the ETAM and the MMSE would be around .5 because the two tests measure the progression of the same disease, whereas the correlations between the ETAM and the other tests were expected to be low (.2 or lower).

Criterion-related validity The variable nursing care needs is an appropriate independent external criterion that was used to assess criterion-related validity. It is determined by external raters working for the "Medical Service of Health Insurances" and is a health measure with relevance to a person's economic standing because it determines the amount of access a person has to financial assistance. We wanted to test the hypothesis that participants achieve significantly different ETAM scores depending on their care level. We computed a one-way ANOVA with the ETAM score at baseline as the dependent variable and nursing care needs as the independent variable. For a post hoc analysis, we computed Hochberg's GT2 because the population variances were equal but the sample sizes were very different.

Sensitivity to change: Subgroup analysis of the control group We wanted to assess the ETAM's sensitivity to reflect change in cognitive abilities that occurred over six months in the subgroup of participants in the control group ($n = 151$) from the "DeTaMAKS" project. We expected that participants with larger decreases in their cognitive abilities as measured with the MMSE would also show larger decreases in their IADL capacities as measured with the ETAM. A regression analysis was computed with the ETAM score at follow-up (t1) as the criterion and the ETAM score at baseline (t0) and the MMSE change score from t0 to t1 as predictors.

The analyses were computed on the baseline data for the sample consisting of participants with MCI, mild dementia, or moderate dementia ($N = 443$) and for the subgroups with MCI (MMSE score 24–30 and MoCA ≤ 22), mild dementia (MMSE score 18–23), and moderate dementia (MMSE score 10–17). For reasons of comparability, we also report results for the original group that was targeted by the ETAM (i.e. persons with MCI or mild dementia; $n = 277$) when similar analyses were carried out in the first validation study [22].

IBM SPSS Statistics 21 was used for most of the statistical analyses. Stata 13.1 was used for the confirmatory factor analysis.

Results

Reliability and item analysis

For the total sample consisting of participants with MCI, mild dementia, or moderate dementia ($N = 443$), the mean ETAM score was 17.3 points with a standard deviation of 7.2. The median was 18.0 points. The distribution had a skewness of $-.264$ and a kurtosis of $-.852$. The maximum range of 0 to 30 points was completely covered. Cronbach's alpha was .79. For the group comparisons, the following Cohen's d values were found: $d = 0.84$ for MCI ($n = 91$) versus mild dementia ($n = 186$), $d = 1.70$ for MCI versus moderate dementia ($n = 166$), and $d = 0.85$ for mild versus moderate dementia. For the original target group of participants with MCI or mild dementia ($n = 277$), the mean ETAM score was 20.0 points ($SD = 6.2$) with a Cronbach's alpha of .74. The mean ETAM scores differed significantly between MCI, mild dementia, and moderate dementia, $F(2, 440) = 87.85$, $p < .001$. A post hoc Games-Howell test revealed that all ETAM scores differed significantly from each other at $p < .001$: Participants with MCI (n = 91) scored on average 23.2 points (95% CI 22.2–24.2), participants with mild dementia (n = 186) scored 18.4 points (95% CI 17.5–19.3), and participants with moderate dementia ($n = 166$) scored 12.9 points (95% CI 11.9–14.0); see Fig. 2.

The overall discriminatory powers were high, ranging from .49 to .64. Only in the subgroup of persons with MCI did the item "alarm clock" have a low discriminatory power of .25. Other items in this subgroup had moderate discriminatory powers ranging from .35 to .44. In the subgroup of persons with mild dementia, the discriminatory power ranged from .45 to .56, and in the subgroup of persons with moderate dementia, from .39

to .63. Overall, the most difficult item was "phone call" (.25), whereas "making tea" (.67) was the easiest item. Again, only for the subgroup of persons with MCI, the easiest items were "pill organizer" and "alarm clock" (both .83) for which the difficulties ranged from .44 to .83. In the subgroup of persons with mild dementia, the difficulties ranged from .25 to .71. In the subgroup of persons with moderate dementia, the difficulties ranged from .13 to .56. Item characteristics are presented in Table 2.

Confirmatory factor analysis

We hypothesized a one-factor model. For the extended total sample of persons with MCI, mild dementia, or moderate dementia, the model indicated a good fit to the data, χ^2 (9, $N = 443$), $p = .088$. The ratio of χ^2 to df was 1.68. The CFI was .975, the TLI was .959, and the RMSEA was .039. Similar results were found for the original target group of participants with MCI or mild dementia: χ^2 (9, $n = 277$), $p = .359$. The ratio of χ^2 to df was 1.10. The CFI was .991, the TLI was .985, and the RMSEA was .019. These values indicate a good fit between the model and the observed data.

Validity

Discriminant validity

Overall, the correlation of the ETAM total score with the MMSE was .59; for the subgroups, the correlations were .20 for MCI, .24 for mild dementia, and .40 for moderate dementia. For the original target group of participants with MCI or mild dementia, the correlation with the MMSE was .43. The ETAM total score was hardly correlated with the other items of the EQ-5D:

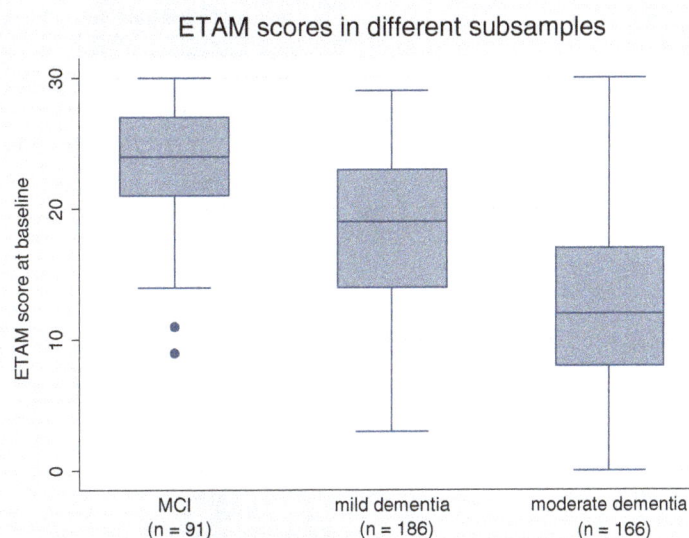

Fig. 2 Boxplots of the ETAM scores in persons with MCI, mild dementia, or moderate dementia

Table 2 Item characteristics of the ETAM

Characteristics	Making tea	Alarm clock	Pill organizer	Finances	Traffic situations	Phone call	ETAM total score
Score Range	0–3	0–3	0–6	0–6	0–6	0–6	0–30
Mean (SD)							
Total	2.3 (1.0)	2.2 (0.9)	3.7 (2.3)	3.6 (2.0)	3.3 (1.9)	2.4 (1.8)	17.3 (7.2)
MCI	2.5 (0.8)	2.7 (0.6)	5.3 (1.4)	5.0 (1.5)	4.2 (1.6)	3.6 (1.7)	23.2 (4.7)
Mild dementia	2.4 (0.9)	2.3 (0.9)	4.0 (2.1)	3.7 (1.9)	3.5 (1.7)	2.5 (1.7)	18.4 (6.2)
Moderate dementia	2.0 (1.1)	1.7 (1.0)	2.5 (2.3)	2.7 (2.0)	2.5 (1.9)	1.6 (1.5)	12.9 (6.7)
Discriminatory power							
Total	.49	.53	.59	.61	.54	.64	
MCI	.37	.25	.35	.44	.42	.40	
Mild dementia	.50	.45	.46	.46	.51	.56	
Moderate dementia	.45	.42	.50	.59	.39	.63	
Difficulty							
Total	.67	.61	.53	.47	.39	.25	
MCI	.77	.83	.83	.44	.57	.44	
Mild dementia	.71	.66	.58	.48	.42	.25	
Moderate dementia	.56	.43	.31	.31	.27	.13	
Cronbach's alpha if item deleted							
Total	.78	.77	.75	.74	.76	.73	
MCI	.60	.62	.59	.55	.56	.57	
Mild dementia	.69	.70	.70	.69	.67	.65	
Moderate dementia	.72	.72	.70	.66	.73	.66	

$N = 443$; n(MCI) = 91; n(mild dementia) = 186; n(moderate dementia) = 166
MCI: MMSE score 24–30; mild dementia: MMSE score 18–23; moderate dementia: MMSE score 10–17

Mobility –.00, Self-Care –.23, Usual Activities –.20, Pain/Discomfort .15, Anxiety/Depression .01. The correlation with the Social Behavior scale from the NOSGER was –.11. The correlations between the ETAM total score and the scores from these instruments are presented in Table 3 in detail.

Criterion-related validity

We computed a one-way ANOVA to test the hypothesis that participants would receive different ETAM scores depending on their care level. The independent variable care level had three factor levels: no care level, care level 1, and care level 2+. We combined participants with care levels 2 and 3 because there were only four participants with care level 3. The results showed that the ETAM scores differed significantly from each other depending on the participants' nursing care needs, $F(2, 440) = 8.660$, $p < .001$, as shown in Table 4. Hochberg's GT2 post hoc test showed that there were significant differences in ETAM scores between participants with no care level and care level 2+ ($p < .001$) and participants with care level 1 and care level 2+ ($p = .015$). Participants with

Table 3 Discriminant validity

	Total	MCI	Mild dementia	Moderate dementia
MMSE	.59[**]	.20	.24[**]	.40[**]
Social Behavior (NOSGER)	–.11[*]	.03	–.04	–.01
EQ-5D items				
Mobility	–.01	.12	–.08	–.07
Self-Care	–.23[**]	–.10	–.18[*]	–.18[*]
Usual Activities	–.20[**]	–.14	–.20	–.08
Pain/Discomfort	.15[**]	.17	.05	.05
Anxiety/Depression	.01	.03	.03	–.03

[*]$p < .05$; [**]$p < .01$

Table 4 Criterion-related validity

	Number	M	SD	p, Hochberg's GT2 post hoc test	
				Care level 1	Care level 2+
No care level	71	19.70	6.18	.11	< .001
Care level 1	232	17.69	7.08		< .05
Care level 2+	140	15.55	7.57		

no care level and care level 1 did not differ significantly in their ETAM scores ($p = .11$).

Sensitivity to change: Subgroup analysis of the control group

In a regression analysis, when predicting the ETAM score at t1, we found that the ETAM score at t0 (b = 0.83, p < .001) and the change in MMSE from t0 to t1 (b = − 0.37, p < .001) were significant predictors; see Table 5. R^2 was 0.65. This supports our hypothesis that when a person's MMSE score had declined after six months, the person also achieved fewer points on the ETAM after six months.

Discussion

In this study, we examined the reliability and validity of the ETAM and confirmed that the ETAM can be used not only with people with MCI and mild dementia but also with people with moderate dementia. We showed that ETAM scores differed between the level of cognitive impairment with people with MCI achieving the best results, people with mild dementia second best, and people with moderate dementia the worst. In addition, we confirmed that the ETAM is able to detect change over time. Also, a confirmatory factor analysis supported the postulated single factor structure of IADLs.

The present study supports the application of the ETAM for persons with MCI or mild dementia. In addition, the ETAM can also be recommended for assessing the subgroup of persons with moderate dementia. This is meaningful because functional assessment becomes more important when the degree of cognitive impairment increases [5]. Our analyses showed that persons with MCI achieved the best results, persons with mild dementia scored on average five points lower, and persons with moderate dementia scored another six points lower. Thus, these results show that as the dementing disease progresses, participants find it increasingly difficult to carry out the IADL-oriented tasks

of the ETAM, thus providing support for the ETAM's reliability and validity.

Further support for the validity of the ETAM was provided by care level, which is primarily related to BADL capacities. We found that participants who had not yet qualified for a care level achieved the most points (i.e. they showed a better performance on the ETAM), and with a higher care level, participants achieved fewer points on the ETAM. Persons with no care level and persons with care level 1 did not show significantly different ETAM scores, which might be due to the different sample sizes that were used or the fact that care level is more strongly related to BADL capacities than to IADL capacities. This finding is especially interesting because care level is an external criterion that was rated by independent testers who were not involved in the study.

We were able to confirm the discriminant validity of the ETAM as predicted in our hypotheses (moderate overall correlation with the MMSE; low correlations with all other tests). Whereas the ETAM scores of people with MCI were barely correlated with the MMSE, the correlation increased when we analyzed the subgroup of persons with mild or moderate dementia. This finding is consistent with Giebel et al.'s [46] results in suggesting that with the progression of the dementing disease, cognition is increasingly affected, and people have more trouble mastering IADLs. Further support for the association between cognitive levels and functional abilities such as IADLs was found, for example, by Njegovan [47], who showed that progressive cognitive decline is associated with a specific pattern of loss of functional tasks. All in all, these findings appear to suggest that activities of daily living and cognitive tasks are increasingly associated as cognitive impairment progresses. This means that the relationship between IADL capacities and performance on cognitive tasks increases as cognitive impairment progresses. A similar yet weaker pattern was found for the correlation between the ETAM and the Self-Care item from the EQ-5D, which can be applied to assess BADLs to a certain extent. Again, as the dementing condition progressed, the correlation with the ETAM increased.

In addition, we used the five EQ-5D items to compute correlation coefficients with dimensions such as pain, anxiety, etc. Aside from Self-Care, we found no meaningful correlation or pattern of correlations across the three subgroups of participants with MCI, mild dementia, or

Table 5 Sensitivity to Change: Subgroup Analysis of the Control Group: Regression Analysis

	Estimate (b)	SE	p	95% CI	
				lower limit	upper limit
ETAM score at t0	0.83	0.05	< .001	.721	.937
MMSE change score t0-t1	−0.37	0.10	< .001	−.566	−.181

moderate dementia, thus providing support for the discriminant validity of the ETAM.

Another important relationship between the ETAM and the MMSE concerns sensitivity to change. For this purpose, we analyzed whether the ETAM was sensitive to other (cognitive) changes over a period of six months. We found that the change in MMSE over a period of six months turned out to be a significant predictor of the ETAM score after six months: When a person's MMSE score had declined after six months, the person also achieved fewer points on the ETAM after six months. This is an important aspect of validity and it demonstrates that the ETAM is able to measure change over time. Thus, we recommend its use in intervention studies.

Similar to the first validation study, the item "phone call" turned out to be the most difficult item by far. The authors of the first validation study argued that how a person handles the phone is an important and sensitive indicator of incipient dementia processes [22]. The item "traffic situations" was the second most difficult item. Apart from these findings, there were some differences in the order of items in comparison with the first validation study. This was most likely due to a smaller sample size in the previous study as well as less variation (the difficulties of the remaining four items ranged only from .47 to .67). In the current study, there was a consistent pattern of difficulty indices with one small exception. For the MCI subgroup, "pill organizer" and "alarm clock" were the easiest items (both .83), and "making tea" was the third easiest item (.77). Because it is common practice to arrange the items on a test in order of increasing difficulty, we propose that the order of the ETAM items be rearranged and adjusted to reflect the difficulties found in the current study. Specifically, we suggest the following order when carrying out the ETAM: 1) "making tea," 2) "alarm clock," 3) "pill organizer," 4) "finances," 5) "traffic situations," 6) "phone call." When the items are administered in this order, the participant is encouraged to continue the test, and this will also ensure that weaker candidates will not become discouraged.

Limitations

Some limitations of the current study should be mentioned. Because the lack of high-quality performance-based assessments for measuring IADL capabilities was the reason we developed the ETAM, we cannot provide convergent validity with other instruments that measure IADL capacities. To date, there is no gold standard for measuring IADL capacities especially by means of a performance-based assessment. Existing performance-based assessments are very time-consuming, taking up to 1.5 h [48] in only very small groups [24], or they seem to measure cognition rather than

IADL functioning [49] (for an overview, see [22]). Because the ETAM already showed acceptable convergent validity with the informant-based Bayer Activities of Daily Living Scale [50] in the first validation study [22], we decided to focus on discriminant validity and sensitivity to change.

In addition, one should consider that differentiating between MCI, mild dementia, and moderate dementia can be performed only with the mean ETAM scores. This is because there is high between-subject variability on the ETAM in the three levels of cognitive impairment. Thus, ETAM scores should not be used to diagnose MCI, mild dementia, or moderate dementia.

Another limitation of the present study was that we used the NOSGER subscale Social Behavior and the EQ-5D items to analyze discriminant validity. However, a measure of mood would have been desirable because depressive mood is associated with a decline in cognitive abilities.

Future research perspectives

In our study, the categorization of MCI, mild dementia, and moderate dementia was solely based on the cognitive tests of the MMSE and the MoCA, which can be influenced by age and education [51, 52]. Thereby, we defined cognitive impairment psychometrically and assessed clinical symptoms. In practice, the MMSE is one of the most commonly used screening tools for cognitive impairment [32], and our analyses also showed that this categorization was successful. For a more accurate categorization for persons with MCI and different stages of dementia, future studies could focus on the use of other instruments besides the MMSE as well (e.g. the Consortium to Establish a Registry for Alzheimer's Disease [CERAD], neuroimaging, and biomarkers). Especially in the preclinical and prodromal stages (MCI) of Alzheimer's disease, biomarker assessments are very informative [5].

Conclusions

There is further evidence for the ETAM as a feasible, reliable, and valid instrument for the measurement of IADL capacities in persons with MCI or mild dementia. In addition, the ETAM can be recommended for the assessment of the IADL capacities of persons with moderate dementia. It shows good discriminant validities with other measures (e.g. Social Behavior, Mobility, Pain/Discomfort, and Anxiety/Depression). The ETAM is sensitive to change, and thus, we recommend its use for intervention studies.

Abbreviations

ADLs: Activities of daily living; BADLs: Basic activities of daily living; CATI: Computer-assisted telephone interview; CFA: Confirmatory factor analysis; CFI: Comparative fit index; CI: Confidence interval; DAFA: Direct assessment of functional abilities; DAFS: Direct assessment of functional status; E-ADL: Erlangen test for activities of daily living; EQ-5D: EuroQol five dimensions questionnaire; ETAM: Erlangen test of activities of daily living in persons with mild dementia or mild cognitive impairment; FLSA: Functional living skills assessment; IADLs: Instrumental activities of daily living; ICF: International classification of functioning, disability, and health; MCI: Mild cognitive impairment; MMSE: Mini-mental status examination; MoCA: Montreal cognitive assessment; NOSGER: Nurses' observation scale for geriatric patients; RMSEA: Root mean square error of approximation; SD: Standard deviation; TLI: Tucker-Lewis index; WHO: World Health Organization

Acknowledgments

We acknowledge receiving funding for the study from the German National Association of the Statutory Health Insurance and Long-Term Care Insurance Funds (GKV-Spitzenverband) (Germany) and the Bavarian State Ministry of Health and Care (Germany). We would like to thank the Friedrich-Alexander-Universität Erlangen-Nürnberg within the funding program Open Access Publishing. We would also like to thank our language editor, Dr. Jane Zagorski. The present work was conducted in partial fulfillment of the requirements for obtaining the degree "Dr. rer. biol. hum." by Stephanie Book.

Authors' contributions

SB drafted the manuscript, performed the data analysis, and developed the structure of the paper. MS provided important information about data analysis and interpretation. KL designed and supervised the study. SM provided important suggestions about the statistical analyses. EG designed the study, supervised the study design and data analysis, and drafted parts of the manuscript. All authors have read and approved the final version of the manuscript

Consent for publication

Not applicable.

Competing interests

The authors declare that they have no competing interests.

Author details

[1]Center for Health Services Research in Medicine, Department of Psychiatry and Psychotherapy, Friedrich-Alexander Universität Erlangen-Nürnberg, Schwabachanlage 6, 91054 Erlangen, Germany. [2]Institute of Psychology, Friedrich-Alexander-Universität Erlangen-Nürnberg, Nägelsbachstr. 49c, 91052 Erlangen, Germany. [3]Institute of Medical Informatics, Biometry, and Epidemiology, Friedrich-Alexander-Universität Erlangen-Nürnberg, Waldstraße 6, 91054 Erlangen, Germany.

References

1. Lawton M, Brody E. Assessment of older people: self-maintaining and instrumental activities of daily living. Gerontologist. 1969;9:179–86.
2. World Health Organization. Dementia: a public health priority. Geneva: World Health Organization; 2012.
3. Dubois B, Feldman HH, Jacova C, Dekosky ST, Barberger-Gateau P, Cummings J, Delacourte A, Galasko D, Gauthier S, Jicha G, et al. Research criteria for the diagnosis of Alzheimer's disease: revising the NINCDS-ADRDA criteria. Lancet Neurol. 2007;6(8):734–46.
4. Sperling RA, Aisen PS, Beckett LA, Bennett DA, Craft S, Fagan AM, Iwatsubo T, Jack CR Jr, Kaye J, Montine TJ, et al. Toward defining the preclinical stages of Alzheimer's disease: recommendations from the National Institute on Aging-Alzheimer's Association workgroups on diagnostic guidelines for Alzheimer's disease. Alzheimers Dement. 2011;7(3):280–92.
5. Ritchie CW, Russ TC, Banerjee S, Barber B, Boaden A, Fox NC, Holmes C, Isaacs JD, Leroi I, Lovestone S, et al. The Edinburgh consensus: preparing for the advent of disease-modifying therapies for Alzheimer's disease. Alzheimers Res Ther. 2017;9(1):85.
6. Sikkes SA, Rotrou J. A qualitative review of instrumental activities of daily living in dementia: what's cooking? Neurodegenerative Disease Management. 2014;4(5):393–400.
7. Farias ST, Mungas D, Reed BR, Harvey D, Cahn-Weiner D, Decarli C. MCI is associated with deficits in everyday functioning. Alzheimer Dis Assoc Disord. 2006;20(4):217–23.
8. Nygard L. Instrumental activities of daily living: a stepping-stone towards Alzheimer's disease diagnosis in subjects with mild cognitive impairment? Acta Neurol Scand Suppl. 2003;179:42–6.
9. Perneczky R, Pohl C, Sorg C, Hartmann J, Komossa K, Alexopoulos P, Wagenpfeil S, Kurz A. Complex activities of daily living in mild cognitive impairment: conceptual and diagnostic issues. Age Ageing. 2006;35(3): 240–5.
10. Perneczky R, Pohl C, Sorg C, Hartmann J, Tosic N, Grimmer T, Heitele S, Kurz A. Impairment of activities of daily living requiring memory or complex reasoning as part of the MCI syndrome. Int J Geriatr Psychiatry. 2006;21(2): 158–62.
11. Overdorp EJ, Kessels RP, Claassen JA, Oosterman JM. The combined effect of neuropsychological and Neuropathological deficits on instrumental activities of daily living in older adults: a systematic review. Neuropsychol Rev. 2016;26(1):92–106.
12. Boyle PA, Cohen RA, Paul R, Moser D, Gordon N. Cognitive and motor impairments predict functional declines in patients with vascular dementia. Int. J. Geriatr. Psychiatry. 2002;17(2):164–9.
13. Peres K, Helmer C, Amieva H, Orgogozo JM, Rouch I, Dartigues JF, Barberger-Gateau P. Natural history of decline in instrumental activities of daily living performance over the 10 years preceding the clinical diagnosis of dementia: a prospective population-based study. J Am Geriatr Soc. 2008; 56(1):37–44.
14. Petersen RC. Mild cognitive impairment as a diagnostic entity. J Intern Med. 2004;256(3):183–94.
15. Palmer K, Backman L, Winblad B, Fratiglioni L. Mild cognitive impairment in the general population: occurrence and progression to Alzheimer disease. J Am Geriatr Soc. 2008;16(7):603–11.
16. Winblad B, Palmer K, Kivipelto M, Jelic V, Fratiglioni L, Wahlund LO, Nordberg A, Backman L, Albert M, Almkvist O, et al. Mild cognitive impairment-beyond controversies, towards a consensus: report of the international working group on mild cognitive impairment. J Intern Med. 2004;256(3):240–6.
17. Jekel K, Damian M, Wattmo C, Hausner L, Bullock R, Connelly PJ, Dubois B, Eriksdotter M, Ewers M, Graessel E, et al. Mild cognitive impairment and deficits in instrumental activities of daily living: a systematic review. Alzheimers Res Ther. 2015;7(1):17.
18. Kim KR, Lee KS, Cheong HK, Eom JS, Oh BH, Hong CH. Characteristic profiles of instrumental activities of daily living in different subtypes of mild cognitive impairment. Dement Geriatr Cogn Disord. 2009;27(3): 278–85.
19. Sikkes SAM, de Lange-de Klerk ESM, Pijnenburg YAL, Scheltens P, Uidehaag BMJ. A systematic review of instrumental activities of daily living scales in dementia: room for improvement. J Neurol Neurosurg Psychiatry. 2009;80:7–12.
20. Graessel E, Viegas R, Stemmer R, Küchly B, Kornhuber J, Donath C. The Erlangen test of activities of daily living: first results on reliability and validity of a short performance test to measure fundamental activities of daily living in dementia patients. International Psychogeriatrics / IPA. 2009;21(1):103–12.
21. Luttenberger K, Schmiedeberg A, Graessel E. Activities of daily living in dementia: revalidation of the E-ADL test and suggestions for further development. BMC Psychiatry. 2012;12(1):208.
22. Luttenberger K, Reppermund S, Schmiedeberg-Sohn A, Book S, Graessel E. Validation of the Erlangen test of activities of daily living in persons with mild dementia or mild cognitive impairment (ETAM). BMC Geriatr. 2016;16(1):12.
23. Farina E, Fioravanti R, Pignatti R, Alberoni M, Mantovani F, Manzoni G, Chiacari L, Imbornone E, Villanelli F, Nemni R. Functional living skills

assessment: a standardized measure of high-order activities of daily living in patients with dementia. Eur J Phys Rehabil Med. 2010;46:73–80.

24. Karagiozis H, Gray S, Sacco J, Shapiro M, Kawas C. The direct assessment of functional abilities (DAFA): a comparison to an indirect measure of instrumental activities of daily living. Gerontologist. 1998;38:113–21.

25. McDougall G, Becker H, Vaughan P, Acee TW, Delville CL. The revised direct assessment of functional status of independent older adults. Gerontologist. 2010;50:363–70.

26. World Health Organization: International Classification of Functioning, Disability and Health (ICF). Geneva: World Health Organization; 2001.

27. Graessel E, Stemmer R, Eichenseer B, Pickel S, Donath C, Kornhuber J, Luttenberger K. Non-pharmacological, multicomponent group therapy in patients with degenerative dementia: a 12-month randomised, controlled trial. BMC Med. 2011;9(1):129.

28. Straubmeier M, Behrndt EM, Seidl H, Oezbe D, Luttenberger K, Graessel E: Effekte einer nichtpharmakologischen Mehrkomponententherapie in Tagespflege-Einrichtungen auf Menschen mit kognitiven Einschränkungen – Ergebnisse der randomisierten kontrollierten „German Day-Care Study". Deutsches Ärzteblatt (accepted).

29. World Health Organization. The international classification of functioning, disability and health: ICF. Geneva: World Health Organization; 2001.

30. Muò R, Schindler A, Vernero I, Schindler O, Ferrario E, Frisoni GB. Alzheimer's disease-associated disability: an ICF approach. Disabil Rehabil. 2005;27:1405–13.

31. Folstein M, Folstein S, Mc Hugh P. "Mini-mental state": a practical method for grading the cognitive state of patients for the clinician. J Psychiatr Res. 1975;12(3):189–98.

32. Arevalo-Rodriguez I, Smailagic N, Roque IFM, Ciapponi A, Sanchez-Perez E, Giannakou A, Pedraza OL, Bonfill Cosp X, Cullum S. Mini-mental state examination (MMSE) for the detection of Alzheimer's disease and other dementias in people with mild cognitive impairment (MCI). Cochrane Database Syst Rev. 2015;3:CD010783.

33. Tombaugh TN, McIntyre NJ. The mini-mental state examination: a comprehensive review. J Am Geriatr Soc. 1992;40(9):922–35.

34. Nasreddine ZS, Phillips NA, Bedirian V, Charbonneau S, Whitehead V, Collin I, Cummings JL, Chertkow H. The Montreal cognitive assessment, MoCA: a brief screening tool for mild cognitive impairment. J Am Geriatr Soc. 2005; 53(4):695–9.

35. Freitas S, Simoes MR, Alves L, Santana I. Montreal cognitive assessment: validation study for mild cognitive impairment and Alzheimer disease. Alzheimer Dis Assoc Disord. 2013;27(1):37–43.

36. Larner AJ. Screening utility of the Montreal cognitive assessment (MoCA): in place of - or as well as - the MMSE? Int Psychogeriatr. 2012;24(3):391–6.

37. Dong Y, Lee WY, Basri NA, Collinson SL, Merchant RA, Venketasubramanian N, Chen CL. The Montreal cognitive assessment is superior to the mini-mental state examination in detecting patients at higher risk of dementia. Int Psychogeriatr. 2012;24(11):1749–55.

38. The EuroQol Group. EuroQol - a new facility for the measurement of health-related quality of life. Health Policy. 1990;16:199–208.

39. Spiegel R, Brunner C, Ermini-Fünfschilling D, Monsch A, Notter M, Puxty J, Tremmel L. A new behavioral assessment scale for geriatric out- and in-patients: the NOSGER (nurses' observation scale for geriatric patients). J Am Geriatr Soc. 1991;39(4):339–47.

40. Ihl R, Frolich L, Dierks T, Martin EM, Maurer K. Differential validity of psychometric tests in dementia of the Alzheimer type. Psychiatry Res. 1992; 44(2):93–106.

41. Peterson RA. A meta-analysis of Cronbach's coefficient alpha. J Consum Res. 1994;21(2):381–91.

42. Fisseni HJ. Lehrbuch der psychologischen Diagnostik. Göttingen: Hogrefe; 1997.

43. Bortz J, Döring N. Forschungsmethoden und Evaluation: für Human- und Sozialwissenschaftler. Berlin, Heidelberg: Springer; 2006.

44. Brown TA. Confirmatory factor analysis for applied research. New York: The Guilford Press; 2006.

45. Schreiber JB, Nora A, Stage FK, Barlow EA, King J. Reporting structural equation modeling and confirmatory factor analysis results: a review. J Educ Res. 2006;99(6):323–37.

46. Giebel CM, Challis DJ, Montaldi D. A revised interview for deterioration in daily living activities in dementia reveals the relationship between social activities and well-being. Dementia (London). 2014:1–14.

47. Giebel CM, Challis, DJ, Montaldi D: A revised interview for deterioration in daily living activities in dementia reveals the relationship between social activities and well-being. Dementia 2016, 15(5):1068–81.

48. Moore DJ, Palmer BW, Patterson TL, Jeste DV. A review of performance-based measures of functional living skills. J Psychiatr Res. 2007;41(1–2):97–118.

49. Cullum CM, Saine K, Chan L, Martin-Cook K, Gray K, Weiner M. Performance-based instrument to assess functional capacity in dementia: the Texas functional living scale. Neuropsychiatry Neuropsychol Behav Neurol. 2001; 14:103–8.

50. Hindmarch I, Lehfeld H, Jongh P, Erzigkeit H. The Bayer activities of daily living scale (B-ADL). Dement Geriatr Cogn Disord. 1998;9:20–6.

51. Crum RM, Anthony JC, Bassett SS, Folstein MF. Population-based norms for the mini-mental state examination by age and educational level. Jama. 1993;269(18):2386–91.

52. Freitas S, Simoes MR, Alves L, Santana I. Montreal cognitive assessment: influence of sociodemographic and health variables. Arch Clin Neuropsychol. 2012;27(2):165–75.

6

Patient preferences concerning the efficacy and side-effect profile of schizophrenia medications: a survey of patients living with schizophrenia

Eric Achtyes[1]*(iD), Adam Simmons[2], Anna Skabeev[2], Nikki Levy[2], Ying Jiang[2], Patricia Marcy[3] and Peter J. Weiden[2]

Abstract

Background: Despite the availability of numerous antipsychotic medications, many patients with schizophrenia continue to experience side effects that contribute to the overall burden of the illness. The present survey of patients with schizophrenia and schizoaffective disorder aimed to assess patient attitudes toward antipsychotic treatment, and understand key factors about willingness to try a new medication.

Methods: A cross-sectional survey was administered to 250 patients with a primary clinical diagnosis of a schizophrenia spectrum disorder across five outpatient clinics in the United States. The survey included self-reported gender, age, weight, and height, and questions about the importance of efficacy and side effects on the decision to take a prescribed antipsychotic medication.

Results: Patients rated efficacy and side effects as important attributes of antipsychotic treatment, with 93.6% and 83.6% of patients listing these as "very" or the "most" important factors in taking prescribed medication. A total of 87.6% of respondents identified the ability to think more clearly as an important property of their medication. Patients identified weight gain, physical restlessness, and somnolence as important side effects of current treatments ("very" or "most" important by 61.6%, 60.8%, and 58.8%, respectively). When asked about willingness to change antipsychotic medication, anticipated weight gain had a negative influence on willingness to try the new treatment, with 22.0% declining to try a medication that would lead to weight gain of 2.7–4.5 kg (6–10 lb), 34.0% declining for anticipated weight gain of 5.0–9.1 kg (11–20 lb), and 52.4% declining for anticipated weight gain greater than 9 kg (20 lbs).

Conclusion: Patients living with schizophrenia spectrum disorders are influenced by many factors when considering whether to take their medication, including efficacy and side effects. It is important for clinicians to assess specific patient concerns to develop a comprehensive treatment plan that maximizes adherence to the prescribed therapy.

Keywords: Adherence, Antipsychotics, Weight, Side effects

* Correspondence: achtyes@msu.edu; ericachtyes@cherryhealth.com
Previous presentation: The study has been presented in part as a poster at the American Psychiatric Association Annual Meeting, May 5–9, 2018, New York City, USA
[1]Cherry Health and Michigan State University College of Human Medicine, Grand Rapids, MI, USA
Full list of author information is available at the end of the article

Background

Despite improvements in the side-effect profile of anti-psychotic medications brought on by the development of atypical antipsychotics, many patients with schizophrenia continue to experience side effects that contribute to the overall burden of the illness [1]. Historically, the most significant side effects, associated with typical antipsychotics, were movement disorders such as antipsychotic-induced Parkinsonism, dystonia, akathisia, and tardive dyskinesia [2, 3]. Although the introduction of atypical antipsychotics lowered the burden of movement disorders, other side effects such as sedation, weight gain, and metabolic dysregulation have become prominent and problematic [1–4]. Weight gain as a side effect is particularly significant in schizophrenia because of the dual challenges of patients' reluctance to take or remain on a medication that causes weight gain, and of elevated cardiovascular risk in this population [4, 5]. The combined influence of inadequate treatment efficacy and side effects contributes to high rates of treatment discontinuation and frequent switching between medications in patients with schizophrenia [6]. In the Clinical Antipsychotic Trials of Intervention Effectiveness (CATIE) study of 1493 patients with schizophrenia, 74% discontinued their initially assigned study medication before 18 months [1].

Current strategies for the design of clinical trials in schizophrenia are based on clinically determined outcomes for efficacy and safety. However, many factors impact adherence to medication, including patient expectations, perceived benefit of treatment, current phase of illness, and the side-effect profile of current and past medications; particularly weight gain, movement disorders, and sedation [7, 8]. Formal randomized controlled trials that factor in these patient-reported outcomes are rare despite their importance in psychiatry because they allow subjective insight into the impact of a treatment on symptoms, tolerability to medication, and quality of life [9]. Therefore, to improve adherence, it is critical that the development of new treatments is based on efficacy and side-effect profiles that are deemed acceptable to patients.

The objective of this study was to evaluate the self-reported reasons for continuing or discontinuing antipsychotic medication in outpatients with schizophrenia spectrum disorders receiving services across five treatment sites in the United States. A survey was designed to ascertain the preferences of patients with schizophrenia spectrum disorders, evaluating the relative importance of medication efficacy and perceived side-effect burden and their impact on the patient's decision to take antipsychotic medication.

Methods

Survey design

The survey was developed with input from the patient advocacy community and from patients living with schizophrenia to ensure the design of a short, easy-to-administer scale designed to assess patient preferences. Insights and feedback from mental health advocates and patients were sought to support the design of a questionnaire aimed at understanding patient preferences regarding the importance of common side effects in treatment decision-making. Feedback on the design and language of the initial draft of the questionnaire led to three valuable insights that were incorporated into the final version: 1) patients found the initial pilot survey too long and confusing, leading to a revised survey that was shortened to focus only on specific side effects judged to be common and associated with adherence challenges [10]; 2) the survey format, which was initially designed to include several question types, was deemed too complex; a straightforward and parallel-constructed Likert-type scale design was subsequently implemented; 3) the symptom descriptions (originally based on the Positive and Negative Syndrome Scale [PANSS]) were considered too technical and not easily understood (e.g., 'Medicines that make the hallucinations or paranoia go away'); on that basis, wording changes suggested by the reviewers were incorporated.

The sample size (250 patients across five clinics) was selected from four states to achieve a geographically-by-region diverse representation. Five community clinics from four states provided a representation of urban (2), suburban (2), and rural (1) communities. Individual clinics used a sample of convenience based on patient flow in order to identify individuals willing to participate in the survey. All clinics were able to complete 25 to 75 surveys, between October 15, 2016 and December 21, 2016.

Study design

This cross-sectional survey was administered to 250 patients aged ≥18 years with a primary clinical diagnosis of schizophrenia or schizoaffective disorder, according to the *Diagnostic and Statistical Manual of Mental Disorders* (Fifth Edition) (DSM-5) [11]. No additional inclusion or exclusion criteria were applied. Patients were recruited from five outpatient clinics across the United States, including community mental health clinics that provide primary treatment to patients with severe mental illness. Recruitment methods varied across clinics, but generally patients were approached at check-in or before meeting with their healthcare provider, if they met the diagnostic criteria. The paper-based survey was completed in the clinic by the patient with assistance from staff, if needed, and each patient was given a $25 gift card upon completion of the survey.

The survey included self-reported gender, age, weight, and height as well as six questions regarding the importance of efficacy and side effects when taking a prescribed medication. Here, findings from the first five items of the six item survey, pertaining to patient medication preferences, are reported. The final survey question is not reported as it is unrelated to that objective. The full questionnaire is provided in the Additional file 1.

Data analysis
Data analysis of non-descriptive measurements was performed using SAS software (SAS Institute, Cary, NC).

Results
Patients
Two hundred and fifty patients completed the survey; of these, 64.0% were male (n = 160) and 2.0% did not include data on gender (n = 4). The mean age of the survey respondents was 43 years (range, 18–72 years), mean weight was 91 kg (200 lb) (range, 49–182 kg [107–402 lb]), and mean body mass index (BMI) was 30 kg/m² (range, 15–63 kg/m²) (Table 1).

Key survey findings
Patients identified both efficacy and side effects as important attributes of medications for the treatment of schizophrenia. Based on a 5-point scale, from "I don't have this problem" to "most important," most patients

Table 1 Patient characteristics

Characteristics	N = 250
Age, years (range)	43 (18–72)
Gender, n (%)	
Male	160 (64)
Female	86 (34)
Missing gender data	4 (2)
Weight, total	
kg (range)	91 (49–182)
lb (range)	200 (107–402)
Weight, male	
kg (range)	92 (49–182)
lb (range)	204 (109–402)
Weight, female	
kg (range)	87 (49–159)
lb (range)	192 (107–350)
BMI, kg/m² (range)	
Total population	30 (15–63)
Males	29 (15–51)
Female	33 (18–63)

All values are means
Abbreviation: *BMI* body mass index

reported the ability to think more clearly as an important reason to take their medication (87.6% rated it as "most important" or "very important"). Most patients also reported the ability to stop hallucinations or paranoia as important (76.4% rated it as "most important" or "very important") and the ability to have fewer side effects than they experienced with their current treatment as important (71.6% rated it as "most important" or "very important") (Survey Question 1).

When considering adherence to medication, efficacy and side effects were identified as the most important drivers for patients to take their prescribed medicine (93.6% and 83.6% rated it as "most important" or "very important," respectively) (Table 2). The presence of active symptoms of schizophrenia was an important factor for 80.4% of patients. Slightly more than half the patients (54.8%) reported that someone reminding them to take their medication was "most important" or "very important," and ease of medication administration was "most important" or "very important" for 67.6% of patients.

When asked about the side effects of current treatments for schizophrenia, 61.6% of patients rated weight gain as "most important" or "very important", compared with 60.8% for restlessness or akathisia and 58.8% for somnolence. The perceived importance of side effects of schizophrenia medication varied with gender; female patients rated all the side effects included in the survey as of greater importance than did male patients (Fig. 1). Considering the perceived importance of side effects according to gender, weight gain was considered to be "most important" or "very important" for 70.9% of female patients and 56.3% of male patients. Feeling tired or drowsy was viewed as being "most important" or "very important" for 61.6% of female patients and 56.9% of male patients. Female patients also assigned feeling restless or having uncontrollable movement slightly greater importance than did male patients (64.0% of females and 59.4% of males rated this as "most important" or "very important," respectively) (Fig. 1).

The presence of anticipated weight gain had a significant impact on self-reported willingness to accept a change in antipsychotic medication. The absolute amount of anticipated weight gain was associated with reluctance to change, with 73.6% of patients indicating that a weight gain of > 9 kg (> 20 lbs) "Would influence my decision a lot" or "I would not take this medicine" compared with 67.2% who were influenced by a weight gain of 5.0–9.1 kg (11–20 lb), 44.0% who were influenced by a weight gain of 2.7–4.5 kg (6–10 lb) and 29.6% who were influenced by a weight gain of < 2.3 kg (< 5 lb) (Fig. 2).

Across all ranges of weight gain, female patients rated the influence of weight gain higher in their decision to take medication than did male patients (Fig. 3). For an anticipated weight gain of 5.0–9.1 kg (11–20 lb), 73.3%

Table 2 Degree of helpfulness of a new medication for the treatment of patients with schizophrenia

Quality	N	Most important, %	Very important, %	Somewhat important, %	Not important, %
How well medication treats my schizophrenia	250	66.0	27.6	4.4	2.0
If I'm actively having symptoms	250	49.6	30.8	10.4	9.2
Side effects of medication	250	45.6	38.0	12.8	3.6
How easy the medication is to take	250	38.4	29.2	21.2	11.2
Somebody reminds me or gives me the medication	250	29.6	25.2	20.4	24.8

Source: Survey Question 4. When you are deciding whether to take a medicine that has been prescribed to you, how important is each of the following factors?

of female patients, compared with 63.8% of male patients, indicated that this would influence their decision to take a medicine. A total of 81.4% of female patients, compared with 71.6% of male patients, reported that an anticipated weight gain of > 9 kg (> 20 lb) would influence their decision to take a medicine. Although patients with a BMI ≥ 27 kg/m^2 viewed gaining weight as a more important side effect than those with a BMI < 27 kg/m^2 (64.9% and 53.4% rated it "most important" or "very important," respectively), the level of influence of different degrees of weight gain on the patient's decision to take a medicine was similar.

When asked about their interest in new medications for the treatment of schizophrenia, 49.4% of patients expressed a likelihood they would try a new medicine (responded "very likely" or "likely"). The most common reasons for responding with an interest in a new medication were to see whether a new medication would have better efficacy and allow them to achieve their personal goals. Those who reported that they were "somewhat likely," "unlikely," "very unlikely," or "not sure" about trying a new medication cited good efficacy of their current treatment or fear of unknown side effects as the rationale for their choice. Patients who considered gaining weight to be an important side effect were more likely to indicate an interest in trying a new medication (56% of patients who indicated that gaining weight was "most important" or "very important" were "very likely" or "likely" to try a new medication vs. 38% who reported gaining weight as "somewhat important" or "not important").

Discussion

From the present survey of patients with schizophrenia spectrum disorders, attitudes toward antipsychotic medication are influenced by both efficacy and side effect profile. The efficacy of medication therapy (ability to think clearly and reduce positive symptoms, such as voices and paranoia) was the most important factor for

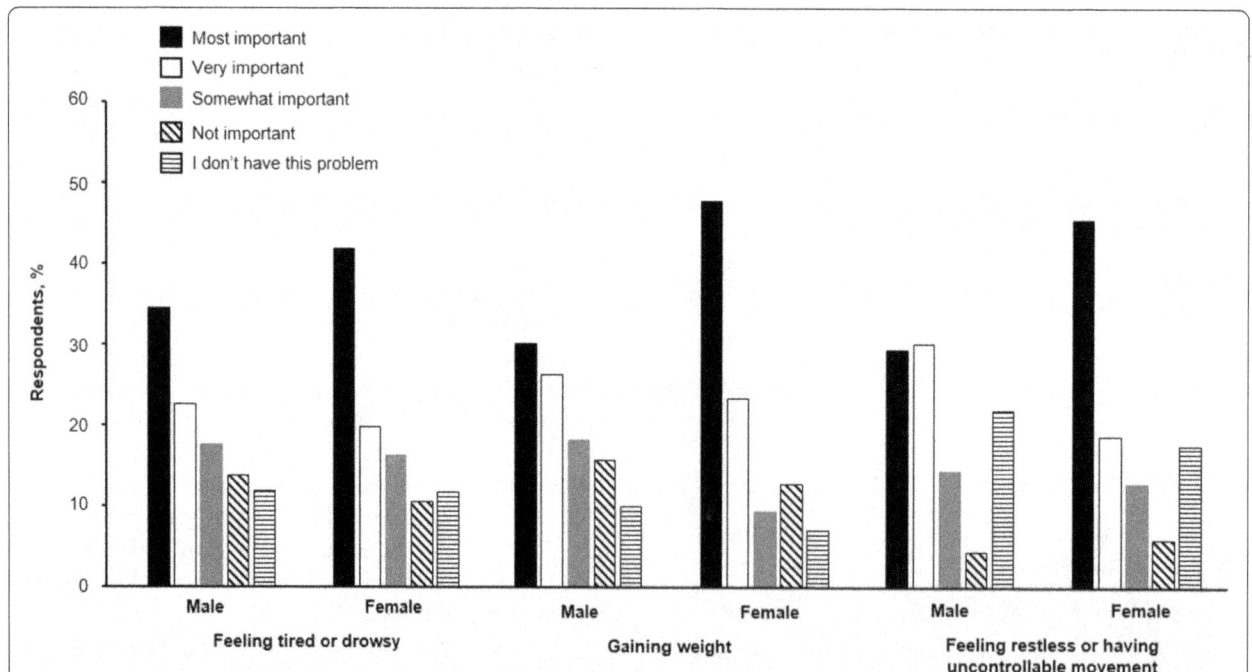

Fig. 1 Importance of common side effects of schizophrenia treatments by gender*. Source: Survey Question 2. Many current treatments for schizophrenia have side effects. How important are these side effects to you? *Data not included for patients who did not self-report gender (n = 4)

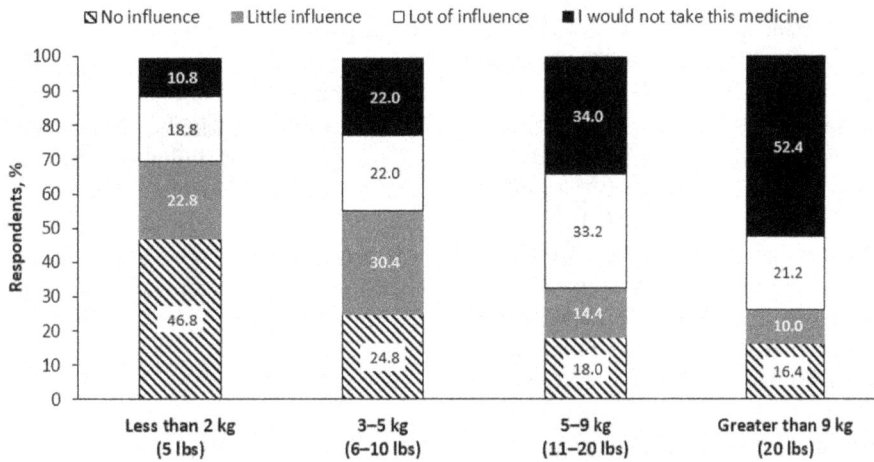

Fig. 2 Influence of anticipated weight gain on patient's decision to take medicine*. *The number (percentage) of patients with missing responses in each weight gain category are: less than 2 kg, $n = 2$ (0.8%); 3–5 kg, $n = 2$ (0.8%); 5–9 kg, $n = 1$ (0.4%). Source: Survey Question 3. One side effect of many medicines for schizophrenia is weight gain. How much would gaining weight influence your decision to take a medicine?

most patients. Side effects, including weight gain, were identified as important factors in determining willingness to take antipsychotic medications, with the level of influence on the decision to take a medicine increasing as anticipated weight gain increased – a finding that was particularly pronounced in female patients. Previous studies have highlighted the importance of weight gain as a cause for both patient distress and nonadherence to prescribed medications [10, 12, 13], as well as poor health outcomes [14]. Individual patient thresholds for side effects such as weight gain are therefore an important consideration when selecting medication or switching medication for schizophrenia.

There was variability in the perceived importance of side effects according to the baseline characteristics of the patients who responded, with female patients rating all side effects included in the survey as of greater importance than did male patients. In a previous patient survey designed to examine the relationship between self-reported side effects and adherence in schizophrenia, patient-reported side effects were strongly associated with self-reported nonadherence; only 42.5% of 876 patients with schizophrenia reported complete adherence to their antipsychotic medication [7]. Findings also suggest that, beyond efficacy and safety assessments, the success of treatment in schizophrenia depends on patient-reported tolerability to

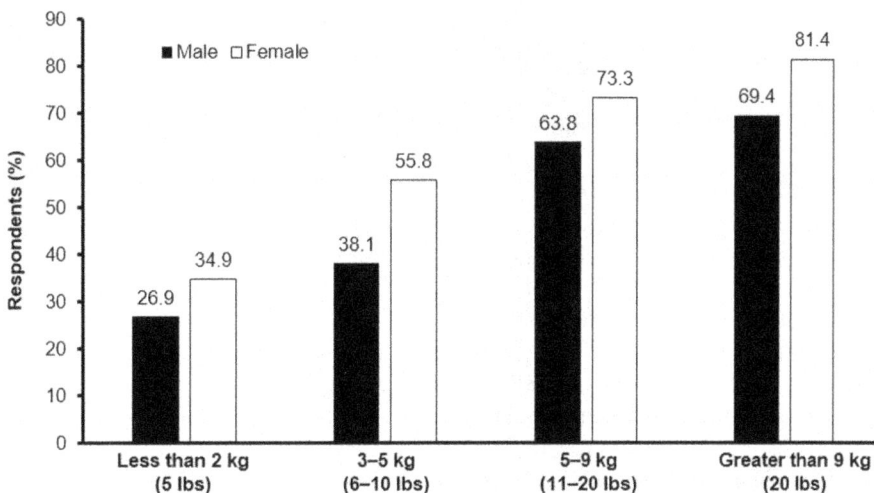

Fig. 3 Patients who would not take a medication or who said their decision would be greatly influenced by the anticipated range of weight gain (by gender)*,†. *Data not included for patients who did not self-report gender ($n = 4$). †210 patients (84%) surveyed had responses that did not change or increased across increasing categories of weight gain. 40 (16%) surveyed had inconsistent responses across weight gain categories. Source: Survey Question 3. One side effect of many medicines for schizophrenia is weight gain. How much would gaining weight influence your decision to take a medicine?

medications, a key factor impacting treatment adherence [15]. It is therefore important that clinicians working with patients who take antipsychotics adopt a mutually agreed decision-making framework where the selection of antipsychotic medication is guided by both efficacy and associated side effects, thereby addressing patients' concerns, and permitting the development of an effective and well-tolerated treatment strategy [2, 16].

Given that the classification of antipsychotics into typical and atypical may not be a helpful distinction [17, 18], antipsychotic selection should be based on an individual risk-benefit assessment that evaluates the psychopathology, the patient's medical comorbidities, and potential medication side effects. Inclusion of patient-reported outcomes in the design of clinical trials is required to ensure the development of treatment options that allow patients to achieve their personal goals [15, 19]. Determining and incorporating these patient goals and thresholds are of particular importance for clinical trial design in psychiatry, an area in which endpoints are based on subjective interpretation by trial investigators, patients, or both. Patient-reported outcomes can also be used to help inform the development of systems to reduce nonadherence to medication, such as medication reminder systems, to improve accuracy of administration, thereby improving patient outcomes [20, 21].

This study has several limitations. Because all data were garnered through self-reported responses to a cross-sectional survey, no baseline demographic characteristics and medical history were collected; hence, patients' ages at diagnosis, current treatment, and treatment histories were not reported. Because age at diagnosis was not reported, it was not possible to determine the chronicity of schizophrenia among the survey respondents and the impact of duration of illness on attitudes towards antipsychotic medication. We recognize that this makes interpreting the study more difficult for clinicians treating patients with varying lengths of illness. However, we think the central theme that patient input should be considered when selecting antipsychotic medication treatment remains relevant. Not all subjective side effects were assessed in this short form, although the ones selected were guided by stakeholder input. The survey required patients to imagine the impact of a side effect they may or may not have experienced, which could have influenced the importance they attributed to the side effects. For example, patients who experienced extrapyramidal symptoms might have placed greater importance on those side effects because of first-hand experience in daily life. Patients' perceptions of the importance of efficacy and side effects could also have been biased if they previously experienced inadequate treatment response or treatment switching. Conversely, by basing the study on a population of outpatients capable and willing to participate in a survey,

bias could have been introduced toward patients experiencing reasonably good efficacy with their current treatments.

Conclusions
When considering whether to take a medication, schizophrenia patients are influenced by many factors, including medication efficacy and side effects. It is important for clinicians to assess all concerns patients may have and to incorporate these into a comprehensive treatment plan designed to maximize adherence to the prescribed therapy.

Abbreviations
BMI: Body mass index; CATIE: Clinical Antipsychotic Trials of Intervention Effectiveness; PANSS: Positive and Negative Syndrome Scale

Acknowledgments
We thank all our collaborators and consultants for their invaluable contributions; without them, this study would not have been possible. We thank the patient advocacy groups consulted: Mental Health America, Schizophrenia and Related Diseases Association of America and the National Alliance on Mental Illness. We are indebted to the many clinicians, research assistants, and administrators at the participating sites within the Vanguard Research Group for their enthusiasm and excellent work and the patients and families who made the study possible with their time, trust, and commitment. We thank Anna Legedza (Alkermes, US) for her assistance with the data analysis. Medical writing and editorial support for the preparation of this manuscript (under the guidance of the authors) was provided by Kate Weatherall (ApotheCom, UK). We also thank Mark S. Todtenkopf, PhD (Alkermes, US) for his assistance in preparing and proofreading the manuscript.

Funding
This study was sponsored by Alkermes, Inc., Waltham, MA, USA. Funding for editorial support was provided by Alkermes, Inc., Waltham, MA, USA. The study sponsor was involved in the design, collection, and analysis of the data.

Authors' contributions
Conception and design: AS1, AS2, NL, YJ, PM. Data acquisition: EA, AS1, AS2, NL, YJ, PM. Data analysis and interpretation: EA, AS1, YJ, AS2, NL, PM, PJW. Drafting the article or critically revising it for important intellectual content: All authors. Final approval of the version to be published: All authors. Agreement to be accountable for all aspects of the work: All authors.

Consent for publication
Not applicable

Competing interests
EA (MD), has received research support from Alkermes, AssurEx, Avanir, Boehringer Ingelheim, Janssen, Neurocrine Biosciences, Novartis, Otsuka, Pfizer, Pine Rest Foundation, Priority Health, Network180, and Vanguard Research Group and has served on advisory panels for Roche, Janssen, Neurocrine Biosciences and the Vanguard Research Group. PM is the executive director of the Vanguard Research Group, which has received

research support from Otsuka, Alkermes, Lundbeck, and Janssen. PJW (MD), A Simmons (MPH), NL, and YJ (PhD), are employees of Alkermes, Inc. A Skabeev (MD), was employed by Alkermes at the time of the study.

Author details

[1]Cherry Health and Michigan State University College of Human Medicine, Grand Rapids, MI, USA. [2]Alkermes, Inc., Waltham, MA, USA. [3]Vanguard Research Group, Northwell Health System, Manhasset, NY, USA.

References

1. Lieberman JA, Stroup TS, Mcevoy JP, Swartz MS, Rosenheck RA, Perkins DO, Keefe RS, Davis SM, Davis CE, Lebowitz BD, et al. Effectiveness of antipsychotic drugs in patients with chronic schizophrenia. New Engl J Med. 2005;353(12):1209–23.
2. Hasan A, Falkai P, Wobrock T, Lieberman J, Glenthoj B, Gattaz WF, Thibaut F, Moller HJ. World federation of societies of biological psychiatry (WFSBP) guidelines for biological treatment of schizophrenia, part 2: update 2012 on the long-term treatment of schizophrenia and management of antipsychotic-induced side effects. World J Biol Psychiatry. 2013;14(1):2–44.
3. Leucht S, Cipriani A, Spineli L, Mavridis D, Orey D, Richter F, Samara M, Barbui C, Engel RR, Geddes JR, et al. Comparative efficacy and tolerability of 15 antipsychotic drugs in schizophrenia: a multiple-treatments meta-analysis. Lancet. 2013;382(9896):951–62.
4. Weiden PJ. Long-term treatment of schizophrenia: minimizing side effect burden to improve patient outcomes. Curr Psychiatr Ther. 2010;9(11)
5. Brown S, Inskip H, Barraclough B. Causes of the excess mortality of schizophrenia. Br J Psychiatry. 2000;177:212–7.
6. Kishimoto T, Agarwal V, Kishi T, Leucht S, Kane J, Correll C. Relapse prevention in schizophrenia: a systematic review and meta-analysis of second-generation antipsychotics versus first-generation antipsychotics. Mol Psychiatry. 2013;18(1):53–66.
7. Dibonaventura M, Gabriel S, Dupclay L, Gupta S, Kim E. A patient perspective of the impact of medication side effects on adherence: results of a cross-sectional Nationwide survey of patients with schizophrenia. Bmc Psychiatry. 2012;12:20.
8. Weiden PJ, Mackell JA, Mcdonnell DD. Obesity as a risk factor for antipsychotic noncompliance. Schizophr Res. 2004;66(1):51–7.
9. Correll CU, Kishimoto T, Nielsen J, Kane JM. Quantifying clinical relevance in the treatment of schizophrenia. Clin Ther. 2011;33(12):B16–39.
10. Weiden PJ, Miller AL. Which side effects really matter? Screening for common and distressing side effects of antipsychotic medications. J Psychiatr Pract. 2001;7(1):41–7.
11. Association Psychiatric Association. Schizophrenia spectrum and other psychiatric disorders. In: Diagnostic and statistical manual of mental disorders, fifth edition (DSM-5). Washington: Dc. p. 2013.
12. Covell NH, Weissman EM, Schell B, Mccorkle BH, Summerfelt WT, Weiden PJ, Essock SM. Distress with medication side effects among persons with severe mental illness. Admin Pol Ment Health. 2007;34(5):435–42.
13. Llorca PM, Lancon C, Hartry A, Brown TM, Dibenedetti DB, Kamat SA, Francois C. Assessing the burden of treatment-emergent adverse events associated with atypical antipsychotic medications. Bmc Psychiatry. 2017;17(1):67.
14. McIntyre RS. Understanding needs, interactions, treatment, and expectations among individuals affected by bipolar disorder or schizophrenia: the unite global survey. J Clin Psychiatry. 2009;70(Suppl 3):5–11.
15. Fleischhacker WW, Rabinowitz J, Kemmler G, Eerdekens M, Mehnert A. Perceived functioning, well-being and psychiatric symptoms in patients with stable schizophrenia treated with long-acting risperidone for 1 year. Br J Psychiatry. 2005;187:131–6.
16. Kuipers E, Yesufu-Udechuku A, Taylor C, Kendall T. Management of psychosis and schizophrenia in adults: summary of updated nice guidance. BMJ. 2014;348:G1173.
17. Correll CU, De Hert M. Antipsychotics for acute schizophrenia: making choices. Lancet. 2013;382(9896):919–20.
18. Hasan A, Falkai P, Wobrock T, Lieberman J, Glenthoj B, Gattaz WF, Thibaut F, Möller H-J. World federation of societies of biological psychiatry (WFSBP) task force on treatment guidelines for schizophrenia. World federation of societies of biological psychiatry (Wfsbp) guidelines for biological treatment of schizophrenia, part 1: update 2012 on the acute treatment of schizophrenia and the management of treatment resistance. World J Biol Psychiatry. 2012;13(5):318–78.
19. Mccabe R, Saidi M, Priebe S. Patient-reported outcomes in schizophrenia. Br J Psychiatry. 2007;50:S21–8.
20. Baumhauer JF. Patient-reported outcomes - are they living up to their potential? New Engl J Med. 2017;377(1):6–9.
21. Velligan DI, Weiden PJ, Sajatovic M, Scott J, Carpenter D, Ross R, Docherty JP. The expert consensus guideline series: adherence problems in patients with serious and persistent mental illness. J Clin Psychiatry. 2009;70(Suppl 4):1–46.

7

Community based telepsychiatry service for older adults residing in a rural and remote region- utilization pattern and satisfaction among stakeholders

Pallavi Dham[1,2,4*] (iD), Neeraj Gupta[3], Jacob Alexander[3], Warwick Black[3], Tarek Rajji[1,2] and Elaine Skinner[3]

Abstract

Background: Evaluation of telepsychiatry (via videoconference) for older adults is mostly focussed on nursing homes or inpatients. We evaluated the role of a community based program for older adults in rural and remote regions of South Australia.

Method: The utilization pattern was studied using retrospective chart review of telepsychiatry assessments over 24 months (2010–2011). Satisfaction was evaluated through prospective post-consultation feedback (using a 5-point Likert scale), from patients, community based clinicians and psychiatrist participating in consecutive assessments from April–November 2012. Descriptive analysis was used for the utilization. Mean scores and proportions were calculated for the feedback. Mann Whitney U test was used to compare patient subgroups based on age, gender, prior exposure to telepsychiatry services and inpatient/ outpatient status. Feedback comments were analysed for emerging themes.

Results: On retrospective review of 134 consults, mean age was 75.89 years (SD 7.55), 60.4% (81) were females, and 71. 6% (96) lived independently. Patients had a broad range of psychiatric disorders, from mood disorders to delirium and dementia, with co-morbid medical illness in 83.5% (112). On feedback evaluation ($N = 98$), mean scores ranged from 3. 88–4.41 for patients, 4.36–4.73 for clinicians and 3.67–4.45 for psychiatrists. Feedback from inpatients (14 out of 37) was significantly lower compared to outpatients (37 out of 61) (chi sq. $= 0.808$, $p < 0.05$), and they were significantly less satisfied with the wait time ($U = 163.0$, $p < 0.05$) and visual clarity ($U = 160.5$, p < 0.05). Audio clarity was the most common aspect of dissatisfaction (mean score less than 3) among patients (6, 11%). Psychiatrists reported a preference for telepsychiatry over face to face in 55.4% (46) assessments. However, they expressed discomfort in situations of cognitive or sensory disabilities in patients.

Conclusions: In rural and remote areas, community-based telepsychiatry program can be a useful adjunct for psychiatrist input in the care of older adults. Innovations to overcome sensory deficits and collaboration with community services should be explored to improve its acceptance among the most vulnerable population.

Keywords: Telepsychiatry, Elderly, Utilization, Satisfaction, Community

* Correspondence: P_dham77@yahoo.com
[1]Division of Geriatric Psychiatry, Centre for Addiction and Mental Health, Toronto, Canada
[2]Department of Psychiatry, University of Toronto, Toronto, Canada
Full list of author information is available at the end of the article

Background

Psychiatric disorders among older adults are often complicated by comorbid medical illnesses and disability [1]. Specialist psychiatry input becomes essential in these situations but is often difficult to access, especially among older adults residing in rural and remote regions [2]. One of the key modalities evaluated to meet this need is video-conferencing, also referred to as tele-medicine. It is now a reliable and accepted mode of assessment and treatment in geriatric medicine [3, 4]. In psychiatry, its use is well established among adults and youth in the community setting [5], but among older adults, the evaluation of telepsychiatry is focused on feasibility and diagnostic accuracy in nursing homes and inpatient settings, rather than utilization or satisfaction in the community [6]. It is evaluated to be comparable to face to face evaluation in terms of diagnostic accuracy and is acceptable among the nursing home population [6]. Surprisingly, only one community based telepsychiatry program has been evaluated among older adults [7], utilized mostly by patients with dementia and it showed a high degree of satisfaction among various stakeholders. We lack an understanding about the use of telepsychiatry among older adults for psychiatric disorders other than dementia, especially in the community setting. We do not know if a community based tele-psychiatry program would be widely used, if it would be acceptable to the various stakeholders and what barriers one may face. Evaluation of community-based telepsychiatry programs for this population is essential to get a better understanding of the role of telepsychiatry in mental health service delivery among older adults, especially in rural and remote regions, which can then help guide models of care.

The program we evaluate here differs from the previously evaluated community based telepsychiatry program [7] in its use of high-speed internet at 768 kbps, and a wider coverage of 13 community mental health teams across an area of 980,000 sq. km. It is embedded within an overarching mental health service in the region with a hub of psychiatrists (geriatric psychiatrists; sub-specialty geriatric psychiatry trainee) and mental health nurses in Adelaide. A clinician (nursing or allied health), trained in old age mental health, is embedded in each of the community mental health teams in the rural and remote regions of South Australia and functions as a link between the primary care services in the community and the central hub. Psychiatrist support in assessment and treatment is provided by a combination of community visits by psychiatrists every 4–6 weeks and via telepsychiatry.

The evaluation objective was to describe the pattern of utilization of the telepsychiatry program over 2 years and assess the acceptance and satisfaction among various stakeholders.

Methods

Study design

This is a cross-sectional cohort study design with a retrospective chart review component and a prospective feedback survey of stakeholders including the patient, the referring clinician/nurse involved in the patient's care and the psychiatrist. South Australian Health Ethics committee approved the study.

Study sample

To assess the pattern of utilization, the sample included consecutive patients, 65 years and over, with mental health problems, resident in rural and remote South Australia, referred to the service for a tele-psychiatry assessment from January 2010–December 2011.

To assess acceptance and satisfaction, feedback about the tele-psychiatry consultation was sought prospectively from patients, referring nurse/clinician and psychiatrist involved in the tele-psychiatry consultation from April to November 2012. The feedback was voluntary and anonymous. Return of the feedback forms was accepted as consent.

Telepsychiatry setup and process of consultation

Telepsychiatry assessment is provided using a secure broadband network at 768 kbps via video conferencing equipment at the Adelaide hub linked to the video-conferencing equipment in community hospitals and health centers in rural and remote regions of South Australia.

Referral from the local General Practitioners (GP) is triaged and a time is booked for an assessment. Referred patient could be residing in the community or nursing home or could be admitted in community hospitals at the time of the assessment. Those residing in the community or nursing homes travel to the nearest community hospital or health center with the videoconferencing equipment. Those admitted to the community hospitals have access to video-conferencing equipment in the hospital premises, but it is not a mobile equipment. A member involved in the patient's care (nurse or community mental health team clinician) accompanies the patient, and family members are encouraged to attend. Following an assessment by a psychiatrist, the diagnosis and proposed management plan are conveyed to the patient/family member and the accompanying clinician, and a typed report is sent to the referring GP and the local mental health team. While majority are one time consults, a patient may be reviewed on a repeat request.

Data collection

To assess the utilization pattern of telepsychiatry services for older patients We retrospectively gathered information regarding demographics (age, gender, type of residence), physical disability (visual/hearing/physical), Standardised Mini-Mental State Examination (SMMSE) score [8], reason for the referral as mentioned in the referral form, person accompanying the patient (clinician/nurse/family member), comorbid medical illness, psychiatric diagnosis based on the DSM IV criteria and recommendations made, from three sources: client records, telepsychiatry referral form and assessment report sent to the GP. Author PD, using a de-identified standard chart review form approved by the ethics committee collected data on each consultation.

To assess acceptance and satisfaction with the service
We prospectively sought post-session feedback from patients, referring clinicians and psychiatrist involved in consecutive telepsychiatry consults from April to November 2012. This was done using standard feedback forms developed for the study and approved by the ethics committee. Telemedicine satisfaction questionnaires have been validated in other areas of medicine [9, 10] and previously used for telepsychiatry among children and adolescents [11] with a primary focus on patient satisfaction. In the absence of validated satisfaction assessment tools in the elderly population, and since we were exploring satisfaction among various stakeholders, we decided to adapt the previously used satisfaction scales to suit the needs of our population and service. The satisfaction questionnaire included questions regarding the referral process, technical aspects, comfort with the use of the medium and satisfaction with the assessment and recommendations (questions detailed in Tables 3 & 5). While the areas covered were similar across the stakeholders, individual questions were modified as relevant to the stakeholders. Each question was rated on a five-point Likert scale with options ranging from "strongly agree" to "strongly disagree". An open comment section titled "Comments" with 3 lined space allowed provision of additional feedback. The forms were made available to the clinicians and specialists prior to the consult. Accompanying clinician provided the feedback form to the patient at the end of the consult. These were filled in soon after the consult to avoid any recall bias and faxed to the central service after completion. If a patient was unable to provide feedback because of illness severity or cognitive impairment, their significant other (usually a family member) if accompanying the patient, was encouraged to do so.

Data analysis

Utilization pattern of telepsychiatry services Descriptive analysis was used to describe the utilization pattern using means with standard deviation (SD) and percentages.

Acceptance and satisfaction
Survey respondent and non-respondent patient groups were compared using t test or Pearson's chi-square Test for any statistical differences in age, gender, living situation, primary psychiatric issue, prior exposure to our telepsychiatry service and inpatient/outpatient status at the time of the assessment.

Responses on each feedback statement were given numerical values from 1 to 5 with 1 representing 'strongly disagree' and 5 representing 'strongly agree'. Mean scores were calculated for each statement. We also calculated the percentage of responses which suggested satisfaction i.e. ≥ 4, ('agree' or 'strongly agree') or dissatisfaction i.e. ≤ 2 ('disagree' or 'strongly disagree') on each statement. Mann-Whitney Rank Sum Test was used to compare feedback scores on each question based on gender, previous experience with telepsychiatry, independent living/nursing home and inpatient/outpatient status. All analyses were performed using SPSS version 23.0.0.0.

We manually analyzed feedback comments received from each group to look for emerging themes. This was done by NG and verified by PD. The comments were first classified as positive (if the feedback was favorable) or negative (if the feedback was unfavorable). The content of the individual comments was categorized into sub-categories or themes, such that one or more sub-category might apply to each comment. Three sub-categories were identified: a) corresponding to the items covered in the feedback form; b) global themes not linked to a specific item on the feedback form; and c) other statements which could not be reconciled with the feedback form items or global themes. They were then expressed as counts (Table 6) and selected verbatim quotes are mentioned in the results section.

Results
Profile of older adult seen via telepsychiatry in 2010–2011
In 2010–11, 140 telepsychiatry consults were performed, of which we analyzed the data from 134 consults of 101 patients, averaging 1.32 consult per patient. The missing data relates to deceased patients whose files were not accessible.

The demographic details and clinical profile of the patients seen via telepsychiatry are described in Table 1. **Their** mean age was 75.89 years (SD 7.55), majority were females (81, 60.4%) and most lived independently (96, 71.6%). Up to 90 patients (67.2%) had no documented disability (defined as visual/hearing/physical/speech). Mean SMMSE [8] score was 24.4 (SD 4.98). Majority had two or more medical conditions (96, 71.6%), including hypertension, diabetes, infections, hypothyroidism, renal failure, cardiac disease, cerebrovascular accidents, seizure, pain, and cancer.

Table 1 Profile of patients seen via tele-psychiatry from January 2010 to 2011

Consumer profile	Jan 2010 to Dec 2011 (N = 134)
Mean Age (SD)	75.89 (SD 7.55)
Female (n, %)	81 (60.4%)
Place of residence (n, %)	
Private own/rental, Independent house	96 (71.6%)
Residential Age Care Facility (RACF)	25 (18.7%)
Hospital	7 (5.2%)
Not stated	6 (4.5%)
Physical disability (n, %)	
No disability	90 (67.2%)
Visual/hearing impaired	21 (15.7%)
Unsteady gait/ restricted mobility	17 (12.7%)
Not stated	6 (4.5%)
Difficult Speech/aphasia	2 (1.5%)
Medical Illnesses (eg: hypertension, diabetes, infections, renal impairment, cancers) (n, %)	
2 or more medical conditions	96 (71.6%)
Single medical condition	16 (11.9%)
No medical illness	17 (12.7%)
Not stated	5 (3.7%)
Standard Mini Mental State Examination (SMMSE)	
Mean score (SD)	24.44 (SD 4.98)
Not mentioned (n, %)	61 (45.5%)
Reason for referral (n, %)	
Depression/anxiety	58 (43.3%)
Difficult-behaviors (odd/confused/paranoid/manic/aggression/uncooperative)	26 (19.4%)
Not specified	28 (20.9%)
Self-harm ideation/attempt	16 (11.9%)
Others (alcohol use, medication side effects, capacity)	6 (4.5%)
Person accompanying the patient (n, %)	
Member of the Community Mental Health Team (CMHT) /clinician	69 (51.5%)
Clinical nurse (RACF/hospital/practice)	56 (41.8%)
Family (spouse/son/daughter)	53 (39.6%)
Not stated	9 (6.3%)
GP	5 (3.7%)
DSM IV diagnosis (n, %)	
Major Depressive Disorder	51 (38.1%)
Bipolar Disorder	20 (14.9%)
Dementia	18 (13.4%)
Schizophrenia/Schizo-affective disorder/Delusional Disorder/Psychotic Disorder NOS	14 (10.5%)

Table 1 Profile of patients seen via tele-psychiatry from January 2010 to 2011 (Continued)

Consumer profile	Jan 2010 to Dec 2011 (N = 134)
Anxiety disorders (PTSD, Panic Disorder, NOS)	11 (8.2%)
Adjustment Disorder	11 (8.2%)
Delirium	9 (6.7%)
Medication side effects	7 (5.2%)
No axis 1 diagnosis	3 (2.2%)
Substance dependence/abuse	2 (1.5%)
Recommendations provided (n, %)	
Medication recommendation only	55 (41.0%)
Medication recommendation + psychosocial supports and services	32 (23.9%)
Recommended further medical evaluation/ inpatient admission+/− medication recommendation	34 (25.4%)
No further changes	13 (9.7%)

Depression and anxiety were the most common reasons for referral to the telepsychiatry service (58, 43.3%). Difficult behaviors (odd, confused, paranoid, aggressive or uncooperative) and self-harm formed a smaller percentage of the referrals (26, 19.4% and 16, 11.9% respectively, Table 1). Major Depressive Disorder was the most common psychiatric diagnosis (51, 38.1%), although the list of psychiatric disorders was diverse including adjustment disorder, bipolar disorder, psychotic disorder, dementia and delirium (Table 1). A clinician from the community team accompanied 69 (51.5%) patients and a family member accompanied 53 (39.6%) consults. In 87 consults (64.9%), recommendations included medication changes with or without other psychosocial assessment/treatments and 34 (25.4%) patients were recommended inpatient treatment or further medical evaluation.

Prospective feedback from patients, clinicians, and psychiatrists for telepsychiatry consultations

The sample population providing the feedback was very similar in terms of mean age (75.89, SD 7.55 and 75.68, SD 6.39) and gender distribution (60–65% females) to the sample used for evaluation of the utilization pattern. Further, depression and anxiety disorders were the most prevalent diagnosis in both populations and severe mental illness, dementia and delirium had a lower prevalence (Tables 1 and 2). The details of the feedback are described below.

Feedback from patients

Table 2 describes the profile of patients who participated in the feedback survey between April to November 2012 (N = 98). Their mean age was 75.68 years (SD 6.39) and 64 (65.5%) were females. Majority were new consults

Table 2 Profile of patients seen via tele-psychiatry seen during the period of feedback review in 2012

	Total (N=98)	Feedback received ($N=51$)	Feedback not received ($N=47$)	Statistical significance
Mean age in years (SD)	75.68 (6.39)	75.94 (6.45)	75.40 (6.39)	$t=0.414$, $p=0.860^a$
Gender				
Females (N, %)	64 (65.3%	34 (66.7%)	30 (63.8%)	$\chi^2=0.087$ $p=0.833^b$
Males (N,%)	34 (34.7%)	17 (33.3%)	17 (36.2%)	
Prior tele-psychiatry contact with the service (N, %)				$\chi^2=1.791$ $p=0.216^b$
Yes	38 (38.8%)	23 (45.1%)	15 (31.9%)	
No	60 (61.2%)	28 (54.9%)	32 (68.1%)	
Primary Psychiatry Diagnosis made at the assessment (N, %)				
Depression or anxiety	51 (52.0%)	30 (58.8%)	21 (44.7%)	$\chi^2=9.107$ $p=0.168^b$
Mania	10 (10.2%)	5 (9.8%)	5 (10.6%)	
Psychotic illness	21 (21.4%)	12 (23.5%)	9 (19.1%)	
Delirium	6 (6.1%)	1 (2.0%)	5 (10.6%)	
Organic mood disorder	2 (2.0%)	1 (2.0%)	1 (2.1%)	
Dementia	7 (7.1%)	1 (2.0%)	6 (12.8%)	
Unclear	1 (1%)	1 (2.0%)	0 (0.0%)	
Living Situation (N, %)				
Independent living (Home or Retirement home)	82 (83.7%)	41 (80.4%)	41 (87.2%)	$\chi^2=1.229$ $p=0.420^b$
Nursing Home	16 (16.3%)	10 (19.6%)	6 (12.8%)	
Status at consultation (N, %)				
Inpatient (admitted in community hospital)	37 (37.8%)	14 (27.5%)	23 (48.9%)	$\chi^2=0.838$ **$p=0.037^{*b}$**
Outpatient	61 (62.2%)	37 (72.5%)	24 (51.1%)	

^{a} = t test; ^{b} = Chi Square test, *significance at $p< 0.05$

(60, 61.2%). Feedback was received from 51 patients (52%), of which family members provided the feedback in 5 consults. The respondents and non-respondent patient groups did not differ statistically based on mean age, gender, previous contact with the service, primary psychiatric diagnosis or independent living versus residence in a nursing home. The feedback however was significantly lower among patients admitted in community hospitals (inpatients) compared to outpatients ($\chi^2=$ 0.808 $p=0.037$, Table 2). Feedback rates were also low in dementia and delirium (provided by significant other), but the difference based on diagnosis was not statistically significant (Table 2).

Table 3 outlines the mean scores on feedback ranging between 3.88–4.41, mean scores greater than 4 on ten out of twelve feedback questions across the domains of process of referral and wait times, technical aspects, comfort and satisfaction with the consultation and recommendations. Satisfaction with the consultation was high with a mean score of 4.14 ± 0.75. While overall expression of dissatisfaction was minimal (2% to 11.8%), most common dissatisfaction was on question 5 i.e. "I was able to hear clearly" (6, 11.8%, Table 3). On most questions they were decisive regarding their satisfaction or dissatisfaction, but a few were unsure if the recommendations

were useful on question 9 (12, 23.5%) or if their needs were met on question 8 (14, 27.5%).

A subgroup analysis of the patient feedback scores using Mann Whitney U test (Table 4) did not show statistically significant differences in satisfaction on any of the questions based on gender, living situation or prior exposure to our telepsychiatry service. However, satisfaction among outpatients was significantly greater than inpatients on question 1 i.e. 'The waiting period (time between making contact with the service and appointment for consultation) was satisfactory' (U = 163.0, $p=0.028$) and question 4 i.e. 'I was able to see clearly' (U = 160.5, $p=0.019$).

Feedback data from clinician's/ nurses

As shown in Table 5; the mean score of the feedback from clinicians/nurses ($N=59$, response rate 57.8%) ranged from 4.36–4.73 on all of the 11 questions with over 90% satisfaction. The lowest rates of satisfaction (88%) with a mean score of 4.36 ± 0.78 was for "process of referral was convenient".

Feedback from the psychiatrists/sub-specialty trainee

Table 5 describes the psychiatrist feedback ($N=80$, response rate: 81.3%). Over the study period, 4 psychiatrists and 1 sub-specialty geriatric psychiatry trainee

Table 3 Feedback scores for patients seen via tele-psychiatry in 2012 (N = 51)

Feedback Question	Mean ± SD	Percentage satisfied[a] (n)	Percentage unsure[a] (n)	Percentage dissatisfied[a] (n)
1. The waiting period for the consultation was satisfactory (i.e The time interval between making contact with the service and appointment for consultation)	4.14 ± 0.94	84.4 (43)	7.8 (4)	7.8 (4)
2. Sufficient explanation was provided regarding the process	4.18 ± 0.71	86.2 (44)	11.8 (6)	2.0 (1)
3. My privacy and confidentiality was respected	4.41 ± 0.61	98.0 (50)	0 (0)	2.0 (1)
4. I was able to see clearly	4.24 ± 0.79	92.2 (47)	3.9 (2)	3.9 (2)
5. I was able to hear clearly	4.00 ± 1.00	80.4 (41)	7.8 (4)	11.8 (6)
6. I was able to express myself adequately using this mode of assessment	4.20 ± 0.78	86.3 (44)	9.8 (5)	3.9 (2)
7. I felt comfortable discussing my problems using this mode of assessment	4.22 ± 0.78	90.2 (46)	3.9 (2)	5.9 (3)
8. The assessment addressed my needs	3.90 ± 0.83	68.6 (35)	27.5 (14)	3.9 (2)
9. The recommendations made were useful	3.88 ± 0.77	72.5 (37)	23.5 (12)	3.9 (2)
10. I am satisfied with the consultation	4.14 ± 0.75	86.3 (44)	9.8 (5)	3.9 (2)
11. I would prefer to use it again?	4.02 ± 0.81	76.5 (39)	19.6 (10)	3.9 (2)
12. I would recommend it to others?	4.08 ± 0.85	86.3 (44)	7.8 (4)	5.9 (3)

Likert Scale: 1-strongly disagree, 2- disagree, 3-neither agree nor disagree, 4- agree, 5- strongly agree
[a]Satisfied: agree or strongly agree, Dissatisfied: disagree or strongly disagree, Unsure: Neither agree nor disagree

performed consults. The mean scores on the feedback ranged between 3.67–4.45. The highest mean score was 4.45 ± 0.8 for "I would encourage its use". The lowest mean score, 3.67 ± 1.39, was for "I prefer it to face to face consultation" but in 46 (55.4%) consults, they agreed with the statement. In 14 (16.9%) consults, psychiatrists did not feel comfortable participating in the assessment.

Feedback comments

In the free text comment section of the feedback form, we received 32 comments from patients/significant others, 23 from clinicians/nurses and 38 from psychiatrists. The themes and content are detailed in Table 6.

Positive themes from patients described the service as useful and time-saving (e.g. *"we are happy to use it as it saves us a lot of time and traveling", "very very helpful", "fantastic)"*. They mentioned that they were treated respectfully (e.g. *"the people were good and understanding"*). Negative themes were predominantly related to audio-visual difficulties (e.g. *"TV (visual) not working", "forgot my hearing aids and eyes were blurry", "couldn't hear clearly"*). Mixed comments had elements of uncertainty (e.g. *"Unsure, but every effort is being made to help me"*).

Positive themes from clinicians made references to telepsychiatry as helpful, educational and easy to access (e.g. *"fantastic service for rural and remote people", "great to have a discussion/ educational opportunity at the end"*). They also valued the support and the time saved (e.g. *"thank you for support and advice", "Telepsychiatry has meant a greatly reduced waiting time for this consult"*). Some clinicians expressed concerns regarding the information required for the referral (e.g. *"the referral process took a while as I had to wait for the GP and*

then had to include the other assessment tools") and audio-visual issues, *"visual not working", "I had not anticipated the hearing problem for the client. Repeating the questions was awkward and made the consultation difficult for both parties"*).

Psychiatrists also found telepsychiatry to be useful and time-saving for rural patients (e.g. *"was very useful to do telemed consultation in this patient- a lot quicker"*). Negative themes mentioned difficulties due to patient-related issues such as disabilities and poor engagement (*eg. "Advanced dementia precluded the assessment but it was still helpful", "patient was not engaging and so the assessment was difficult"*) or technical aspects like audio-visual difficulties, noise, cold and privacy issues (e.g. *"visual not clear", "too cold in the room- uncomfortable", "there was a lot of background noise at the far end"*).

Discussion

This study focuses on the clinical role of telepsychiatry for older adults, when embedded within a larger psychiatry service. It is a crucial adjunct to the visiting service in the region which is infrequent and cost intensive, often unable to cater for all needs of the community [12]. It is also the only service evaluated which caters to older adults resident in the community, nursing homes and those admitted in community hospitals providing a unique opportunity to compare satisfaction in different settings within the rural and remote community.

Utilization patterns

The pattern of utilization shows that in remote areas, where psychiatry services may not be readily accessible, a community-based telepsychiatry program is applicable in a broad range of psychiatric disorders from adjustment

Table 4 Differences in patient feedback scores based on their previous contact with the service, gender, living situation and inpatient or outpatient status at the time of the assessment

Questions[a]	Prior telepsychiatry contact with the service			Gender			Living Situation			Status at the time of the assessment		
	Yes = 23 Mean, SD	No = 28 Mean, SD	U, 2 tailed P value	Male = 17 Mean, SD	Female = 34 Mean, SD	U, 2 tailed P value	Independent living = 41 Mean, SD	Nursing Home = 10 Mean, SD	U, 2 tailed P value	Inpatient = 14 Mean, SD	Outpatient = 37 Mean, SD	U, 2 tailed P value
Q1	4.30, 0.765	4.0, 1.054	275.5, 0.339	4.24, 0.831	4.09, 0.996	271.0, 0.696	4.15, 1.014	4.10, 0.568	174.5, 0.432	3.64, 1.324	4.32, 0.784	163.0, 0.028*
Q2	4.30, 0.765	4.07, 0.663	253.5, 0.150	4.12, 0.781	4.21, 0.687	270.0, 0.674	4.22, 0.759	4.00, 0.471	160.5, 0.242	4.07, 0.616	4.22, 0.750	222.0, 0.386
Q3	4.43, 0.507	4.39, 0.685	319.0, 0.948	4.41, 0.507	4.41, 0.657	277.0, 0.783	4.41, 0.631	4.40, 0.516	195.0, 0.786	4.36, 0.497	4.43, 0.647	230.0, 0.483
Q4	4.26, 0.689	4.21, 0.876	321.0, 0.983	4.06, 0.966	4.32, 0.684	246.5, 0.337	4.20, 0.843	4.40, 0.516	186.0, 0.612	3.71, 1.139	4.43, 0.502	160.5, 0.019*
Q5	3.83, 1.072	4.14, 0.932	269.0, 0.279	4.24, 0.664	3.88, 1.122	253.5, 0.444	4.07, 0.985	3.70, 1.059	160.0, 0.249	3.93, 1.141	4.03, 0.957	252.0, 0.873
Q6	4.17, 0.937	4.21, 0.630	307.0, 0.755	4.29, 0.588	4.15, 0.857	274.0, 0.742	4.27, 0.708	3.90, 0.994	162.5, 0.268	3.93, 0.829	4.30, 0.740	192.5, 0.123
Q7	4.26, 0.752	4.18, 0.819	307.5, 0.759	4.18, 0.728	4.24, 0.819	268.0, 0.639	4.22, 0.822	4.20, 0.632	189.5, 0.681	3.86, 0.949	4.35, 0.676	181.5, 0.067
Q8	3.87, 0.869	3.93, 0.813	309.5, 0.801	3.88, 0.781	3.91, 0.866	276.5, 0.790	3.93, 0.848	3.80, 0.789	183.0, 0.579	3.86, 0.770	3.92, 0.862	242.5, 0.711
Q9	4.00, 0.798	3.79, 0.738	269.5, 0.276	3.82, 0.728	3.91, 0.793	261.5, 0.547	3.90, 0.800	3.80, 0.632	185.0, 0.603	4.00, 0.679	3.84, 0.800	234.0, 0.563
Q10	4.13, 0.757	4.14, 0.756	319.5, 0.958	4.24, 0.562	4.09, 0.830	272.0, 0.705	4.17, 0.771	4.00, 0.667	171.0, 0.368	4.07, 0.616	4.16, 0.800	229.0, 0.480
Q11	4.17, 0.650	3.89, 0.916	271.0, 0.299	4.00, 0.707	4.03, 0.870	273.5, 0.739	4.05, 0.835	3.90, 0.738	178.0, 0.491	3.71, 0.681	4.14, 0.787	186.0, 0.097
Q12	4.22, 0.600	3.96, 0.999	293.0, 0.537	4.00, 0.935	4.12, 0.808	271.5, 0.694	4.10, 0.889	4.00, 0.667	176.0, 0.439	3.86, 0.770	4.16, 0.866	194.5, 0.126

*2 tailed p value significance < 0.05; U: Mann Whitney U test statistics

[a]Feedback Questions: Q1:The waiting period for the consultation was satisfactory, Q2: Sufficient explanation was provided regarding the process,Q3: My privacy and confidentiality was respected, Q4: I was able to see clearly, Q5: I was able to hear clearly, Q6:I was able to express myself adequately using this mode of assessment, Q7: I felt comfortable discussing my problems using this mode of assessment, Q8: The assessment addressed my needs, Q9: The recommendations made were useful, Q10: I am satisfied with the consultation, Q11: I would prefer to use it again, Q12.I would recommend it to others

Table 5 Feedback for tele-psychiatry consults in 2012 from clinicians/nurses and psychiatrists

Clinicians/Nurses (N = 59)

Feedback Question	Mean ± SD	Satisfied[a] % (n)	Unsure[b] % (n)	Dissatisfied[c] % (n)
The waiting period of the consultation was satisfactory (ie, from the time of referral to consultation)	4.53 ± 0.68	93.2 (55)	5.1 (3)	1.7 (1)
The process of referral was convenient	4.36 ± 0.78	88.1 (52)	8.5 (5)	3.4 (2)
Adequate privacy and confidentiality was provided during the consultation	4.58 ± 0.91	93.2 (55)	1.7 (1)	5.1 (3)
The video was clear	4.56 ± 0.90	93.2 (55)	1.7 (1)	5.1 (3)
The audio was clear	4.71 ± 0.53	96.6 (57)	3.4 (2)	0 (0)
I felt comfortable participating in the Telemed assessment process	4.68 ± 0.54	96.6 (57)	3.4 (2)	0 (0)
The assessment confirmed to our desired outcomes as mentioned on the referral	4.54 ± 0.65	91.5 (54)	8.5 (5)	0 (0)
The recommendation for management was useful	4.51 ± .65	91.5 (54)	8.5 (5)	0 (0)
I am satisfied with the consultation	4.63 ± 0.52	98.3 (58)	1.7 (1)	0 (0)
I would use it again	4.71 ± 0.46	100 (59)	0 (0)	0 (0)
I would recommend it to others	4.73 ± 0.45	100 (59)	0 (0)	0 (0)

Psychiatrist (N = 80)

Feedback Question	Mean ± SD	Satisfied[a] % (n)	Unsure[b] % (n)	Dissatisfied[c] (n)
I was able to fit the referral in my existing time schedule	4.13 ± 0.88	86.7 (72)	3.6 (3)	9.6 (8)
The referral had adequate information	4.19 ± 0.96	83.1 (69)	8.4 (7)	8.4 (7)
Adequate privacy and confidentiality was provided	4.08 ± 0.94	81.9 (68)	7.2 (6)	10.8 (9)
The video was clear	4.24 ± 1.07	85.5 (71)	3.6 (3)	10.8 (9)
The audio was clear	4.25 ± 1.03	72 (86.7)	3.6 (3)	9.6 (8)
I felt comfortable participating in the Tele-med assessment process	3.78 ± 1.12	66.2 (54)	16.9 (14)	16.9 (14)
The time was sufficient to do the assessment and make recommendation	4.36 ± 0.77	94.0 (78)	3.6 (3)	2.4 (2)
The recommendations can be followed up in the community	4.04 ± 0.99	79.5 (66)	10.8 (9)	9.6 (8)
It was a useful adjunct to my routine work	4.25 ± 0.88	85.6 (71)	10.8 (9)	3.6 (3)
I preferred it to face to face consultation	3.67 ± 1.39	55.4 (46)	15.7 (13)	28.9 (24)
I would encourage its use	4.45 ± 0.80	92.7 (77)	4.8 (4)	2.4 (2)

Likert Scale: 1-strongly disagree, 2- disagree, 3-neither agree nor disagree, 4- agree, 5- strongly agree
[a]Satisfied: agree or strongly agree (1,2), [c]Dissatisfied: disagree or strongly disagree (4,5), [b]Unsure: Neither agree nor disagree (3)

Table 6 Themes from feedback comments by consumers, clinicians/referrers and specialists for tele-psychiatry consults in 2012

Themes	Patients		Nurses/Clinicians		Psychiatrist	
	Positive	Negative	Positive	Negative	Positive	Negative
Referral process/information	0	0	Referral process (2)	Referral information requirements (3)	0	Lack of adequate information (2); Difficulty accommodating the referral (2)
Privacy (not sound proof/ external noise/intrusions)	0	0	0	Background noise (2)	0	Background noise (5); Intrusions (1)
Audio-visual	0	Audio visual issues (5)	0	Audio-visual issues (5)	0	Technical issues- audio-visual, (5)
Comfort	Comfortable (3)	Daunting (1)	0	0	0	Cold/uncomfortable (3)
Recommendations	Useful recommendations (1)	0	0	0	0	Deficient community resources (1)
Global	Good/Helpful (14)	Unsure (1)	Helpful (4)	0	Useful (4); Suitable (2)	0
Others	Saved time travelling (4); Staff helpful (2); Treated respectfully (1)	0	Educational (2); Supportive (2); Saved time (1)	Interruption by a Medical emergency (2)	Time saving (3)	Patient related issues-behaviour/ cognition/hearing (10)

disorders to severe mental illnesses apart from dementia. This is in contrast to most other telepsychiatry programs evaluated among older adults, where the most common diagnosis is dementia [6, 7]. Moreover, a high proportion of patients (71.6%) also had 2 or more medical conditions, emphasizing the need for a specialist input in assessment and management of psychiatric disorders. Thus, telepsychiatry can be used to bridge the gap in specialist psychiatry services for older adults resident in rural and remote communities, not only for dementia, but also for other psychiatric disorders.

Telepsychiatry can be a useful means of providing a cohesive management plan with the psychiatrist input as evident by the recommendations for psychosocial interventions. On the other hand, it also allowed evaluation of patients admitted in community general hospitals and severely ill patients in the community who needed urgent intervention such as specialist inpatient transfer or further medical evaluation as evident in the recommendations made (Table 1).

Majority of the patients reside independently in the community, similar to the rates in a psychogeriatric outpatient clinic where only about 14% were in nursing homes [13]. Telepsychiatry in nursing homes is feasible and acceptable [6, 14], however, compared to patients living independently in the community, its use by patients in nursing homes was lower. A community based program expectedly has a different pattern of utilization but one of the factors possibly hampering its use by the nursing home population in this program was the lack of mobile telepsychiatry set-up within the nursing homes linked to the secure video-conferencing system. Patient disabilities make transport to the nearest facility with a secure network challenging. A qualitative evaluation of satisfaction with mental health service delivery among patients with dementia and their care givers found that services within the home setting were less distressing and more empowering than being transported to a clinic which is not only onerous but also worsens the confusion and distress [15]. To improve the reach of a community-based service in nursing homes, or even among the more disabled population in the community, it may help to use compatible mobile video-conferencing units which bring the equipment to their place of residence than having to transport them. Another factor could be the limitation of its use in patients with sensory or cognitive disabilities common in the nursing home population, a point raised by all stakeholders in their feedback comments. It may help to support the assessment by hearing and visual aids in the presence of trained staff to facilitate the process. This would help to improve the access and overcome the challenges to its use among older adults with cognitive or sensory disabilities. Another option for the more disabled populations is to focus the visiting service on this

population and use telepsychiatry for urgent support. This can help with efficient use of resources and maximize the access.

Acutely unwell patients with difficult behaviors formed a small percentage (31.3%) of the assessments (Table 1), similar to another community-based program [7]. Telepsychiatry may not be appropriate for violent, unstable, or impulsive individuals [16], though the most recent guidelines [17] do not discourage its use in acutely disturbed patients. In their feedback comments, psychiatrists mentioned the difficulty engaging with patients with behavioral symptoms or cognitive difficulties (Table 6). The concerns in a in-person consult may be similar where it becomes important to assess non-verbal behaviors and obtain collateral information. In telepsychiatry, these barriers can be overcome by involving the clinicians and patients' family along with improved visual and audio quality.

Feedback on acceptance and satisfaction

Though the population sample used for evaluating the satisfaction was different from the one used for the utilization pattern, the two samples were very similar in their mean age, gender distribution, as well as their primary psychiatric diagnoses. Thus, even though two different samples were used, the two findings tie in together to tell a coherent story.

Patient satisfaction

Mean scores ranging from 3.88–4.41 is suggestive of comparable acceptability to other population groups and specialties [18–20]. The overall satisfaction with the consultation was highly rated. In case of severe dementia, delirium and severe psychotic illness, we received feedback from 5 family members which provides some input on behalf of the patients. Eventhough overall satisfcation was high, patients admitted in community hospitals at the time of telepsychiatry assessment were significantly less satisfied with wait times and visual clarity compared to outpatients and this could be because of subjective differences in needs/expectations or illness severity. A study on an acute inpatient unit showed lower satisfaction across all domains in patients with a psychotic illness compared to those without psychosis [21]. Since inpatient admissions are primarily to safely manage difficult behaviors and acute disturbances, some of which may be psychotic symptoms, this difference may not be unusual. A comparison of inpatient and outpatient community setting has never been done and may need further evaluation.

The feedback response rate among patients (52%) is lower than most other studies (60%) [20]. The feedback response rate was significantly low among inpatients in community hospitals. We postulate that this was possibly because of illness severity and non-availability of a family member as these consults are done as a priority, which may not provide sufficient time to engage the family. Also, administratively, it was challenging to make the feedback forms available in a timely manner given the multiple sites. Our study did not have an alternative if the feedback forms were missed at the end of the consult, for example, if the patient left before providing the feedback.

Satisfaction among clinicians/nurses
The mean score of 4.36–4.74 is similar to some other studies [7, 22]. Telepsychiatry appears to be a well-accepted mode of assisting our clinicians/nurses in their clinical work. As reflected in their comments, telepsychiatry was seen as an important support and an opportunity for enhancing clinical skills (Table 6). Some expressed their displeasure with the referral process, needing much information and referral signed by the GP, which is similar to the experience of the community program at Baycrest [7].

Satisfaction among psychiatrists
Our findings on psychiatrist satisfaction feedback were similar to another study where they were keen to encourage its use in older adults but in some scenarios, they expressed doubts regarding telepsychiatry over an in-person consultation [23].

Psychiatrists expressed a high level of satisfaction with the technical aspects, time available and feasibility of the recommendations in the community. Some of their comments revealed concerns regarding the physical environment (e.g. noise and temperature) and lack of comfort in situations where cognitive or sensory disabilities and behavioural symptoms were prominent (Table 6). This is an important aspect to consider in resource allocation and structuring of services. In severely ill or disabled older adults, telepsychiatry can be used for urgent review and support, but more detailed assessment could be the focus of the visiting service. Given that all psychiatrists were from the same service and there was only one trainee, any comparison within the group was not done.

Technical challenges
The dissatisfaction with the audio among patients (6, 11%) was higher than what is seen among younger adults (less than 5%) [24, 25]. Means scores for satisfaction with the audio were lower among patients compared to other stakeholders (psychiatrists and clinicians/nurses, Tables 3 & 5). Both these observations reflect possible sensorineural deficits among older adults. The psychiatrists and clinicians expressed a sense of discomfort when patients had hearing difficulties. Use of hearing devices or noise cancellation could improve the satisfaction but has never been assessed. Some of the

challenges can be overcome by involving the family and clinicians in the process as observed in another study in a memory clinic [18]. This is a crucial aspect for application of telepsychiatry in this population.

This evaluation was carried out a few year ago and while the data may be old, not much has changed over the years. There have been no further studies published in the field of community based telepsychiatry service models for the elderly. The service under evaluation continues to use the hub and spoke model with the use of telepsychiatry as an adjunct to the visiting service. Data derived from this evaluation has helped the service review its processes and resource allocation. Listening devices were introduced but were perceived to be complex and often not used. With advancing technology, it may be possible to develop better listening devices which could be used with ease. Usability and usefulness of the equipment has been identified as one of the important barriers in adoption of technology in one qualitative study which in turn stresses on the need for innovation [26]. Synchronizing mobile devices to a secure network such that the video and audio quality remains reliable has been a challenge. This is especially so in terms of meeting the confidentiality and privacy requirements of the health system. Given the challenges of incorporating technology in day to day mental health service delivery, especially for elderly with significant cognitive and sensory deficits, the service has reorganized its visiting service as a means of assessment of more disabled population in the community and nursing homes, while telepsychiatry continues to be used for specialist input in cases of less disabled population and for urgent support to the clinicians and nursing home staff. Over the past few years, the use of telemedicine as a means of education and support to the staff in rural and remote has gained momentum through the Extended Community Health Outcomes (ECHO) platform [27] and the current service uses videoconferencing as a means of education and support to the clinicians in the community, though not as part of the formal ECHO platform. Thus, the findings and recommendations remain equally relevant and raise important questions about future direction of community based telepsychiatry services for elderly.

Strengths and limitations
Our study is the only one in Australia evaluating a community-based telepsychiatry program for older adults and only second to the one evaluated at Baycrest, Toronto. The greater area of coverage and population with diverse diagnoses, besides dementia, represents the strength of a community-based service.

However, there are various limitations. Firstly, this is a descriptive study. Secondly, the time frame for feedback evaluation is brief, but the large numbers of consults, make it comparable to other studies. Thirdly, being a single Centre study, the findings may be limited to the service under evaluation and should be generalized with care. Fourthly, the feedback tools used were not standardized or validated. They were adapted from other telepsychiatry surveys and reviewed internally. This was done as there are no standardized feedback surveys in telepsychiatry that could be used across various stakeholders. Fifthly, the results regarding satisfaction were limited by a low response rate from patients and clinicians. This raises questions about the representativeness of our sample. Comparison of the survey responders and non-responders among the patient group did not reveal any significant differences except lower feedback from in-patients. Future studies should incorporate alternative strategies such as mailing the feedback if it is missed or follow up over the phone so as to maximize the feedback. We also do not have a follow up of the telepsychiatry consults to measure the outcomes. Never the less, it does provide a direction for future studies in this area.

Conclusions

In rural and remote areas:

1. A community-based telepsychiatry program can be useful for assessment and input in a broad range of psychiatric disorders among older adults.
2. It is well accepted by various stakeholders and can be a useful means of supporting the community services.
3. Satisfaction among patients admitted in hospital was lower than those seen as outpatients.
4. Sensory disabilities and illness related deficits were a major area of dissatisfaction among all stakeholders even with the use of high speed internet and advanced equipment.

Future directions and recommendations for the use of telepsychiatry among older adults

1. Use of community-based telepsychiatry programs for a broad range of psychiatric disorders can help to close the gap in rural and remote regions and expand the reach of psychiatrist services.
2. Given the limitation with the use of telepsychiatry in patients with disability, telepsychiatry should be used as a means of collaboration with existing community services and support the visiting service to enable efficient use of resources. This seems to concur with previous studies [5] .
3. Further evaluation is needed for difference in satisfaction with the use of telepsychiatry among

inpatients compared to outpatients and implicating factors.
4. More robust research is needed on technological innovations specific to tele-psycho-geriatrics such as using portable devices, hearing or visual aids and background noise cancellation strategies.

Acknowledgements

We acknowledge the support of Elizabeth Davison, Lorraine Hall, and Felicity Green during the data collection and evaluation.

Author's contributions

PD, JA and ES were involved in the initial design of the study. PD and NG worked on data acquisition and analysis. All authors were involved with the preparation of the manuscript. All authors have seen and approved the final version of this article.

Competing interest

Authors have no potential conflict of interest.

Consent for publication

Not applicable.

Author details

[1]Division of Geriatric Psychiatry, Centre for Addiction and Mental Health, Toronto, Canada. [2]Department of Psychiatry, University of Toronto, Toronto, Canada. [3]Departments of Psychiatry, Rural and Remote Mental Health Services, Adelaide, South Australia. [4]Address on submission: Centre for Addiction and Mental Health, 80 Workman Way, 6th floor, Room 6312, Toronto, ON M6J1H4, Canada.

References

1. Barnett K, Mercer SW, Norbury M, Watt G, Wyke S, Guthrie B. Epidemiology of multimorbidity and implications for health care, research, and medical education: a cross-sectional study. Lancet (London, England) 2012 Jul 07; 380(9836):37–43. PubMed PMID: 22579043. Epub 2012/05/15. eng.
2. Sumner CR. Telepsychiatry: challenges in rural aging. The Journal of rural health : official journal of the American Rural Health Association and the National Rural Health Care Association. 2001 Fall;17(4):370–3. PubMed PMID: 12071564 Epub 2002/06/20. eng.
3. Brignell M, Wootton R, Gray L. The application of telemedicine to geriatric medicine. Age Ageing 2007 Jul;36(4):369–374. PubMed PMID: WOS: 000248723500006. English.
4. Jhaveri D, Larkins S, Sabesan S. Telestroke, tele-oncology and teledialysis: a systematic review to analyse the outcomes of active therapies delivered with telemedicine support. J Telemed Telecare 2015 Jun;21(4):181–188. PubMed PMID: 25680389. Epub 2015/02/15. eng.
5. Hilty DM, Ferrer DC, Parish MB, Johnston B, Callahan EJ, Yellowlees PM. The effectiveness of Telemental health: a 2013 review. Telemed e-Health 2013 Jun;19(6):444–454. PubMed PMID: WOS:000319395100004. English.
6. Ramos-Rios R, Mateos R, Lojo D, Conn DK, Patterson T. Telepsychogeriatrics: a new horizon in the care of mental health problems in the elderly. Int

Psychogeriatr 2012 Nov;24(11):1708–1724. PubMed PMID: WOS: 000308857900002. English.

7. Conn DK, Madan R, Lam J, Patterson T, Skirten S. Program evaluation of a telepsychiatry service for older adults connecting a university-affiliated geriatric center to a rural psychogeriatric outreach service in Northwest Ontario, Canada. Int Psychogeriatr 2013 Nov;25(11):1795–1800. PubMed PMID: WOS:000325491400006. English.

8. Molloy DW, Alemayehu E, Roberts R. Reliability of a standardized mini-mental state examination compared with the traditional mini-mental state examination. Am J Psychiatry. 1991 Jan;148(1):102–5. PubMed PMID: 1984692 Epub 1991/01/01. eng.

9. Bakken S, Grullon-Figueroa L, Izquierdo R, Lee NJ, Morin P, Palmas W, et al. Development, validation, and use of English and Spanish versions of the telemedicine satisfaction and usefulness questionnaire. J Am Med Inform Assoc : JAMIA. 2006 Nov-Dec;13(6):660–667. PubMed PMID: 16929036. Pubmed Central PMCID: PMC1656962. Epub 2006/08/25. eng.

10. Yip MP, Chang AM, Chan J, MacKenzie AE. Development of the telemedicine satisfaction questionnaire to evaluate patient satisfaction with telemedicine: a preliminary study. J Telemed Telecare 2003;9(1):46–50. PubMed PMID: 12641893. Epub 2003/03/19. eng.

11. Myers KM, Valentine JM, Melzer SM. Feasibility, acceptability, and sustainability of telepsychiatry for children and adolescents. Psychiatr Serv (Washington, DC). 2007 Nov;58(11):1493–1496. PubMed PMID: 17978264. Epub 2007/11/06. eng.

12. Kavanagh S, Hawker F. The fall and rise of the south Australian telepsychiatry network. J Telemed Telecare 2001;7 Suppl 2:41–43. PubMed PMID: 11747655. Epub 2001/12/19. eng.

13. Holroyd S, Duryee JJ. Characteristics of persons utilizing a geriatric psychiatry outpatient clinic. J Geriatr Psychiatry Neurol 1997 Oct;10(4):136–141. PubMed PMID: 9453678. Epub 1998/02/07. eng.

14. Rabinowitz T, Murphy KM, Amour JL, Ricci MA, Caputo MP, Newhouse PA. Benefits of a Telepsychiatry consultation Service for Rural Nursing Home Residents. Telemed J e-Health 2010;16(1):34–40. PubMed PMID: WOS: 000274181600007. English.

15. Gibson G, Timlin A, Curran S, Wattis J. The impact of location on satisfaction with dementia services amongst people with dementia and their informal carers: a comparative evaluation of a community-based and a clinic-based memory service. International psychogeriatrics / IPA 2007 Apr;19(2):267–277. PubMed PMID: 16973102. Epub 2006/09/16. eng.

16. Gilles Pineau KM, St-Hilaire C, Perreault R, Levac É, Hamel B. Telehealth: Clinical Guidelines andTechnological Standards for Telepsychiatry. Montreal. 2006.

17. RANZCP. Professional Practice standards and guides for telepsychiatry: RANZCP; 2013 [updated 2013]. Available from: https://www.ranzcp.org/Files/Resources/RANZCP-Professional-Practice-Standards-and-Guides.aspx.

18. Morgan DG, Crossley M, Kirk A, McBain L, Stewart NJ, D'Arcy C, et al. Evaluation of telehealth for Preclinic assessment and follow-up in an Interprofessional rural and remote memory clinic. J Appl Gerontol 2011 Jun; 30(3):304–331. PubMed PMID: WOS:000290100600004. English.

19. Urness D, Wass M, Gordon A, Tian E, Bulger T. Client acceptability and quality of life - telepsychiatry compared to in-person consultation. J Telemed Telecare 2006;12(5):251–254. PubMed PMID: WOS: 000239690600007. English.

20. Williams TL, May CR, Esmail A. Limitations of patient satisfaction studies in telehealthcare: a systematic review of the literature. Telemed J e-Health. 2001 Win;7(4):293–316. PubMed PMID: WOS:000174083300005. English.

21. Grady B, Singleton M. Telepsychiatry "coverage" to a rural inpatient psychiatric unit. Telemedicine journal and e-health : the official journal of the American Telemedicine Association 2011 Oct;17(8):603–608. PubMed PMID: 21939381. Epub 2011/09/24. eng.

22. Hilty DM, Yellowlees PM, Nesbitt TS. Evolution of telepsychiatry to rural sites: changes over time in types of referral and in primary care providers' knowledge, skills and satisfaction. Gen Hosp Psych 2006 Sep-Oct;28(5):367–373. PubMed PMID: WOS:000240693500001. English.

23. Modai I, Jabarin M, Kurs R, Barak P, Hanan I, Kitain L. Cost effectiveness, safety, and satisfaction with video telepsychiatry versus face-to-face care in ambulatory settings. Telemed J E Health 2006 Oct;12(5):515–520. PubMed PMID: 17042703.

24. Mucic D. International telepsychiatry: a study of patient acceptability. J Telemed Telecare 2008;14(5):241–243. PubMed PMID: 18632998.

25. Simpson J, Doze S, Urness D, Hailey D, Jacobs P. Telepsychiatry as a routine service--the perspective of the patient. J Telemed Telecare 2001;7(3):155–160. PubMed PMID: 11346475. Epub 2001/05/11. eng.

26. Cook EJ, Randhawa G, Sharp C, Ali N, Guppy A, Barton G, et al. Exploring the factors that influence the decision to adopt and engage with an integrated assistive telehealth and telecare service in Cambridgeshire, UK: a nested qualitative study of patient 'users' and 'non-users'. BMC Health Serv Res 2016 Apr 19;16:137. PubMed PMID: 27095102. Pubmed Central PMCID: PMC4837551. Epub 2016/04/21. eng.

27. Komaromy M, Duhigg D, Metcalf A, Carlson C, Kalishman S, Hayes L, et al. Project ECHO (extension for community healthcare outcomes): a new model for educating primary care providers about treatment of substance use disorders. Subst Abus 2016;37(1):20–24. PubMed PMID: 26848803. Pubmed Central PMCID: PMC4873719. Epub 2016/02/06. eng.

8

Extending research on Emotion Regulation Individual Therapy for Adolescents (ERITA) with nonsuicidal self-injury disorder: open pilot trial and mediation analysis of a novel online version

Johan Bjureberg[1]* [iD], Hanna Sahlin[1], Erik Hedman-Lagerlöf[2], Kim L. Gratz[3], Matthew T. Tull[3], Jussi Jokinen[1,4], Clara Hellner[1] and Brjánn Ljótsson[1,2]

Abstract

Background: Nonsuicidal self-injury (NSSI) is common among adolescents and associated with negative outcomes. However, treatments developed specifically for NSSI and the proposed NSSI disorder (NSSID) are scarce, and access to empirically supported treatments for NSSI in many areas is limited. Online treatments carry the potential to increase the availability of evidence-based treatments. Emotion regulation individual therapy for adolescents (ERITA) has shown promise in the treatment of adolescents with NSSID.

Method: The present study examined the feasibility, acceptability, and utility of an online version of ERITA. Twenty-five adolescents (aged 13–17) with NSSID and their parents were included in an uncontrolled open trial. Self-report and clinician-rated assessments of outcomes such as NSSI, self-destructive behaviors, emotion dysregulation, and global functioning were administered at pre-treatment, post-treatment, 3- and 6- month follow-up. Measures of NSSI, self-destructive behaviors, and emotion dysregulation were also assessed weekly during treatment.

Results: Ratings of treatment credibility, expectancy, and satisfaction were acceptable, and the therapeutic alliance and treatment completion rate (96%) were high. Adolescent participation in the treatment was associated with a statistically significant increase in past-month NSSI abstinence ($p = .007$), large-sized improvements in past-month NSSI frequency (55% reduction, 95% confidence interval [CI]: 29, 72; Cohen's $d = 0.88$, 95% CI: 0.73, 1.06) and global functioning ($d = 1.01$, 95% CI: 0.77, 1.32), and medium-sized improvements in emotion dysregulation ($d = 0.75$, 95% CI: 0.59, 0.90) and NSSI versatility ($d = 0.63$, 95% CI: 0.54, 0.77) from pre- to post-treatment. These improvements were further strengthened at 3-month follow-up and maintained at 6-month follow-up. The online therapist-guided parent program was associated with small- to large-sized ($ds = 0.47–1.22$) improvements in adaptive parent behaviors, and these improvements were maintained or further improved upon at 6-month follow-up. Moreover, in line with the theoretical model underlying ERITA, change in emotion dysregulation mediated changes in both NSSI frequency and self-destructive behaviors over the course of treatment.

Conclusions: Together, results suggest that online ERITA is an acceptable, feasible, and promising low-intensity treatment for adolescents with NSSID. The results of this open trial must be replicated in controlled studies.

(Continued on next page)

* Correspondence: Johan.Bjureberg@ki.se
[1]Centre for Psychiatry Research, Department of Clinical Neuroscience, Karolinska Institutet, & Stockholm Health Care Services, Stockholm County Council, Norra stationsgatan 69, SE-11364 Stockholm, Sweden
Full list of author information is available at the end of the article

(Continued from previous page)

Keywords: Nonsuicidal self-injury disorder, Self-injurious behavior, Emotion regulation individual therapy, Emotion regulation, Online treatment, Internet-based treatment

Background

Nonsuicidal self-injury (NSSI) is defined as the deliberate self-inflicted destruction of body tissue without suicidal intent and for purposes not socially sanctioned [1]. NSSI disorder (NSSID) was introduced in the most recent version of the Diagnostic and Statistical Manual of Mental Disorders (DSM-5 [2]) as a disorder for further study. NSSID has a prevalence of 3.1 to 6.7% in adolescent community samples [3, 4], and both NSSI and NSSID have been associated with a variety of negative outcomes, including general psychopathology and suicide attempts [5, 6]. Despite the potentially severe consequences of NSSI and NSSID, there are few publications on interventions specifically designed to treat NSSI [7–10]. Moreover, although a recent review of treatments for suicidal and nonsuicidal self-injurious behaviors among adolescents [9] identified three treatments as promising (including dialectical behavior therapy [11, 12], mentalization-based treatment [13], and cognitive behavior therapy [CBT; [14, 15]), the authors concluded that no treatment for NSSI in adolescents (when analyzed separately from suicide attempts) is superior to treatment as usual.

To address the relative lack of effective treatments for youth with NSSI, we developed emotion regulation individual therapy for adolescents (ERITA [16]). ERITA is a 12-week, acceptance-based behavioral individual therapy adapted from emotion regulation group therapy (ERGT) for NSSI in adults [17, 18]. Similar to ERGT, ERITA was developed specifically to decrease NSSI among adolescents by improving emotion regulation skills. In the initial pilot study of ERITA, this treatment was delivered to adolescents in a traditional face-to-face format. The parents also participated in a parallel online parent program developed to increase their ability to interact effectively with their adolescents to decrease their child's NSSI. The utility, acceptability, and feasibility of face-to-face ERITA for NSSID was supported in the open pilot trial including 17 adolescents (aged 13–17 years) and their parents [16]. Participants rated the treatment as credible, and both the treatment completion rate (88%) and treatment attendance were high. Intent-to-treat analyses revealed large-sized uncontrolled effects from pre- to post-treatment in past-month NSSI frequency, emotion dysregulation, self-destructive behaviors, and global functioning, as well as a medium-sized effect in past-month NSSI versatility. All of these improvements were either maintained or further improved upon at 6-month follow-up. Moreover, change in emotion dysregulation mediated the observed improvements in NSSI during treatment, providing preliminary support for the theoretical model underlying ERITA [16].

ERITA was developed to provide a targeted and effective intervention that could be easily and widely implemented at a low cost. However, Internet-delivered CBT (ICBT) has the potential to further increase accessibility to evidence-based treatments by eliminating the effects of geographical distances between patients and providers, allowing for less therapist time per patient, and facilitating flexible scheduling at times that are convenient for families [19]. Therapist-guided ICBT has been shown to be effective for several psychiatric and physical disorders in adolescents (for a review, see [20]). There is also research indicating that ICBT is at least as efficacious as face-to-face CBT for a range of psychiatric disorders in adults [21]. Further, given research indicating that individuals with stigmatizing illnesses are more likely to use the Internet than traditional health care services to seek help [22], online treatment may be particularly suitable for the treatment of NSSI, given its association with shame [23] and low levels of disclosure [24]. Nonetheless, although there have been some efforts to develop web-based interventions for suicidal behaviors (e.g. [25]), online interventions have not (to our knowledge) been evaluated specifically for individuals who engage in NSSI.

Thus, given both evidence for the utility and feasibility of ERITA delivered face-to-face and the advantages of the ICBT format, we adapted ERITA to an online intervention. Following recommendations for early research on novel interventions [26, 27], the present pilot study examined the feasibility, acceptability, and utility of this online ERITA in an uncontrolled open pilot trial. We expected high levels of treatment module completion, low treatment attrition, and high treatment credibility and satisfaction. Further, we expected to find significant improvements from pre- to post-treatment in adolescent NSSI, emotion regulation difficulties, psychological inflexibility, global functioning, and symptoms of borderline personality disorder (BPD), as well as parents' ability to respond effectively to their children's negative emotions. We also anticipated that these improvements would be maintained or further improved upon at 3- and 6-month follow up periods. Finally, we hypothesized that change in emotion dysregulation would mediate improvements in NSSI and self-destructive behaviors during treatment.

Method

Design

This study employed an uncontrolled open trial design evaluating online ERITA for NSSID among adolescent participants in Stockholm, Sweden. Participants were either self-referred or referred from child and adolescent mental health services (CAMHS). Referring clinics received information about the trial through written information distributed via emails and the Stockholm County Council's internal website. Self-referred participants were recruited through advertisements in the local newspaper and through information posted on social media and the Swedish National Self-Injury Project's website. The adolescent treatment included 11 online modules adapted from the ERITA manual [16]. As in the previous ERITA trial [16], parents were enrolled in a parent program also delivered via the Internet. Demographic, diagnostic, and baseline data were collected through self-report measures and via interviews conducted by licensed psychologists. Self-report measures were also administered weekly beginning 2 weeks prior to treatment and continuing throughout treatment. Post-treatment and follow-up assessments were administered directly after treatment completion (i.e., 11 weeks after treatment start) and at 3 and 6 months post-treatment completion. These included both clinician administered interviews and self-report measures. The self-report measures used in the study were administered online which has been shown to be a reliable and valid method [28].

The study was registered on Clinicaltrials.gov (Identifier NCT02697019), and the TREND Statement guidelines for nonrandomized interventions [29] were followed when reporting the trial.

Participants

A total of 60 families were screened by telephone for eligibility between March 2016 and March 2017. Thirty-six of these families were assessed face-to-face, and 25 met inclusion criteria. Of these, 19 (76%) were self-referred and six (24%) were referred from CAMHS. The inclusion criteria for the adolescents were: (a) 13–17 years of age; (b) meeting diagnostic criteria for NSSID [2]; (c) having engaged in ≥1 NSSI episode during the past month; (d) having at least one parent who committed to participate in the parent program; and (e) stability of psychotropic medications (if any) for at least 2 months. Exclusion criteria for the adolescents were: (f) severe suicidal ideation; (g) a diagnosis of psychotic or bipolar I disorder or ongoing (past month) substance dependence; (h) ongoing dialectical behavioral therapy or mentalization-based treatment; and (i) insufficient understanding of the Swedish language. Of the enrolled participants, 92% met diagnostic criteria for at least one psychiatric disorder other than NSSID, and the median length of previous

psychological treatment was 9 months. Demographic and diagnostic data are described in Table 1, and participant flow through the trial is presented in Fig. 1.

Measures

Diagnostic assessments

A full diagnostic interview was conducted using the MINI-KID International Neuropsychiatric Interview, version 6 [30]. The Clinician-Administered Nonsuicidal Self-Injury Disorder Index [31] was used to determine if participants met criteria for NSSID, and the Structured Clinical Interview for DSM-IV Personality Disorders BPD Module [32] was used to assess diagnostic criteria for BPD.

Adolescent-rated outcome measures

Acceptability measures Perceived credibility and expectancy of the treatment was measured using the Credibility/Expectancy Scales [33]. Higher scores indicate greater credibility (range 1–9) and expectancy (range 0–100%). Evidence for the reliability and predictive validity of this measure has been provided [34]. This measure was administered after the first treatment module. Satisfaction with the treatment was measured using the self-report measure, Client Satisfaction Questionnaire – 8 item version [35]. Scores on this measure range from 8 and 32, with higher scores indicating greater treatment satisfaction. Internal consistency of this measure in the adolescent sample was excellent ($\alpha = .92$). Aspects of therapeutic alliance were measured using the 12-item version of the Working Alliance Inventory – Revised Short Version [36], which has demonstrated sound psychometric properties [36]. Scores range between 12 and 84, with higher scores indicating better therapeutic alliance. This measure was administered after the third treatment module, and internal consistency in the present sample was excellent ($\alpha = .95$). At the post-treatment assessment, participants completed a self-report measure of the occurrence of any potential adverse events associated with the online intervention.

Primary outcome measure The primary outcome of NSSI frequency was measured using the 9-item Deliberate Self Harm Inventory (DSHI-9 [37]). The DSHI-9 assesses the presence and frequency of the most common forms of NSSI, including cutting, burning, severe scratching, self-biting, carving, sticking sharp objects into the skin, self-punching, and head banging. For this study (and consistent with the pilot study on ERITA [16]), the item assessing presence and frequency of preventing wounds from healing was not included, as this behavior is considered to be relatively normative and a less severe form of self-injury. Evidence for the test-retest reliability and concurrent validity of the DSHI-9 has been provided among

Table 1 Sociodemographic, clinical, and diagnostic data of the sample (N = 25)

Age (years)	M (SD)	15.7 (1.3)	
	Min-max	13.4–17.7	
Gender	Female	19	76%
	Male	1	4%
	Other (non-binary)	5	20%
Country of birth	Sweden	24	96%
	Other European country	1	4%
Gender of treatment responsible parent	Female	22	88%
	Male	3	12%
Treatment responsible parent's educational level	Primary	1	4%
	Secondary	7	28%
	University	17	68%
Ongoing psychotropic medication	Yes	8	32%
Earlier psychological treatments	Yes	15	60%
	Mean length in months (SD)	11.9 (16.4)	
Meeting full diagnostic criteria for BPD	Yes	5	20%
Mean number of BPD criteria		3.2 (1.6)	
Adolescent's report on age of NSSI onset	M (SD)	13.3 (1.3)	
Parent's report on age of their child's NSSI onset	M (SD)	14.1 (1.6)	
NSSI frequency past 12 months	Median	103	
	IQR	25–197	
Frequency of co-occurring disorders	Depression	13	52%
	Panic disorder	9	36%
	ADHD	3	12%
	Social anxiety disorder	13	52%
	Separation anxiety	1	4%
	Specific phobia	2	8%
	Bulimia nervosa	1	4%
	GAD	7	28%
	BDD	5	20%
Number of participants with 0 - ≥5 co-occurring disorders	None	2	8%
	One	3	12%
	Two	9	36%
	Three	5	20%
	Four	2	8%
	≥Five	5	16%

Note. ADHD Attention deficit hyperactivity disorder, BDD Body dysmorphic disorder, BPD Borderline personality, GAD Generalized anxiety disorder, IQR Interquartile range, NSSI Nonsuicidal self-injury

adolescents [37]. The DSHI-9 was also used to assess past month NSSI versatility (i.e., the number of different types of NSSI behaviors), which has been shown to be a marker of NSSI severity [38]. The DSHI-9 was administered at pre-treatment, post-treatment, and 3- and 6-month follow-up to assess past month engagement in NSSI. The DSHI-9 was also administered weekly during treatment to measure past week engagement in NSSI.

Secondary outcome measures Participants' emotion regulation difficulties were assessed using the 36-item Difficulties in Emotion Regulation Scale (DERS [39]). Scores on this scale range from 36 to 180, with higher scores indicating greater difficulties in emotion regulation. The DERS has demonstrated good reliability and construct and convergent validity in adolescents [40]. The DERS was administered at pre-treatment, post-treatment, and 3- and 6-month follow-up. Internal consistency in this sample was excellent ($\alpha = .90$). Emotion regulation difficulties were also measured weekly during treatment using the 16-item version of the DERS, the DERS-16 [41]. Scores on this scale range from 16 to 80, with higher scores indicating greater emotion regulation difficulties. The DERS-16 has been found to demonstrate good test-retest reliability and construct and predictive validity among adults [41–43]. Internal consistency in this sample was good ($\alpha = .89$).

Past week engagement in a variety of risky, self-destructive behaviors (e.g., risky sexual behavior, binge eating, substance misuse) was measured using the 11-item behavior supplement to the Borderline Symptom List (BSL [44]). Scores on this measure range from 0 to 55. The BSL-supplement was administered weekly during treatment. BPD features were measured using the Borderline Personality Feature Scale for Children (BPFS-C [45]). The BPFS-C is a 24–item self-report measure with scores ranging from 24 to 120; higher scores indicate greater BPD features. The BPFS-C has demonstrated adequate construct validity among youth [45]. The BPFSC was administered at pre-treatment, post-treatment, and 3- and 6-month follow-up. Internal consistency in this sample was good ($\alpha = .84$). Finally, psychological inflexibility was measured using the 7-item Acceptance and Action Questionnaire (AAQ-II [46]). Scores on the AAQ-II range from 7 to 49, with higher scores indicating less psychological flexibility. Evidence has been provided for the test-retest reliability and concurrent, predictive, and discriminant validity of this measure [46]. The AAQ-II was administered at pre-treatment, post-treatment, and 3- and 6-month follow-up. Internal consistency in the present sample was excellent ($\alpha = .90$).

Clinician-rated outcome measure Global functioning was assessed using the Children's Global Assessment Scale (CGAS [47]). Scores on this measure range from 0 to 100, with higher scores indicating better functioning.

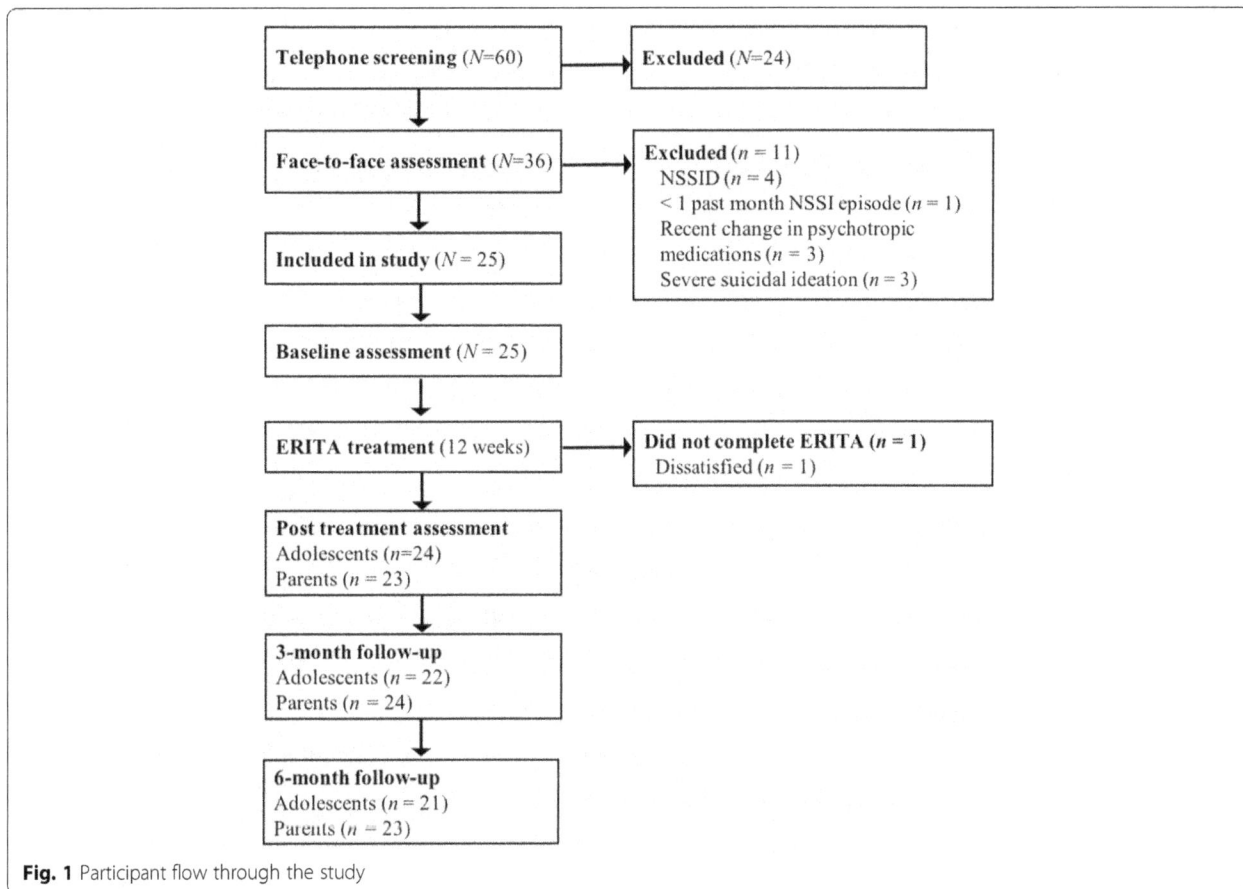

Fig. 1 Participant flow through the study

Evidence for moderate to excellent inter-rater reliability, good stability over time, and good concurrent and discriminant validity has been provided [47, 48]. The CGAS was administered at pre-treatment, post-treatment, and 3- and 6-month follow-up.

Parent-rated outcome measures

Parents' perceived ability to cope with and respond effectively to their children's negative emotions was assessed with the Coping with Children's Negative Emotions Scale – Adolescent version (CCNES-A [49]). Parents rate 36 items on a seven-point Likert type scale ranging from 1 (very unlikely) to 7 (very likely). The CCNES-A version used in this study consists of nine hypothetical scenarios accompanied by four types of responses. The responses assessed for each scenario include distress reactions, punitive reactions, and minimization reactions (for which lower scores indicate more effective responses) and expressive encouragement (for which higher scores indicate more effective responses). The CCNES has demonstrated good test-retest reliability and construct validity [50]. Internal consistency in this sample was adequate for each dimension (αs = .68–.80).

Treatment

ERITA is an individual therapy for adolescents that was adapted from the original ERGT manual used in several trials of adult women with NSSI [17, 18, 51, 52]. The utility of ERITA as a face-to-face treatment was examined in a previous study, and a detailed description of the treatment is available in that article [16]. In the present study, some modifications were made to both the adolescent treatment and the parent program in response to therapist and participant feedback from the previous study. Specifically, modifications to the adolescent treatment included: (1) combining the four sessions on emotional acceptance, awareness, and clarity into two modules; (2) combining the two sessions on emotional unwillingness and willingness into one module; (3) moving information on valued directions and actions to the first module (vs. the end of treatment) to provide a rationale for approaching emotions early in treatment; and (4) incorporating a greater emphasis on the practice of emotional approach strategies throughout treatment. Table 2 provides an overview of the structure and specific topics addressed in the 11 treatment modules. The modifications to the parent program aimed to increase the emphasis on emotional awareness and validation by replacing the conflict management and problem solving

Table 2 An overview of the content of the online ERITA

Adolescent treatment (Module) Content	Parent program (Module) Content
(1) Functions of NSSI and valued directions	(1) Psychoeducation
(2) Impulse control	(2) Emotional awareness
(3) Functionality of emotions and emotional awareness	(3) Validation and invalidation
(4) Primary vs. secondary emotions	(4) Self-validation and self- invalidation
(5) Emotional avoidance / unwillingness vs. emotional acceptance / willingness	(5) How to improve parenting in the long run / behavioral activation
(6) Emotional willingness / approach	(6) Summary and evaluation
(7) Emotional willingness / approach	
(8) Non-avoidant emotion regulation strategies	
(9) Validation and emotional approach	
(10) Repetition	
(11) Relapse prevention	

session with one module on the function and awareness of emotions and two modules on validation and invalidation [53]; An outline of the structure and topics addressed in the parent program is available in Table 2.

The treatment platform was completely web-based and designed with age-appropriate appearance, animations, and interactive scripts (see Additional file 1: Figure A.1–3). It has previously been tested in several online treatments for a range of mental and medical disorders (e.g., [54–56]). The treatment includes educational texts, animated films, illustrations, case examples, and interactive exercises. For this study, a mobile app was developed to complement the adolescent online treatment. This app provided the adolescents with the opportunity to report on both self-destructive behaviors and impulses to engage in these behaviors on a daily basis. If the participant had neither engaged in a self-destructive behavior nor experienced impulses to do so, they were instructed to report on potential protective factors. Furthermore, the mobile app (see Additional file 1: Figure A. 4) included reminders of homework assignments and several built-in programs providing assistance in the skills acquired in the online treatment (e.g., impulse control strategies, emotional awareness and clarity, and distraction and approach strategies). Moreover, the individualized crisis plan (see "Participant safety") could easily be accessed through the app.

During the 12-week treatment period, both adolescents and parents had online contact with an assigned clinical psychologist. The adolescents completed one

module every week (i.e., they had one extra week to complete the 11 modules) and the parents completed a module every other week. The psychologist reviewed the participants' responses and provided written feedback through the platform. In the case of participant inactivity, the psychologist reminded the participant through text messages or telephone calls. Further, the psychologist helped problem solve, guide participants through the program, and assist with the homework assignments when necessary. The amount of therapist time spent with each adolescent and parent was measured.

Participant safety

In order to ensure participant safety and facilitate detection of sudden deterioration, participants were instructed to complete online weekly assessments of NSSI and suicidal ideation. An individualized crisis plan was established prior to treatment start, which contained necessary contact information to acute health care services. If increased suicidality was observed, the adolescent and/or parent were immediately contacted.

Statistical analysis

Statistical analyses were conducted using R version 3.3.1 [57]. Generalized estimation equations (GEE) with exchangeable working correlation structure along with robust error estimations were used to model change in outcome measures across the treatment and follow up periods (from pre-treatment to post-treatment to 3- and 6-month follow-up), as well as for the weekly measures administered before and during treatment. The GEE models for the count variables (i.e., NSSI frequency and self-destructive behaviors) used a negative binomial distribution with a log link function, and the remaining outcomes were analyzed using GEE models with a normal distribution.

Consistent with the use of an intent-to-treat sample, all models included all available data for each outcome. We estimated separate coefficients for the change from pre- to post-treatment, post-treatment to 3-month follow-up, 3-month follow-up to 6-month follow-up, and pre-treatment to 6-month follow-up. We included regression weights in the GEE models that were inversely related to the probability of a value being observed as a function of time (which gives unbiased estimation under the assumption of data missing at random [58, 59]. Ordinal variables were analyzed using Wilcoxon signed ranks test. Effect sizes were calculated for changes between all assessment points. The average percentage change across time for the count variables (i.e., NSSI frequency and BSL) was calculated from the GEE models with 95% confidence intervals. The effect size Cohen's d was calculated for the remaining continuous outcomes by dividing the estimated means derived from the GEE models by the baseline standard deviation. For comparative reasons (with previous studies), Cohen's d was also calculated for the count data based on log-transformed NSSI frequency and BSL scores (these analyses were used only for effect size estimation, and not to draw inferences about statistical significance or percentage change). The 95% confidence intervals for effect sizes were calculated using 5000 bootstrap replications [60] clustered on participants [61]. Finally, we calculated the number of participants who reported no (zero) NSSI episodes at pre-treatment, post-treatment, and 3- and 6-month follow-up and used McNemar's mid-p test [62] to analyze the changes between the assessment points (list-wise deletion was used in these specific analyses when data were missing).

We also examined change in emotion regulation difficulties as a mediator of improvements in NSSI and self-destructive behaviors during treatment in two sets of mediation analyses (with NSSI and self-destructive behaviors coded as the dependent variable in the first and second analysis, respectively). In both sets, two regression equations were estimated [63]. First, the relationship between the independent variable (i.e., time in treatment) and the dependent variable (i.e., c-path) was examined to see if time in treatment was associated with frequency of NSSI or self-destructive behaviors. Second, the association between the independent variable and the mediator (i.e., a-path) was investigated to test if emotion regulation difficulties decreased as a function of week in treatment. Second, the relationship between the mediator and the dependent variable (i.e., b-path) was examined to see if emotion regulation difficulties were associated with NSSI or self-destructive behavior frequency (controlling for time in treatment). The first and third regression equations used a negative binomial distribution with a log link function [64], and the second equation used a normal distribution. The indirect relations of time in treatment to improvements in the dependent variables through improvements in emotion regulation difficulties were calculated as the product of the a- and b-path estimates, denoted ab. A 95% confidence interval (CI) was obtained by 5000 bootstrap replications using the bias-corrected and accelerated method around the ab-product, and the criterion for mediation was that the CI for ab did not contain zero [65].

Results

Feasibility: Treatment completion rates and attrition

Of the 25 participants who started treatment, only one (4%) dropped out of treatment (after the second module, see Fig. 1). The average number of completed treatment modules was 9.7 ($SD = 2.1$; median = 11) out of 11 modules for all included adolescent participants, and 5.2 ($SD = 1.6$; median = 6) out of six modules for the parents. All enrolled adolescents and 24 parents (96%) completed at least one follow-up assessment (see Fig. 1). Mean therapist time for the whole treatment (including reading patient exercises

and written feedback) was 309.6 min ($SD = 133.1$) per family (the adolescent and parent), with an average of 238.5 ($SD = 115.4$) and 93.9 ($SD = 44.2$) minutes for the adolescents and parents, respectively. The therapist had additional contact outside of the platform with five of the participants (20%) and their parents through phone calls ($M = 37$ min; $SD = 13.6$ min). At post-treatment, ten participants (40%) reported having some form of treatment contact (e.g., a social worker, psychologist, or medical doctor) while engaged in the online ERITA. However, five of these reported that they had only met with their treatment provider once or twice a month (with the remaining five reporting they had met with their treatment provider once a week during the course of treatment).

Acceptability: Treatment satisfaction, credibility, and adverse events

Mean ratings of treatment credibility ($M = 6.5$, $SD = 1.1$) and expectancy ($M = 55.6\%$, $SD = 21.4$) completed after the first session were satisfactory and very similar to the face to face ERITA trial [16]. In general, participants also rated their alliance with their therapist as very high ($M = 59.8$, $SD = 15.2$). At post-treatment, mean ratings of treatment satisfaction were acceptable for both adolescents ($M = 17.3$, $SD = 4.6$) and parents ($M = 17.8$; $SD = 3.6$).

Eight adolescents reported experiencing one or more adverse events during the treatment, including increased distress ($n = 7$), lack of time for school homework and other obligations ($n = 3$), and feeling depressed when having difficulties practicing the treatment skills ($n = 1$).

Utility: Outcome analyses

Medians, inter quartile range, means, standard deviations, percentage change, and Cohen's d for the adolescent outcomes are presented in Table 3 and for the parent outcomes in Table 4.

Primary outcomes

There was a significant 55% reduction in NSSI frequency from pre-treatment to post-treatment. Additionally, results revealed a further 52% significant reduction from post-treatment to 3-month follow-up, which was maintained at 6-month follow-up. The overall change in NSSI frequency between pre-treatment and 6-month follow-up was associated with a significant 69% reduction. The observed means for NSSI frequency were 10.0 ($SD = 9.3$), 4.5 ($SD = 4.8$), 2.2 ($SD = 3.2$), and 3.1 ($SD = 4.7$) at pre-treatment, post-treatment, and 3- and 6-month follow-ups, respectively. Effect sizes (Cohen's d) based on log-transformed data on past month NSSI frequency showed a large reduction from pre- to post-treatment ($d = 0.88$, 95% CI: 0.73, 1.06), a medium reduction from post-treatment to 3-month follow-up ($d = 0.57$, 95%

Table 3 Adolescent treatment outcome variables at pre-treatment, post-treatment, 3- and 6-month follow-up

Outcome	Pre-treatment	Post-treatment	3-mo f-u	6-mo f-u	Pre- to post-treatment		Post- to 3-mo f-u		3-mo f-u- to 6-mo f-u		Pre to to 6-mo f-u	
Count- data	Median (IQR)	Median (IQR)	Median (IQR)	Median (IQR)	Z	% change [95% CI]	Z	% change [95% CI]	Z	% change [95% CI]	Z	% change [95% CI]
DSHI-9-f	9 (3–15)	2 (0–8)	0 (0–3)	1 (0–6)	3.43***	55 [29–72]	3.34***	52 [26–69]	−1.35	−44 [− 144–15]	3.95***	69 [45–83]
Continuous	Mean (SD)	Mean (SD)	Mean (SD	Mean (SD)	Z	Cohen's d [95% CI]	Z	Cohen's d [95% CI]	Z	Cohen's d [95% CI]	Z	Cohen's d [95% CI]
DSHI-9-v	2.2 (1.2)	1.4 (1.3)	0.8 (1.0)	0.9 (1.0)	2.33*	0.63 [0.54,0.77]	2.97**	0.54 [0.47,0.66]	−0.36	−0.06 [−0.5,-0.08]	4.73***	1.11 [0.96,1.35]
DERS	125.6 (20.1)	110.6 (27.2)	101.3 (23.3)	99.7 (26.8)	3.14**	0.75 [0.59,0.90]	2.07*	0.39 [0.31,0.47]	0.34	0.06 [0.05,-0.08]	4.40***	1.20 [0.95,1.44]
AAQ	31.4 (9.3)	29.0 (9.8)	27.8 (7.8)	27.6 (9.3)	2.28*	0.27 [0.22,0.31]	0.42	0.06 [0.05,0.07]	0.21	0.03 [0.03,-0.04]	2.07*	0.36 [0.30,0.43]
BPFSC	67.1 (12.9)	67.3 (13.9)	65.0 (14.1)	64.4 (12.2)	0.16	0.02 [0.02,0.03]	1.73	0.18 [0.15,0.20]	0.23	0.03 [0.02,-0.04]	1.51	0.23 [0.19,0.27]
CGAS	52.4 (7.1)	60.0 (9.8)	64.6 (8.3)	63.2 (10.6)	3.79***	1.01 [0.77,1.32]	3.76***	0.53 [0.40,0.70]	0.51	−0.10 [−0.14,-0.08]	4.59***	1.44 [1.09,1.88]

Note. Count data. Test statistics are based on generalized estimation equation models using either a negative binomial or normal distribution for count and continuous data, respectively. Confidence intervals for effect sizes are based on 5000 bootstrap replications

Abbreviations: AAQ acceptance and action questionnaire, BPFSC borderline personality feature scale for children, CGAS Children's Global Assessment Scale, DERS difficulties in emotion regulation scale, DSHI-9-f deliberate self-harm inventory – frequency past month, DSHI-9-v deliberate self-harm inventory – versatility past month

*p < .05; **p < .01; ***p < .001

CI: 0.46, 0.68), and no change from 3- to 6-month follow-up ($d = - 0.09$, 95% CI: -0.10, – 0.07). Finally, between pre-treatment and 6-month follow-up, the overall change in NSSI frequency was associated with a large effect size ($d = 1.36$, 95% CI: 1.12, 1.63). The GEE models revealed a significant, medium-sized reduction in past-month NSSI versatility from pre- to post-treatment, with additional significant improvements in NSSI versatility from post-treatment to 3-month follow-up, and no significant changes from 3- to 6-month follow-up. Finally, the proportion of participants with past month NSSI abstinence increased significantly ($p = .007$) from 0% at pre-treatment to 28% at post-treatment, and remained stable from

post-treatment to 3- and 6-month follow-ups (48 and 40%, respectively).

Secondary outcomes

Results revealed significant medium-sized improvements in emotion regulation difficulties (on the DERS) and large improvements in global functioning (on the CGAS) from pre- to post-treatment, both of which were further improved upon at 3-month follow up and maintained at 6-month follow-up. Likewise, results revealed significant improvements (associated with a small effect size) in psychological flexibility on the AAQ from pre- to

Table 4 Parent treatment outcome variables at pre-treatment, post-treatment, 3- and 6-month follow-up

Outcome	Pre-treatment	Post-treatment	3-mo f-u	6-mo f-u	Pre- to post-treatment		Post- to 3-mo f-u		3-mo f-u- to 6-mo f-u		Pre to 6-mo f-u	
Continuous	Mean (SD)	Mean (SD)	Mean (SD	Mean (SD)	Z	Cohen's d [95% CI]	Z	Cohen's d [95% CI]	Z	Cohen's d [95% CI]	Z	Cohen's d [95% CI]
CCNES-DR	2.0 (0.8)	1.9 (0.8)	1.9 (1.0)	1.9 (1.1)	0.54	0.11 [0.09,0.15]	−0.36	−0.05 [− 0.6,-0.04]	0.30	0.09 [0.07,0.11]	0.54	0.15 [0.12,0.19]
CCNES-PR	1.5 (0.5)	1.3 (0.3)	1.1 (0.2)	1.3 (0.4)	2.27*	0.47 [0.35,0.60]	3.31***	0.34 [0.25,0.43]	−1.84	−0.26 [0.20,0.34]	4.37***	0.55 [0.41,0.70]
CCNES-EE	5.4 (0.9)	5.9 (0.7)	5.8 (1.1)	5.8 (1.0)	3.31***	0.58 [0.49,0.68]	−0.46	−0.10 [0.08,0.11]	0.00	0.0 [0.00,0.00]	2.81**	0.48 [0.41,0.57]
CCNES-MR	2.9 (0.9)	1.8 (0.6)	1.6 (0.6)	1.7 (0.6)	6.54***	1.22 [0.99,1.44]	2.03*	0.21 [0.17,0.25]	−0.24	−0.05 [0.01,0.02]	9.08***	1.39 [1.15,1.67]

Note. Test statistics are based on generalized estimation equation models using normal distribution. Confidence intervals for effect sizes are based on 5000 bootstrap replications

Abbreviations: EE expressive encouragement, DR distress reactions, MR minimization reactions, PR punitive reactions

*p < .05; **p < .01; ***p < .001

post-treatment, which were maintained throughout the follow up period. Notably, however, BPD symptoms did not change significantly during treatment or follow-up.

Weekly measures

Difficulties in emotion regulation (on the DERS-16) decreased significantly throughout treatment ($d = 0.62$; 95% CI: 0.51, 0.75; $p = .002$). Similarly, the GEE analyses revealed that NSSI frequency (on the DSHI-9) and self-destructive behaviors (on the BSL) decreased significantly across treatment, with estimated mean week-to-week reductions of 10.1% (95% CI: 3.8, 15.1; $p = .001$) and 5.2% (95% CI: 1.1, 8.8; $p = .01$), respectively (see Fig. 2).

Parent outcomes

Parents' distress reactions to their children's expression of negative emotions (on the CNNES-DR) did not improve during treatment or follow-up. However, parental punitive reactions to their children's expressions of negative emotions (on the CNNES-PR) decreased significantly from pre- to post-treatment and were further improved upon during follow-up. Parental support and encouragement of children's emotional expressions (on the CCNES-EE) also improved during the treatment period, and these improvements were maintained at the 3- and 6-month follow-ups. Finally, parental minimization of children's negative emotions (on the CCNES-MR) also improved significantly from pre- to post-treatment, with further improvements in this outcome from post-treatment to 3-month follow up (and maintenance of these gains at the 6-month follow-up).

Mediation analysis

The relations between time in treatment and improvements in both NSSI frequency ($c\text{-}path = -0.101$; 95% CI: -0.161, -0.046) and emotion regulation difficulties ($a\text{-}path = -0.657$; 95% CI: -1.056, -0.278) were significant, as was the association between emotion regulation

difficulties and NSSI improvements during treatment, controlling for time in treatment ($b\text{-}path = 0.029$; 95% CI: 0.005, 0.052). Likewise, the indirect relation of time in treatment to NSSI improvement through change in emotion regulation difficulties was significant ($ab = -0.019$; 95% CI: - 0.045, - 0.003). The corresponding GEE analyses for self-destructive behaviors showed a significant $c\text{-}path$ (- 0.052; 95% CI: -0.086, - 0.008), $a\text{-}path$ (- 0.657; 95% CI: -1.056, - 0.278), and a near significant $b\text{-}path$ (0.016; 95% CI: -0.004, 0.031). Finally, the indirect relation of time in treatment to improvement in self-destructive behaviors through change in emotion regulation difficulties was also significant ($ab = 0.011$; 95% CI: 0.025, 0.001).

Discussion

NSSID is common among adolescents and associated with a wide variety of negative outcomes. However, treatments developed specifically for NSSI are scarce, and access to empirically-supported treatments for this behavior is limited [9]. Online treatments carry several advantages compared to traditional face-to-face psychological treatments and may be particularly useful for treating NSSI, as this behavior is associated with high levels of shame and non-disclosure [23, 24]. Support for the feasibility and acceptability of online ERITA was provided by findings of high levels of treatment module completion and low treatment attrition, acceptable ratings of treatment credibility, expectancy, and satisfaction (by adolescents and their parents), as well as strong ratings of therapeutic alliance. Providing initial support for the utility of this online treatment for NSSI, participation in the study was associated with significant, medium- to large-sized improvements in past-month NSSI frequency and versatility, emotion regulation difficulties, and global functioning from pre- to post-treatment. Moreover, all of these improvements were either maintained or further improved upon at 3- and 6-month follow-ups. Not only are

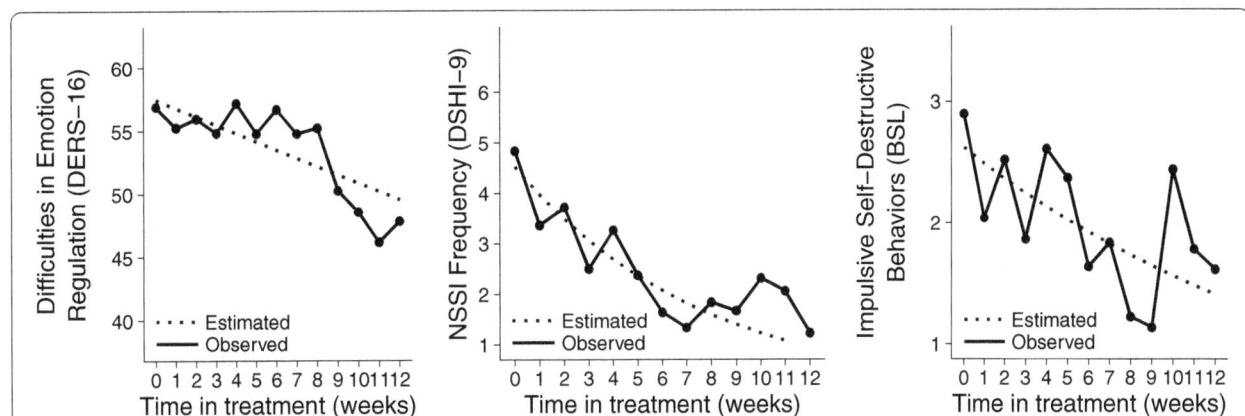

Fig. 2 Observed means and estimated regression lines show a significant decrease in difficulties in emotion regulation ($p = .001$), NSSI frequency ($p < .001$), and other self-destructive behavior ($p = .012$) during the course of treatment

these findings promising and suggestive of the utility of this online treatment, they are comparable to the findings obtained in previous trials of face-to-face versions of ERITA and ERGT [16–18, 51, 52]. Notably, however, the mean therapist time per family in the current study was approximately one third of the time required in brief face-to-face treatments for NSSI (e.g., [16, 66]) and this substantial reduction in therapist time was managed without a related loss in the feasibility, acceptance, or utility of the intervention. Moreover, consistent with past research on ICBT for adults [67], the therapeutic alliance was strong and comparable to the ratings obtained in the face-to-face trial of ERITA [16]. This is notable given that most therapist support was only provided online; although telephone contact was allowed between therapists and participants, this option was not used for most participants. Even so, participant enrollment in the treatment was associated with durable improvements in behavioral problems, emotion regulation difficulties, and global functioning.

The high treatment completion rates and overall positive findings obtained in this study may be due, in part, to some of the advantages of online interventions in general, such as the structured treatment format, lesser impact of therapist drift, lack of a need to schedule appointments, and greater access to the treatment material. It may also reflect the particular utility of the method of communication inherent to online treatment for individuals with stigmatizing behaviors (e.g., secure self-disclosure [68]). In order to further develop and refine online treatments, future research should include qualitative interviews exploring the experience of participating in online treatments for NSSI.

Despite the positive results found in many domains, only small non-significant improvements were found in BPD symptoms at follow-up. These findings suggest that this brief treatment may not be sufficient to address BPD symptoms beyond emotion dysregulation, NSSI, and other self- destructive behaviors, and that this online treatment may be needed to be incorporated into an overall treatment approach for individuals with BPD for long term remission. However, only 20% of the participants in the present sample met diagnostic criteria for BPD at baseline; thus, replication in larger samples, including larger proportions of adolescents with BPD, is needed before any conclusions regarding the treatment's utility for BPD symptoms can be drawn.

Family support is important in the treatment of adolescents with self-injurious behaviors [69]. Consistent with both expectations and the intended purpose of the parent program, the online ERITA parent program was associated with small- to large-sized improvements in parental punitive and minimizing responses to adolescents' expressions of negative emotions and parental encouragement of their children's emotional expressions.

Given past findings that parental invalidation is associated with higher levels of adolescent externalizing problem behaviors, and parental validation is associated with lower levels of emotion dysregulation [70], these findings may, at least in part, account for some of the observed improvements in adolescent NSSI and emotion dysregulation. Contrary to expectations, however, no improvements were found for parental distress reactions to children's negative emotions. These results suggest that behavioral responses to children's emotions may be more amenable to brief interventions (and easier to change) than emotional reactions, highlighting the utility of teaching parents' adaptive ways of responding to children's distress regardless of their own emotional reactions to that distress. Indeed, even with increased knowledge about the function of and motivations for NSSI, it is reasonable to expect that parents still experience strong emotional reactions to the occurrence of NSSI in their child. However, our findings suggest that, even in the context of high levels of emotional distress, parents can respond behaviorally in an effective manner, possibly due to the emotional awareness and validation skills taught in the parent course. Overall, these findings are encouraging and highlight the utility of further research examining the role of changes in parental behaviors and parents' own emotion regulation skills in treatment outcomes among adolescents with NSSI and other maladaptive behaviors.

Consistent with past research on both ERGT [71, 72] and ERITA [16], results of the present trial provided further support for the mediating role of change in emotion regulation difficulties in NSSI improvements during treatment. Change in emotion regulation difficulties also mediated improvements in self-destructive behaviors during treatment. These findings provide further support for the underlying role of emotion regulation difficulties in the maintenance of self-destructive behaviors, as well as for emotion regulation as a key mechanism of change in ERGT-based treatments.

Several limitations warrant mention. First, the absence of a control group and/or randomized controlled design precludes any conclusions regarding the effects of this treatment versus the passage of time or other factors. Likewise, ten participants (40%) reported having some form of face to face treatment contact while engaged in the online ERITA. However, it is important to note that five of these reported minimal contact with this treatment provider over the course of treatment. Thus, it is unlikely that the observed improvements in this trial were the result of these additional treatment contacts alone. Nonetheless, further research examining the effects of this treatment in a randomized controlled trial is needed. Second, the majority of participants were self-referred and highly educated, potentially limiting the generalizability of this sample to more complex or severe patient populations. However, findings that 60% of the adolescents in this sample had a history of psychological treatment and rates of co-occurring psychiatric disorders were high suggest that the sample may be representative of a clinical sample in terms of treatment history and psychological burden. Third, the relatively small sample size limits the generalizability of our findings and reduces our statistical power. Finally, the sample largely consisted of girls, limiting our ability to generalize our results to boys.

Conclusions

The present study provides preliminary support for the acceptability, feasibility, and utility of an online version of ERITA for adolescents with NSSID and their parents, as well as the theory underlying the treatment. Given the benefits of an online treatment format, particularly with regard to therapist time, patient ease and flexibility of scheduling, access to treatment in underserved areas, and its usefulness for stigmatized behaviors, further research examining the efficacy of online ERITA in a larger-scale randomized controlled trial is needed.

Abbreviations

AAQ: Acceptance and action questionnaire; ADHD: Attention deficit hyperactivity disorder; BPD: Borderline personality disorder; BPFS-C: Borderline personality feature scale for children; BSL: Borderline symptom list; CBT: Cognitive behavior therapy; CGAS: Children's global assessment scale; CI: Confidence interval; DERS: Difficulties in emotion regulation scale; DR: Distress reactions; DSHI: Deliberate self-harm inventory; DSM: Diagnostic and statistical manual of mental disorders; EE: Expressive encouragement; ERGT: Emotion regulation group therapy; ERITA: Emotion regulation individual therapy; GEE: Generalized estimation equation; ICBT: Internet-delivered cognitive behavior therapy; MR: Minimization reactions; NSSI: Nonsuicidal self-injury; NSSID: Nonsuicidal self-injury disorder; PR: Punitive reactions

Acknowledgements

We thank Professor Lars-Gunnar Lundh and Dr. Jonas Bjärehed for scientific advice; Olivia Simonsson, Julia Stensils, and Linn Bjureberg for help with study administration; Gunnar Dagnå for support in graphical design of the web platform and app; and the team at BarnInternetPsykiatrin at the Child and Adolescent Mental Health Service in Stockholm for invaluable support and know-how when treating adolescents over the Internet.

Author contributions

JB, HS, EHL, KLG, MTT, JJ, CH, and BL were involved in the design of the study. JB, HS, CH, and BL were responsible for data collection. JB and HS treated all patients. JB and BL analyzed the patient data and JB, CH, and BL interpreted the results. JB drafted the initial manuscript and all authors provided critical feedback on and revisions to manuscript content. All authors read and approved the final version of the manuscript.

Funding

This project was supported by the National Self Injury Project in Sweden, grant 2014–1008 from the Swedish Research Council, grant MAW 2014.0021 from the Markus and Amelia Wallenberg Foundation, Fredrik och Ingrid Thurings Stifelse, L. J., the Sven Jerring Foundation, the Kempe-Carlgrenska Foundation, and Bror Gadelius minnesfond. None of the funding organizations had any influence on study design; in the collection, analysis, or interpretation of the data; or in the preparation, review, or approval of the manuscript.

Consent for publication

No individual details, images, or videos of participants were included in this manuscript; thus, specific consent for publication was not deemed necessary.

Competing interests

JB, HS, KLG, MTT, JJ, and CH report no competing interests. EHL and BL are shareholders of DahliaQomit, a company specializing in online psychiatric symptom assessment.

Author details

[1]Centre for Psychiatry Research, Department of Clinical Neuroscience, Karolinska Institutet, & Stockholm Health Care Services, Stockholm County Council, Norra stationsgatan 69, SE-11364 Stockholm, Sweden. [2]Division of Psychology, Department of Clinical Neuroscience, Karolinska Institutet, Nobels väg 9, SE-171 65 Stockholm, Sweden. [3]Department of Psychology, University of Toledo, 2801 W. Bancroft Street, Toledo, OH 43606, USA. [4]Department of Clinical Sciences/Psychiatry, Umeå University, By 23, Enheten för psykiatri, 901 85 Umeå, Sweden.

References

1. International Society for the Study of Self-Injury. Fast facts. httpitriples. orgredesadminfast-facts. 2018 [cited 2018 Feb 4]; Available from: http://www.webcitation.org/query?url=http%3A%2F%2Fitriples.org%2Fredesadmin15%2Ffast-facts&date=2018-02-04

2. American Psychiatric Association. Diagnostic and statistical manual of mental disorders. 5th ed. Washington, DC: Author; 2013.

3. Manca M, Presaghi F, Cerutti R. Clinical specificity of acute versus chronic self-injury: measurement and evaluation of repetitive non-suicidal self-injury. Psychiatry Res. 2014;215:111–9.

4. Zetterqvist M, Lundh L-G, Dahlström Ö, Svedin CG. Prevalence and function of Non-Suicidal Self-Injury (NSSI) in a community sample of adolescents, using suggested DSM-5 criteria for a potential NSSI disorder. J Abnorm Child Psychol. 2013;41:759–73.

5. Bjureberg J, Ohlis A, Ljótsson B, D'Onofrio BM, Hedman-Lagerlöf E, Jokinen J, et al. Adolescent self-harm with and without suicidality: cross-sectional and longitudinal analyses of a Swedish regional register. J Child Psychol Psychiatr. 2018. https://doi.org/10.1111/jcpp.12967. [Epub ahead of print].

6. Glenn CR, Klonsky ED. Nonsuicidal self-injury disorder: an empirical investigation in adolescent psychiatric patients. J Clin Child Adolesc Psychol. 2013;42:496–507.

7. Glenn CR, Franklin JC, Nock MK. Evidence-based psychosocial treatments for self-injurious thoughts and behaviors in youth. J Clin Child Adolesc Psychol. 2014;44:1–29.

8. Hawton K, Witt KG, Taylor Salisbury TL, Arensman E, Gunnell D, Townsend E, et al. Interventions for self-harm in children and adolescents. Cochrane Database Syst Rev. 2015:CD012013.

9. Ougrin D, Tranah T, Stahl D, Moran P, Asarnow JR. Therapeutic interventions for suicide attempts and self-harm in adolescents: systematic review and meta-analysis. J Am Acad Child Adolesc Psychiatry. 2015;54:97–107.e2.

10. Turner BJ, Austin SB, Chapman AL. Treating nonsuicidal self-injury: a systematic review of psychological and pharmacological interventions. Can J Psychiatr. 2014;59:576–85.

11. Mehlum L, Tørmoen AJ, Ramberg M, Haga E, Diep LM, Laberg S. Dialectical behavior therapy for adolescents with repeated suicidal and self-harming behavior: a randomized trial. J Am Acad Child Adolesc Psychiatry. 2014;53.

12. McCauley E, Berk MS, Asarnow JR, Adrian M, Cohen J, Korslund K, et al. Efficacy of dialectical behavior therapy for adolescents at high risk for suicide. JAMA Psychiatry. 2018;75:777–9.

13. Rossouw TI, Fonagy P. Mentalization-based treatment for self-harm in adolescents: a randomized controlled trial. J Am Acad Child Adolesc Psychiatry. 2012;51:1304–1313.e3.

14. Esposito-Smythers C, Spirito A, Kahler CW, Hunt J, Monti P. Treatment of co-occurring substance abuse and suicidality among adolescents: a randomized trial. J Consult Psychol. 2011;79:728–39.

15. Slee N, Garnefski N, van der Leeden R, Arensman E, Spinhoven P. Cognitive-behavioural intervention for self-harm: randomised controlled trial. Br J Psychiatry. 2008;192:202–11.

16. Bjureberg J, Sahlin H, Hellner C, Hedman-Lagerlöf E, Gratz KL, Bjärehed J, et al. Emotion regulation individual therapy for adolescents with nonsuicidal self-injury disorder: a feasibility study. BMC Psychiatry. 2017;17:411.

17. Gratz KL, Gunderson JG. Preliminary data on an acceptance-based emotion regulation group intervention for deliberate self-harm among women with borderline personality disorder. Behav Ther. 2006;37:25–35.

18. Gratz KL, Tull MT, Levy R. Randomized controlled trial and uncontrolled 9-month follow-up of an adjunctive emotion regulation group therapy for deliberate self-harm among women with borderline personality disorder. Psychol Med. 2014;44:2099–112.

19. Andersson G. Internet-delivered psychological treatments. Annu Rev Clin Psychol. 2016;12:157–79.

20. Vigerland S, Lenhard F, Bonnert M, Lalouni M, Hedman E, Ahlen J, et al. Internet-delivered cognitive behavior therapy for children and adolescents: a systematic review and meta-analysis. Clin Psychol Rev. 2016;50:1–10.

21. Carlbring P, Andersson G, Cuijpers P, Riper H, Hedman-Lagerlöf E. Internet-based vs. face-to-face cognitive behavior therapy for psychiatric and somatic disorders: an updated systematic review and meta-analysis. Cogn Behav Ther. 2017;47:1–21.

22. Berger M, Wagner TH, Baker LC. Internet use and stigmatized illness. Soc Sci Med. 2005;61:1821–7.

23. Lloyd-Richardson EE, Perrine N, Dierker L, Kelley ML. Characteristics and functions of non-suicidal self-injury in a community sample of adolescents. Psychol Med. 2007;37:1183–92.

24. Armiento JS, Hamza CA, Willoughby T. An examination of disclosure of nonsuicidal self-injury among university students. J Community Appl Soc Psychol. 2014;24:518–33.

25. Hetrick SE, Yuen HP, Bailey E, Cox GR, Templer K, Rice SM, et al. Internet-based cognitive behavioural therapy for young people with suicide-related behaviour (Reframe-IT): a randomised controlled trial. Evid Based Ment Health. 2017;20:76–82.

26. Leon AC, Davis LL, Kraemer HC. The role and interpretation of pilot studies in clinical research. J Psychiatr Res. 2011;45:626–9.

27. Rounsaville BJ, Carroll KM, Onken LS. A stage model of behavioral therapies research: getting started and moving on from stage I. Clin Psychol Sci Pract. 2001;8:133–42.

28. Hedman E, Ljótsson B, Rück C, Furmark T, Carlbring P, Lindefors N, et al. Internet administration of self-report measures commonly used in research on social anxiety disorder: a psychometric evaluation. Comput Hum Behav. 2010;26:736–40.

29. Jarlais Des DC, Lyles C, Crepaz N, the TREND Group. Improving the reporting quality of nonrandomized evaluations of behavioral and public health interventions: the TREND statement. Am J Public Health. 2004;94:361–6.

30. Sheehan DV, Lecrubier Y, Sheehan KH, Amorim P, Janavs J, Weiller E, et al. The Mini-International Neuropsychiatric Interview (M.I.N.I.): the development and validation of a structured diagnostic psychiatric interview for DSM-IV and ICD-10. J Clin Psychiatry. 1998;59(Suppl 20):22–33 quiz34–57.

31. Gratz KL, Dixon-Gordon KL, Chapman AL, Tull MT. Diagnosis and characterization of DSM-5 nonsuicidal self-injury disorder using the clinician-administered nonsuicidal self-injury disorder index. Assessment. 2015;22:527–39.

32. First MB, Gibbon M, Spitzer RL, Williams JB, Benjamin L. Structured clinical interview for DSM-IV personality disorders (SCID-II): interview and questionnaire. Washington, DC: APA; 1997.

33. Borkovec TD, Nau SD. Credibility of analogue therapy rationales. J Behav Ther Exp Psychiatry. 1972;3:257–60.

34. Devilly GJ, Borkovec TD. Psychometric properties of the credibility/expectancy questionnaire. J Behav Ther Exp Psychiatry. 2000;31:73–86.

35. Attkisson CC, Zwick R. The client satisfaction questionnaire. Psychometric properties and correlations with service utilization and psychotherapy outcome. Eval Program Plann. 1982;5:233–7.

36. Hatcher RL, Gillaspy JA. Development and validation of a revised short version of the working alliance inventory. Psychother Res. 2006;16:12–25.

37. Bjärehed J, Lundh L-G. Deliberate self-harm in 14-year-old adolescents: how frequent is it, and how is it associated with psychopathology, relationship variables, and styles of emotional regulation? Cogn Behav Ther. 2008;37:26–37.

38. Turner BJ, Layden BK, Butler SM, Chapman AL. How often, or how many ways: clarifying the relationship between non-suicidal self-injury and suicidality. Arch Suicide Res. 2013;17:397–415.

39. Gratz KL, Roemer L. Multidimensional assessment of emotion regulation and dysregulation: development, factor structure, and initial validation of the difficulties in emotion regulation scale. J Psychopathol Behav Assess. 2004;26:41–54.

40. Neumann A, van Lier PAC, Gratz KL, Koot HM. Multidimensional assessment of emotion regulation difficulties in adolescents using the difficulties in emotion regulation scale. Assessment. 2010;17:138–49.

41. Bjureberg J, Ljótsson B, Tull MT, Hedman E, Sahlin H, Lundh L-G, et al. Development and validation of a brief version of the difficulties in emotion regulation scale: the DERS-16. J Psychopathol Behav Assess. 2016;38:284–96.

42. Shahabi M, Hasani J, Bjureberg J. Psychometric properties of the brief Persian version of the difficulties in emotion regulation scale (the DERS-16). Assess Eff Interv. https://doi.org/10.1177/1534508418800210. [Epub ahead of print].

43. Miguel FK, Giromini L, Colombarolli MS, Zuanazzi AC, Zennaro A. A Brazilian investigation of the 36- and 16-item difficulties in emotion regulation scales. J Clin Psychol. 2016:1–14.

44. Bohus M, Limberger MF, Frank U, Sender I, Gratwohl T, Stieglitz RD. Development of the borderline symptom list. Psychother Psychosom Med Psychol. 2001;51:201–11.

45. Crick NR, Murray-Close D, Woods K. Borderline personality features in childhood: a short-term longitudinal study. Dev Psychopathol. 2005;17:1051–70.

46. Bond FW, Hayes SC, Baer RA, Carpenter KM, Guenole N, Orcutt HK, et al. Preliminary psychometric properties of the acceptance and action questionnaire-II: a revised measure of psychological inflexibility and experiential avoidance. Behav Ther. 2011;42:676–88.

47. Shaffer D, Gould MS, Brasic J, Ambrosini P, Fisher P, Bird H, et al. A children's global assessment scale (CGAS). Arch Gen Psychiatry. 1983;40:1228–31.

48. Lundh A, Kowalski J, Sundberg CJ, Gumpert C, Landen M. Children's Global Assessment Scale (CGAS) in a naturalistic clinical setting: inter-rater reliability and comparison with expert ratings. Psychiatry Res. 2010;177:206–10.

49. Fabes RA, Eisenberger N. The Coping with Children's Negative Emotions Scale Adolescent Version: Procedures and Scoring. 1998.

50. Fabes RA, Poulin RE, Eisenberg N, Madden-Derdich DA. The Coping with Children's Negative Emotions Scale (CCNES): psychometric properties and relations with children's emotional competence. Marriage Fam Rev. 2002;34:285–310.

51. Gratz KL, Tull MT. Extending research on the utility of an adjunctive emotion regulation group therapy for deliberate self-harm among women with borderline personality pathology. Personal Disord. 2011;2:316–26.

52. Sahlin H, Bjureberg J, Gratz KL, Tull MT, Hedman E, Bjärehed J, et al. Emotion regulation group therapy for deliberate self-harm: a multi-site evaluation in routine care using an uncontrolled open trial design. BMJ Open. 2017;7:e016220–12.

53. Linehan M. Cognitive-behavioral treatment of borderline personality disorder. New York: Guilford press; 1993.

54. Bonnert M, Olén O, Lalouni M, Benninga MA, Bottai M, Engelbrektsson J, et al. Internet-delivered cognitive behavior therapy for adolescents with irritable bowel syndrome: a randomized controlled trial. Am J Gastroenterol. 2016;112:152–62.

55. Lenhard F, Andersson E, Mataix-Cols D, Rück C, Vigerland S, Högström J, et al. Therapist-guided, internet-delivered cognitive-behavioral therapy for adolescents with obsessive-compulsive disorder: a randomized controlled trial. J Am Acad Child Adolesc Psychiatry. 2017;56:10–2.

56. Vigerland S, Ljótsson B, Thulin U, Öst L-G, Andersson G, Serlachius E. Internet-delivered cognitive behavioural therapy for children with anxiety disorders: a randomised controlled trial. Behav Res Ther. 2016;76:47–56.

57. R Core Team. R: A language and environment for statistical computing. 2016; Available from: https://www.R-project.org/.

58. Preisser JS, Lohman KK, Rathouz PJ. Performance of weighted estimating equations for longitudinal binary data with drop-outs missing at random. Stat Med. 2002;21:3035–54.

59. Robins JM, Rotnitzky A. Semiparametric efficiency in multivariate regression models with missing data. J Am Stat Assoc. 1995;90:122–9.

60. Kelley K. The effects of nonnormal distributions on confidence intervals around the standardized mean difference: bootstrap and parametric confidence intervals. Educ Psychol Meas. 2005;65:51–69.

61. Ren S, Lai H, Tong W, Aminzadeh M, Hou X, Lai S. Nonparametric bootstrapping for hierarchical data. J Appl Stat. 2010;37:1487–98.

62. Fagerland MW, Lydersen S, Laake P. The McNemar test for binary matched-pairs data: mid-p and asymptotic are better than exact conditional. BMC Med Res Methodol. 2013;13:91.

63. MacKinnon DP, Fairchild AJ, Fritz MS. Mediation analysis. Annu Rev Psychol. 2007;58:593–614.

64. Geldhof GJ, Anthony KP, Selig JP, Mendez-Luck CA. Accommodating binary and count variables in mediation. Int J Behav Dev. 2017:016502541772787–9.

65. Preacher KJ, Hayes AF. Asymptotic and resampling strategies for assessing and comparing indirect effects in multiple mediator models. Behav Res Methods. 2008;40:879–91.

66. Andover MS, Schatten HT, Morris BW, Holman CS, Miller IW. An intervention for nonsuicidal self-injury in young adults: a pilot randomized controlled trial. J Consult Psychol. 2017;85:620–31.

67. Andersson G, Paxling B, Wiwe M, Vernmark K, Felix CB, Lundborg L, et al. Therapeutic alliance in guided internet-delivered cognitive behavioural treatment of depression, generalized anxiety disorder and social anxiety disorder. Behav Res Ther. 2012;50:544–50.

68. Lenhard F, Vigerland S, Engberg H, Hallberg A, Thermaenius H, Serlachius E. "On my own, but not alone" - adolescents' experiences of internet-delivered cognitive behavior therapy for obsessive-compulsive disorder. PLoS One. 2016;11:e0164311–4.

69. Brent DA, McMakin DL, Kennard BD, Goldstein TR, Mayes TL, Douaihy AB. Protecting adolescents from self-harm: a critical review of intervention studies. J Am Acad Child Adolesc Psychiatry. 2013;52:1260–71.

70. Shenk CE, Fruzzetti AE. Parental validating and invalidating responses and adolescent psychological functioning. Fam J. 2013;22:43–8.

71. Gratz KL, Bardeen JR, Levy R, Dixon-Gordon KL, Tull MT. Mechanisms of change in an emotion regulation group therapy for deliberate self-harm among women with borderline personality disorder. Behav Res Ther. 2015;65:29–35.

72. Gratz KL, Levy R, Tull MT. Emotion regulation as a mechanism of change in an acceptance-based emotion regulation group therapy for deliberate self-harm among women with borderline personality pathology. J Cogn Psychother. 2012;26:365–80.

9

Cytokine profiles and diagnoses in elderly, hospitalized psychiatric patients

Erlend Bugge[1][*] [iD], Rolf Wynn[2], Tom Eirik Mollnes[3,4,5,6,7], Solveig Klæbo Reitan[8] and Ole Kristian Grønli[1]

Abstract

Background: There is a paucity of studies on inflammatory markers in elderly psychiatric patients. Hence, our study was undertaken to investigate cytokines as biomarkers in diagnostically unselected elderly patients admitted to a psychiatric hospital.

Methods: Demographic data, clinical data and blood samples, including 27 cytokines, were collected from 98 patients above 60 years, consecutively admitted to a psychiatric hospital in Tromsø, Norway (69°N).

Results: The most common diagnosis was Recurrent depressive disorder (26.5%), the second most common was dementia in Alzheimer's disease (20.4%). The most frequent somatic disease was cardiovascular disease (28%). No statistical association ($p < 0.01$) was found between cytokines and gender, age, BMI, anti-inflammatory drugs, psychotropic drugs, reason for admittance, smoking, vitamin supplements, alcohol consumption, length of stay, somatic disease (present/not-present) or psychiatric diagnoses. However, when allocating patients to two groups, *depression* and *no depression*, we found higher levels of 10 cytokines in the *no depression* group (FDR-*p* < 0.0044). Possibly, this could in part be explained by the higher prevalence of cardiovascular disease (CVD) and dementia in the no depression group, as these factors were significant predictors of patients being categorized as not depressed in a logistic regression. In addition, other unknown factors might have contributed to the association between no depression and elevated cytokines. On the other hand, the high level of psychiatric and somatic comorbidity in the study population may have led to increased levels of cytokines in general, possibly diluting the potential effect of other factors, depression included, on the cytokine levels.

The size of the study, and particularly the size of the subgroups, represents a limitation of the study, as do the general heterogeneity and the lack of a control group.

Conclusions: There was no significant difference in cytokine levels between various psychiatric diagnoses in hospitalized elderly psychiatric patients. This indicates that previous findings of correlations between cytokines and various psychiatric disorders in highly selected adult cases might not be applicable to elderly psychiatric inpatients. Further immunological studies are needed on gerontopsychiatric patients in general and gerontopsychiatric patients with specific disorders, preferably with patients that are physically healthy.

Keywords: Psychogeriatric, Gerontopsychiatric, Cytokine, Depression, Neuroimmunology

* Correspondence: erlend.bugge@unn.no
[1]Division of Mental Health and Addictions, University Hospital of North Norway, N-9037 Tromsø, Norway
Full list of author information is available at the end of the article

Background

Several studies have demonstrated an association between psychiatric disorders and biomarkers of inflammation, particularly cytokines. Primarily, these studies have focused on specific disorders and selected sets of cytokines. Depression and schizophrenia seem to dominate this research, both disorders repeatedly demonstrating elevated levels of pro-inflammatory cytokines such as IL-1β, IL-2, IL-6, and TNF [1–3]. Though some of these studies include elderly patients [4–6], most studies have been conducted on younger adults. Thus, there is a paucity of studies on elderly psychiatric patients and particularly elderly psychiatric in-patients. Besides the fact that populations are ageing in most countries [7], the elderly are of particular interest because they are more likely to represent biological diversity due to age-related neuroimmunological changes [8] and higher frequencies of comorbid conditions. Consequently, findings of cytokine changes in younger adults do not readily translate to elderly psychiatric patients. Hence, our study was undertaken to investigate cytokines as biomarkers in diagnostically unselected elderly patients admitted to a psychiatric hospital.

Methods

Population

The population has been described in a previous publication [9]. Demographic data, clinical data and blood samples were collected from 98 patients, 60 years and older, consecutively admitted to a psychiatric hospital in Tromsø, Norway (69°N). The catchment area of the hospital was approximately 250,000 citizens. Exclusion criteria comprised inability to communicate and cooperate, e.g. due to a severe psychiatric condition like severe dementia or confusion/delirium, or a medical condition likely to significantly affect the blood/plasma analysis like severe dehydration or ongoing infection. The reasons for referral included a variety of psychiatric conditions, spanning from anxiety to psychosis, with depression (42%) and dementia (26%) being the most common. In terms of gender, age and diagnostic distribution, the study population was quite similar to the general population of patients admitted to gerontopsychiatric units in Norway [10], the possible exception being a lower proportion of dementia. However, the Norwegian national data included patients with severe dementia, whereas these patients were excluded from our study.

Clinical assessment

The following instruments were applied to assess the psychiatric and cognitive status of the participants (N = number of patients): the MINI International Neuropsychiatric Interview, $N = 43$ [11], the Montgomery and Aasberg Depression Rating Scale, $N = 76$ [12], the Cornell Scale for Depression in Dementia, $N = 22$ [13], the Mini-Mental State Examination, $N = 92$ [14] and the Clockdrawing Test, $N = 90$ [15]. In addition, clinical interviews and reviews of medical records were undertaken by experienced clinicians in assessment and diagnostics, according to ICD-10 research criteria. Interview of next of kin was also undertaken when appropriate.

Blood samples

During the first 3 days of admittance, morning blood samples (before 10 AM) were obtained for a range of analyses, e.g. electrolytes, liver enzymes, blood cells and thyroid hormones. In addition, plasma samples from EDTA-tubes were successively and rapidly frozen to – 70 °C, until analysed for cytokines in one batch. The analyses were performed by multiplex technology on a Multiplex Analyser with a predefined kit, according to the instructions of the manufacturer (Bio-Plex Human Cytokine 27-Plex Panel; Bio-Rad Laboratories Inc., Hercules, CA, USA). The assay was set up to detect the following interleukins, chemokines and growth factors: IL-1β, IL-1 receptor antagonist (IL1-ra), IL-2, IL-4, IL-5, IL-6, IL-7, IL-8, IL-9, IL-10, IL-12 (p70), IL-13, IL-15, IL-17, eotaxin, basic fibroblast growth factor (bFGF), granulocyte-colony stimulating factor (G-CSF), granulocyte macrophage colony stimulating factor (GM-CSF), interferon (IFN)-γ, interferon-inducible protein (IP-10), monocyte chemotactic protein (MCP-1), macrophage inflammatory protein (MIP-1α, MIP-1β), platelet derived growth factor-BB (PDGF-BB), regulated upon activation T cell expressed and secreted (RANTES), tumor necrosis factor (TNF), and vascular endothelial growth factor (VEGF).

GM-CSF and IL-15 had a high frequency of non-detectable levels, i.e. below the lower detection limit, and were therefore excluded in the statistical analyses. Another eight cytokines had a small number of patients with cytokine levels below the lower detection limit (number of patients with non-detectable levels): IL-2 (4), IL-10 (11), IL-13 (1), IL-17 (4), bFGF (2), G-CSF (2), PDGF-BB (2), and VEGF (4). Data for these patients were imputed using SPSS, see Statistical analyses section.

Statistical analyses

Most of the data were not strictly normally distributed, as demonstrated by the Kolmogorov-Smirnov test, and several groups had unequal variances. Thus, nonparametric tests were applied. The Spearman rank correlation coefficient and Kendall Tau coefficient were used to analyse differences between the rankings of two variables. The Mann-Whitney U or the Kruskal-Wallis tests were applied when comparing ranks of two or several subgroups, subsequently. Goodness of fit was assessed by binary logistic regression. To examine whether the raised cytokine levels and the other variables could predict depression, we performed logistic regression analyses with depression/no depression as dependent variable. Patients were allocated to the depression group if they had been given depression as a primary or secondary diagnosis, or the no depression group if they had not been given a depression analysis.

Due to multiple statistical analyses, 0.01 was selected as significance level. In addition, false detection rate adjusted p-value (FDR-p) was calculated and applied to all analyses related to the cytokines. IBM Statistical Package for the Social Sciences, Version 23 (SPSS Inc., Chicago, Illinois, USA) software was used in the statistical analysis.

A small group of patients had no or very low levels of certain cytokines (which is a common finding for most cytokines in healthy adults), but the actual value could not be computed by the instrumentation; they are so-called non-detects (NDs). Accordingly, data from the NDs could hold valuable information, and in order to include them in the statistical analyses, we did single imputations, i.e. the NDs were substituted with a random value between zero and the lower detection limit, with a uniform distribution, using the random number generator of SPSS [16].

Results

Population characteristics
Population characteristics are presented in Table 1.

Diagnoses
The main diagnostic groups are presented in Table 2. The most common diagnosis was Recurrent depressive disorder (26.5%), the second most common was dementia in Alzheimer's disease (20.4%). Considering depression as a separate clinical entity, depending on whether the patients had been given depression as a primary or secondary diagnosis or not, the majority of patients could be allotted to the depression group, see Table 2. Selected features of the groups depression and no depression are presented in Table 3.

Distribution and correlation analysis
The cytokine values of the patients are presented in Table 4. In this group of diagnostically unselected elderly in-patients, no statistical correlation or unequal distribution was found between cytokines and gender, age, BMI, anti-inflammatory drugs, psychotropic drugs, reason for admittance, smoking, vitamin supplements, alcohol consumption, length of stay, somatic disease (present/not-present) or psychiatric diagnoses, dementia included. However, a correlation (FDR-p < 0.0044) was found

Table 1 In-patients' characteristics

Characteristics	
Age, median/SD (years)	76/7.3
80 years and older (%)	39.8
Women (%)	61.2
Men (%)	38.8
Length of stay, median/SD (days)	34/25
Living alone (%)	53
Previous hospitalization (%) [a]	49
Two or more previous hospitalizations (%) [a]	38
No known somatic disease (%)	21
Cardiovascular disease (%)	28
Pulmonary disease (%)	10
Thyroid disease (%)	10
Previous stroke (%)	10
Rheumatic disease (%)	3.5
Other somatic diseases (%)	17.5
Potentially anti-inflammatory drug (%) [b]	55.1
Daily smokers (%)	29.6
BMI, median/SD (kilos)	24/5.3

[a] Psychiatric hospitalization
[b] The most common drug in this category is acetylsalicylic acid in low dose as prevention of cardiovascular events (N = 30/68.2%)

between *no depression* (N = 39) and raised levels of several cytokines, see Table 5.

While none of the raised cytokine levels predicted depression in a logistic regression model, cardiovascular disease (CVD) and dementia were predictors of patients being categorized as not depressed/no depression (Table 6). However, none of the cytokines came out as predictive in logistic regression models with CVD/no CVD, or dementia/no dementia, as dependent variables.

Looking at distributional data, CVD and dementia were more prevalent in the no depression group, compared to the depression group, 46.2% versus 15.3%, and 51.3% versus 22.0%, respectively.

Table 2 Distribution of diagnoses

Diagnoses	ICD-10	%
Organic, including symptomatic, mental disorders	F00–09	37.8
Mental and behavioural disorders due to psychoactive substance abuse	F10–19	1
Schizophrenia, schizotypal and delusional disorders	F20–29	12.2
Affective disorders	F30–39	41.8
Neurotic, stress-related and somatoform disorders	F40–48	7.2
Depression/No depression		60.2/39.8

Table 3 Selected features of depressed and non-depressed patients

Comorbidities/features	Depression (%)	No depression (%)
Somatic disease (any)	76.3	82.1
Cardiovascular disease	15.3	46.2
Dementia	22.0	51.3
Antidepressants	74.6	25.6

Discussion

To our knowledge, this is the first study to explore cytokine levels in diagnostically unselected elderly psychiatric in-patients. Using an immunoassay method, we analysed 27 plasma cytokines in 98 patients, 60 years and older, admitted to a gerontopsychiatric unit.

The results demonstrated that cytokine levels did not correlate with variables such as age, gender, psychiatric diagnoses, somatic disease (present/not present), and the use of anti-inflammatory and psychotropic drugs. Considering each of these factors separately, this does not seem to match previous findings, as prior studies

have shown positive associations between for instance Alzheimer's disease and increased levels of several cytokines [17], and between aging and increased levels of IL-6 and TNF-α [18]. Then again, our heterogeneous study population differs substantially from most of the diagnostically uniform populations previously studied.

The high frequency of somatic and psychiatric comorbidity in the study population may have contributed to the increased levels of cytokines in general, masking possible correlations between any single factor and changes in levels of cytokines. On the other hand, there is a possibility that altered immune activity in psychiatric patients is a general phenomenon, not restricted to specific diagnoses. Such a hypothesis can be bolstered by the fact that research has shown raised levels of inflammatory markers in several psychiatric disorders, ranging from schizophrenia to anxiety disorders [19, 20].

Contrary to some prior studies, we did not find any correlation between cytokines and depression. Given the fact the majority of our depressed patients were diagnosed with recurrent depressive disorder, it could be

Table 4 Serum levels of cytokines (pg/ml) in elderly psychiatric in-patients

Cytokine	Median	SD*	Minimum	Maximum	P 25**	P 75***
IL-1b	3.00	4.65	0.53	38.00	1.58	5.00
IL-1ra	158.00	769.64	31.00	7396.00	84.00	268.75
IL-2	9.00	17.97	0.01	147.00	3.00	16.00
IL-4	3.00	2.55	1.00	13.00	2.00	4.00
IL-5	5.00	5.65	0.73	28.00	3.00	9.00
IL-6	11.00	15.39	3.00	119.00	7.00	18.75
IL-7	21.00	22.83	0.25	104.00	11.00	36.00
IL-8	13.00	9.35	3.00	47.00	8.00	19.00
IL-9	18.00	47.03	3.00	441.00	11.00	28.00
IL-10	8.50	16.92	0.01	102.00	2.00	16.00
IL-12	27.00	51.60	0.05	381.00	11.00	46.75
IL-13	7.00	15.51	0.50	96.00	4.00	14.00
IL-17	42.50	66.57	0.35	371.00	15.25	88.25
Eotaxin	93.00	257.20	28.00	2286.00	65.50	157.75
bFGF	46.00	48.58	1.16	259.00	21.00	79.75
G-CSF	52.00	52.92	1.53	316.00	29.25	82.75
INF-g	184.00	217.26	20.00	1179.00	94.75	280.75
IP-10	1015.50	744.58	216.00	5075.00	762.25	1338.00
MCP-1	19.00	16.04	4.00	128.00	13.25	26.00
MIP-1a	10.00	9.82	2.00	58.00	6.00	15.00
MIP-1b	44.00	24.77	17.00	198.00	34.00	56.00
PDGF-BB	137.50	325.59	1.03	1651.00	34.25	308.00
RANTES	6642.00	12,393.18	532.00	60,319.70	2876.00	16,859.75
TNF-a	92.00	137.85	8.00	1173.00	43.50	127.25
VEGF	21.50	25.94	1.90	130.00	10.00	36.00

* Standard deviation. ** 25-percentile. *** 75-percentile

Table 5 Correlation between cytokines and *No depression* (p-level > 0.01 excluded)

Cytokine	Correlation coefficient*	p	FDR-p**	Significant***	Eta²****
IL-2	0.268	0.008	0.0060	No	0.072
bFGF	0.271	0.008	0.0056	No	0.074
IL-1ra	0.271	0.008	0.0052	No	0.074
IL-1b	0.283	0.005	0.0048	No	0.080
IL-5	0.288	0.004	0.0044	Yes	0.083
IL-12	0.289	0.004	0.0040	Yes	0.083
IL-6	0.290	0.004	0.0036	Yes	0.084
TNF-a	0.295	0.004	0.0028	Yes	0.087
IL-7	0.306	0.002	0.0024	Yes	0.093
IL-10	0.321	0.001	0.0020	Yes	0.103
G-CSF	0.322	0.001	0.0016	Yes	0.104
INF-g	0.334	0.001	0.0012	Yes	0.111
IL-4	0.348	0.001	0.0008	Yes	0.121
IL-8	0.349	0.000	0.0004	Yes	0.122

*Spearman Rho; **False detection rate adjusted p-value, q-level 0.01, based on p-values of all 25 cytokines; ***FDR-adjusted p-criterion of 0.0044 ****Effect size. Based on Mann-Whitney Z-statistics of all 25 cytokines

hypothesized that relapsing depression in the elderly represents a somewhat different immunological process compared to depression in younger patients, on whom most studies have been conducted. On the other hand, our intra-group comparison could be the main explanation why the depressed patients did not have comparably higher levels of cytokines, considering that the overall level of cytokines was high regardless of diagnosis.

One relevant point to consider is that anti-depressants have exhibited anti-inflammatory properties in both clinical and experimental studies [21, 22]. Accordingly, the high percentage of antidepressant use in the depression group (74.6% versus 25.6% in the no depression group) might have been a factor in terms of lowering the cytokine levels amongst the depressed patients, cancelling out the association between depression and cytokine levels.

We did observe a correlation between *no depression*, a term denoting patients without significant depression irrespective of other clinical features, and several cytokines (FDR-p < 0.0044). Presumably, this correlation is not explained by the lack of depression per se. Rather, it is more likely that other factors contribute to increased

cytokines in the no depression group. CVD and dementia are two possible contributing factors, as they are more prevalent in the no depression group, hence becoming predictors in a binary logistic model. Both CVD and dementia have been linked to increased levels of cytokines [23–26]. Yet, the fact that none of the cytokines correlated with dementia or CVD, in addition to the absence of predictive power of any of the cytokines for both dementia and CVD in binary logistic regression, indicate that other, unrecognized factors also contribute to the association between no depression and elevated cytokines.

Finally, it should be taken into account that the total level of psychiatric morbidity in the no depression group (e.g. organic mental disorders) was probably just as high, perhaps higher, than in the depression group, hence diluting the potential effect of depression on the cytokine levels. There might also be a proportion of the no depression patients with dementia that actually was depressed, as it cannot be ruled out that patients with dementia express depressive symptoms in a way that is less likely to be recognized by the clinician. Then again, altered cytokine levels in psychiatric patients

Table 6 Logistic regression model assessing predictors of patients categorized as *no depression*[a]

Predictors of *no depression*	Log odds	SE[b]	Wald Chi²	P-value	Odds ratio	95% CI[c] for OR Lower - Upper
Dementia (*N* = 20)	1.422	0.484	8.651	0.003	4.147	1.607–10.700
Cardiovascular disease (*N* = 18)	1.664	0.515	10.441	0.001	5.279	1.924–14.479
Constant	−1.409	0.344	16.745	0.000	0.244	

[a]Nagelkerke R Square 0.253, Cox & Snell R Square 0.187
[b]SE: Standard error
[c]CI: Confidence interval

may be a general phenomenon, possibly being primarily dependent on the severity of the disorder, and not the diagnosis.

When interpreting the result of our study, we need to be cautious, given the size of the study, and particularly the size of the subgroups. It should also be noted that though we chose 0.01 as significance levels due to multiple comparisons, and calculated FDR-p for the cytokine statistics, the risk of spurious correlations is still present. On this point, it worth mentioning that a Bonferroni correction would have required a significance threshold of 0.002. Moreover, applying few exclusion criteria may have provided a study population that resembled real-life gerontopsychiatric in-patients, but heightened the risk of confounders due to the general heterogeneity of the group, i.e. differences in age, socioeconomic background, lifestyle factors etc. Adding to this risk was the possibility of greater variability in health status, including immunological functioning, in the elderly compared to younger adults. Another possible source of cytokine variability could be that not all blood samples were fasting (35.7% non-fasting). Though the studies are somewhat conflicting, most seem to indicate that fasting has a certain anti-inflammatory effect [27–29]. A correlational analysis between fasting and cytokine levels in our population demonstrated nevertheless no correlation. Furthermore, a control group of healthy elderly would have made a statistical comparison possible, but at the time, we did not have such data available. Finally, it should be mentioned that single imputation of data to remedy NDs (see section Statistical analysis) may confer a risk of distorting the statistics, in particular when the number of NDs are high. In our study, the number of NDs are small (four at the most) and running the statistics without the NDs did not produce any significant change.

The plasma levels of cytokines observed in this group of elderly patients were the results of complex immunological processes, where different cytokines might have played different roles at different stages. Several interplaying factors, such as age, life style factors, somatic health, genetics, drugs and the psychiatric disorders per se, may have contributed in these processes. Besides, it is still unclear how an increased level of cytokines in systemic circulation relates to neuroimmunological processes in psychiatric disorders. Adding to the complexity is the application of various methods of cytokine analysis and methodological issues [30, 31]. Hence, caution should be exercised when interpreting data and making inferences about cytokine profiles and biomarkers in psychiatry, and perhaps particularly in the elderly population. This also begs the question as to what extent findings in younger adults, with uniform diagnostic profiles and no comorbidity, have bearings on real-life elderly patients.

Though the field of old age neuroimmunology has made great advances in the last decade, there is still a lot to be learned about the immunology of gerontopsychiatry. Further studies are needed on gerontopsychiatric patients in general and gerontopsychiatric patients with specific disorders, preferably with patients that are physically healthy. Clinical studies are necessary to gauge the immunological effects, both cellular and humoral, of various forms of treatment. As for our patients, the question is if psychiatric treatment can impact the high, probably multi-etiological, levels of cytokines. Finally, genomic and proteomic studies are required to uncover the immunological underpinnings of psychiatric disorders affecting the elderly, including longitudinal studies of healthy populations at risk.

Conclusions

There was no significant difference in cytokine levels between various psychiatric diagnoses in elderly psychiatric in-patients. However, when patients were allocated to two groups, *depression* and *no depression*, irrespective of diagnoses and other clinical features, we found higher levels of certain cytokines in the *no depression* group compared to the *depression* group. This might be due to a higher frequency of CVD and dementia in the *no depression* group, as well as other unknown factors.

Abbreviations

BMI: Body mass index; CVD: Cardiovascular disease; EDTA: Ethylenediaminetetraacetic acid; FDR: False detection rate; ICD-10: International classification of diseases version 10; NDs: Non-detects; SPSS: Statistical package for the Social Sciences

Acknowledgments

We thank the laboratory staff at the Department of Laboratory Medicine, University Hospital of North Norway for their contributions to this study. We also thank the participating patients.

Funding

This project is financed by the Northern Norway Regional Health Authority, grant number PFP1298–16. The recipients are EB and OKG. The funding institution had no role in the study design, data collection and analysis, decision to publish, or preparation of the manuscript. The publication charges for this article have been funded by a grant from the publication fund of UiT The Arctic University of Norway.

Authors' contributions

EB designed the study, analyzed the data, drafted the manuscript, revised the manuscript, and approved the final version. OKG designed the study, analyzed the data, drafted the manuscript, revised the manuscript, and approved the final version. RW designed the study, analyzed the data, drafted the manuscript, revised the manuscript, and approved the final version. TEM analyzed the data, drafted the manuscript, revised the manuscript, and approved the final version. SKR analyzed the data, drafted the manuscript, revised the manuscript, and approved the final version. All authors have agreed to be accountable for all aspects of the work in ensuring that questions related to the accuracy or integrity of any part of the work are appropriately investigated and resolved.

Consent for publication
Not applicable.

Competing interests
The authors declare that they have no competing interests.

Author details
[1]Division of Mental Health and Addictions, University Hospital of North Norway, N-9037 Tromsø, Norway. [2]Department of Clinical Medicine, UiT The Arctic University of Norway, N-9038 Tromsø, Norway. [3]UiT The Arctic University of Norway, K.G. Jebsen TREC, N-9038 Tromsø, Norway. [4]Research Laboratory, Nordland Hospital, Bodø, Norway. [5]Faculty of Health Sciences, K.G. Jebsen TREC, University of Tromsø, Tromsø, Norway. [6]Department of Immunology, Oslo University Hospital, and University of Oslo, Oslo, Norway. [7]Centre of Molecular Inflammation Research, Norwegian University of Science and Technology, Trondheim, Norway. [8]Norwegian University of Science and Technology, Faculty of Medicine and Health Sciences, N-7491 Trondheim, Norway.

References

1. Rosenblat JD, Cha DS, Mansur RB, McIntyre RS. Inflamed moods: a review of the interactions between inflammation and mood disorders. Prog Neuro-Psychopharmacol Biol Psychiatry. 2014;53:23–34.
2. Upthegrove R, Manzanares-Teson N, Barnes NM. Cytokine function in medication-naive first episode psychosis: a systematic review and meta-analysis. Schizophr Res. 2014;155(1–3):101–8.
3. Na KS, Jung HY, Kim YK. The role of pro-inflammatory cytokines in the neuroinflammation and neurogenesis of schizophrenia. Prog Neuro-Psychopharmacol Biol Psychiatry. 2014;48:277–86.
4. Gaarden TL, Engedal K, Benth JS, Larsen M, Lorentzen B, Mollnes TE, et al. Exploration of 27 plasma immune markers: a cross-sectional comparison of 64 old psychiatric inpatients having unipolar major depression and 18 non-depressed old persons. BMC Geriatr. 2018;18(1):149.
5. Brambilla F, Maggioni M. Blood levels of cytokines in elderly patients with major depressive disorder. Acta Psychiatr Scand. 1998;97(4):309–13.
6. Thomas AJ, Davis S, Morris C, Jackson E, Harrison R, O'Brien JT. Increase in interleukin-1beta in late-life depression. Am J Psychiatry. 2005;162(1):175–7.
7. WHO. World Report on Ageing and Health. 2015.
8. Schwartz M, London A, Lindvall O. Neuroimmunity : a new science that will revolutionize how we keep our brains healthy and young, vol. xxix. New Haven: Yale University Press; 2015. p. 283.
9. Gronli O, Kvamme JM, Jorde R, Wynn R. Vitamin D deficiency is common in psychogeriatric patients, independent of diagnosis. BMC Psychiatry. 2014;14:134.
10. Sørensen L. In: NDo H, editor. Rapport fra kartlegging av tilbud ved alderspsykiatriske avdelinger og DPSer. Oslo: Norwegian Directorate of Health; 2012.
11. Sheehan DV, Lecrubier Y, Sheehan KH, Amorim P, Janavs J, Weiller E, et al. The Mini-International Neuropsychiatric Interview (M.I.N.I.): the development and validation of a structured diagnostic psychiatric interview for DSM-IV and ICD-10. J Clin Psychiatry. 1998;59(Suppl 20):22–33 quiz 4–57.
12. Montgomery SA, Asberg M. A new depression scale designed to be sensitive to change. Br J Psychiatry. 1979;134:382–9.
13. Alexopoulos GS, Abrams RC, Young RC, Shamoian CA. Cornell scale for depression in dementia. Biol Psychiatry. 1988;23(3):271–84.
14. Folstein MF, Folstein SE, McHugh PR. "Mini-mental state". A practical method for grading the cognitive state of patients for the clinician. J Psychiatr Res. 1975;12(3):189–98.
15. Tuokko H, Hadjistavropoulos T, Miller JA, Beattie BL. The clock test: a sensitive measure to differentiate normal elderly from those with Alzheimer disease. J Am Geriatr Soc. 1992;40(6):579–84.
16. Uh HWHF, Yazdanbakhsh M, Houwing-Duistermaat JJ. Evaluation of regression methods when immunological measurements are constrained by detection limits. BMC Immunol. 2008;9:59.
17. Heppner FL, Ransohoff RM, Becher B. Immune attack: the role of inflammation in Alzheimer disease. Nat Rev Neurosci. 2015;16(6):358–72.
18. Singh T, Newman AB. Inflammatory markers in population studies of aging. Ageing Res Rev. 2011;10(3):319–29.
19. Vogelzangs N, Beekman AT, de Jonge P, Penninx BW. Anxiety disorders and inflammation in a large adult cohort. Transl Psychiatry. 2013;3:e249.
20. Rodrigues-Amorim D, Rivera-Baltanas T, Spuch C, Caruncho HJ, Gonzalez-Fernandez A, Olivares JM, et al. Cytokines dysregulation in schizophrenia: A systematic review of psychoneuroimmune relationship. Schizophr Res. 2017.
21. Hashioka S, Miyaoka T, Wake R, Furuya M, Horiguchi J. Glia: an important target for anti-inflammatory and antidepressant activity. Curr Drug Targets. 2013;14(11):1322–8.
22. Hashioka S, McGeer PL, Monji A, Kanba S. Anti-inflammatory effects of antidepressants: possibilities for preventives against Alzheimer's disease. Cent Nerv Syst Agents Med Chem. 2009;9(1):12–9.
23. Kaptoge S, Seshasai SR, Gao P, Freitag DF, Butterworth AS, Borglykke A, et al. Inflammatory cytokines and risk of coronary heart disease: new prospective study and updated meta-analysis. Eur Heart J. 2014;35(9):578–89.
24. Hansson GK. Inflammation, atherosclerosis, and coronary artery disease. N Engl J Med. 2005;352(16):1685–95.
25. Clough Z, Jeyapaul P, Zotova E, Holmes C. Proinflammatory cytokines and the clinical features of dementia with lewy bodies. Alzheimer Dis Assoc Disord. 2015;29(1):97–9.
26. Angelopoulos P, Agouridaki H, Vaiopoulos H, Siskou E, Doutsou K, Costa V, et al. Cytokines in Alzheimer's disease and vascular dementia. Int J Neurosci. 2008;118(12):1659–72.
27. Traba J, Geiger SS, Kwarteng-Siaw M, Han K, Ra OH, Siegel RM, et al. Prolonged fasting suppresses mitochondrial NLRP3 inflammasome assembly and activation via SIRT3-mediated activation of superoxide dismutase 2. J Biol Chem. 2017;292(29):12153–64.
28. Faris MA, Kacimi S, Al-Kurd RA, Fararjeh MA, Bustanji YK, Mohammad MK, et al. Intermittent fasting during Ramadan attenuates proinflammatory cytokines and immune cells in healthy subjects. Nutr Res. 2012;32(12):947–55.
29. Aliasghari F, Izadi A, Gargari BP, Ebrahimi S. The effects of Ramadan fasting on body composition, blood pressure, glucose metabolism, and markers of inflammation in NAFLD patients: an observational trial. J Am Coll Nutr. 2017; 36(8):640–5.
30. Zhou X, Fragala MS, McElhaney JE, Kuchel GA. Conceptual and methodological issues relevant to cytokine and inflammatory marker measurements in clinical research. Curr Opin Clin Nutr Metab Care. 2010; 13(5):541–7.
31. Biancotto A, Wank A, Perl S, Cook W, Olnes MJ, Dagur PK, et al. Baseline levels and temporal stability of 27 multiplexed serum cytokine concentrations in healthy subjects. PLoS One. 2013;8(12):e76091.
32. Pedersen R, Hofmann B, Mangset M. Patient autonomy and informed consent in clinical practice. Tidsskr Nor Laegeforen. 2007;127(12): 1644–7.

10

Effects of stress on behavior and resting-state fMRI in rats and evaluation of Telmisartan therapy in a stress-induced depression model

Junling Li[1,2], Ran Yang[3], Kai Xia[2], Tian Wang[2], Binbin Nie[4], Kuo Gao[2], Jianxin Chen[2], Huihui Zhao[2], Yubo Li[5] and Wei Wang[2*]

Abstract

Background: The etiology of depression and its effective therapeutic treatment have not been clearly identified. Using behavioral phenotyping and resting-state functional magnetic resonance imaging (r-fMRI), we investigated the behavioral impact and cerebral alterations of chronic unpredictable mild stress (CUMS) in the rat. We also evaluated the efficacy of telmisartan therapy in this rodent model of depression.

Methods: Thirty-two rats were divided into 4 groups: a control group(C group), a stress group(S group), a stress + telmisartan(0.5 mg/kg)group (T-0.5 mg/kg group) and a stress + telmisartan(1 mg/kg) group (T-1 mg/kg group). A behavioral battery, including an open field test (OFT), a sucrose preference test (SPT), and an object recognition test (ORT), as well as r-fMRI were conducted after 4 weeks of CUMS and telmisartan therapy. The r-fMRI data were analyzed using the amplitude of low-frequency fluctuations (ALFF) and regional homogeneity (ReHo) approach. The group differences in the behavior and r-fMRI test results as well as the correlations between these 2 approaches were examined.

Results: CUMS reduced the number of rearings and the total moved distance in OFT, the sucrose preference in SPT, and novel object recognition ability in ORT. The telmisartan treatment (1 mg/kg) significantly improved B-A/B + A in the ORT and improved latency scores in the OFT and SPT. The S group exhibited a decreased ReHo in the motor cortex and pons, but increased ReHo in the thalamus, visual cortex, midbrain, cerebellum, hippocampus, hypothalamus, and olfactory cortex compared to the C group. Telmisartan (1 mg/kg)reversed or attenuated the stress-induced changes in the motor cortex, midbrain, thalamus, hippocampus, hypothalamus, visual cortex, and olfactory cortex. A negative correlation was found between OFT rearing and ReHo values in the thalamus. Two positive correlations were found between ORT B-A and the ReHo values in the olfactory cortexand pons.

Conclusions: Telmisartan may be an effective complementary drug for individuals with depression who also exhibit memory impairments. Stress induced widespread regional alterations in the cerebrum in ReHo measures while telmissartan can reverse part of theses alterations. These data lend support for future research on the pathology of depression and provide a new insight into the effects of telmisartan on brain function in depression.

Keywords: Chronic stress, Telmisartan, fMRI, Resting state, Behavioral test, Reho, ALFF

* Correspondence: wangwei26960@126.com
[2]Beijing University of Chinese Medicine, Beijing 100029, China
Full list of author information is available at the end of the article

Background

Depression is a complex psychiatric disorder characterized by anhedonia and feelings of sadness [1]. It is not only life threatening but also has a negative impact on cognitive processes, especially learning and memory [2]. Stress is known to be a key factor in the development of depression and memory impairment. However, the pathogenes of stress leading to depression and its effective therapeutic strategies have not been clearly identified.

There are many limitations in conducting research on the etiology of depression and the efficacy of new drugs on individuals with depression due to ethical reasons. Therefore, it is imperative to use reliable preclinical animal models in order to evaluate effective therapies prior to implementing these strategies in the clinic. One rat model of depression, which was initially described by Willner [3], uses a regimen of chronic unpredictable mild stress (CUMS) to mimic the daily hassles and stress levels in humans. It has been commonly used to study the etiology of depression and antidepressant efficacy [4, 5].

Resting-state functional magnetic resonance imaging (r-fMRI), a promising neuroimaging technique that measures intrinsic or spontaneous neural activity in vivo [6], has been increasingly used to study neuropsychiatric disorders, including mild cognitive impairment (MCI) [7], depression [8], Alzheimer's disease (AD) [9], schizophrenia [10] and medial temporal lobe epilepsy [11]. In contrast to task-based experimental paradigms, r-fMRI is another way to capture brain activity from rodents that are unable to complete functional tasks due to the anesthesia and/or restraint used during traditional fMRI data acquisition [12]. Analysis of the amplitude of the low-frequency fluctuations (ALFF) and the regional homogeneity (ReHo) are two methods that investigate the resting-state activity in regions across the brain [13, 14]. These two methods have been successfully applied to detect alterations in subjects with various mental disorders [7, 8, 15, 16]. ALFF measures the amplitude of the regional spontaneous neuronal activity [17]. The ReHo method, developed by Zang et al. [14], focuses on the similarities or the coherence of intraregional spontaneous low-frequency activity, measuring the level of coordination in regional neural activity. Hence, ALFF and ReHo, which provide different types of information regarding neuronal activity, are two complementary methods that investigate alterations in the activity of the entire brain. The combination of ALFF and ReHo may provide a more comprehensive pathophysiological assessment of brain dysfunction than either method alone, especially in exploratory research.

Angiotensin type 1 receptor (AT1 receptor) blockers have attracted much attention for their possible antidepressant effects. The renin-angiotensin system (RAS) is one of the critical body reaction systems in response to stress [18]. The pathophysiological response to stressful stimuli that exceeds the body's adaptive mechanisms include increased brain Angiotensin II (Ang II) activity, amplified AT1 receptor expression, which is associated with higher hypothalamic-pituitary-adrenal (HPA) axis activation, and enhanced peripheral RAS activity [19]. In addition, excessive brain AT1 receptor activity is associated with brain inflammation [20], which is involved in the pathogenesis of emotional and cognitive impairments [21]. Telmisartan, a commonly used angiotensin receptor blockers (ARBs), is very lipophilic, which allows it to readily cross the brain-blood barrier (BBB). Because telmisartan induces central AT1 receptor blockade [22], this compound can be used as a potential oral antidepressant. Several studies have demonstrated that telmisartan is neuroprotective [23] and can attenuate cognitive impairments induced by chronic stress in rats [24]. However, there are few reports to explore which brain regions telmisartan's possible antidepressant effect is related to.

Based on the previous reports, we hypothesized that telmisartan could alleviate the depressive and cognitive dysfunction symptoms caused by chronic stress. The related brain regions could be explored by the ALFF and Reho analysis for r-fMRI. Hence, we employed the two analyses to directly compare the resting-state brain activity among normal rats, rats that were exposed to chronic stress, and rats exposed to chronic stress and administered telmisartan. In addition, the open field test (OFT), the sucrose preference test (SPT), and the object recognition test (ORT) were conducted to evaluate locomotor activity, anhedonia, and cognition in the experimental animals.

Methods

Animals

These experiments were conducted in male Sprague-Dawley rats (5 weeks), provided by Beijing Weitong Lihua Experimental Animal Technology Co., Ltd. (experimental animal production license: SCXK Beijing 2012–0001). The rats were housed 4 per cage in a temperature-(18–24 °C) and humidity-(40–60%) controlled room on a 12 h light/dark cycle (lights on at 7:00 a.m.). The rats had free access to standard laboratory food and tap water. Animal maintenance was performed according to the National Institutes of Health Guidelines for the Care and Use of Laboratory animals [25].The experimental protocols were approved by the Beijing University of Chinese Medicine Institutional Animal Care and Use Committee (Ethics number: 2013BZHYLL1001B). All efforts were made to minimize animal suffering. All animals were decapitated after anesthetized deeply with isoflurane.

Drug administration and experimental groups

After 2 weeks of acclimation, 32 rats were randomly divided into 4 groups with 8 animals per group including: (1) a Control group (C group)that was administered distilled water as a vehicle; (2) a Stress group (S group)that underwent the CUMS procedure and was administered distilled water; (3) a Stress + Telmisartan group (T-0.5 mg/kg group) that underwent the CUMS procedure and was administered telmisartan (0.5 mg/kg) dissolved in distilled water; (4) a Stress + Telmisartan group (T-1 mg/kg group) that underwent the CUMS procedure and was administered telmisartan (1 mg/kg) dissolved in distilled water. The telmisartan dose of 1 mg/kg is considered to be a nonhypotensive dose in rats [26, 27]. The rats received either telmisartan or vehicle by oral gavage each day immediately before the stress procedure.

Chronic unpredictable mild stress (CUMS) procedures

The rats in the C group were housed in groups of 4, while the rats in the S and T groups were singly housed in isolation. The following stimulations were applied to the experimental animals, according to previous CUMS rat model methods. These included 12 h food deprivation, 12 h water deprivation, overnight wet housing, forced swimming (4 °C for 5 min), 2.5 h restraint, overnight illumination, 45°cage tilt for 12 h, and 36 sessions of inescapable foot shock (1.5 mA intensity; 30 shocks in 1 min, with an inter-session interval of 30s). The rats were exposed to a random selection of 2 stressors per day, with no repetition of the same type on continuous days, in order to have the stimulation remain unpredictable. The CUMS process lasted for 4 continuous weeks. The behavioral experimental tests were performed 24 h after the last stimulation. There were no rats injured or ill during the experiment.

Open field test (OFT)

The open field test was performed to assess the rats' spontaneous exploratory activity. The open field arena was a square 100 cm × 100 cm black floor divided by 8 lines into 25 equal squares, surrounded by a 35 cm high wall. A digital camera was placed 2 m above the open field to capture the whole field. During OFT, the rats were placed in the center of the field and recorded using a small animal behavior recorder for 3 min. The rearings were counted manually during the recording. An animal behavior analysis system was used to analyze the total moved distance during the 3 min.

Sucrose preference test (SPT)

The sucrose preference test evaluated potential anhedonia in the experimental animals. The rats were trained for the SPT by providing a continuous choice of 2 bottles, which contain 2% sucrose, for 24 h. Afterwards, one of the bottles was replaced with water for 24 h. During this 24-h period, the bottles were switched after 12 h to control for any side bias. Following this adaptation procedure, the rats were deprived of water and food for 12 h. The SPT was conducted at 9:00 a.m. The rats were housed in individual cages and given free access to the 2 bottles of water and sucrose, which were weighed in advance. After 4 h, the weight of both the consumed sucrose solution and water was recorded. The sucrose preference was calculated as sucrose preference (%) = sucrose consumption (g)/(sucrose consumption (g) + water consumption (g)) × 100%.

Object recognition test (ORT)

Object recognition was evaluated in a plastic box 62 cm long, 40 cm wide and 45 cm high. The objects, which were in duplicate, were made of glass, and did not appear to have any innate significance for the subject animals. The rats were naïve to the objects, which were weighted so they could not be displaced by the test subject. ORT was performed as described previously [28]. Briefly, all rats underwent 2 habituation sessions with a 1 h inter-session interval. During habituation, the animals were allowed to freely explore the apparatus for 3 min. After 24 h, the rats returned to the testing apparatus for the experimental session. The experimental session consisted of 2 trials, which were 3 min and 5 min in duration, respectively. During the first trial (T1), the rats were exposed to 2 identical objects, A1 and A2. During the second trial (T2) 60 min later, the rats were exposed to 2 objects, a duplicate of either A1 or A2, and a new object, B. The position of the 2 objects was counter balanced and randomly permuted during T2 in order to reduce any bias due to object and place preference. Object recognition was assessed by the subject rat's T2 object exploration time. The object exploration was defined as the subject touching the object with its nose. Turning around or sitting on the object was not considered to be exploratory behavior. The time spent in exploring the 2 different objects in T2 was recorded. Object recognition was defined as variable B-A, and B-A/B + A.

fMRI acquisition

fMRI measurements were conducted on a 7.0 T /16US MRI scanner (Bruker), using a radiofrequency transmission coil (300 1H 089/072 QUAD TO AD) and a 38 mm rat head surface coil for receiving. The rats were anesthetized with isoflurane/O2 (5% for induction and 1–1.5% for maintenance) and prostrated on a custom-made holder to minimize any head motion. The respiration was monitored at a rate of 40–50 breaths per min. First, the T2-weighted data were acquired for the localization of the functional scans. Then, the resting-state functional images were recorded axially over 13 min and 26 s with the following parameters: repetition time (TR) = 3280 ms, Matrix = 128*128, echo time (TE) = 27.6 ms, flip angle = 90°, 20slices ,thickness/gap = 1.0 mm/0.2 mm, field of vision (FOV) =2.5 cm × 2.0 cm.

Statistical analysis
Behavior test data analysis
SPSS 17.0 software (SPSS v.17.0 for Windows; SPSS Inc., Chicago, IL, USA) was used to analyze the data. A Shapiro-Wilk test was used to examine the normality of the data. If the data fit a normal distribution, a one-way analysis of variance (ANOVA) was used to compare the 4 groups. For a comparison of 2 selected groups, an LSD post-hoc test was used for data with a homogeneity of variance, and a Tamhane's T2 test was used for those with a heterogeneity of variance. If the data did not have a normal distribution, a Kruskal-Wallis H test was used. A $p \leq 0.01$ was considered significant.

fMRI data analysis
The data were pre-processed using spmratIHEP based on the statistical parametric mapping (SPM8) software and Resting-State fMRI Data Analysis Toolkit (REST) software, and statistically analyzed by spmratIHEP based on SPM8. The ReHo and ALFF measures were analyzed and compared between the C, S, and T groups.

All the functional images post-processing was performed by a single experienced observer, unaware to whom the scans belonged. The pre-processing and data analysis were performed using spmratIHEP [29, 30], based on SPM8 (Welcome Department of Imaging Science; http://www.fil.ion.ucl.ac.uk/spm) and REST software (http://restfmri.net/forum/index.php?q=rest).

The voxel size of the functional datasets of all individuals were first multiplied by a factor of 5 to better approximate human dimensions, and then pre-processed using the following main steps. (1) Slice timing: the differences of slice acquisition times of each individual were corrected using slice timing. (2) Realign: the temporal processed volumes of each subject were re-aligned to the first volume to remove any head motion, and a mean image was created over the 180 re-aligned volumes. All participants had less than 1 mm of translation in the x, y, or z axis and a 1° of rotation in each axis. (3) Spatial normalization: the re-aligned volumes were spatially standardized into the Paxinos & Watson space [31] by normalizing with the EPI template via their corresponding mean image. Subsequently, all the normalized images were re-sliced by $1.0 \times 1.5 \times 1.0$ mm^3 voxels (after zooming). (4) Smooth: the normalized functional series were smoothed with a Gaussian kernel of 2mm^3 Full Width at Half-maximum (FWHM). (5) Removal of

the linear trend: the smoothed images had any systematic drift or trend removed using a linear model. (6) ALFF: the filtered estimated the value of LFF. (7) ReHo: It was calculated based on the step (3). In detail, the normalized images had any systematic drift or trend removed using a linear model. Then, the temporal band-pass filtering was performed in order to reduce the effects of low-frequency drift and high-frequency. Finally, the Kendall's coefficient was calculated to examine the degree of regional synchronization, including the 27 pixels of the fMRI time courses.

The pre-processed images were analyzed within spmratIHEP in SPM8 based on the framework of the general linear model. In order to identify the differences of the ALFF and ReHo measures between the C,S and T groups, a one-way ANOVA was performed. The cerebral regions with significant ALFF and ReHo values between 2 chosen groups were yielded based on a voxel-level height threshold of $p < 0.001$ (uncorrected) and a cluster-extent threshold of 20 voxels.

Correlations between behavior and fMRI
In order to examine the associations between the evaluated behaviors and the cerebral alterations caused by stress and telmisartan administration, we performed Pearson (data fit a normal distribution) or Spearman (data did not have a normal distribution) correlation analyses between the behavioral test indices and ALLF/ReHo values in the brain regions that exhibited significant differences between the S and C groups, as well as between the S and T groups. A $p \leq 0.05$ was considered significant. The ALLF and ReHo values were comprised of the mean value of the selected cerebral regions extracted from the smoothed individual images, which were also in the Paxinos & Watson space.

Results
The effects of stress and telmisartan on the OFT
The number of rearings in all groups fit a normal distribution with heterogeneity of variance. The Tamhane's T2 test was used to compare the 2 chosen groups. The data of total moved distance was converted to log10 format to make each group fit a normal distribution with homogeneity of variance. The LSD post-hoc test was used to compare the 2 chosen groups. The total distance was significantly decreased in the S group compared to the C group, while the number of rearings showing a decreased trend (Figs. 1 and 2, Table 1). However, there were no significant differences between theT-1 mg/kg and C groups (Figs. 1 and 2, Table 1). The T-1 mg/kg group exhibited a much higher number of rearings and moved a greater distance than the S group, although these measures were not significant between the two

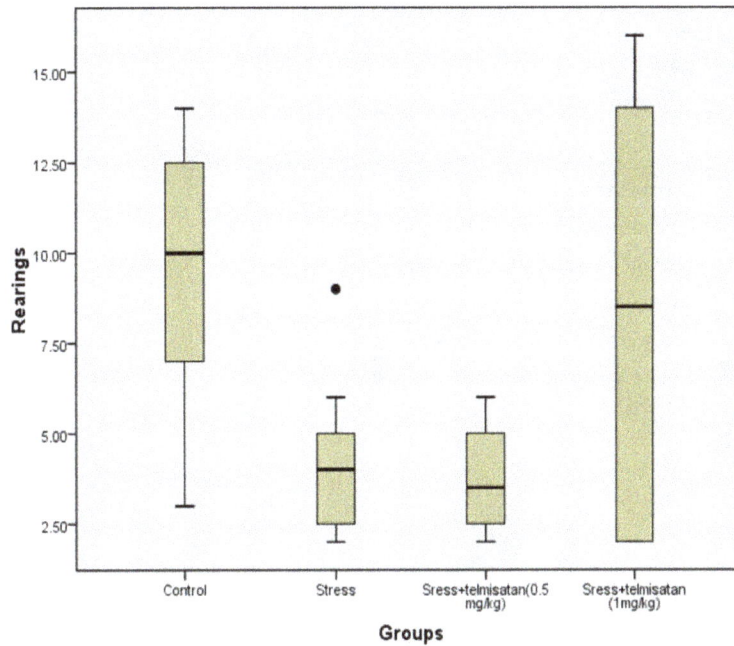

Fig. 1 Effects of stress and telmisartan on rearings (outliers)

groups (Figs. 1 and 2, Table 1). The T-0.5 mg/kg group only exhibited a much greater moved distance than the S group with no significant difference (Fig. 2, Table 1).

The effects of stress and telmisartan on the SPT
The sucrose preference measures from all groups fit a normal distribution pattern with a homogeneity of variance. The LSD was then used to compare the 2 chosen groups, followed by the ANOVA. The sucrose preferences were significantly lower in the S, T-0.5 mg/kg, and T-1 mg/kg groups than in the C group (Fig. 3). The telmisartan administration tended to improve sucrose preference, but this was not significant when compared to the S group.

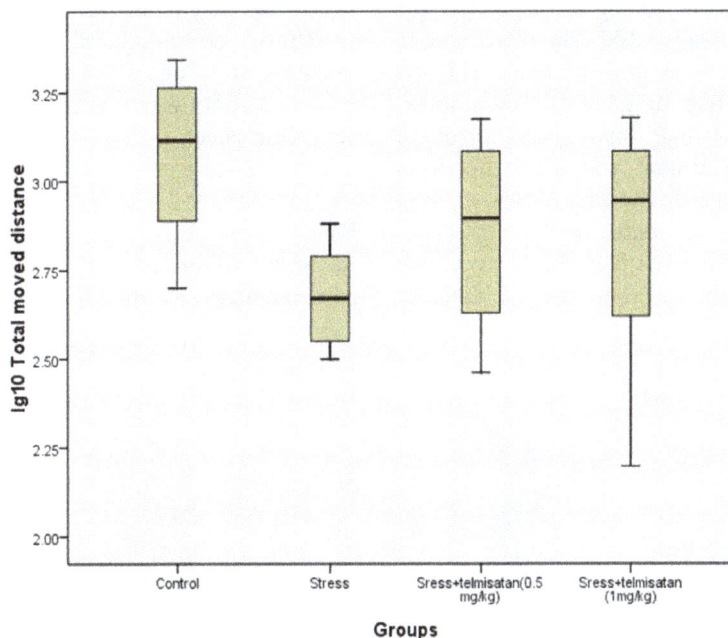

Fig. 2 Effects of stress and telmisartan on the total moved distance (unit: centimeter)

Table 1 Effects of stress and telmisartan on the OFT

Rearings		F value		P value	
		5.976		0.00	
			Effect size	Standard error of effect size	P value
	Control-Stress		5.25	1.54	0.03
	Control-Sress+telmisatan (0.5 mg/kg))		5.75	1.42	0.02
	Control-Sress+telmisatan (1 mg/kg))		1.13	2.51	1.00
	Stress-Sress+telmisatan (0.5 mg/kg))		0.50	1.00	1.00
	Stress-Sress+telmisatan (1 mg/kg))		−4.13	2.29	0.49
	Sress+telmisatan (0.5 mg/kg)-Sress+telmisatan (1 mg/kg)		−4.63	2.21	0.35
Lg10 (Total moved distance)		F value		P value	
		3.28		0.04	
			Effect size	Standard error of effect size	P value
	Control-Stress		0.40*	0.13	0.00
	Control-Sress+telmisatan (0.5 mg/kg))		0.22	0.13	0.10
	Control-Sress+telmisatan (1 mg/kg))		0.24	0.13	0.07
	Stress-Sress+telmisatan (0.5 mg/kg))		−0.18	0.13	0.16
	Stress-Sress+telmisatan (1 mg/kg))		−0.16	0.13	0.22
	Sress+telmisatan (0.5 mg/kg)-Sress+telmisatan (1 mg/kg)		0.02	0.13	0.86

Note: *$P \leq 0.01$

The effects of stress and telmisartan on the ORT

A Shapiro-Wilk test indicated that the B-A data in the S group was not normally distributed. A Kruskal-Wallis H test compared the B-A values among the 4 groups. The result was that the $x^2 = 11.96, p = 0.00$. The mean rank in each group (from high to low) was as follows: T-1 mg/kg > C > T-0.5 mg/kg > S (Fig. 4, Table 2). To some extent, these results suggest that stress caused an object recognition memory impairment and that telmisartan can attenuate this impairment. The data of B-A/A + B in each group was normally distributed, and had a homogeneity of variance. The B-A/A + B in the S group was significantly lower than the C group (Fig. 5, Table 2).

The B-A/A + B of the T-1 mg/kg group was not significantly different from the C group (Table 2), but was significantly higher than that of the S group (Table 2), suggesting that telmisartan at the dose of 1 mg/kg reversed the stress-induced object recognition memory impairment. The T-0.5 mg/kg group exhibited a higher B-A/B + A than S group but with no significant difference.

fMRI

According to the result of behavior tests, the telmisartan administration at the dose of 1 mg/kg significantly

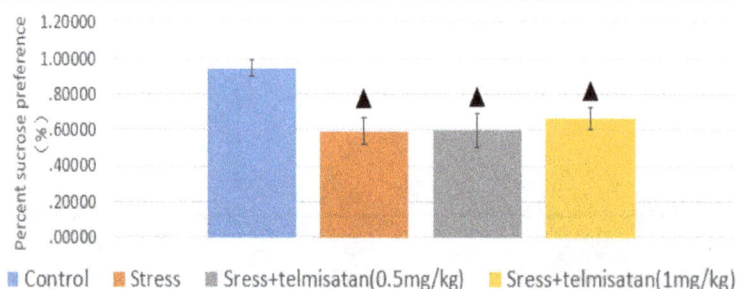

Fig. 3 Effects of stress and telmisartan on the SPT. ▲ $p \leq 0.01$ in comparison to C group, values are means±standard deviation (unit: %)

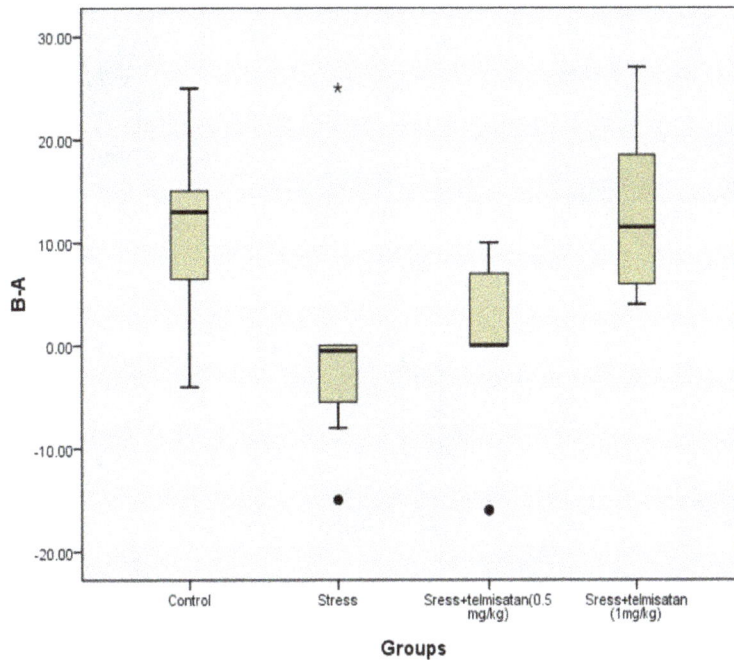

Fig. 4 Effects of stress and telmisartan on the B-A (outliers, *extreme values)

improved the behavior changes caused by stress, while the effect of telmisartan administration at the dose of 0.5 mg/kg was weak. Hence, the r- fMRI was conducted on the rats in the C, S and T-1 mg/kg groups to investigate the effects of stress and telmisatan administration on the brain.

ALFF

There were no significant alterations in ALFF between the C and S groups. The T group exhibited an increased ALFF in the insular cortex compared with the S group, and a decreased ALFF in the hypothalamus compared with the C group (Fig. 6).

Table 2 Effects of stress and telmisartan on the ORT

B-A/B + A	F value			P value	
	6.5			0.02	
			Effect size	Standard error of effect size	P value
	Control-Stress		0.71*	0.22	0.00
	Control-Sress+telmisatan (0.5 mg/kg))		0.39	0.22	0.08
	Control-Sress+telmisatan (1 mg/kg))		−0.15	0.22	0.48
	Stress-Sress+telmisatan (0.5 mg/kg))		−0.32	0.22	0.15
	Stress-Sress+telmisatan (1 mg/kg))		−0.87*	0.22	0.00
	Sress+telmisatan (0.5 mg/kg)-Sress+telmisatan (1 mg/kg)		−0.55	0.22	0.02
B-A	x2 value			P value	
	11.99			0.01	
				Mean Rank	
	Control			21.25	
	Stress			9.56	
	telmisatan (0.5 mg/kg)			12.25	
	telmisatan (1 mg/kg			22.94	

Note: *$P \leq 0.01$

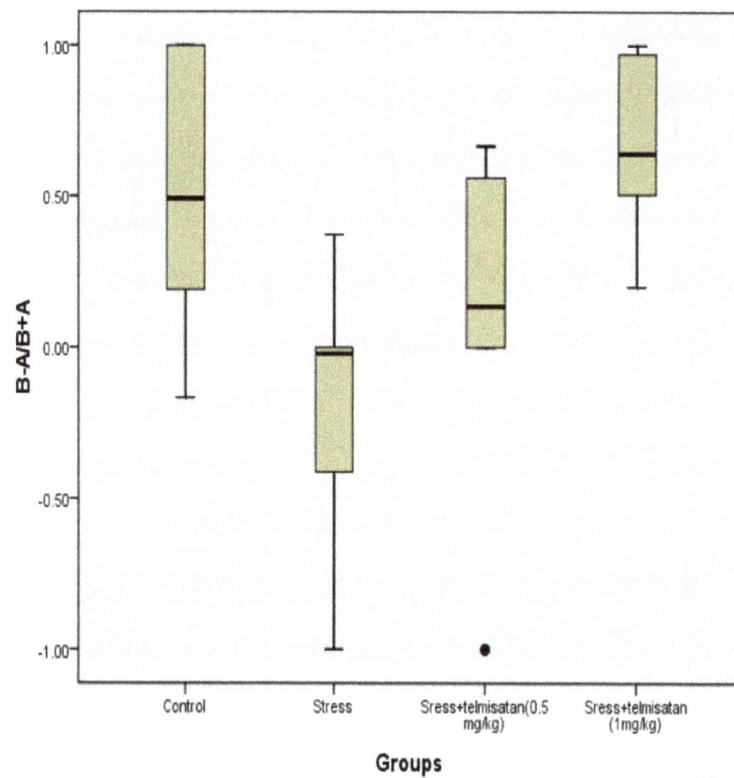

Fig. 5 Effects of stress and telmisartan on the B-A/B + A (outliers)

ReHo

There were widespread cerebral region alterations in the ReHo measures between the C, S, and T-1 mg/kg groups (Fig. 6). The S group demonstrated a decreased ReHo in the motor cortex and pons, an increased ReHo in the thalamus, visual cortex, midbrain, cerebellum, hippocampus, hypothalamus, and olfactory cortex compared to the C group. Conversely,the motor cortex in the T-1 mg/kg group displayed an increased ReHo compared with the S and C groups, suggesting that telmisartan reversed the stress-induced alterations in the motor cortex. The midbrain, thalamus, hippocampus, hypothalamus, visual cortex, and olfactory cortex in the T-1 mg/kg group exhibited a decreased ReHo compared to the S group, and an increased ReHo or no change compared to the C group, suggesting that telmisartan attenuated or eliminated the corresponding cerebral alterations caused by stress. The other cerebral regions, including the insular cortex, sensory cortex, orbital cortex, and amygdaloid body, were significantly different in their ReHo measures between the T-1 mg/kg and S groups but were not different between the C and S groups.

Correlations between behavior and fMRI

The regions with significant group differences (S vs. C) in ReHo included the motor cortex, pons, thalamus, visual cortex, midbrain, cerebellum, hippocampus, hypothalamus, and olfactory cortex. The brain regions showing significant difference between the T-1 mg/kg and S groups in ALFF or ReHo included the insular cortex, sensory cortex, orbital cortex and amygdaloid body. We analyzed the correlations between the OFT and ORT's indices and the ALLF and Reho values in the altered brain regions. The significant correlations were between the number of rearings in the OFT and the ReHo values in the thalamus ($r = -0.446$, $p = 0.029$), the value of B-A and the ReHo values in the olfactory cortex($r = 0.501$, $p = 0.013$) and pons($r = .413$, $p = 0.045$).

Discussion

The present study investigated the behavioral and cerebral alterations induced by chronic stress and telmisartan administration. To the best of our knowledge, this is the first study using ALFF and ReHo methods in a rat model of depression to examine whole brain r-fMRI alterations caused by stress and telmisartan administration.

According to our behavioral results, chronic stress decreased locomotor activity, sucrose preference and impaired ability of novel object recognition, which is in line with the results of previous studies, and suggests that we successfully established a rat model of

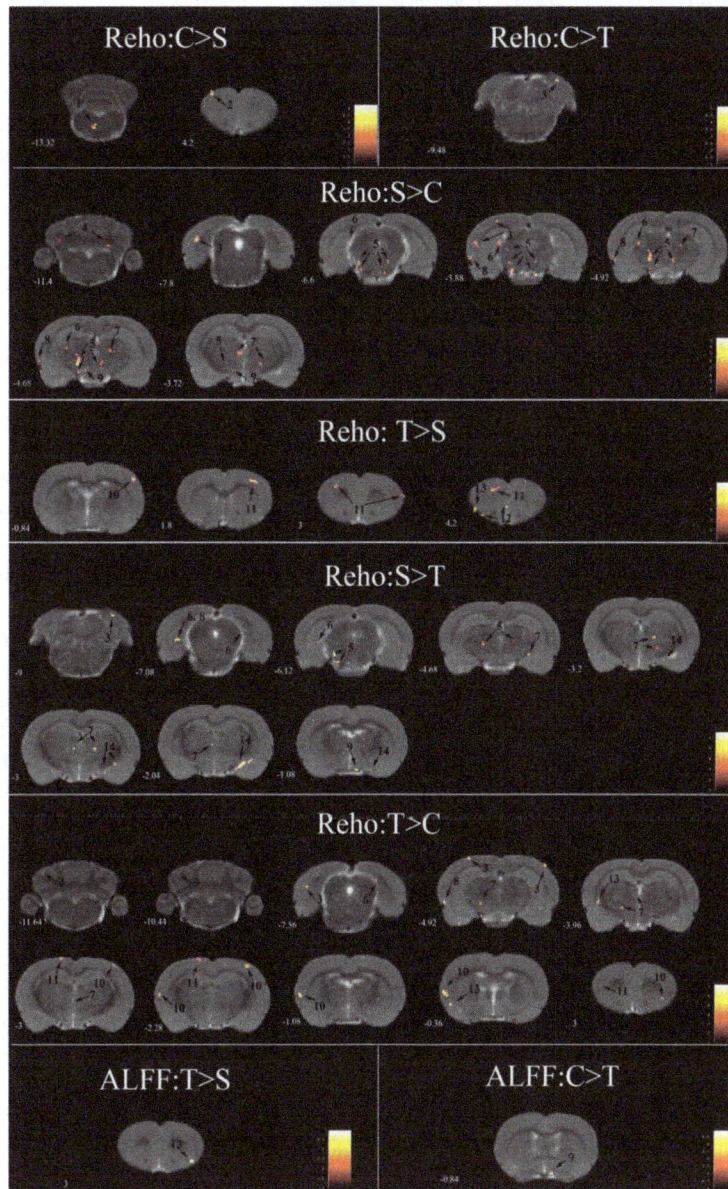

Fig. 6 Statistical maps of voxel t values of ReHo and ALFF comparisons of two chosen groups. The numbers at the bottom left of each image refer to the z coordinates in the stereotaxic space of Paxinos and Watson. The color bars were used to signify the t-value of the group analysis(the color is brighter, the t value is higher). The left side of the images corresponds to the left side of the brain, and vice versa. The numbers on each brain image stand for the different brain regions as follows: 1. pons 2. motor cortex 3.visual cortex 4. cerebellum 5. midbrain 6. hippocampus 7. dorsal thalamus 8. olfactory cortex 9. hypothalamus 10. sensory cortex 11.motor cortex 12.orbital cortex 13. insular cortex 14. amygdaloid body

depression [24, 32]. Since the dose of 1 mg/kg/day telmisartan has been proven nonhypotensive for mice [26], we applied two doses' (1 mg/kg/day and a lower dose, 0.5 mg/kg/day) telmisartan on the model. We found that the telmisartan of 1 mg/kg /day could significantly improve the impaired ability of novel object recognition, while the effect of 0.5 mg/kg/day was weak. Since the ORT indicating a kind of cognitive function, it's worth conducting additional experiments such as Morris water maze to evaluate telmisartan's potential effect on the cognitive function more comprehensively. For the tests of OFT and SPT, we found a trend for telmisartan to improve the decreased locomotor activity and sucrose preference, although these were not significant. A previous study showed that the treatment with telmisartan of 1 mg/kg for five weeks could notably improve the depressive symptoms in the stress mouse model [33]. Hence, the not significant effect may be due to the short treatment time and a relatively small dose for rats. Taken together, these data demonstrated a possible antidepressant effect with telmisartan. It's worth performing further analyses to look into the potential of telmisartan in alleviation of symptoms of depression.

We observed no significant alterations in ALFF in the chronically stressed rat compared to the normal rat. However, there were widespread cerebral region alterations in ReHo between the two groups. To some extent, it can be concluded that the coordination of regional neural activity, rather than its amplitude, may be more easily disrupted by chronic stress.

In the present study, we observed that the rats in the S group had increased ReHo in some limbic system regions, including the hippocampus, hypothalamus, thalamus, and olfactory cortex. The hippocampus, a critical structure in the limbic system, is well-known for its important role in the formation of depression [34] and cognitive decline [35]. The result of increased ReHo value in the hippocampus is consistent with a previous study on the later adult onset depression patients, supporting the validity of our findings [36]. There were rare clinical reports about the altered ReHo in the hypothalamus, though hypothalamus' pathological alterations have been widely reported in depression and cognitive impairment [37–39]. Hence, there may be differences between the rat model and patients with depression in the Reho signal of hypothalamus. Thalamus has been well positioned for an involvement in major depressive disorder pathophysiology, earning its name as the limbic thalamus [40]. Previous study has showed that cognitive decline may be related to the volume of thalamic atrophy [41]. In the present study, we found increased Reho within the thalamus in the S group, and notably, a significant negative correlation between the number of rearings in the OFT and the ReHo within the thalamus. Since OFT rearings negatively correlated with the emotionality and anxiety level in rats [42], our study demonstrated that increased Reho within the thalamus could be served as a potential neuroimaging marker for the depression. It has been found that the dysfunction of olfactory cortex was closely related with the cognitive impairment [43]. This study also found a significant positive correlation between the value of B-A and the ReHo values in the olfactory cortex, further confirmed the important role of olfactory cortex in the cognitive function.

In addition to a direct involvement of limbic system, our results demonstrated stress-induced ReHo alterations in other cerebral regions, including the cerebellum, pons, motor cortex, visual cortex, and midbrain. Previous studies have demonstrated ReHo alterations in the pons and cerebellum in depressed patients [15, 44–46], which is consistent with our study. Together, these data suggest that the pons and cerebellum are associated with

depression. These abnormalities could serve as markers for the diagnosis of depression and are worth exploring further for their role in the etiology of depression. Besides, since a significant positive correlation was found between the B-A value and the ReHo within the pons, the decreased ReHo in pons could also be a marker of cognitive impairment. The function of the motor cortex has been shown altered in depression [47], and a decreased ReHo within motor cortex was found in the generalized anxiety disorder patients [48]. Hence, the result of decreased ReHo within motor cortex in the present study may be a neuroimaging reflection of anxiety. Although several studies have demonstrated abnormal cerebral connectivity involving the visual cortex and midbrain in depression [49, 50], rare clinical studies reported altered ReHo in the two regions. Since the pathological alterations of the visual cortex and midbrain exist in depression [51–53], there may be also differences between the rat model and patients with depression in the visual cortex and midbrain Reho signal.

Telmisartan has strong anti-inflammatory effects on the brain [23, 54] and neuroprotective effects in cultured primary neurons [55], suggesting that telmisartan may be a novel therapeutic approach for the treatment of depression. Some studies suggest that telmisartan can ameliorate memory deficits through beneficially effects on the hippocampus [56, 57], little is known about which other brain regions are affected by telmisartan. Using ALFF and ReHo, our study demonstrated that stress-induced alterations in multiple brain regions were partly reversed or attenuated by telmisartan. In addition to decreased ReHo measures in the motor cortex and pons due to stress, the motor cortex in the T-1 mg/kg group displayed an increased ReHo compared to the S and C groups, suggesting that telmisartan reversed the motor cortex changes caused by stress. Increased ReHo in the midbrain, thalamus, hippocampus, hypothalamus, visual cortex, and olfactory cortex caused by stress was identified. However, the T-1 mg/kg group exhibited a decreased ReHo in these regions compared to the S group, and increased or unchanged ReHo in these regions compared to the C group. Hence, telmisartan also attenuated or eliminated these stress-induced brain region changes. Besides, since a significant negative correlation was found between the number of rearings in the OFT and the ReHo within the thalamus, telmisartan may attenuate the anxiety symptoms by decreasing the hypercoordination of neural activity within the thalamus. Thalamus could be an important brain region to investigate further in the future study. Other brain regions, including the insular cortex, the sensory cortex, the orbital cortex, and the amygdaloid body, also showed significant differences between the T-1 mg/kg and S groups. However, because there were no significant differences between the S and C groups, it is difficult to determine whether telmisartan had positive or negative effect on these brain regions. Together, our study demonstrated that telmisartan may be a potential antidepressant by beneficially affected a series of brain regions. Future research is required to determine the extent of telmisartan's effects on the brain in depression.

In conclusion, our study demonstrated widespread alterations in brain regions in a rat model of depression using the ReHo method. These regions consist of some components of the limbic system that contribute to the formation of depression, but also some other regions, such as the motor cortex, visual cortex, midbrain, cerebellum and pons, which are rarely intensively studied for their role in depression. Combined with previous clinical studies, this study revealed that the Reho alterations in several brain rigions could be potential markers for depression and cognitive impairment. Hence, this study suggests future areas for the pathological research of depression. This study also demonstrated that telmisartan can be a complementary medicine for patients with depression, and affects several brain regions. To our best knowledge, this is the first study of the telmisartan's antidepressant effect on the whole brain in a rat model of depression.

There were several limitations in our study. Firstly, the rats we used are outbred. Since genetic differences may contribute to the behavioral effects of rodents in models of depression [58], it would be more ideal to use inbred strains in the future. Secondly, we were unable to have a pre- and post-stress brain comparison due to laboratory regulations limiting the physical movement of the animals after r-fMRI. Thirdly, we only observed telmisartan's effect on the stress model due to our strict animal ethic regulations of limiting the animal number. It will be more rigorous to conduct additional groups to explore whether telmisartan could alter behavior, cognitive function or brain activity in the absence of stress for further study.

Conclusions

Despite these limitations, this study has demonstrated a series of brain regions involved in depression and telmisartan administration. We believe that this finding has instructive significance for future pathological research of depression and can provide important insight into the effects of telmisartan on nervous system function in depression.

Abbreviations
AD: Alzheimer's disease; ALFF: amplitude of low-frequency fluctuations; AngII: Angiotensin II; ANOVA: Analysis of variance; ARBs: Angiotensin receptor blockers; AT1 receptor: Angiotensin type 1 receptor; BBB: Brain-blood barrier;

C group: Control group; CUMS: Chronic unpredictable mild stress; FOV: Field of vision; FWHM: Full Width at Half-maximum; HPA: Hypothalamic-pituitary-adrenal; MCI: Mild cognitive impairment; OFT: Open field test; ORT: Object recognition test; RAS: Renin-angiotensin system; ReHo: Regional homogeneity; r-fMRI: Resting-state functional magnetic resonance imaging; S group: Stress group; SNc: Substantia nigra pars compacta; SPT: Sucrose preference test; T-0.5 mg/kg group: Telmisartan(0.5 mg/kg)group; T-1 mg/kg group: Telmisartan(1 mg/kg)group; T1: The first trial; T2: The second trial; TE: Echo time; TR: Repetition time; VAT: Ventral tegmental area

Acknowledgements
We would like to thank Jianfeng Lei in the nuclear magnetic laboratory for assisting with fMRI acquisition.

Funding
Supported by National Natural Science Foundation of China (No. 81470191), National Natural Science Foundation of China (No. 81703863), and a Grant from the National Basic Research Program of China (973 Program No. 2011CB505106).

Authors' contributions
JL, RY, and WW conceived and designed the experiments; JL, KX, TW and YL performed the experiments; BN, JC and HZ analyzed and discussed the data. JL and KG wrote the manuscript; All authors read and approved the final manuscript.

Consent for publication
Not applicable.

Competing interests
Author Wei Wang is currently acting as a Section Editor for BMC Psychiatry. The authors declare that they have no competing interests.

Author details
[1]School of Traditional Chinese Medicine, Capital Medical University, Beijing 100069, China. [2]Beijing University of Chinese Medicine, Beijing 100029, China. [3]Cardiovascular department of Guang'anmen Hospital, China Academy of Chinese Medical Sciences, Beijing 100053, China. [4]Key Laboratory of Nuclear Analytical Techniques, Institute of High Energy Physics, Chinese Academy of Sciences, Beijing 100049, China. [5]Institute of Basic Theory for Chinese Medicine, China Academy of Chinese Medical Sciences, Beijing 100700, China.

References
1. Gronli J, Murison R, Fiske E, Bjorvatn B, Sorensen E, Portas CM, Ursin R. Effects of chronic mild stress on sexual behavior, locomotor activity and consumption of sucrose and saccharine solutions. Physiol Behav. 2005;84(4):571–7.
2. Hui J, Zhang J, Pu M, et al. Modulation of GSK-3beta/beta-Catenin Signaling Contributes to Learning and Memory Impairment in a Rat Model of Depression[J]. Int J Neuropsychopharmacol. 2018;21(9):858–70.
3. Willner P. Validity, reliability and utility of the chronic mild stress model of depression: a 10-year review and evaluation. Psychopharmacology. 1997;134(4):319–29.
4. Segev A, Rubin AS, Abush H, Richter-Levin G, Akirav I. Cannabinoid receptor activation prevents the effects of chronic mild stress on emotional learning and LTP in a rat model of depression. Neuropsychopharmacology. 2014;39(4):919–33.

5.   Xing Y, He J, Hou J, Lin F, Tian J, Kurihara H. Gender differences in CMS and the effects of antidepressant venlafaxine in rats. Neurochem Int. 2013;63(6):570-5.

6.   Fox MD, Raichle ME. Spontaneous fluctuations in brain activity observed with functional magnetic resonance imaging. NAT REV NEUROSCI. 2007;8(9):700-11.

7.   Han Y, Wang J, Zhao Z, Min B, Lu J, Li K, He Y, Jia J. Frequency-dependent changes in the amplitude of low-frequency fluctuations in amnestic mild cognitive impairment: a resting-state fMRI study. NEUROIMAGE. 2011;55(1):287-95.

8.   Liu CH, Li F, Li SF, Wang YJ, Tie CL, Wu HY, Zhou Z, Zhang D, Dong J, Yang Z, et al. Abnormal baseline brain activity in bipolar depression: a resting state functional magnetic resonance imaging study. Psychiatry Res. 2012;203(2-3):175-9.

9.   He Y, Wang L, Zang Y, Tian L, Zhang X, Li K, Jiang T. Regional coherence changes in the early stages of Alzheimer's disease: a combined structural and resting-state functional MRI study. NEUROIMAGE. 2007;35(2):488-500.

10. Hoptman MJ, Zuo XN, Butler PD, Javitt DC, D'Angelo D, Mauro CJ, Milham MP. Amplitude of low-frequency oscillations in schizophrenia: a resting state fMRI study. Schizophr Res. 2010;117(1):13-20.

11. Zhang ZQ, Lu GM, Zhong Y, Tan QF, Zhu JG, Jiang L, Chen ZL, Wang ZQ, Shi JX, Zang YF, et al. Application of amplitude of low-frequency fluctuation to the temporal lobe epilepsy with bilateral hippocampal sclerosis: an fMRI study. Zhonghua Yi Xue Za Zhi. 2008;88(23):1594-8.

12. Gass N, Cleppien D, Zheng L, Schwarz AJ, Meyer-Lindenberg A, Vollmayr B, Weber-Fahr W. Sartorius: functionally altered neurocircuits in a rat model of treatment-resistant depression show prominent role of the habenula. Eur Neuropsychopharmacol. 2014;24:381-90.

13. Zang YF, He Y, Zhu CZ, Cao QJ, Sui MQ, Liang M, Tian LX, Jiang TZ, Wang YF. Altered baseline brain activity in children with ADHD revealed by resting-state functional MRI. Brain and Development. 2007;29(2):83-91.

14. Zang Y, Jiang T, Lu Y, He Y, Tian L. Regional homogeneity approach to fMRI data analysis. NEUROIMAGE. 2004;22(1):394-400.

15. Wang L, Li K, Zhang Q, Zeng Y, Dai W, Su Y, Wang G, Tan Y, Jin Z, Yu X, et al. Short-term effects of escitalopram on regional brain function in first-episode drug-naive patients with major depressive disorder assessed by resting-state functional magnetic resonance imaging. Psychol Med. 2014;44(7):1417-26.

16. Yang H, Long X, Yang Y, Yan H, Zhu C, Zhou X, Gong Q. Amplitude of low frequency fluctuation within visual areas revealed by resting-state functional MRI. Neuroimage. 2007;36(1):144-52.

17. Liu CH, Ma X, Li F, Wang YJ, Tie CL, Li SF, Chen TL, Fan TT, Zhang Y, Dong J, et al. Regional homogeneity within the default mode network in bipolar depression: a resting-state functional magnetic resonance imaging study. PLOS ONE. 2012;7(11):e48181.

18. Yang G, Wan Y, Zhu Y. Angiotensin II--an important stress hormone. Biol Signals. 1996;5(1):1-8.

19. Saavedra JM, Sanchez-Lemus E, Benicky J. Blockade of brain angiotensin II AT1 receptors ameliorates stress, anxiety, brain inflammation and ischemia: therapeutic implications. PSYCHONEUROENDOCRINO. 2011;36(1):1-18.

20. Saavedra JM. Angiotensin II AT(1) receptor blockers as treatments for inflammatory brain disorders. Clin Sci (Lond). 2012;123(10):567-90.

21. Castanon N, Luheshi G, Laye S. Role of neuroinflammation in the emotional and cognitive alterations displayed by animal models of obesity. Front Neurosci. 2015;9:229.

22. Wang JM, Tan J, Leenen FH. Central nervous system blockade by peripheral administration of AT1 receptor blockers. J Cardiovasc Pharmacol. 2003;41(4):593-9.

23. Pang T, Wang J, Benicky J, Sanchez-Lemus E, Saavedra JM. Telmisartan directly ameliorates the neuronal inflammatory response to IL-1beta partly through the JNK/c-Jun and NADPH oxidase pathways. J Neuroinflammation. 2012;9:102.

24. Wincewicz D, Braszko JJ. Telmisartan attenuates cognitive impairment caused by chronic stress in rats. Pharmacol Rep. 2014;66(3):436-41.

25. National Research Council. Guide for the care and use of laboratory animals (8th edition). Washington DC: National Academies; 2011.

26. Washida K, Ihara M, Nishio K, Fujita Y, Maki T, Yamada M, Takahashi J, Wu X, Kihara T, Ito H et al. Nonhypotensive dose of telmisartan attenuates cognitive impairment partially due to peroxisome proliferator-activated receptor-gamma activation in mice with chronic cerebral hypoperfusion. Stroke. 2010;41(8):1798-806.

27. Wienen W, Hauel N, Van Meel JC, Narr B, Ries U, Entzeroth M. Pharmacological characterization of the novel nonpeptide angiotensin II receptor antagonist, BIBR 277. Br J Pharmacol. 1993;110(1):245-52.

28. Wincewicz D, Braszko JJ. Telmisartan attenuates cognitive impairment caused by chronic stress in rats. PHARMACOL REP. 2014;66(3):436-41.

29. Nie B, Chen K, Zhao S, Liu J, Gu X, Yao Q, Hui J, Zhang Z, Teng G, Zhao C, et al. A rat brain MRI template with digital stereotaxic atlas of fine anatomical delineations in paxinos space and its automated application in voxel-wise analysis. HUM BRAIN MAPP 2013. 34(6):1306-18.

30. Nie B, Liu H, Chen K, Jiang X, Shan B. A statistical parametric mapping toolbox used for voxel-wise analysis of FDG-PET images of rat brain. PLoS One. 2014;9(9):e108295.

31. Watson C, Paxinos G. The rat brain in stereotaxic coordinates. 5th ed. edition. Amsterdam: Elsevier Academic Press; 2005.

32. Ding L, Zhang X, Guo H, Yuan J, Li S, Hu W, Golden T, Wu N. The functional study of a Chinese herbal compounded antidepressant medicine--Jie Yu Chu fan capsule on chronic unpredictable mild stress mouse model. PLoS One. 2015;10(7):e133405.

33. Li Y, Cheng KC, Liu KF, Peng WH, Cheng JT, Niu HS. Telmisartan activates PPARdelta to improve symptoms of unpredictable chronic mild stress-induced depression in mice. Sci Rep. 2017;7(1):14021.

34. Lorenzetti V, Allen NB, Fornito A, Yucel M. Structural brain abnormalities in major depressive disorder: a selective review of recent MRI studies. J Affect Disord. 2009;117(1-2):1-17.

35. Neumeister A, Charney DS, Drevets WC. Hippocampus, VI. Depression and the Hippocampus. Am J Psychiatry. 2005;162(6):10.

36. Shen Z, Jiang L, Yang S, Ye J, Dai N, Liu X, Li N, Lu J, Liu F, Lu Y, et al. Identify changes of brain regional homogeneity in early and later adult onset patients with first-episode depression using resting-state fMRI. PLoS One. 2017;12(9):e184712.

37. Wang SS, Kamphuis W, Huitinga I, Zhou JN, Swaab DF. Gene expression analysis in the human hypothalamus in depression by laser microdissection and real-time PCR: the presence of multiple receptor imbalances. Mol Psychiatry. 2008;13(8):786-799, 741.

38. Mironova VI, Rybnikova EA, Rakitskaya VV. Expression of vasopressin in the hypothalamus of active and passive rats with poststress depression. Bull Exp Biol Med. 2005;140(6):668-71.

39. Liu X, Chen W, Tu Y, Hou H, Huang X, Chen X, Guo Z, Bai G, Chen W. The abnormal functional connectivity between the hypothalamus and the temporal gyrus Underl ying depression in Alzheimer's disease patients. Front Aging Neurosci. 2018;10:37.

40. Cardoso EF, Maia FM, Fregni F, Myczkowski ML, Melo LM, Sato JR, Marcolin MA, Rigonatti SP, Cruz AJ, Barbosa ER, et al. Depression in Parkinson's disease: convergence from voxel-based morphometry and functional magnetic resonance imaging in the limbic thalamus. NEUROIMAGE. 2009; 47(2):467-72.

41. Bivard A, Lillicrap T, Marechal B, Garcia-Esperon C, Holliday E, Krishnamurthy V, Levi CR, Parsons M. Transient ischemic attack results in delayed brain atrophy and cognitive decline. STROKE. 2018;49(2):384-90.

42. Grabovskaya SV, Salyha YT. Do results of the open field test depend on the arena shape? NEUROPHYSIOLOGY. 2014;46(4):376-80.

43. Vasavada MM, Martinez B, Wang J, Eslinger PJ, Gill DJ, Sun X, Karunanayaka P, Yang QX. Central olfactory dysfunction in Alzheimer's disease and mild cognitive impairment: a functional MRI study. J Alzheimers Dis. 2017;59(1):359-68.

44. Liang MJ, Zhou Q, Yang KR, Yang XL, Fang J, Chen WL, Huang Z. Identify changes of brain regional homogeneity in bipolar disorder and unipolar depression using resting-state FMRI. PLoS One. 2013;8(12):e79999.

45. Guo WB, Sun XL, Liu L, Xu Q, Wu RR, Liu ZN, Tan CL, Chen HF, Zhao JP. Disrupted regional homogeneity in treatment-resistant depression: a resting-state fMRI study. Prog Neuro-Psychopharmacol Biol Psychiatry. 2011;35(5):1297-302.

46. Li J, Li GX, Guo Y, Lu XQ, Li L, Ding JP. Regional homogeneity in the patients of irritable bowel syndrome complicated with depression: a resting-state functional magnetic resonance imaging study. Zhonghua Yi Xue Za Zhi. 2018;98(3):196-201.

47. Maeda F, Keenan JP, Pascual-Leone A. Interhemispheric asymmetry of motor cortical excitability in major depression as measured by transcranial magnetic stimulation. Br J Psychiatry. 2000;177:169-73.

48. Xia L, Li S, Wang T, Guo Y, Meng L, Feng Y, Cui Y, Wang F, Ma J, Jiang G. Spontaneous alterations of regional brain activity in patients with adult generalized anxiety disorder. Neuropsychiatr Dis Treat. 2017;13:1957-65.

49. Samara Z, Evers E, Peeters F, Uylings H, Rajkowska G, Ramaekers JG, Stiers P. Orbital and medial prefrontal cortex functional connectivity of major depression vulnerability and disease. Biol Psychiatry Cogn Neurosci Neuroimaging. 2018;3(4):348–57.

50. Kumar P, Goer F, Murray L, Dillon DG, Beltzer ML, Cohen AL, Brooks NH, Pizzagalli DA. Impaired reward prediction error encoding and striatal-midbrain connectivity in depression. NEUROPSYCHOPHARMACOL. 2018; 43(7):1581–8.

51. Homberg JR, Lesch KP. Looking on the bright side of serotonin transporter gene variation. Biol Psychiatry. 2011;69(6):513–9.

52. Hsieh PC, Chen KC, Yeh TL, Lee IH, Chen PS, Yao WJ, Chiu NT, Chen CC, Liao MH, Yang YK. Lower availability of midbrain serotonin transporter between healthy subjects with and without a family history of major depressive disorder - a preliminary two-ligand SPECT study. Eur Psychiatry. 2014;29(7):414–8.

53. Dahlstrom M, Ahonen A, Ebeling H, Torniainen P, Heikkila J, Moilanen I. Elevated hypothalamic/midbrain serotonin (monoamine) transporter availability in depressive drug-naive children and adolescents. Mol Psychiatry. 2000;5(5):514–22.

54. Xu Y, Xu Y, Wang Y, Wang Y, He L, Jiang Z, Huang Z, Liao H, Li J, Saavedra JM, et al. Telmisartan prevention of LPS-induced microglia activation involves M2 microglia polarization via CaMKKbeta-dependent AMPK activation. Brain Behav Immun. 2015;50:298–313.

55. Wang J, Pang T, Hafko R, Benicky J, Sanchez-Lemus E, Saavedra JM. Telmisartan ameliorates glutamate-induced neurotoxicity: roles of AT(1) receptor blockade and PPARgamma activation. NEUROPHARMACOLOGY. 2014;79:249–61.

56. Du GT, Hu M, Mei ZL, Wang C, Liu GJ, Hu M, Long Y, Miao MX, Chang LJ, Hong H. Telmisartan treatment ameliorates memory deficits in streptozotocin-induced diabetic mice via attenuating cerebral amyloidosis. J Pharmacol Sci. 2014;124(4):418–26.

57. Shindo T, Takasaki K, Uchida K, Onimura R, Kubota K, Uchida N, Irie K, Katsurabayashi S, Mishima K, Nishimura R, et al. Ameliorative effects of telmisartan on the inflammatory response and impaired spatial memory in a rat model of Alzheimer's disease incorporating additional cerebrovascular disease factors. Biol Pharm Bull. 2012;35(12):2141–7.

58. Jung YH, Hong SI, Ma SX, Hwang JY, Kim JS, Lee JH, Seo JY, Lee SY, Jang CG. Strain differences in the chronic mild stress animal model of depression and anxiety in mice. Biomol Ther (Seoul). 2014;22(5):453–9.

11

Prevalence of post-traumatic stress disorder, acute stress disorder and depression following violence related injury treated at the emergency department

Robbin H. Ophuis[*] [iD], Branko F. Olij, Suzanne Polinder and Juanita A. Haagsma

Abstract

Background: In order to gain insight into the health impact of violence related injury, the psychological consequences should be taken into account. There has been uncertainty regarding the prevalence of posttraumatic stress disorder (PTSD), acute stress disorder (ASD), and depression among patients with violence related injury. An overview of prevalence rates may inform our understanding of both prognosis and recovery for these patients. Therefore, we aim to provide an overview of the published literature reporting the prevalence rates and trajectories of PTSD, ASD, and depression following violence related injury, and to assess the quality of the studies included.

Methods: A systematic review was conducted in order to provide an overview of the published literature reporting the prevalence of PTSD, ASD and depression following violence related injury treated at the emergency department or hospital. The EMBASE, MEDLINE, Cochrane Central, PubMed, and PsycINFO databases were searched systematically. The quality of the included studies was assessed.

Results: We included sixteen studies reporting the prevalence rates of PTSD, ASD, or depression. Clear prevalence trajectories could not be identified because the range of prevalence rates was diverse at each time point. Heterogeneity resulting from the use of different diagnostic instruments limited comparability. The included studies were susceptible to bias due to low response rates and loss to follow-up.

Conclusions: The differences in diagnostic instruments limited comparability of the prevalence rates. Therefore, clear prevalence trajectories could not be identified. Study participation and loss to follow-up require more attention in future studies. Uniformity in diagnostic procedures is needed in order to draw general conclusions on the prevalence of PTSD, ASD, and depression following violence related injury.

Keywords: Depression, Post-traumatic stress disorder, Trauma, Violence, Injury, Emergency department, Prevalence

* Correspondence: r.ophuis@erasmusmc.nl
Department of Public Health, Erasmus University Medical Center, PO Box 2040, 3000, CA, Rotterdam, The Netherlands

Background

More than 1.5 million people worldwide die from violence related injury every year, and even more people suffer from non-fatal injury caused by violence [1]. Approximately 1.4 million non-fatal violence related injuries are treated annually in hospital emergency departments (ED) in the US [2]. In Western Europe, 670,000 violence related injuries require medical treatment each year [3]. According to the diagnostic and statistical manual for mental disorders (DSM), exposure to serious injury is an example of a traumatic event [4]. Longitudinal studies of responses to traumatic events show that mental disorders such as post-traumatic stress disorder (PTSD), acute stress disorder (ASD), and depression frequently occur after experiencing a traumatic event, although the course can be variable [5].

PTSD and ASD are trauma and stressor-related psychiatric disorders that could occur after experiencing or witnessing events involving physical injury, death, or other threats to the physical integrity [4]. Re-experience of the traumatic event and avoidance of trauma-related stimuli are the main symptoms of trauma and stressor-related disorders [4]. Unlike PTSD and ASD, depression is a mental disorder that is not directly linked to a traumatic event. However, substantial depression prevalence rates have been reported among patients who experienced a traumatic event such as interpersonal violence [6, 7]. A depressive episode is characterized by a constant depressed mood, loss of interest, or loss of pleasure [4].

A systematic review by Santiago et al. [5] reported that PTSD trajectories differ between patients exposed to intentional and non-intentional traumatic events. The PTSD prevalence among patients exposed to non-intentional traumatic events decreased in time, whereas the prevalence among patients exposed to intentional traumatic events increased. This might suggest that the PTSD trajectory of patients with violence-related injury differs from patients with non-intentional injury. However, Santiago et al. [5] also included studies on victims of terroristic attacks, war, and hostage situations in their systematic review. These participants did not necessarily sustain injury. It therefore remains unclear what the specific trajectories are for patients with violence related injury. Furthermore, little is known about the prevalence and trajectories of ASD and depression in this specific population.

In order to gain insight into the total health impact of injury following violence, the psychological consequences should be taken into account given the high prevalence rates of PTSD, ASD, and depression that have been reported post-injury [5, 8–10]. This paper provides PTSD, ASD, and depression prevalence estimates among patients with violence related injury, which may inform our understanding of both prognosis and recovery for these patients.

An overview of prevalence rates provides insight into the public health treatment needs. Targeted interventions can be provided when the PTSD, ASD and depression trajectories of patients who sustained violence related injury are known. Therefore, we aim to (1) provide an overview of the published literature reporting the prevalence rates and trajectories of ASD, PTSD, and depression following violence related injury, and (2) to assess the quality of the studies included.

Methods

In order to identify studies reporting the prevalence rates of ASD, PTSD, and depression among patients who sustained violence related injury, a systematic literature review was conducted. The methods and reporting of this systematic review are in concordance with the PRISMA statement on reporting standards for systematic reviews [11]. The study protocol is registered in the PROSPERO international prospective register of systematic reviews (registration number CRD42016043167).

Literature search

Relevant studies were identified through systematic literature searches in the EMBASE, MEDLINE, Cochrane Central, PubMed, and PsycINFO databases. The search strategies were developed in consultation with a medical librarian. A detailed description of the search strategy can be found in the Additional file 1. Reference lists and citation indices of the included papers were inspected to identify additional relevant citations. We restricted searches to English-language papers, published in peer-reviewed journals before November 2017.

Study selection

Studies reporting the prevalence of PTSD, ASD, or depression after ED or hospital treated injury following interpersonal violence were included in this review. We defined the following inclusion and exclusion criteria:

Participants

Studies were included if the injury was intentionally caused by another person or persons, such as (sexual) assault or stabbing. Studies on violent incidents that not necessarily involve injury, such as hostage situations or witnessing terroristic attacks, were excluded. Studies on a mixed population, e.g. all trauma patients, were only included if they reported separate prevalence rates for injury caused by intentional violence (excluding self-harm). We only included studies on patients who have been treated at the ED or hospital in order to maintain comparability in terms of injury severity. We did not apply restrictions on countries or regions in which studies were conducted. Studies on adults, children, and adolescents were included.

Outcome

We included studies in which the prevalence rates of PTSD, ASD or depression were reported directly or indirectly (i.e. by reporting the number of cases and the total number of patients) based on a validated questionnaire or diagnostic interview. We applied the case definitions and diagnostic thresholds as reported in the individual studies.

Study design

Prospective and retrospective cohort studies, longitudinal studies, cross-sectional studies, time series, and clinical trials were included. We excluded reviews, qualitative studies, case reports, editorials, and study protocols.

Data extraction

Titles and abstracts of all identified studies were screened for relevance by one reviewer (RO, BO, or JH). After initial selection, the remaining records were independently read in full-text by two reviewers (RO and BO) for the eligibility assessment. Discrepancies were discussed and resolved by consulting a third reviewer (JH). Two reviewers (RO and BO) extracted data on the study populations, study setting, injury details, prevalence rates, diagnostic instruments, and follow-up. If possible, we provided prevalence rates at different points in time. We used approximations when specific time points were not reported. For example, when 'within two weeks after ED admission' was reported as time indication, the midpoint (one week) was used. We reported gender-specific prevalence rates and measures of injury severity if provided.

Quality assessment

A quality assessment in terms of risk of bias was performed with the Quality in Prognosis Studies (QUIPS) tool [12], which was developed for assessing the risk of bias of prognostic studies. Although the current systematic review does not focus on prognostic studies, we used the QUIPS tool because it covers general quality criteria on risk of bias. We considered these general criteria as appropriate because of the variety of study designs included in our study. The following domains of the QUIPS were selected in order to assess the risk of bias: study participation, study attrition, outcome measurement, and statistical analysis. Two reviewers (RO and BO) independently used the QUIPS tool to assess the risk of bias. Each domain was scored as 'low risk', 'moderate risk' or 'high risk'. Any discrepancies in the domain scores were resolved via discussion until consensus was reached.

Results

Literature search

In total, the literature search yielded 3556 articles. After excluding 1537 duplicates, the titles and abstracts of 2019 articles were screened for relevance. The screening of titles and abstracts resulted in the exclusion of 1979 articles. Forty studies were left for full-text eligibility assessment, of which 24 were excluded for several main reasons: no prevalence reported, no violence related injury, no ED or hospital admission, literature review. Finally, sixteen studies were included in the systematic review. A flow chart of the study identification process is presented in Fig. 1.

Study characteristics

The majority of the studies were conducted in the United States (*n* = 10) [13–22] (Table 1). The remaining studies were conducted in the United Kingdom (*n* = 3) [23–25], Denmark (*n* = 1) [26], and Norway (*n* = 2) [27, 28]. Seven studies included patients aged eighteen years and older [14, 20–22, 26–28] and two studies included patients aged sixteen years and older [23, 25]. In two studies [13, 24], the age of the participants was not specified. The remaining five studies applied different age criteria (Table 1) [15, 19].

All studies included patients who presented to the ED, trauma center, or hospital with injury following intentional violence. Alarcon et al. [13] included patients with the ICD-9-CM injury codes 800–995, covering injury such as open wounds and fractures. Injury related to sexual assault was excluded in three studies [14, 15, 19] and injury caused by domestic violence was excluded in four studies [19, 24, 27, 28]. In four studies on children and adolescents, injury caused by child abuse was excluded [15, 16, 18, 19].

Diagnostic instruments

A full structured clinical interview was used as diagnostic instrument in four out of sixteen studies [15, 20, 22, 24]. All DSM IV or V diagnostic criteria for PTSD (*n* = 4) and depression (*n* = 1) were met in these studies (Table 2). The Child and Adolescents Trauma Survey for assessing PTSD symptoms was used as diagnostic instrument in two studies [16, 18]. In both studies, patients were considered having PTSD when they scored 27 or higher. The Immediate Stress Response Checklist for ASD was used in the same studies [16, 18], although one of these studies did not report a cut-off score [18]. The diagnostic instruments used in the other studies were all different from each other. Twelve out of sixteen studies (75%) used brief questionnaires based on self-report or screening measures to obtain probable diagnoses. Therefore, these studies may have included individuals who would not have met the diagnostic criteria for ASD, PTSD, or depression if a

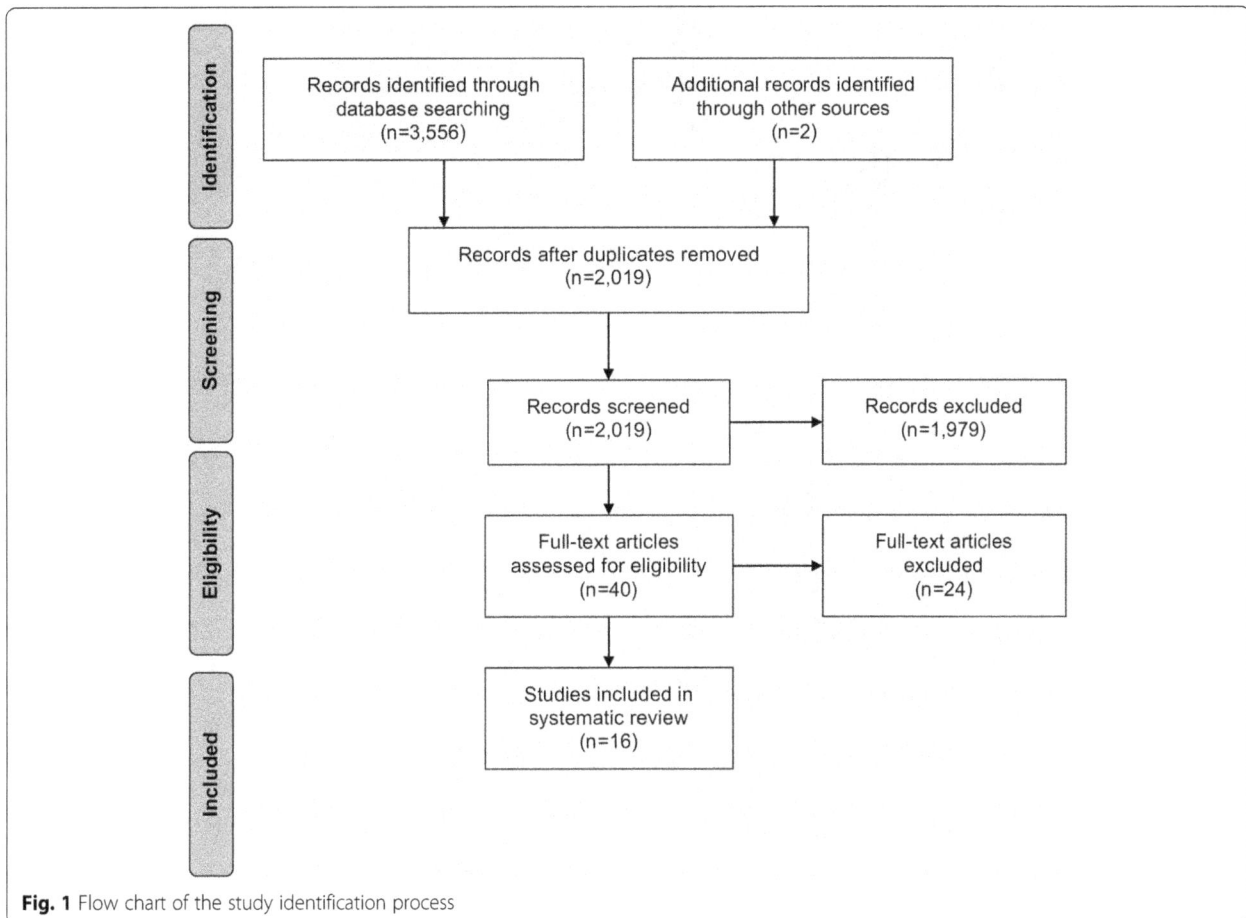

Fig. 1 Flow chart of the study identification process

full diagnostic interview would have been conducted. Brief questionnaires are mainly focused on symptoms whereas in a full diagnostic interview impairment is assessed as well.

Prevalence rates

The PTSD, ASD, and depression prevalence rates at different points in time are reported in Table 2. Fifteen studies reported the prevalence of PTSD following violence related injury [13, 15–28], five studies reported the prevalence of ASD [14, 16, 18, 24, 26], and five studies reported the prevalence of depression [14, 15, 17, 18, 21]. The PTSD prevalence at 1, 3, 6, and 12 months post-injury ranged between 11.0–60.9%, 5.8–30.4%, 1.9–23.9%, and 16.3–27.1% respectively. The following range of ASD prevalence rates were reported < 1 week post-injury and 1–2 weeks post-injury: 24.0–24.6% and 11.7–40.6%. Four studies reported depression prevalence rates < 1 month post-injury ranging between 3.0 and 35.3%. Beyond one month post-injury, a prevalence rate of 16.8% was reported. Heterogeneity resulting from the use of different diagnostic instruments strongly limited the comparability of the reported prevalence rates of PTSD, ASD, and depression. In total, one study reported injury severity of

the target population [26] and one study reported gender-specific prevalence rates [27] (Table 2).

Quality assessment

Of all 64 possible scoring options (four quality domains times sixteen studies), the reviewers disagreed on five scoring options resulting in a disagreement rate of 7.8%. Two of the disagreements belonged to the study participation domain and three to the outcome measurement domain. Disagreements were resolved after discussion. Table 3 describes the risk of bias per domain (study participation, study attrition, outcome measurement, and statistical analysis) for all studies included. The study by Pailler et al. [18] was the only study with a low risk of bias on all four domains. The study attrition domain was mainly scored as high risk (83%) because of low participation rates and/or poor descriptions of the patients lost to follow-up. One study scored 'low risk' in this domain [18]. The statistical analyses and the presentation of the results were adequate in all studies. Therefore, all studies scored 'low risk' on the statistical analyses domain. The outcome measurement domain was mainly scored as low risk (67%). The majority had a low risk score for the study participation domain (67%), but one study had a

Table 1 Overview of the study characteristics reporting the prevalence of ASD, PTSD, or depression following violence related injury

Authors, year, country, ref.	Study population	Setting details	Violence and injury details	Disorder	DSM criteria[a]
Alarcon et al., 2012, USA, [13]	Injured patients treated at the ED, age not specified	Urban level I trauma center	Assault	PTSD	No
Bisson et al., 2010, UK, [23]	Patients aged over 16 years, treated at the ED following physical assault	ED	Assault	PTSD	No
Boccelari et al., 2007, USA, [14]	Patients aged 18 years and older who are victims of violent crime treated at the ED, with and without hospitalization	Urban hospital	All types of violence, sexual assault excluded	Depression, ASD	No
Cunningham et al., 2015, USA, [15]	Patients aged between 14 and 24 years treated at the ED following assault	Urban public ED, high crime rates in region	Assault, sexual assault and child abuse excluded	Depression, PTSD	Yes, DSM-IV
Elklit et al., 2003, Denmark, [26]	Patients aged 18 years and older who are victims of physical assault, treated at the ED	ED	Assault, mean Injury Severity Score 1.47, two-third of the sample had head and face injuries	ASD, PTSD	No
Fein et al., 2002, USA, [16]	Patients aged between 12 and 24 years treated at the ED for intentional violence	Urban EDs	Assault/fights, child abuse and domestic violence excluded	ASD, PTSD	No
Hunt et al., 2016, USA, [20]	Injured trauma survivors aged 18 years and older, admitted to trauma center, 8.6% of the patients were victims of intentional stabbing	Two level I trauma centers	Stabbing	PTSD	Yes, DSM-V
Johansen et al., 2006, Norway, [27]	Patients aged over 18, treated at the ED following assault	ED	Assault, domestic violence excluded	PTSD	No
Johansen et al., 2007, Norway, [28]	Patients aged 18 years and older, treated at the ED following physical assault	ED	Assault, domestic violence excluded	PTSD	No
Kleim et al., 2007, UK, [24]	Patients treated at the ED following assault, mean age 35 years	ED	Assault, domestic violence excluded	ASD, PTSD	PTSD only, DSM-IV
McCart et al., 2005, USA, [17]	Patients aged 9–18 years, treated at the ED following assault	ED	Assault, with and without weapons	Depression, PTSD	No
Pailler et al., 2007, USA, [18]	Patients aged between 12 and 17, treated at the ED following a violence-related event	ED	Violent event, child abuse excluded	Depression, ASD, PTSD	No
Purtle et al., 2014, USA, [19]	Patients aged between 7 and 17 years who sustained intentional interpersonal injury treated at the ED	Urban level I trauma center	Violent event, child abuse, domestic violence, and sexual assault excluded	PTSD	No
Roy-Byrne et al., 2004, USA, [22]	Patients aged 18 years and older, admitted to ED following sexual or physical assault, not requiring hospitalization	Urban level I trauma center	Sexual or physical assault	PTSD	Yes, DSM-IV
Sullivan et al., 2017, USA, [21]	Patients aged 18 years and older, admitted to the trauma service for at least 24 h following aggravated assault	Urban level I trauma center	Aggravated assault and gunshot wounds	Depression, PTSD	No
Walters et al., 2007, UK, [25]	Patients aged over 16 years, treated at the ED following assault	ED	Assault, no further exclusion criteria	PTSD	No

ASD acute stress disorder, *ED* emergency department, *PTSD* post-traumatic stress disorder
[a]Are all DSM-IV or DSM-V diagnostic criteria for ASD, PTSD, or depression met, e.g. assessed by means of a structured clinical interview?

Table 2 Overview of PTSD, ASD, and depression prevalence rates and diagnostic instruments

PTSD (n = 15)	Instrument, cut-off	No./total no.	Prevalence in % (95% CI)				
			< 1 month	1 month	3 months	6 months	12 months
Alarcon et al. [13]	PCL-C, ≥35	7/16	–	43.7 (11.4–76.2)	–	–	–
Bisson et al. [23]	TSQ, ≥6	338/3349	59.1 (52.8–65.4)	–	–	–	–
Cunningham et al. [15]	MINI, DSM-IV criteria	30/184	–	–	–	–	16.3 (10.5–22.1)
Elklit et al. [26]	HTQ, ≥3 on all scales	26/118	–	–	–	22.0 (13.5–30.5)	–
Fein et al. [16]	CATS, ≥27	4/96	–	–	5.8 (0.12–11.5)	–	–
Hunt et al. [20]	CAPS, DSM-V criteria	7/12	–	58.3 (15.1–100)	–	–	–
Johansen et al. [27]	PTSS-10[a,b]	46/138	–	33.3 (23.7–43.0)[c]	–	–	–
Johansen et al. [28]	PTSS-10[a,b]	20/70, 17/70, 19–70	–	28.6 (16.0–41.1)	24.3 (12.7–35.8)	–	27.1 (14.9–39.3)
Kleim et al. [24]	SCID, DSM-IV criteria	49/205	–	–	–	23.9 (17.2–30.6)	–
McCart et al. [17]	TSCC, NR	7/89	7.1 (1.85–12.4)	–	–	–	–
Pailler et al. [18]	CATS, ≥27	3/158	–	–	–	1.9 (3.8–12.7)	–
Purtle et al. [19]	CTSQ, ≥5	31/47	66.0 (42.7–89.2)	–	–	–	–
Roy-Byrne et al. [22]	CAPS, DSM-V criteria	14/23, 7/23	–	60.9 (29.0–92.8)	30.4 (7.9–53.0)	–	–
Sullivan et al. [21]	PC-PTSD, ≥3	33/87	37.9 (25.0–50.9)	–	–	–	–
Walters et al. [25]	DTS[d]	NR	–	11 (NR)	–	7.7 (NR)	–

ASD (N = 5)	Instrument, cut-off	No./total no.	Prevalence in % (95% CI)		
			< 1 week	1 week	> 1 week
Boccelari et al. [14]	ASDS, > 36	221/541	–	40.9 (35.5–46.2)	–
Elklit et al. [26]	HTQ, ≥2	47/196	24.0 (17.1–30.8)	–	–
Fein et al. [16]	ISRC[e]	17/69	24.6 (12.9–36.3)	–	–
Kleim et al. [24]	ASDS, NR	37/222	–	–	16.7 (11.3–22.0)
Pailler et al. [18]	ISRC, NR	46/394	–	11.7 (8.3–15.0)	–

Depression (N = 5)	Instrument, cut-off	No./total no.	Prevalence in % (95% CI)	
			< 1 month	≥ 1 month
Boccelari et al. [14]	PHQ, NR	191/541	35.3 (30.3–40.3)	–
Cunningham et al. [15]	MINI, DSM-IV criteria	31/184	–	16.8 (10.9–22.8)
McCart et al. [17]	TSCC, NR	5/89	5.1 (0.6–9.6)	–
Pailler et al. [18]	CDI-SF, > 65	12/394	3.0 (1.3–4.8)	–
Sullivan et al. [21]	PHQ-8, ≥10	36/87	41.4 (27.9–54.9)	–

ASD acute stress disorder, *ASDS* Acute Stress Disorder Scale, *CAPS* Clinician Administered PTSD Scale, *CATS* Child and Adolescents Trauma Survey, *CDI-SF* Children's Depression Inventory Short Form, *CTSQ* Child Trauma Screening Questionnaire, *DTS* Davidson Trauma Scale, *HTQ* Harvard Trauma Questionnaire, *ISRC* Immediate Stress Response Checklist, *MINI* Mini International Neuropsychiatric Interview, *NR* not reported, *PC-PTSD* Primary Care PTSD, *PCL-C* PTSD Checklist-Civilian, *PHQ(– 8)* Patient Health Questionnaire (8), *PTSD* post-traumatic stress disorder, *PTSS-10* Post Traumatic Symptom Scale 10, *SCID* Structured Clinical Interview for DSM-IV, *TSCC* Trauma Symptom Checklist for Children, *TSQ* Trauma Screening Questionnaire
[a]Cut-off: a score of four or more on six or more items indicating PTSD
[b]IES-15 (Impact of Event Scale 15) was used as a secondary instrument, prevalence rates: 25.7% 1 month, 30.0% 3 months, 31.4% 12 months
[c]Males: 33/110 (30%), females: 13/28 (46%)
[d]Cut-off: at least one re-experiencing, three avoidance and two hyperarousal symptoms at a frequency of at least twice in the previous week
[e]Cut-off: at least one significant symptom in every category

high risk of bias because the recruitment process, inclusion criteria, and baseline characteristics were not reported adequately [26].

Discussion

This systematic review provides an overview of the published literature reporting the prevalence rates and trajectories of PTSD, ASD, and depression following violence

related injury treated at the ED or hospital. The quality of the included studies was assessed. We identified sixteen studies reporting the prevalence of ASD, PTSD, or depression. The reported prevalence rates were diverse across different follow-up points resulting in a wide range. The quality assessment indicated that almost all studies were susceptible to bias due to low response rates and loss to follow-up.

Table 3 QUIPS risk of bias assessment

Study	Study participation	Study attrition	Outcome measurement	Statistical analysis and presentation
Alarcon et al. [13]	Low	High	Low	Low
Bisson et al. [23]	Moderate	High	Low	NA
Boccelari et al. [14]	Moderate	High	Moderate	Low
Cunningham et al. [15]	Low	High	Moderate	Low
Elklit et al. [26]	High	High	Low	Low
Fein et al. [16]	Low	Moderate	Moderate	Low
Hunt et al. [20]	Low	Moderate	Low	Low
Johansen et al. [27]	Low	High	Moderate	Low
Johansen et al. [28]	Low	High	Moderate	Low
Kleim et al. [24]	Low	High	Low	Low
McCart et al. [17]	Moderate	High	Low	Low
Pailler et al. [18]	Low	Low	Low	Low
Purtle et al. [19]	Low	High	Low	Low
Roy-Byrne et al. [22]	Low	High	Low	Low
Sullivan et al. [21]	Low	High	Low	Low
Walters et al. [25]	Low	High	Low	Low

NA not applicable

In a previous meta-analysis on the prevalence of PTSD among trauma-exposed children and adolescents, an overall pooled prevalence rate of 15.9% was reported [29]. The pooled prevalence rate for victims of interpersonal violence was 25.2%. The time of diagnosis was not specified, however. We found prevalence rates ranging from 1.9% (3 months) to 66% (< 1 month) among children and adolescents. It is not warranted to aggregate these prevalence rates given the differences in the timing of the diagnosis and diagnostic instruments. White et al. [30] reported a PTSD prevalence of 14.3% among an adult sample that experienced a traumatic event. Again, this finding is difficult to compare with our results as the PTSD prevalence ranged from 7.7% (6 months) to 60.9% (< 1 month). Brewin et al. [31] reported an ASD prevalence estimate of 19% among adult violent crime victims who were not necessarily treated for injury. This prevalence rate is comparable with the ASD prevalence rates reported in four included studies (11.7–24.6%), but one study reported a prevalence rate of 41% [14]. These findings suggest that ASD is highly prevalent in patients with violence related injury and that the prevalence is comparable to populations consisting of injured and non-injured violence victims.

Four studies reported PTSD prevalence rates before one month after the traumatic event [17, 19, 21, 23], which is not in accordance with the DSM (IV and V) criteria. It could be possible that these PTSD symptoms resulted from other traumatic events. Data on pre-existing PTSD, ASD, and depression among the study samples were not available, however. Consequently, it is unclear whether mental disorders were already present prior to the injury. This limitation is common in violence and injury research, but has to be taken into account when interpreting the results. It is also possible that people who already have PTSD, ASD or depression are more likely to be involved in interpersonal violence. It is known that PTSD is associated with more risk behavior [32] which could increase the likelihood of involvement in violence. Information regarding the diagnostic status before the injury is therefore valuable for interpreting the prevalence rates.

All studies were conducted in high-income countries, of which the vast majority in the United States. The findings of this review are therefore limited to these countries. Health care systems in high-income countries are relatively well established, which facilitates recognition, prevention, and treatment. It is therefore likely that the prevalence rates and trajectories of PTSD, ASD, and depression are different in middle and low-income countries.

Strengths and limitations

One of the strengths of our study is that standard methods for conducting and reporting systematic reviews were followed [11]. Furthermore, psychological, medical, and other relevant literature databases were searched exhaustively. Another strength is that we assessed the quality of the included studies. A limitation of our review is that the search was restricted to studies published in scientific peer-reviewed journals in English language. We did not consider dissertations, unpublished material or studies in non-English language, which could have biased our findings.

Recommendations

For future research, we recommend uniformity in diagnostic procedures. Structured diagnostic interviews by a clinician are preferred, but this is often not feasible. These interviews are time consuming and costly as they require involvement of trained professionals. Nevertheless, validated questionnaires can be used as an approximation. Our findings show that a large variety of questionnaires are available, however. Estimates of PTSD prevalence tend to vary according to the diagnostic criteria used, which underpins the need for uniformity in diagnostic procedures. These differences in diagnostic procedures could be reduced by establishing international guidelines on assessing mental health problems among trauma patients. Although international uniformity in diagnostic procedures would increase the comparability of PTSD, ASD and depression estimates, one should pay attention to ethnocultural differences. The validity of responses to measures may vary between populations, cultures, and countries [33]. Values and norms associated with culture guide perception and individual responses, including psychiatric symptoms [34]. Marshall et al. [35] investigated posttraumatic stress among a sample of Hispanic, non-Hispanic Caucasian, and African American survivors of physical injury. They found that the Hispanic group reported different symptoms and higher levels of overall posttraumatic distress. Such results raise questions regarding whether certain cultures truly experience higher levels of distress after experiencing a traumatic event, or whether cultural factors have an impact on the symptom manifestation only.

One of the sixteen included studies reported gender-specific prevalence rates. We recommend to report gender specific prevalence rates, since it is known that women are more likely to develop PTSD after trauma than men [29, 36]. Trajectories of PTSD, ASD, and depression can be better understood when distinguishing gender specific prevalence rates.

Prevalence rates should also be reported separately for injury types, such as sexual versus physical assault injuries and injuries caused by strangers versus family. The studies in the current review included patients with different injury types but prevalence rates were not reported separately. Identifying injury types that are associated with higher rates of PTSD, ASD, or depression may lead to earlier identification of high risk patients. Furthermore, ethnocultural differences in prevalence estimates should be considered in future studies. Cultural factors shape the subjective meaning of traumatic events, which in turn influences symptom expression [37].

Only few studies had follow-up measurements beyond one year after the violent incident. Previous studies suggest that the course of PTSD may vary over time. Prospective assessments are required to study the course of mental disorders following violence related injury treated at the ED or hospital. Since there are indications that the prevalence of PTSD among victims of intentional violence increases over time [5] it is relevant to know what the trajectories of PTSD and other mental disorders are for individuals who sustained injury following violence. For future research, extending the follow-up could contribute to better understanding of mental disorder trajectories following violence related injury.

Conclusions

Heterogeneity resulting from the use different diagnostic instruments limited the comparability of the ASD, PTSD, and depression prevalence rates. The reported prevalence rates should be interpreted carefully as almost all studies were susceptible to bias due to low response rates. Definitive or broad statements on the prevalence rates and trajectories are therefore not warranted. Study participation and loss to follow-up require more attention in future studies. Uniformity in diagnostic procedures is needed for future studies on mental disorders following violence related injury.

Abbreviations

ASD: acute stress disorder; DSM: Diagnostic and Statistical Manual of Mental Disorders; ED: emergency department; PTSD: post-traumatic stress disorder; QUIPS: Quality in Prognosis Studies

Acknowledgements

The authors thank W. Bramer for his contributions to the development of the literature search strategy and E. van Beeck for reviewing the manuscript.

Funding

The authors did not receive funding for this work.

Authors' contributions

Study design: RO, SP, JH. Eligibility assessment and data extraction: RO, BO, JH. Writing the manuscript: RO. Editing and revising the manuscript: BO, SP, JH. All authors read and approved the final manuscript.

Consent for publication
Not applicable.

Competing interests
The authors declare that they have no competing interests.

References
1.   World Health Organization: World Report on Violence and Health. 2002.
2.   Lipsky S, Caetano R, Field CA, Bazargan S. Violence-related injury and intimate partner violence in an urban emergency department. J Trauma. 2004;57(2):352–9.
3.   GBD 2016 Disease and Injury Incidence and Prevalence Collaborators. Global, regional, and national incidence, prevalence, and years lived with disability for 328 diseases and injuries for 195 countries, 1990-2016: a systematic analysis for the global burden of disease study 2016. Lancet. 2017;390(10100):1211–59.
4.   American Psychiatric Association. Diagnostic and statistical manual of mental disorders. 5th ed. Washington: DC; 2013.
5.   Santiago PN, Ursano RJ, Gray CL, Pynoos RS, Spiegel D, Lewis-Fernandez R, Friedman MJ, Fullerton CS. A systematic review of PTSD prevalence and trajectories in DSM-5 defined trauma exposed populations: intentional and non-intentional traumatic events. PLoS One. 2013;8(4):e59236.
6.   Ellis A, Stores G, Mayou R. Psychological consequences of road traffic accidents in children. Eur Child Adolesc Psychiatry. 1998;7(2):61–8.
7.   O'Donnell ML, Creamer M, Pattison P, Atkin C. Psychiatric morbidity following injury. Am J Psychiatry. 2004;161(3):507–14.
8.   Haagsma JA, van Beeck EF, Toet H, Polinder S. Posttraumatic stress disorder following injury: trajectories and impact on health-related quality of life. Journal of Depression and Anxiety. 2013;2013.
9.   Harvey AG, Bryant RA. Two-year prospective evaluation of the relationship between acute stress disorder and posttraumatic stress disorder following mild traumatic brain injury. Am J Psychiatry. 2000;157(4):626–8.
10. Koponen S, Taiminen T, Portin R, Himanen L, Isoniemi H, Heinonen H, Hinkka S, Tenovuo O. Axis I and II psychiatric disorders after traumatic brain injury: a 30-year follow-up study. Am J Psychiatry. 2002;159(8):1315–21.
11. Moher D, Liberati A, Tetzlaff J, Altman DG, Group P. Preferred reporting items for systematic reviews and meta-analyses: the PRISMA statement. Int J Surg. 2010;8(5):336–41.
12. Hayden JA, van der Windt DA, Cartwright JL, Cote P, Bombardier C. Assessing bias in studies of prognostic factors. Ann Intern Med. 2013;158(4):280–6.
13. Alarcon LH, Germain A, Clontz AS, Roach E, Nicholas DH, Zenati MS, Peitzman AB, Sperry JL. Predictors of acute posttraumatic stress disorder symptoms following civilian trauma: highest incidence and severity of symptoms after assault. J Trauma Acute Care Surg. 2012;72(3):629–35 discussion 635-627.
14. Boccellari A, Alvidrez J, Shumway M, Kelly V, Merrill G, Gelb M, Smart S, Okin RL. Characteristics and psychosocial needs of victims of violent crime identified at a public-sector hospital: data from a large clinical trial. Gen Hosp Psychiatry. 2007;29(3):236–43.
15. Cunningham RM, Carter PM, Ranney M, Zimmerman MA, Blow FC, Booth BM, Goldstick J, Walton MA. Violent reinjury and mortality among youth seeking emergency department care for assault-related injury: a 2-year prospective cohort study. JAMA Pediatr. 2015;169(1):63–70.
16. Fein JA, Kassam-Adams N, Gavin M, Huang R, Blanchard D, Datner EM. Persistence of posttraumatic stress in violently injured youth seen in the emergency department. Arch Pediatr Adolesc Med. 2002;156(8):836–40.
17. McCart MR, Davies WH, Harris R, Wincek J, Calhoun AD, Melzer-Lange MD. Assessment of trauma symptoms among adolescent assault victims. J Adolesc Health. 2005;36(1):70 e77–13.
18. Pailler ME, Kassam-Adams N, Datner EM, Fein JA. Depression, acute stress and behavioral risk factors in violently injured adolescents. Gen Hosp Psychiatry. 2007;29(4):357–63.
19. Purtle J, Harris E, Compton R, Baccare R, Morris A, Dibartolo D, Campbell C, Vogel K, Schwartz N, Moront M. The psychological sequelae of violent injury in a pediatric intervention. J Pediatr Surg. 2014;49(11):1668–72.
20. Hunt JC, Sapp M, Walker C, Warren AM, Brasel K, deRoon-Cassini TA. Utility of the injured trauma survivor screen to predict PTSD and depression during hospital admission. J Trauma Acute Care Surg. 2017;82(1):93–101.
21. Sullivan E, Shelley J, Rainey E, Bennett M, Prajapati P, Powers MB, Foreman M, Warren AM. The association between posttraumatic stress symptoms, depression, and length of hospital stay following traumatic injury. Gen Hosp Psychiatry. 2017;46:49–54.
22. Roy-Byrne PP, Russo J, Michelson E, Zatzick D, Pitman RK, Berliner L. Risk factors and outcome in ambulatory assault victims presenting to the acute emergency department setting: implications for secondary prevention studies in PTSD. Depress Anxiety. 2004;19(2):77–84.
23. Bisson JI, Weltch R, Maddern S, Shepherd JP. Implementing a screening programme for post-traumatic stress disorder following violent crime. Eur J Psychotraumatol. 2010;1.
24. Kleim B, Ehlers A, Glucksman E. Early predictors of chronic post-traumatic stress disorder in assault survivors. Psychol Med. 2007;37(10):1457–67.
25. Walters JT, Bisson JI, Shepherd JP. Predicting post-traumatic stress disorder: validation of the trauma screening questionnaire in victims of assault. Psychol Med. 2007;37(1):143–50.
26. Elklit A, Brink O. Acute stress disorder as a predictor of post-traumatic stress disorder in physical assault victims. J Interpers Violence. 2004;19(6):709–26.
27. Johansen VA, Wahl AK, Eilertsen DE, Hanestad BR, Weisaeth L. Acute psychological reactions in assault victims of non-domestic violence: peritraumatic dissociation, post-traumatic stress disorder, anxiety and depression. Nord J Psychiatry. 2006;60(6):452–62.
28. Johansen VA, Wahl AK, Eilertsen DE, Weisaeth L. Prevalence and predictors of post-traumatic stress disorder (PTSD) in physically injured victims of non-domestic violence. A longitudinal study. Soc Psychiatry Psychiatr Epidemiol. 2007;42(7):583–93.
29. Alisic E, Zalta AK, van Wesel F, Larsen SE, Hafstad GS, Hassanpour K, Smid GE. Rates of post-traumatic stress disorder in trauma-exposed children and adolescents: meta-analysis. Br J Psychiatry. 2014;204:335–40.
30. White J, Pearce J, Morrison S, Dunstan F, Bisson JI, Fone DL. Risk of post-traumatic stress disorder following traumatic events in a community sample. Epidemiol Psychiatr Sci. 2015;24(3):249–57.
31. Brewin CR, Andrews B, Rose S, Kirk M. Acute stress disorder and posttraumatic stress disorder in victims of violent crime. Am J Psychiatry. 1999;156(3):360–6.
32. Danielson CK, Amstadter AB, Dangelmaier RE, Resnick HS, Saunders BE, Kilpatrick DG. Trauma-related risk factors for substance abuse among male versus female young adults. Addict Behav. 2009;34(4):395–9.
33. Hinton DE, Lewis-Fernandez R. The cross-cultural validity of posttraumatic stress disorder: implications for DSM-5. Depress Anxiety. 2011;28(9):783–801.
34. Schubert CC, Punamaki RL. Mental health among torture survivors: cultural background, refugee status and gender. Nord J Psychiatry. 2011;65(3):175–82.
35. Marshall GN, Schell TL, Miles JN. Ethnic differences in posttraumatic distress: Hispanics' symptoms differ in kind and degree. J Consult Clin Psychol. 2009; 77(6):1169–78.
36. de Vries GJ, Olff M. The lifetime prevalence of traumatic events and posttraumatic stress disorder in the Netherlands. J Trauma Stress. 2009;22(4): 259–67.
37. Stephens KA, Sue S, Roy-Byrne P, Unutzer J, Wang J, Rivara FP, Jurkovich GJ, Zatzick DF. Ethnoracial variations in acute PTSD symptoms among hospitalized survivors of traumatic injury. J Trauma Stress. 2010;23(3):384–92.

12

Substance use disorder and associated factors among prisoners in a correctional institution in Jimma, Southwest Ethiopia

Yimenu Yitayih[1*], Mubarek Abera[1], Eliais Tesfaye[1], Almaz Mamaru[1], Matiwos Soboka[1†] and Kristina Adorjan[2,3,4†]

Abstract

Background: Substance use disorder is an important public health problem and one of the major causes of disability worldwide. Substance use and criminal behavior are closely related and there is a significant association between substance misuse and crime, but little is known about substance use disorder among prisoners, in particular in low-income countries. Therefore, we investigated substance use disorder and associated factors in inmates of a correctional institution in Jimma, Southwest Ethiopia.

Methods: We used a cross-sectional study design to collect data from 336 prisoners from June 5 to July 5, 2017. Study participants were selected from the total of 1460 prisoners eligible for the study by a systematic random sampling technique, i.e., one participant was randomly selected from every four consecutive admissions in the registration book. Alcohol use disorder, nicotine dependence, khat abuse, cannabis use disorder, psychopathy, adverse traumatic life events, and social support were assessed. Data were entered into EpiData version 3.1 and analyzed in bivariate and multivariable logistic regression models with the Statistical Package for Social Science version 21. Variables with a P value < 0.05 in the final fitting model were declared to be associated with the outcome variable.

Results: The overall prevalence of substance use disorder was 55.9%. The prevalence of khat abuse was 41.9%; alcohol use disorder, 36.2%; nicotine dependence, 19.8%; and cannabis use disorder, 3.6%. Poor social support, living in urban areas, psychopathy, and a family history of substance use were positively associated with substance use disorder.

Conclusions: Substance use disorder is prevalent among prisoners. The increased morbidity and unpleasant psychosocial consequences associated with substance use disorder, together with our finding that 66.3% of prisoners with substance use disorder were interested in obtaining treatment, suggest a need to establish prison-based treatment in this correctional institution in Jimma.

Keywords: Crime, Prisoners, Substance use disorder, Alcohol use, Khat abuse, Tobacco dependence

* Correspondence: yemenu2007@gmail.com
†Matiwos Soboka and Kristina Adorjan contributed equally to this work.
[1]Department of Psychiatry, College of Health Sciences, Jimma University, Jimma, Ethiopia
Full list of author information is available at the end of the article

Background

According to a WHO 2014 report, alcohol consumption, accounted for 5.9% of all deaths worldwide in the year 2012 [1]. Also, smoking caused more than one in ten deaths global, killing more than 6 million people in 2015 [2]. The report also found that the global use of these substances is growing rapidly and contributes significantly to the global burden of disease, assessed as disability-adjusted life years [3, 4]. It estimated that substance use accounted for 14.7% of disability-adjusted life years in 2010 (alcohol: 6.9%) [4].

Substance use and criminal behavior are closely related, and a large proportion of substance users commit crimes while under the influence of a substance [5]. Substance use significantly increases the likelihood of arrest because it increases the need to commit crimes to obtain money to buy a particular substance [5]. Furthermore, 37% of almost 2 million convicted offenders currently in jail were drinking at the time of their arrest [6]. According to a U.S. Department of Justice report, in 2004 about one-third (32%) of inmates in state facilities reported that they had committed a crime while under the influence of drugs [6]. Alcohol is a factor in 40% of all violent crimes in the USA [5], and alcohol and other drugs contribute to 78% of violent crimes, 83% of property crimes, and 77% of public order crimes [7]. Inmates with substance abuse problems are more likely to be re-incarcerated, begin their criminal careers at an early age and have more contact with the criminal justice system [7]. Additionally, prisoners with substance abuse problems are four times more likely to receive income through illegal activities [7].

The risk factors for substance use disorder include a family history of substance use; personality traits, such as high impulsivity or sensation seeking; depression and anxiety; exposure to physical, sexual, or emotional abuse or trauma; and starting substance use at an early age [8]. Rounds-Bryant and Baker [9] stated that ongoing substance abuse in prisoners is a concern because if prisoners are not given adequate treatment in prison and supervision is lacking in the community after they are discharged they have a high potential to become re-addicted and commit a crime after their release. Furthermore, community samples do not necessarily reflect samples in custodial settings, where histories of drug and alcohol use are particularly high compared with the general population [9]. Because a better understanding of this situation could help to highlight the need for different services to meet prisoners' needs, a systematic review studied the prevalence of problematic substance use and types of substance use disorder diagnosis among people admitted to prison [10].

The review found that 24% of the studied population met the criteria for alcohol use disorder (AUD) and 30% of male and 51% of female prisoners had a drug use disorder [10].

Prison-based drug treatment is diverse and includes a wide range of treatment programs, such as psychosocial-behavioral interventions, therapeutic communities, and victim impact panels, interventions involving legal sanctions, and group and individual psychotherapy for drug-abusing offenders [11]. One study found that 20.5% of prisoners who had completed in-prison residential treatment used drugs or alcohol compared with 36.7% of untreated prisoners within the first six month after release [12].

Despite the contribution of substance use disorder to the global burden of diseases and the high prevalence among incarcerated people, little attention is given to this disorder in the general population and among prisoners in particular [9]. This is particularly true in low-income countries; in Ethiopia, for example, no study has examined the prevalence of substance use disorder in a prison population. Therefore, this study aimed to assess the prevalence of this disorder and associated factors among prisoners in a correctional institution in Jimma, Southwest Ethiopia.

Methods

Study setting

The prison is managed by the Oromiya Regional Correcting Units Administrative Office. It was put into service after the expulsion of the occupying Italian forces in 1943 and serves the following regions: Oromiya, Southern nations and nationalities, and Gambella region. The facility was built to accommodate 450 prisoners but currently houses about 1460 (1418 male and 42 female). It is designated as a maximum-security facility. The prison population includes offenders on remand and people convicted to a limited or life-long sentence. The prison compound houses a medical clinic and sick bay, in addition to the usual prison facilities. The study was conducted from June 5 to July 5, 2017.

Study design

This was a cross-sectional study conducted in the correctional institution in Jimma, Southwest Ethiopia

Sampling technique

We used a systematic random sampling technique to select participants. The total number of prisoners was used as a sampling frame. About 1460 prisoners were eligible for the study, and the sampling interval was 1460/336 = 4. The first prisoner was randomly selected from the first four prisoners listed in the registration book according to their date of entry into the prison.

We then continued to select one prisoner from every subsequent group of 4 until the required sample size was reached ($n = 336$).

Sample size

The sample size (n) was calculated by the single population proportion formula, $n = (Zalpha/2)^2 * P (1-P)/d^2$ [13], assuming a prevalence (P) of 50%, i.e. 0.5 (because a priori prevalence of 0.5 yields a maximally conservative estimate for the required sample size and no similar study has been performed among a prison population in Ethiopia or any other African country), a 95% confidence interval (CI) of 1.96 (Zalpha/2 = 1.96), a 5% margin of error (d, 0.05), and a non-response rate of 10%.

We applied the single population proportion formula to give $n = (1.96)^2 * [0.5 (1-0.5)]/0.05^2 = 384$. Because the population size is < 10,000, we used the finite population correction formula with the calculated sample size of 384 and the total population of 1460:

$$n_f = \frac{n_i}{1+\dfrac{n_i}{N}} = 384/(1+[384/1460]) = 305$$

Thus, assuming a 10% non-response rate the final sample size was 336.

Study procedures

Data were collected by five Master of Science in Psychiatry students. All data collectors were given two-day training on the study objectives, data collection methods, tools, methods for maintaining confidentiality, acquisition of informed consent, and handling of ethical issues. The five students were supervised by two Master of Science in Public Health students and the principal investigator. A pre-test was conducted on 5% of the sample in the Agaro prison, which is located 45 km from Jimma. On each day of data collection, the completed questionnaires were checked for completeness. The collected data were entered into a computer and processed in a timely fashion.

We assessed the presence of four substance use disorders: AUD, khat abuse, nicotine dependence, and cannabis use disorder. To identify AUD, we used the Alcohol Use Disorders Identification Test (AUDIT) [14]. An AUDIT score ≥ 8 is considered to indicate an AUD. The sensitivity and specificity of AUDIT for AUD are 0.90 and 0.80, respectively [14], and the reliability in this study was 0.87 (Cronbach's α). We assessed nicotine dependence with the Fagerstrom Test for Nicotine Dependence (FTND), in which a score ≥ 1 indicates nicotine dependence [15]. The reliability of the FTND in this study was 0.80 (Cronbach's α). To evaluate khat abuse, we used the Drug Abuse Screening Test (DAST); a score ≥ 3 indicates abuse [16]. The reliability of the

DAST in this study was 0.88 (Cronbach's α). Finally, we used the Cannabis Use Problems Identification Test (CUPIT) to assess cannabis use disorder; a score ≥ 12 indicates a cannabis use disorder [17]. The reliability of CUPIT in this study was 0.87 (Cronbach's α). We chose those tools to assess substance use disorder because they were previously used in similar populations [18].

We used a questionnaire to assess the following potential explanatory variables for substance use disorder: socioeconomic factors (age, sex, marital status, ethnicity, religion, educational status, occupation, income); environmental factors (family history of substance use, social support, immigration history); behavioral and mental health factors (previous known mental illness, perception that substance use does not impair health, start of substance use at an early age, chronic physical illness, suicidal ideation and attempts); and criminal factors (previous arrest, previous substance-related offences, type of crime, committed a crime under the influence of a substance). We chose to explore these variables because an earlier study found that they are relevant for substance use disorder [7, 19]. We also assessed social support with the Oslo 3-item Social Support Scale [20], psychopathy with the Psychopathy Checklist: Screening Version (PCL: SV; cut-off score ≥ 13 [21]; sensitivity, 0.94; specificity, 0.85; reliability in this study: Cronbach's α = 0.86), and adverse traumatic life events with the Life Events Checklist (positive if at least one traumatic event recorded).

Lastly, we used a 4-item questionnaire to gather data on other aspects of substance use: 1. which reason(s) explain(s) why you use the substance? (possible responses: [A] To relax; [B] To relieve stress; [C] To be accepted by peers (peer pressure); [D] To feel normal; [E] For confidence to commit an offence; [F] Others [specify]); 2. Have you been treated for a substance use disorder? ([A]Yes; [B] No); 3. Are you interested in receiving treatment for substance use disorder? ([A] Yes; [B] No); 4. Are you interested in continuing to take the substance after you are released from prison? ([A] Yes; [B] No).

Data processing and analysis

EpiData Version 3.1 was used to enter the data; the mean was used in case of missing data. Then, the data were exported to Statistical Package for Social Science version 21.0 for further analysis. Descriptive statistics, such as the frequency and median, were computed, and bivariate and multivariable analyses were used to identify factors associated with the outcome variable. Factors associated with the outcome variables that had a P value < 0.25 in the bivariate analysis were included in the multivariable analysis. Statistical significance was set at $P < 0.05$. An odds ratio with a 95% CI was computed to assess the level of association and statistical significance.

Ethical considerations

The study protocol was approved by the Research Ethics and Approval Committee of the Jimma University Institute of Health, and the study was performed according to the Declaration of Helsinki. Verbal informed consent was obtained from prisoners. Participants were told that selection for participation in the study was random and that they had the right not to respond to questions they were not comfortable with and to ask questions. After data entry was complete, the questionnaires were kept securely locked away.

Results

Socio-demographic characteristics

A total of 329 prisoners participated in the study. The response rate was 97.9%: of the 336 prisoners approached to participate in the study, $n = 7$ (2.1%) declined to participate because they were unwilling to be interviewed about their substance use histories. The median age of the participants was 26 years (inter-quartile range [IQR] 14). The majorities of participants had been residing in urban areas before imprisonment and were unmarried. The most common ethnicity was Oromo, and the most common religion, Muslim. Detailed information on socio-demographic characteristics is given in Table 1.

Prevalence of substance use disorder

A total of $n = 227$ (69.0%) of the participants had a history of substance use. More than half of all participants ($n = 184/329$, 55.9%) reported a substance use disorder within the 12 months before imprisonment, and half ($n = 165/329$, 50.2%) had used a substance within the 30 days before imprisonment.

Khat was the most commonly used substance in the 12 months before imprisonment, ($n = 138/329$, 41.9%). Among the participants with khat abuse, $n = 81(58.7\%)$ had harmful use, and $n = 57$ (41.3%), khat dependence. The prevalence of AUD within the 12 months before imprisonment was 36.2% ($n = 119/329$). Among the participants with an AUD, $n = 57$ (47.9%) had hazardous drinking; $n = 20$ (16.8%), harmful drinking; and $n = 42$ (35.2%), alcohol dependence. The next most commonly used substance was nicotine: $n = 65/329$ (19.8%) of participants had a history of nicotine dependence within the 12 months before imprisonment (low dependence: $n = 28$, 43.1%; low to moderate dependence: $n = 10$, 15.4%; moderate dependence: $n = 22$ (33.8%); and high dependence: $n = 5$ (7.7%). The prevalence of cannabis use disorder within the 12 months before imprisonment was 3.6% ($n = 13/329$).

A total of $n = 105$ participants (31.9%) had a history of two or more substance use disorders. Among the prisoners with an AUD, $n = 87$ (73.1%) had a history of khat abuse; $n = 41$ (34.5%), a history of nicotine dependence; and $n = 13$ (10.9%), a history of cannabis use disorder. Among the prisoners with khat abuse, $n = 87$ (63%) had a history of AUD; $n = 43$ (31.2%), a history of nicotine dependence; and $n = 13$ (9.4%), a history of cannabis use disorder. Among the prisoners with nicotine dependence, $n = 43$ (66.2%) had a history of khat abuse; $n = 41$ (63.1), a history of AUD; and $n = 12$ (18.5%), a history of cannabis use disorder.

The median age at the first use of a substance was 16 years (IQR 5), and 44% of the participants started using the substance before the age of 15 years. The median duration of substance use was 6 years (IQR 7).

The main reasons for starting substance use reported by participants were peer pressure ($n = 77$, 41.8%), recreational reasons ($n = 63$, 34.2%), and stress relief ($n = 54$, 29.3%). Almost all of the prisoners with a substance use disorder had not received treatment prior to imprisonment ($n = 178$, 96.7%), but $n = 122$ (66.3%) of them were interested in receiving treatment. A third ($n = 62$, 33.7%), however, wanted to continue using the substance after they were released from prison.

Among the prisoners with a substance use disorder, the most common reasons for imprisonment were assault ($n = 65$, 35.3%) and theft ($n = 47$, 25.5%). The most common reasons for imprisonment among participants with an AUD, nicotine dependence, or cannabis use disorder were assault ($n = 42$, 35.3%; $n = 24$, 36.9%; and $n = 5$, 38.5%, respectively) and murder ($n = 28$, 23.5%; $n = 12$, 26.2%; and $n = 4$, 30.8%, respectively), and among prisoners with khat abuse, assault ($n = 48$, 34.8%) and theft ($n = 38$, 27.5%).

Prison history

The median age of participants at the first imprisonment was 24 years (IQR 13). Nearly all of the participants were convicted prisoners. At the time of the study, the median duration of incarceration was 48 months (IQR 90) and the median duration of time spent in prison was 9 months (IQR 20).

Assault and murder were the most common causes of imprisonment. Most of the participants had no previous history of imprisonment, and most of the crimes were not committed under the influence of a substance. Among the crimes that were committed under the influence of a substance ($n = 42/329$), $n = 24$ (57.1%) were committed under the influence of alcohol; $n = 14$ (33.3%), under the influence of khat; and $n = 4$ (9.6%), under the influence of cannabis. Table 2 shows the study participants' forensic history. See (Table 2)

Table 1 Socio-demographic characteristics of prisoners in the correctional institution in Jimma, Southwest Ethiopia, June–July 2017 (n = 329) and bivariate analysis of socio-demographic characteristics

Variables	Category	Frequency	Percentage (%)	Substance use disorder		COR (95% CI)	P value
				No (%)	Yes (%)		
Sex	Male	307	93.3	130 (42.3)	177 (57.7)	2.92 (1.16–7.36)	0.023[a]
	Female	22	6.7	15 (68.2)	7 (31.8)	Reference value	
Age categories	< 30	219	66.6	98 (44.7)	121 (55.3)	1.52 (0.49–4.67)	0.465
	≥ 30	110	33.4	47 (42.7)	63 (57.3)	Reference value	
Place of residence	Rural	106	32.2	60 (56.6)	46 (43.4)	Reference value	
	Urban	223	67.8	85 (38.1)	138 (61.9)	2.12 (1.32–3.39)	0.002[a]
Ethnicity[a]	Oromo	210	63.8	–	–	–	–
	Amhara	51	15.5	–	–	–	–
	Tigray	16	4.9	–	–	–	–
	Gurage	17	5.2	–	–	–	–
	Dawuro	17	5.2	–	–	–	–
	Yem	16	4.9	–	–	–	–
	Other[b]	2	0.6	–	–	–	–
Educational status	No formal education	27	8.2	11 (40.7)	16 (59.3)	Reference value	
	Primary education	178	54.1	83 (46.6)	95 (53.4)	0.79 (0.35–1.79)	0.568
	Secondary education	94	28.6	41 (43.6)	53 (56.4)	0.89 (0.37–2.12)	0.790
	Tertiary education	30	9.1	10 (33.3)	20 (66.7)	1.38 (0.47–4.05)	0.563
Religion	Muslim	181	55.0	79 (43.6)	102 (56.4)	2.91 (0.86–9.78)	0.085[a]
	Orthodox	97	29.5	40 (41.2)	57 (58.8)	3.21 (0.92–1.14)	0.067[a]
	Protestant	38	11.6	17 (44.7)	21 (55.3)	2.78 (0.73–0.62)	0.135[a]
	Catholic	13	4.0	9 (69.2)	4 (30.8)	Reference value	
Marital status	Married	124	37.7	58 (46.8)	66 (53.2)	Reference value	
	Unmarried	205	62.3	87 (42.4)	118 (57.6)	1.19 (0.76–1.87)	0.443
Occupation	Employed	134	40.7	62 (46.3)	72 (53.7)	Reference value	
	Unemployed	36	10.9	14 (38.9)	22 (61.1)	1.35 (0.64–2.87)	0.430
	Farmer	99	30.1	40 (40.4)	59 (59.6)	1.27 (0.75–2.15)	0.373
	Student	43	13.1	22 (51.2)	21 (48.8)	0.82 (0.41–1.64)	0.576
	Other[c]	17	5.2	7 (41.2)	10 (58.8)	1.23 (0.44–3.43)	0.692
Average monthly income (birr)	< 1200	192	58.4	81 (42.2)	111 (57.8)	Reference value	
	≥1200	137	41.6	64 (46.7)	73 (53.3)	0.83 (0.54–1.29)	0.415

Reference value: In the analysis, this variable indicated lower risk for developing substance use; coded as zero in SPSS logistic regression
[a]Bivariate analysis was not performed for ethnicities
[b]Other ethnicities: kafa, walayita, and silte
[c]Other occupations: retired or homemaker

Factors associated with substance use disorder

Various behavioral, mental health, environmental, and criminal factors were found to be associated with substance use disorder (see Table 3).

Multivariable logistic regression showed that four variables were significantly associated with substance use disorder: poor social support (adjusted odds ratio [AOR]: 4.41; 95% CI, 2.22–8.77), living in an urban setting (AOR: 2.42; 95% CI, 1.33–4.40), psychopathy (AOR: 4.68; 95% CI, 1.71–12.78), and a family history of substance use (AOR: 4.39; 95% CI, 2.49–7.79). Prisoners

with poor social support were more than four times more likely to develop a substance use disorder than prisoners with good social support (AOR:4.41; 95% CI, 2.22–8.77). Also, prisoners living in an urban setting were more than two times more likely to have a substance use disorder than prisoners living in a rural setting (AOR:2.42; 95% CI, 1.33–4.40). Prisoners with psychopathy were nearly five times more likely to develop a substance use disorder than those without psychopathy (AOR: 4.68; 95% CI, 1.71–12.78). Prisoners with a family history of substance use were more than

Table 2 Forensic history of prisoners ($n = 329$) in the correctional institution in Jimma, Southwest Ethiopia, in June–July 2017

Variables		Frequency	Percentage (%)	Substance use disorder	
				No, n (%)	Yes, n (%)
Reason for admission to prison	On remand	25	7.6	15 (60.0)	10 (40.0)
	Convicted	304	92.4	130 (42.8)	174 (57.2)
Type of offence committed	Assault	103	31.3	38 (36.9)	65 (63.1)
	Murder	83	25.2	41 (49.4)	42 (50.6)
	Theft	81	24.6	34 (42.0)	47 (58.0)
	Rape	32	9.7	16 (50.0)	16 (50.0)
	Robbery	12	3.6	5 (41.7)	7 (58.3)
	Other[a]	18	5.4	11 (61.1)	7 (38.9)
Previous imprisonment	No	301	91.5	140 (46.5)	161 (53.5)
	Yes	28	8.5	5 (17.9)	23 (82.1)
Committed crime under the influence of substance	No	287	87.2	140 (48.4)	147 (51.6)
	Yes	42	12.8	5 (11.9)	37 (88.1)

[a]Other types of offence = political offence and offence related to forest destruction

Table 3 Bivariate analysis of behavioral, mental health, environmental, and criminal factors among prisoners in the correctional institution in Jimma, Southwest Ethiopia, June–July 2017 ($n = 329$)

Variable		Substance use disorder		COR (95% CI)	P value
		No (%)	Yes (%)		
Psychopathy	No	139 (48.3)	149 (51.7)	Reference value	
	Yes	6 (14.6)	35 (85.4)	5.44 (2.22–13.34)	0.001*
Adverse traumatic life event	No exposure to traumatic life event	62 (51.7)	58 (48.3)	Reference value	
	One traumatic life event	33 (52.4)	30 (47.6)	0.97 (0.53–1.79)	0.927
	Multiple traumatic life events	50 (34.2)	96 (65.8)	2.05 (1.25–3.37)	0.004*
Mental illness	No	132 (44.3)	166 (55.7)	Reference value	
	Yes	13 (41.9)	18 (58.1)	1.10 (0.52–2.33)	0.801
Social support	Poor	53 (28.8)	131 (71.2)	4.35 (2.42–7.81)	0.001*
	Moderate	48 (63.2)	28 (36.8)	1.03 (0.52–2.02)	0.939
	Strong	44 (63.8)	25 (36.2)	Reference value	
Immigration	No	123 (45.6)	147 (54.4)	Reference value	
	Yes	22 (37.3)	37 (62.7)	1.40 (0.79–2.51)	0.248*
Previous imprisonment	No	140 (46.5)	161 (53.5)	Reference value	
	Yes	5 (17.9)	23 (82.1)	4.00 (1.48–10.80)	0.006*
Family history of substance use	No	110 (57.0)	83 (43.0)	Reference value	
	Yes	35 (25.7)	101 (74.3)	3.82 (2.37–6.17)	0.001
Suicidal ideation and suicide attempt	No	114 (46.9)	129 (53.1)	Reference value	
	Yes	31 (36.0)	55 (64.0)	1.57 (0.94–2.60)	0.082*
Chronic physical illness	No	120 (43.5)	156 (56.5)	Reference value	
	Yes	25 (47.2)	28 (52.8)	0.86 (0.48–1.55)	0.62
Perceived that substance use did not affect health	No	66 (46.5)	76 (53.5)	Reference value	
	Yes	79 (42.2)	108 (57.8)	1.19 (0.77–1.84)	0.444

Reference value: In the analysis, this variable indicated lower risk for developing substance use; coded as zero in SPSS logistic regression
*Identified as factors for multivariable logistic regression analysis ($P < 0.25$)

four times more likely to have a substance use disorder than prisoners with no family history of substance use (AOR: 4.39; 95% CI, 2.49–7.79) (see Table 4).

Discussion

This cross-sectional study assessed the prevalence of substance use disorder among prisoners in a correctional facility in Jimma, Southwest Ethiopia, in the 12 months before imprisonment. The prevalence of substance use disorder was 55.9%, which is similar to a comparable study performed in Australia (66%) [22].

The prevalence of AUD among prisoners in the current study was in line with a similar study performed Sudan (32.2%, $N = 1569$) [23] but lower than the prevalence found in a Finnish study (68%, $N = 610$) [24]. The difference might be due to differences in sample size and the tool used to assess AUD (the Finnish study used a clinical psychiatric interview in a larger sample). A study performed in a prison in Lyon, France, found a lower prevalence of AUD (13.7%, $N = 535$) [25], which may be because it was performed in women only and the participants may have had other differences in socio-demographic characteristics.

The prevalence of khat abuse found in the current study was much higher than that in a study in Uganda (17%) [26]. However, the Ugandan study used a self-report questionnaire, so khat use may have been underreported.

The prevalence of nicotine dependence among the prisoners in the current study in the 12 months before imprisonment was lower than the findings of studies in Kenya (32.7%) [27] and Lyon (37.5%) [25]. The differences might be due to the different tools used to measure nicotine dependence and differences between the study populations (the Kenyan study used a self-report questionnaire, and the study in Lyon was in female participants only).

The presence of psychopathy was significantly associated with substance use disorder. This finding is in line with similar studies performed in England and Wales [28] and Turkey [29], both of which found that psychopathy was associated with substance use disorder. The reason for this association might be that people with psychopathy have an irresponsible lifestyle, are impulsive, curious to try new things and unconventional and show sensation-seeking behavior, which in turn makes them more likely to use a substance as a form of self-medication [28].

In the current study, prisoners who lived in an urban setting had a higher likelihood of developing a substance use disorder than those who lived in a rural setting. This finding is in line with a similar study performed in Kenya [27]. This difference might be explained by various characteristics of urban environments, such as population density, built-up environments, and greater access to substances [30].

Both in our study and in a study performed in incarcerated delinquents in Nigeria [31], a family history of substance use was associated with the prisoners' substance use disorder. Prisoners with a family history of substance use had a more than four times higher likelihood of developing a substance use disorder than those with no such family history. One reason for this association might be that parents with a history of substance use may not be deeply involved in bringing up their family and may be less attached to their family, so that their children have difficulties in learning social behavior patterns and experience more adverse life events [32]. Furthermore, families may have a genetic susceptibility to substance use, and it may also be a learned behavior. The implication of this finding is that substance use awareness campaigns should target not only prisoners but also their parents and relatives.

Prisoners with poor social support were more likely to develop a substance use disorder than those with good

Table 4 Multivariable logistic regression analysis for independent predictors of a substance use disorder among prisoners ($n = 329$) in a correctional institution in Jimma, Southwest Ethiopia, in June–July 2017

Variable		Substance use disorder		AOR (95% CI)
		No, n (%)	Yes, n (%)	
Social support	Poor support	53 (28.8)	131 (71.2)	4.41 (2.22–8.77)
	Moderate support	48 (63.2)	28 (36.8)	1.07 (0.49–2.34)
	Strong support	44 (63.8)	25 (36.2)	Reference value
Family history of substance use	No	110 (57.0)	83 (43.0)	Reference value
	Yes	35 (25.7)	101 (74.3)	4.39 (2.49–7.79)
Psychopathy	No	139 (48.3)	149 (51.7)	Reference value
	Yes	6 (14.6)	35 (85.4)	4.68 (1.71–12.78)
Place of residence	Rural	60 (56.6)	46 (43.4)	Reference value
	Urban	85 (38.1)	138 (61.9)	2.42 (1.33–4.40)

social support. A study performed in Hungary also found that poor social support, in the form of poor support from the father, was a factor for substance use [33]. Social support has been found to help people cope with stress and to reduce the risk for anxiety, depression, and distress, all of which are risk factors for substance use [34]. Thus, people with poor social support might be that at greater risk of using substances. Furthermore, people may be more likely to use substances if they have no one to live for other than themselves. This may also apply to people who do not receive any feedback and criticism from others because such feedback and criticism could help them form socially acceptable behavior.

Our finding that just over half of all prisoners had a substance use disorder within 12 months prior to their imprisonment is alarming in view of the fact that substance use disorder treatment is not accessible in the prison. If current prevalence rates are generalizable to all prisons in Ethiopia, our results suggest that about two thirds of prisoners with substance use disorder are interested in receiving treatment; however, almost no prisoners with substance use disorder have access to such treatment services. With regard to the treatment of substance use disorder in prison, therapeutic community intervention (TCI) and individual and group therapy are methods that can decrease the rates of re-incarceration, drug misuse relapse, and re-arrest [35]. Research has shown that an unfortunate consequence of this shortage of treatment services is that offenders quickly return to drug use and crime after their release from prison [36, 37].

In summary, this study has substantial clinical implications for health services in correctional institutions because it shows the need for management plans for acute substance withdrawal and for recovery and rehabilitation support for prisoners with substance use disorder.

Limitations

This study may have a social desirability bias, i.e. prisoners may have underestimated, underreported or denied their substance use. Also, data on the previous 12 months were collected by interview, which has a risk of recall bias. DAST was not validated in our population, even though it has been shown to be useful in screening for khat abuse across cultures. Another limitation is that prisoners' reports of past or present physical illness and mental illness were not clinically confirmed.

Conclusions

This study found a high prevalence of substance use disorder among prisoners in a correctional institution in Jimma, Southwest Ethiopia, in the 12 months before imprisonment. The most commonly used substance was khat, followed by alcohol, nicotine, and cannabis. Living in an urban setting and having psychopathy, a family history of substance use, and poor social support were positively associated with substance use disorder. Generally, despite the increased morbidity of substance users and unpleasant psychosocial consequences of this habit, most prisoners reported not receiving treatment prior to imprisonment. The large number of prisoners with substance use disorder, the unavailability of treatment in prisons, and the substantial gap in services relative to the need indicate that prisoners are more likely to return to risky substance use after release from prison. Therefore, increasing access to substance use disorder treatment, such as TCI, in prison could have substantial long-term economic and social benefits, e.g. reduced recidivism, easier transition to the community after release, and less drug abuse [38].

Further research is needed into substance abuse in other correctional institutions in Ethiopia and the efficacy of prison-based treatment for substance use disorder.

Abbreviations
AOR: Adjusted odds ratio; AUD: Alcohol use disorder; AUDIT: Alcohol Use Disorders Identification Test; CUPIT: Cannabis Use Problems Identification Test; DAST: Drug Abuse Screening Test; FTND: Fagerstrom Test for Nicotine Dependence; IQR: Interquartile range

Acknowledgments
We would like to thank Jimma University for granting ethical approval and funding the study. Our deep thanks go to all study participants, who spent their valuable time responding to the questions in this study. We also thank Jacquie Klesing, Board-certified Editor in the Life Sciences (ELS), for editing assistance with the manuscript.

Funding
The study was funded by Jimma University. The University had no role in the design of the study; in the collection, analysis, and interpretation of the data; or in writing the manuscript.

Authors' contributions
YY wrote the protocol, participated in data collection, analyzed the data and wrote the manuscript. MS and KA participated in conception of the project, data analysis, reviewing and editing of the manuscript. MA, ET and AM made substantial contributions to data analysis, revising and approving the protocol. All authors read and approved the final manuscript.

Consent for publication
Not applicable.

Competing interests
The authors declare that they have no competing interests.

Author details
[1]Department of Psychiatry, College of Health Sciences, Jimma University, Jimma, Ethiopia. [2]Center for International Health, Ludwig-Maximilians-Universität, Munich, Germany. [3]Department of Psychiatry and Psychotherapy, Medical Center of the University of Munich, Munich, Germany. [4]Institute of Psychiatric Phenomics and Genomics (IPPG), Medical Center of the University of Munich, Munich, Germany.

References
1. World Health Organization, World Health Organization. Management of Substance Abuse Unit. Global status report on alcohol and health, 2014. In: World Health Organization; 2014.
2. Reitsma MB, Fullman N, Ng M, Salama JS, Abajobir A, Abate KH, Abbafati C, Abera SF, Abraham B, Abyu GY, Adebiyi AO. Smoking prevalence and attributable disease burden in 195 countries and territories, 1990–2015: a systematic analysis from the Global Burden of Disease Study 2015. Lancet. 2017;389(10082):1885–906.
3. Charlson FJ, Baxter AJ, Dua T, Degenhardt L, Whiteford HA, Vos T. Excess mortality from mental, neurological and substance use disorders in the global burden of disease study 2010. Epidemiol Psychiat Sci. 2015;24(2):121–40.
4. Whiteford H, Ferrari A, Degenhardt L. Global burden of disease studies: implications for mental and substance use disorders. Health Aff. 2016;35(6):1114–20.
5. National Council on Alcoholism and Drug Dependence, Inc. Alcohol, Drugs and Crime https://www.ncadd.org/about-addiction/alcohol-drugs-and-crime. Accessed 9 Jan 2018.
6. Mumola CJ, Karberg JC. Drug use and dependence, state and Federal Prisoners, 2004. Washington, DC: US Department of Justice, Office of Justice Programs; 2006.
7. The National Center on Addiction and Substance Abuse at Colombia University. Behind Bars II: Substance Abuse and America's Prison Population. https://www.centeronaddiction.org/addiction-research/reports/behind-bars-ii-substance-abuse-and-america%E2%80%99s-prison-population. Accessed 9 Jan 2018.
8. Addiction Risk Factors | The National Center on Addiction and Substance Use. https://www.centeronaddiction.org/addiction/addiction-risk-factors. Accessed 8 Jan 2018.
9. Rounds-Bryant JL, Baker L Jr. Substance dependence and level of treatment need among recently-incarcerated prisoners. Am J Drug Alcohol Abuse. 2007;33:557–61.
10. Fazel S, Yoon IA, Hayes AJ. Substance use disorders in prisoners: an updated systematic review and meta-regression analysis in recently incarcerated men and women. Addiction. 2017;112(10):1725–39.
11. Roberts AJ, Hayes AJ, Carlisle J, Shaw J. Review of drug and alcohol treatments in prison and community settings. In: A systematic review conducted on the behalf of the prison Health Research network. England: Prison Health Research network, Department of Health; 2007.
12. Pelissier B, Wallace S, O'Neil JA, Gaes GG, Camp S, Rhodes W, Saylor W. Federal prison residential drug treatment reduces substance use and arrests after release. Am J Drug Alcohol Abuse. 2001;27(2):315–37.
13. Charan J, Biswas T. How to calculate sample size for different study designs in medical research? Indian J Psychol Med. 2013;35(2):121.
14. Babor TF, Higgins-Biddle JC, Saunders JB, Monteiro MG. AUDIT. The alcohol use disorders identification test. Guidelines for use in primary care. 2nd ed. Geneva: World Health Organization; 2001.
15. Heatherton TF, Kozlowski LT, Frecker RC, Fagerström KO. The Fagerström test for nicotine dependence: a revision of the Fagerström tolerance questionnaire. Br J Addict. 1991;86:1119–27.
16. Wazema DH, Madhavi K. Prevalence of Khat abuse and associated factors among undergraduate students of Jimma University. Ethiopia Int J Res Med Sci. 2017;3:1751–7.
17. Bashford J, Flett R, Copeland J. The Cannabis use problems identification test (CUPIT): development, reliability, concurrent and predictive validity among adolescents and adults. Addiction. 2010;105:615–25.
18. MacAskill S, Parkes T, Brooks O, Graham L, McAuley A, Brown A. Assessment of alcohol problems using AUDIT in a prison setting: more than an'aye or no'question. BMC Public Health. 2011;11(1):865.
19. Kilpatrick DG, Acierno R, Saunders B, Resnick HS, Best CL, Schnurr PP. Risk factors for adolescent substance abuse and dependence: data from a national sample. J Consult Clin Psychol. 2000;68(1):19.
20. Bøen H, Dalgard OS, Bjertness E. The importance of social support in the associations between psychological distress and somatic health problems and socio-economic factors among older adults living at home: a cross sectional study. BMC Geriatr. 2012;12:27.
21. Hart SD, Cox DN, Hare RD. Manual for the hare psychopathy checklist: screening version (PCL: SV). Multi-Heath Systems: Toronto, Canada; 1995.
22. Heffernan E, Davidson F, Andersen K, Kinner S. Substance use disorders among aboriginal and Torres Strait islander people in custody: a public health opportunity. Health Justice. 2016;4:12.
23. Karim E-FIA, Mohamed HM, Mohamed MI, Ahmed AF, Mohammed SAA. Drug use among prisoners in three main prisons in Khartoum, Sudan. La Revue de Santé de la Méditerranée orientale. 1998;4:122–7.
24. Lintonen TP, Vartiainen H, Aarnio J, Hakamäki S, Viitanen P, Wuolijoki T, Joukamaa M. Drug use among prisoners: by any definition, it's a big problem. Subst Use Misuse. 2011;46:440–51.
25. Sahajian F, Lamothe P, Fabry J, Vanhems P. Consumption of psychoactive substances among 535 women entering a Lyon prison (France) between June 2004 and December 2008. Rev Epidemiol Sante Publique. 2012;60:371–81.
26. Uganda Prisons Service. A rapid situation assessment of HIV/STI/TB and drug abuse among prisoners in Uganda prisons service. Kampala: Uganda Prisons Service and United Nations Office on Drugs and Crime; 2009.
27. Kinyanjui DWC, Atwoli L. Substance use among inmates at the Eldoret prison in Western Kenya. BMC Psychiatry. 2013;13:53.
28. Coid J, Yang M, Ullrich S, Roberts A, Moran P, Bebbington P, Brugha T, Jenkins R, Farrell M, Lewis G, Singleton N. Psychopathy among prisoners in England and Wales. Int J Law Psychiatry. 2009;32:134–41.
29. Evren C, Kural S, Erkiran M. Antisocial personality disorder in Turkish substance dependent patients and its relationship with anxiety, depression and a history of childhood abuse. Isr J Psychiatry Relat Sci. 2006;43:40–6.
30. Galea S, Rudenstine S, Vlahov D. Drug use, misuse, and the urban environment. Drug Alcohol Rev. 2005;24:127–36.
31. Ebiti NW, Ike JO, Sheikh TL, Lasisi DM, Babalola OJ, Agunbiade S. Determinants of psychoactive substance use among incarcerated delinquents in Nigeria. Afr J Drug Alcohol Stud. 2012;11(2):122–120.
32. Poikolainen K. Risk factors for alcohol dependence: a case-control study. Alcohol Alcohol. 2000;35:190–6.
33. Piko B. Perceived social support from parents and peers: which is the stronger predictor of adolescent substance use? Subst Use Misuse. 2000;35:617–30.
34. Mulia N, Schmidt L, Bond J, Jacobs L, Korcha R. Stress, social support and problem drinking among women in poverty. Addiction. 2008;103:1283–93.
35. Belenko S, Peugh J. Fighting crime by treating substance abuse. Issues Sci and Technol. 1998;15(1):53–60.
36. Kinner SA. Continuity of health impairment and substance misuse among adult prisoners in Queensland, Australia. Int J Prison Health. 2006;2:101–13.
37. Thomas E, Degenhardt L, Alati R, Kinner S. Predictive validity of the AUDIT for hazardous alcohol consumption in recently released prisoners. Drug Alcohol Depend. 2014;134:322–9.
38. Galassi A, Mpofu E, Athanasou J. Therapeutic community treatment of an inmate population with substance use disorders: post-release trends in re-arrest, re-incarceration, and drug misuse relapse. Int J Environ Res Public Health. 2015;12:7059–72.

13

Short term risk of non-fatal and fatal suicidal behaviours: the predictive validity of the Columbia-Suicide Severity Rating Scale in a Swedish adult psychiatric population with a recent episode of self-harm

Åsa U. Lindh[1][*] ⓘ, Margda Waern[2], Karin Beckman[1], Ellinor Salander Renberg[3], Marie Dahlin[1] and Bo Runeson[1]

Abstract

Background: The Columbia-Suicide Severity Rating Scale (C-SSRS) is a relatively new instrument for the assessment of suicidal ideation and behaviour that is widely used in clinical and research settings. The predictive properties of the C-SSRS have mainly been evaluated in young US populations. We wanted to examine the instrument's predictive validity in a Swedish cohort of adults seeking psychiatric emergency services after an episode of self-harm.

Methods: Prospective cohort study of patients ($n = 804$) presenting for psychiatric emergency assessment after an episode of self-harm with or without suicidal intent. Suicidal ideation and behaviours at baseline were rated with the C-SSRS and subsequent non-fatal and fatal suicide attempts within 6 months were identified by record review. Logistic regression was used to evaluate separate ideation items and total scores as predictors of non-fatal and fatal suicide attempts. Receiver operating characteristics (ROC) curves were constructed for the suicidal ideation (SI) intensity score and the C-SSRS total score.

Results: In this cohort, the median age at baseline was 33 years, 67% were women and 68% had made at least one suicide attempt prior to the index attempt. At least one non-fatal or fatal suicide attempt was recorded during follow-up for 165 persons (20.5%). The single C-SSRS items frequency, duration and deterrents were associated with this composite outcome; controllability and reasons were not. In a logistic regression model adjusted for previous history of suicide attempt, SI intensity score was a significant predictor of a non-fatal or fatal suicide attempt (OR 1.08; 95% CI 1.03–1.12). ROC analysis showed that the SI intensity score was somewhat better than chance in correctly classifying the outcome (AUC 0.62, 95% CI 0.57–0.66). The corresponding figures for the C-SSRS total score were 0.65, 95% CI 0.60–0.69.

Conclusions: The C-SSRS items frequency, duration and deterrents were associated with elevated short term risk in this adult psychiatric cohort, as were both the SI intensity score and the C-SSRS total score. However, the ability to correctly predict future suicidal behaviour was limited for both scores.

Keywords: Self-harm, Suicide, Risk factors, Classification, Outcome

* Correspondence: asa.lindh@ki.se
[1]Centre for Psychiatry Research, Department of Clinical Neuroscience, Karolinska Institutet, & Stockholm Health Care Services, Stockholm County Council, S:t Görans Hospital, Vårdvägen 1, SE-112 81 Stockholm, Sweden
Full list of author information is available at the end of the article

Background

Suicide accounts for more than 1% of all deaths worldwide, making it the 15th leading cause of death. Non-fatal self-harm is more common, with an estimated annual prevalence of 4/1000 adults [1]. People who have self-harmed are at increased risk of future self-harm and of dying by suicide [2–8]. The one-year rate of repetition has been estimated at 16% for non-fatal attempts and 1.6–1.8% for fatal attempts [9, 10].

Given the suffering associated with suicidal behaviours, effort has been put into understanding and predicting the phenomenon, with the ultimate goal of prevention. Risk factors for suicide and suicide attempt have been identified in numerous cohorts, but clinically useful tools for prediction at the individual level have yet to be identified [11–13]. In a recent review of the diagnostic accuracy regarding suicide and suicide attempt for several suicide risk assessment instruments, the Columbia-Suicide Severity Rating Scale (C-SSRS) was highlighted as an instrument in need of testing in larger populations [14]. The C-SSRS is a relatively new instrument designed for classification and grading of suicidal ideation and behaviours [15, 16]. Suicidal ideation (SI) is assessed with regard to severity and intensity. Previous studies performed mainly in the US and in adolescent and young adult age groups suggest that both SI severity [15, 17–20], SI intensity [17, 20, 21] and the C-SSRS total score [19] are predictive of suicidal behaviours. The instrument has solid psychometric properties [15, 19, 22, 23].

We aimed to evaluate the predictive ability of the C-SSRS in a large adult sample of patients seeking or being referred to psychiatric emergency care after an episode of self-harm with or without suicide intent. We chose a follow-up time of six months as this is the period with the highest risk of repetition [7, 24] and a time span relevant for treatment planning [25–27]. Since the cohort had a large proportion of actual suicide attempts at the index episode, we assumed there would be relatively little variation in the ratings on severity of suicidal ideation compared to the intensity, which could make the SI intensity score or the separate intensity items more suited as predictors. To be of predictive use in a population similar to our sample, an item or risk scale must show predictive ability when suicide attempts are adjusted for, since this is already acknowledged as one of the most important risk factors for future suicide attempt and suicide [4, 8, 28, 29]. Therefore, we tested whether the SI intensity score, the separate intensity items and the single item *most severe ideation* would predict a repeated suicide attempt also after adjustment for previous attempts.

Methods

Participants

The present study uses data from a Swedish multi-centre study conducted at S:t Görans Hospital (Karolinska Institutet, Stockholm), Sahlgrenska University Hospital (Gothenburg) and Umea University Hospital (Umeå). Adult patients (aged 18 and above) presenting for or being referred to a psychiatric assessment after an episode of self-harm were considered for participation if they were able to take part in an interview. There were no exclusion criteria regarding specific diagnoses, but patients with symptoms interfering with verbal communication (e g severe psychotic symptoms, aggression, confusion, severe somatic conditions and severe cognitive impairment) were not considered for participation. To enable follow-up by medical records, participants were required to have a Swedish personal identity number and to be a registered resident of the catchment area for psychiatric services at one of the participating hospitals. Participants were interviewed by mental health staff (psychiatrists, psychologist and psychiatric nurses) specially trained in the application of the assessment instrument. All interviews took place daytime from April 25, 2012 to April 6, 2016, in most cases within a couple of days of the index episode.

Scorings and outcome
Patient data

The following variables were collected during the interview: sex, age, current occupation (work/student/unemployed/on sick leave/receiving disability pension/retired), living alone/together with someone, current outpatient treatment for psychiatric disorder (including both primary care and specialized mental health care), psychiatric hospitalization during the past 3 months, previous suicide attempt (SA), previous non-suicidal injury (NSSI) and type of index episode (SA or NSSI). Suicide attempt was defined as a potentially self-injurious act committed with at least some wish to die as a result of the act [15, 30]. The questions from the behavioural part of the C-SSRS were used to assess intent. Non-suicidal self-injury was defined as a self-injurious act with no wish to die as a result [31].

Suicidal ideation and behaviour

We used the clinician-administered version of the C-SSRS (baseline/screening version) to assess suicidal ideation (SI) within the past 30 days, suicidal behaviour for the past three months and lifetime ratings for both ideation and behaviour. Suicidal ideation severity is assessed with five yes/no questions summarized in the single item *most severe ideation*, scored 0–5 where 0 corresponds to no suicidal ideation, 1 to a wish to die and 5 to active suicidal ideation with a specific plan and intent to act. The intensity of suicidal ideation is assessed if some degree of SI severity is endorsed. The SI intensity score was derived from the ratings for the following items: frequency, duration, controllability, deterrents and reasons for ideation. Participants denying any degree of suicidal ideation were given 0 points for each of these items. For the items *frequency* and *duration* (scored 1–5), high ratings correspond to high frequency and long duration. For the items *controllability* and *deterrents* (scored 0–5), high ratings indicate a low level of controllability, and little or no deterring effect of factors that could stop someone from acting on suicidal thoughts. In line with a previous study [21], participants stating that there was nothing deterring them from acting upon suicidal thoughts were given a rating of 5 on this item. For the item *reasons for ideation* (scored 0–5), low ratings indicate that a wish to affect others is the main reason for suicidal ideation whereas a high rating indicates that the motive is to end one's own pain. Ratings for the intensity items were summed to yield a SI intensity score that could range from 0 to 25.

In the subscale assessing suicidal behaviour, the participants state whether or not they have engaged in actual, aborted or interrupted suicide attempts, NSSI or preparatory behaviour. The total number of episodes is recorded for each type of behaviour. For actual suicide attempts, actual lethality/medical damage is scored on a six-point ordinal scale. If actual lethality is rated 0, potential lethality is scored from 0 to 2.

The C-SSRS was constructed as an instrument for classification, and there are thus no instructions for calculating a total score. Regarding the ideation items, we used the above-described values. For the behaviour items, we chose to categorize the number of attempts in three groups: 0 (no attempts), 1 (1–2 attempts) and 2 (three or more attempts). If NSSI and/or preparatory behaviour were recorded, 1 point each was given. Regarding lethality of the attempt, the score for the most recent attempt was used. Using this method, the C-SSRS total score has a possible range of 0–42.

Regarding internal consistency, Cronbach's α was 0.64 for the five initial questions assessing SI severity and 0.49 for the SI intensity score. Inter-rater reliability was assessed using weighted kappa for items with even distribution of responses. Prevalence-adjusted, bias-adjusted kappa (PABAK) was calculated when responses were unevenly distributed. The prevalence-adjusted, bias-adjusted kappa for the items *most severe ideation*, frequency, duration, controllability and reasons for ideation ranged from 0.82–0.95 whereas deterrents had a PABAK of 0.63. The PABAK for the behaviour items ranged from 0.70–0.90.

Outcome

The composite outcome was any non-fatal or fatal suicide attempt within six months of the index episode, as identified by medical record review. All available entries recorded during the follow-up period were examined. An act of self-injury that involved at least some wish to die was classified as a suicide attempt. Fatal attempts were defined as deaths that were specifically identified as suicides in the medical records. The electronic medical record systems used at all three sites are all linked to the Swedish population register. This register includes all Swedish residents and is updated daily, with almost 100% of deaths being registered within 30 days [32]. While the population register does not contain information about cause of death, it does identify persons who are still alive after 6 months, including those with no health care contact after the index episode.

Statistical analysis

Data analyses were conducted using the Statistical Package for the Social Sciences (SPSS) version 22.0. We used past month ratings for all analyses involving suicidal ideation and past three month ratings for those involving suicidal behaviour. Ratings on the single item *most severe suicidal ideation* as well as the SI intensity score and the separate intensity items (frequency, duration, controllability, deterrents and reasons) were entered in separate bivariate and multivariable logistic regression models, as single predictors of the composite outcome (non-fatal or fatal attempt) and adjusted for age, sex and suicide attempt prior to the index episode. The C-SSRS total score was analysed without adjustment for prior suicide attempts as this factor is incorporated in the total score. Those with missing values were excluded from the regression analyses.

Receiving operating characteristic analyses were performed for the SI intensity score as well as the C-SSRS total score to assess the area under the curve and identify potential cut-off scores.

Results

The cohort at baseline

Of 1138 eligible participants, 804 (71%) agreed to participate in the study. Baseline characteristics of the study cohort are shown in Table 1.

Two thirds of the participants were women and the age range was 18–95 years, with a median of 33 years (interquartile range 23–50). Almost half of the participants were either unemployed or had sickness benefits or disability pension, and almost three quarters were already in outpatient treatment for a psychiatric disorder. Two thirds of the participants had a history of at least one previous suicide attempt, and half of them had at least one previous episode of non-suicidal self-injury. Most participants were admitted to psychiatric hospital care after the index episode; median stay was 9 days (range 1–238 days). A clinical diagnosis of mood disorder was recorded in one third of the participants, and one fifth had a substance use disorder.

Table 2 shows the baseline ratings on the C-SSRS. A majority of the participants (*n* = 689, 86%) reported high

Table 1 Baseline characteristics of adults presenting at psychiatric emergency services in connection with an episode of self-harm in a Swedish multicentre study 2012–2016 (N = 804)

	Mean	SD
Age	38 years	18
	N	%
Women	541	67%
Current occupation		
Work/student	325	40%
Unemployed/ sick leave/disability pension	395	49%
Retired	84	10%
Living alone	424	53%
Current mental health treatment[a]	573	71%
Inpatient care past 3 months	231	29%
Previous suicide attempt	544	68%
Previous non-suicidal self-injury	421	53%
Suicide attempt at index	666	83%
Psychiatric hospitalization at index[b]	750	93%
Mood disorder at index (F30–39)[c]	295	37%
Substance use disorder at index (F10–19)[c]	172	21%

[a]: having an ongoing contact with primary or psychiatric care with treatment for a psychiatric condition
[b]: defined as at least one night's admission to inpatient care
[c]: diagnosis in primary or secondary position
SD Standard Deviation

Table 2 Baseline C-SSRS ratings in adults presenting at psychiatric emergency services in connection with an episode of self-harm in a Swedish multicentre study 2012–2016 (N = 804)

C-SSRS ratings, past 30 days	Mean	SD
Most severe ideation, range 0–5	4.5	1.2
Intensity items, range 0–5		
Frequency	3.5	1.6
Duration	2.9	1.5
Controllability	3.2	1.7
Deterrents	3.3	1.7
Reasons	4.4	1.3
SI intensity score, range 0–25	17.2	5.3
C-SSRS total score[a], range 0–42	26	7
C-SSRS ratings, lifetime	Mean	SD
Most severe ideation, range 0–5	4.7	0.9
Intensity items, range 0–5		
Frequency	3.9	1.4
Duration	3.3	3.3
Controllability	3.4	3.4
Deterrents	3.5	3.5
Reasons	4.6	0.9
SI intensity score, range 0–25	18.6	4.8
C-SSRS total score, range 0–42	29	7

C-SSRS Columbia-Suicide Severity Rating Scale, *SD* Standard deviation, *SI* Suicidal ideation
[a]C-SSRS behavioural items are rated for past three months

ratings (4–5) on the C-SSRS item *most severe ideation* during the 30 days before the index episode with a mean score of 4.5 (SD 1.2) for the whole group. Corresponding figures were lower for all intensity items except *reasons for ideation*. Lifetime ratings were very similar to those reported for the past 30 days. Twenty-nine participants, twelve of which had made a suicide attempt at index, denied any suicidal ideation during the past month. Five or more actual suicide attempts (range 5–50) were recorded during the past three months for 19 participants. Six of these stated that they had made many hundreds of actual, aborted and interrupted attempts during their lifetime.

Non-fatal and fatal suicide attempts during follow-up

During the six months follow-up, 165 (20.5%) participants made a non-fatal or fatal suicide attempt. Of these, 159 persons (19.8% of the cohort; 18% of all men, 20.5% of all women) made at least one non-fatal suicide attempt and ten persons (1.2% of the cohort; 1.9% of all men, 0.9% of all women) died by suicide. Four persons made a suicide attempt and survived, but died by suicide later in the follow-up period. Nine persons died from causes other than suicide. No entries appeared in the medical records after the index attempt in 15 persons (1.9% of the total sample), which in most cases was due

to the participant moving from the catchment area. All 15 were still alive at the end of the follow-up period.

Associations between C-SSRS ratings and future suicide attempts

The single item *most severe ideation* was significantly associated with a non-fatal or fatal suicide attempt during the six month follow-up, but this did not withstand adjustment for age, sex and suicide attempt prior to the index episode (Table 3).

The separate intensity items frequency, duration and controllability were significant predictors of a future attempt in unadjusted analyses. After adjustment for sex, age and prior suicide attempt all intensity items except reasons for ideation were significantly associated with the outcome with the odds increasing by 20% for each one-step increment in frequency and duration, and by 10% for each one-step increment in controllability and deterrents. The SI intensity score and the C-SSRS total score were also significantly associated with a future attempt before and after adjustment, with the odds increasing with 7 and 8% for each one-step increment, respectively. Figure 1 shows the ROC curve for the SI

Table 3 C-SSRS items, intensity score and total score as predictors of non-fatal and fatal suicide attempt during six month follow-up among adult patients presenting at psychiatric emergency services in connection with an episode of self-harm in a Swedish multicentre study 2012–2016

Item	N with score (n with outcome)	Actual attempts, non-fatal and fatal, during 6 month follow-up; unadjusted				Actual attempts, non-fatal and fatal, during 6 month follow-up; adjusted models[a]			
		OR (95% CI)	p	C&S R^2	N's R^2	OR (95% CI)	p	C&S R^2	N's R^2
Most severe ideation	801(165)	1.2 (1.001–1.4)	0.048	0.006	0.009	1.2 (0.9–1.4)	0.06	0.051	0.079
SI Intensity score	800 (165)	1.1 (1.04–1.1)	< 0.001	0.020	0.034	1.07 (1.03–1.1)	0.001	0.059	0.093
SI Frequency	798 (165)	1.3 (1.1–1.4)	< 0.001	0.020	0.031	1.2 (1.1–1.4)	0.002	0.057	0.089
SI Duration	798 (165)	1.2 (1.1–1.4)	< 0.001	0.017	0.026	1.2 (1.03–1.3)	0.01	0.053	0.083
SI Controllability	796 (164)	1.2 (1.1–1.3)	0.002	0.013	0.020	1.1 (1.01–1.3)	0.03	0.052	0.081
SI Deterrents	796 (164)	1.1 (0.9–1.2)	0.05	0.005	0.008	1.1 (1.03–1.3)	0.02	0.054	0.084
SI Reasons	794 (162)	1.1 (0.9–1.3)	0.2	0.002	0.003	1.1 (0.9–1.3)	0.3	0.046	0.073
C-SSRS total score	802 (165)	1.08 (1.05–1.1)	< 0.001	0.033	0.052	1.08 (1.04–1.1)	< 0.001	0.049	0.077

[a]Adjusted for age, sex, suicide attempt prior to index episode; C-SSRS total score adjusted for age and sex only
C-SSRS Columbia-Suicide Severity Rating Scale, *SI* Suicidal ideation, *OR* Odds ratio, *CI* Confidence interval, *C&S* Cox & Snell, *N's* Nagelkerke's

intensity score as a predictor of non-fatal or fatal suicide attempt within six months. The area under the curve (AUC) was 0.62 (95% CI 0.57–0.67), $p < 0.001$). A cut-off of 18.5 gave a sensitivity of 59% and a specificity of 57% in predicting a non-fatal or fatal suicide attempt. For the C-SSRS total score (Fig. 2), the AUC was 0.65 (95% CI 0.60–0.69, p < 0.001) and a cut-off of 28.5 gave a sensitivity of 69% and a specificity of 54%. Table 4 shows sensitivity and specificity over a range of cut-off values for the SI intensity score. Corresponding values for the C-SSRS total score are shown in Table 5.

Discussion

One fifth of the participants in this large adult cohort made a non-fatal or fatal suicide attempt during the six-month follow-up. The C-SSRS total score and the SI intensity score were significant predictors of suicide attempt within six months, as were the single intensity items frequency, duration and deterrents after taking prior history of attempt into consideration. The overall ability of the SI intensity score to correctly distinguish between those who would and would not make non-fatal or fatal attempts within six months was only

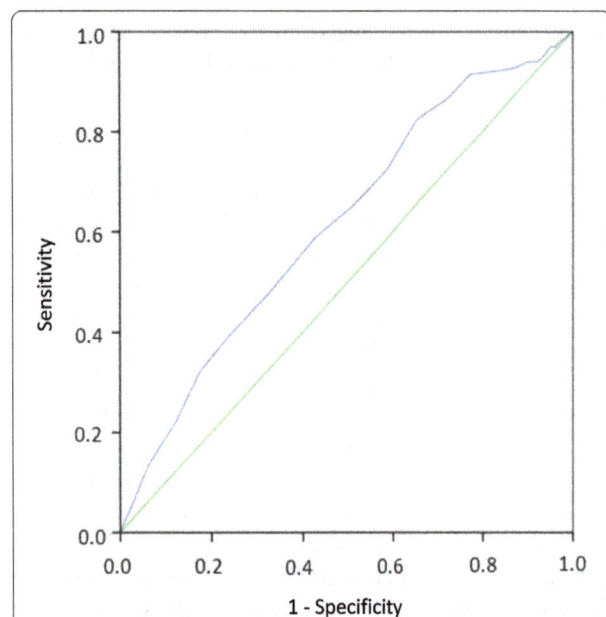

Fig. 1 SI intensity score as predictor of a non-fatal or fatal attempt within 6 months in adult patients presenting at psychiatric emergency services in connection with an episode of self-harm in a Swedish multicentre study 2012–2016. AUC: 0.62 (95% CI 0.57–0.67), *p* < 0.001

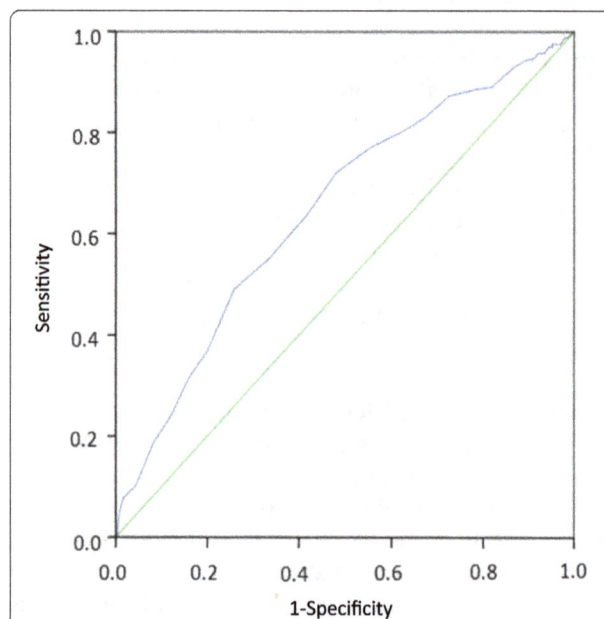

Fig. 2 C-SSRS total score recent time as predictor of a non-fatal or fatal attempt within 6 months in adult patients presenting at psychiatric emergency services in connection with an episode of self-harm in a Swedish multicentre study 2012–2016. AUC 0.65 (95% CI 0.60–0.69), *p* < 0.001

Table 4 Sensitivity and specificity at different cut-off levels for baseline C-SSRS ratings on SI intensity score in predicting non-fatal and fatal suicide attempt during six month follow-up among adult patients presenting at psychiatric emergency services in connection with an episode of self-harm in a Swedish multicentre study 2012–2016

C-SSRS Intensity score, cut-off	Sensitivity	Specificity
15.5	82	34
16.6	73	41
17.5	65	49
18.5	59	57
19.5	47	68

C-SSRS Columbia-Suicide Severity Rating Scale, *SI* Suicidal ideation

somewhat better than chance and the C-SSRS total score performed in a similar fashion.

The ratings on the item *most severe ideation* were high and uniform in this cohort and this item was not a significant predictor of suicide attempt within six months after adjustment for age, sex and prior attempt. This contrasts with results from some previous studies on the C-SSRS. In a treatment study of 124 teenagers who had made an actual or interrupted suicide attempt during the 90 days before inclusion, the most severe suicidal ideation during lifetime (which may or may not coincide with the index episode) predicted suicide attempt during six months follow-up [15]. In a retrospective medical record review of 473 consecutive psychiatric emergency cases with a follow-up time of 18 months, *most severe ideation* was predictive of suicide attempt over and above the impact of a previous suicide attempt [17]. Proportions with suicide attempts during follow-up were lower in these two cohorts (13% and 8%, respectively), suggesting a broader range of psychopathology. Under such circumstances, severe suicidal ideation could constitute a significant marker of risk. This would not be the case, however, in a cohort like ours with a high prevalence of severe ideation.

Table 5 Sensitivity and specificity at different cut-off levels for baseline C-SSRS total score in predicting non-fatal and fatal suicide attempt during six month follow-up among adult patients presenting at psychiatric emergency services in connection with an episode of self-harm in a Swedish multicentre study 2012–2016

C-SSRS total score, cut-off	Sensitivity	Specificity
25.5	77	45
26.5	72	52
27.5	64	58
28.5	55	66
29.5	49	74

C-SSRS Columbia-Suicide Severity Rating Scale

Regarding SI intensity, our finding that frequency, duration and deterrents were predictive of a non-fatal or fatal suicide attempt is in line with previous studies. In the above-cited retrospective study [17], the SI intensity score and the intensity item frequency were predictive of suicide attempt during the 18 month follow-up. In a cohort of 178 consecutive cases of adolescents seeking psychiatric emergency services, the SI intensity score and the intensity item duration were predictive of suicide attempt during 12 month follow-up [21]. Both frequency and duration of ideation have been suggested as markers of a ruminative process [17, 21]. Rumination has been correlated with both suicidal ideation [33] and suicide attempts [34]; the latter however not shown in prospective studies [35]. In a Danish study of 85 teenagers with suicidal behaviour or severe suicide thoughts, the single intensity item deterrents was associated with an actual suicide attempt with an almost three-fold increase in odds during a mean follow-up time of 80 days, when adjusting for actual attempts at baseline [20].

Even though we could demonstrate significant associations between different aspects of the C-SSRS and the outcome, in comparison with previous prediction studies our point estimates for all odds ratios are low, with narrow confidence intervals. In no instance did the upper limit of the 95% confidence interval exceed 1.4. Consequently, there is a low probability of a true population odds ratio greatly exceeding 1. It is unlikely that the factors studied are of major importance for an accurate clinical risk assessment after self-harm. This is also signalled by the fact that the regression models explain a very small proportion of the variance in the outcome.

The ROC curve for the C-SSRS total score as predictor had an AUC of 0.65 in the present study as compared with 0.76 in an adult psychiatric inpatient population [19]. While the same observation period was employed in both studies, comparison is difficult since the outcome of the latter study included also less serious behaviours (aborted and interrupted attempts and preparatory behaviour). Further, the proportion of actual suicide attempts was not presented in that study, nor was the proportion of patients with previous self-harm.

The Cronbach's α for the SI intensity scale was 0.49, indicating limited internal consistency. This finding is similar to that of Youngstrom et al. [22] and might indicate that the SI intensity scale measures more than one underlying construct. These findings, however, contrast with the higher α values (0.73–0.95) presented by Posner and co-workers [15]. The interrater reliability for the different items varied from excellent for the items *most severe ideation*, frequency and duration to moderate/substantial for the item deterrents. This could indicate that the question about deterrents is more complex and that the others are more straightforward and easy to understand for both the patient and the interviewer.

In recent years, several authors have highlighted some problematic aspects of suicide risk assessment in general, e g that suicide risk is largely influenced by factors that are not yet present at the time of assessment [36]. Further, the categorization of patients in high- or low-risk groups is problematic since the incidence of suicide in the high-risk groups, as they have been defined, still is too low to motivate highly interfering interventions (e g involuntary treatment) and the low-risk group is large, meaning that many who die by suicide will have been classified as low-risk [11, 36]. In a recent systematic review of risk scales, even instruments with high sensitivity tended to have a low positive predictive value and no single instrument could be recommended for routine clinical work [37]. Another issue in the field of suicide research has been the lack of uniform terminology [30, 38, 39]. The C-SSRS makes an important contribution to the clarification of suicide-related behaviours. However, it has been argued that the C-SSRS does not cover all possible combinations of ideation and behaviour, and that the questions and instructions could be misinterpreted [40]. For example, a few participants in our study acknowledged some degree of suicidal intention in connection with an attempt that occurred within the past few days, yet negated any suicidal ideation during the past month.

Strengths

This is the first study prospectively evaluating the predictive performance of the C-SSRS in an adult psychiatric population outside the US, contributing to the evidence base for this widely used instrument. The size of the cohort and the small proportion of participants lacking follow-up data are major strengths. The narrow confidence intervals indicate that non-significant results are not likely to be due to insufficient statistical power. The generous inclusion criteria, few exclusion criteria and high participation rate imply adequate external validity. Further, the age range is wide rendering results more relevant to clinical situations involving adult emergency psychiatric populations. The follow-up time of six months is shorter, and thus more clinically relevant, than in most prediction studies published to date [11, 14, 26]. Experienced mental health staff performed the data collection, both the index interview and the follow-up examination of medical records. The quality and quantity of information recorded during the follow-up period is very good since the Swedish personal identity number allows multiple service providers to share the same electronic medical record system, and makes feasible automatic updates from the population register. Age range, gender distribution and repetition rate in the present study population are similar to figures reported from previous studies on adult hospital-presenting self-harm patients [9, 41], which implies that our results might be applicable to similar

clinical populations in other countries. The majority of the participants had inpatient treatment in connection with the index episode, which limits generalizability to hospital-treated self-harm patients. To the best of our knowledge, this is the first prediction study of the C-SSRS in such a population.

Limitations

The number of suicides was not sufficient to analyse suicide as a separate outcome. Some participants may have made suicide attempts during the follow-up period without it coming to the attention of psychiatric services, and in this study, we only have knowledge of those episodes of self-harm that were mentioned in the medical records. Still, this is likely to give a more correct estimate of outcome events than only using data from the national diagnostic registers, since not all self-harm events are registered. While we do know that all patients without follow-up data were still alive six months after the index episode, we lack information on non-fatal suicide attempts for this small group.

Conclusions

In this study of psychiatric patients with self-harm, suicidal ideation intensity and the C-SSRS total score were associated with increasing odds for non-fatal and fatal suicide attempt during a six-month follow-up. The associations, however, are not specific enough to guide treatment. Since the C-SSRS is widely used internationally, further studies could investigate its predictive properties in varied settings and cultures. With the exception of one item, the interrater reliability estimates indicate that the instrument works well for classification, for which it was originally developed.

Abbreviations

AUC: Area under the curve; CI: Confidence interval; C-SSRS: Columbia-Suicide Severity Rating Scale; NSSI: Non-suicidal self-injury; OR: Odds ratio; PABAK: Prevalence-adjusted, bias-adjusted kappa; ROC: Receiver operating characteristic.; SA: Suicide attempt; SD: Standard deviation; SI: Suicidal ideation

Acknowledgements

The authors wish to thank Håkan Källmén who assisted in the statistical analysis of the data.

Funding

The study was supported by grants provided by the Swedish Research Council 521–2011-299, ALFGBG-715841, the Stockholm County Council (ALF project 20120225, ALF project 20150290), Umeå University and Västerbotten County Council (ALF, VLL-549931) and the Bror Gadelius Foundation. The funding bodies were not involved neither in the design of the study nor in collection, analysis, or interpretation of data or in writing the manuscript.

Authors' contributions

ÅL and BR designed the study with input from MW, KB, MD and ESR. ÅL extracted, processed and analysed the data. All authors interpreted the results and ÅL wrote the first draft. All the authors contributed to subsequent drafts and have approved the final version of the manuscript.

Consent for publication

Not applicable.

Competing interests

The authors declare that they have no competing interests.

Author details

[1]Centre for Psychiatry Research, Department of Clinical Neuroscience, Karolinska Institutet, & Stockholm Health Care Services, Stockholm County Council, S:t Görans Hospital, Vårdvägen 1, SE-112 81 Stockholm, Sweden. [2]Department of Psychiatry and Neurochemistry, University of Göteborg, Gothenburg, Sweden. [3]Department of Clinical Sciences, Division of Psychiatry, University of Umeå, Umeå, Sweden.

References

1. WHO: Preventing suicide - A global imperative. 2014.
2. Beghi M, Rosenbaum JF, Cerri C, Cornaggia CM. Risk factors for fatal and nonfatal repetition of suicide attempts: a literature review. Neuropsychiatr Dis Treat. 2013;9:1725–36.
3. Foster T, Gillespie K, McClelland R, Patterson C. Risk factors for suicide independent of DSM-III-R Axis I disorder. Case-control psychological autopsy study in Northern Ireland. Br J Psychiatry. 1999;175:175–9.
4. Hawton K, van Heeringen K. Suicide. Lancet. 2009;373(9672):1372–81.
5. Tidemalm D, Langstrom N, Lichtenstein P, Runeson B. Risk of suicide after suicide attempt according to coexisting psychiatric disorder: Swedish cohort study with long term follow-up. BMJ. 2008;337:a2205.
6. Zahl DL, Hawton K. Repetition of deliberate self-harm and subsequent suicide risk: long-term follow-up study of 11,583 patients. Br J Psychiatry. 2004;185:70–5.
7. Cooper J, Kapur N, Webb R, Lawlor M, Guthrie E, Mackway-Jones K, Appleby L. Suicide after deliberate self-harm: a 4-year cohort study. Am J Psychiatry. 2005;162(2):297–303.
8. Runeson B, Haglund A, Lichtenstein P, Tidemalm D. Suicide risk after nonfatal self-harm: a national cohort study, 2000-2008. J Clin Psychiatry. 2016;77(2):240–6.
9. Owens D, Horrocks J, House A. Fatal and non-fatal repetition of self-harm. Systematic review Br J Psychiatry. 2002;181:193–9.
10. Carroll R, Metcalfe C, Gunnell D. Hospital presenting self-harm and risk of fatal and non-fatal repetition: systematic review and meta-analysis. PLoS One. 2014;9(2):e89944.
11. Large M, Kaneson M, Myles N, Myles H, Gunaratne P, Ryan C. Meta-analysis of longitudinal cohort studies of suicide risk assessment among psychiatric patients: heterogeneity in results and lack of improvement over time. PLoS One. 2016;11(6):e0156322.
12. Chan MK, Bhatti H, Meader N, Stockton S, Evans J, O'Connor RC, Kapur N, Kendall T. Predicting suicide following self-harm: systematic review of risk factors and risk scales. Br J Psychiatry. 2016;209(4):277–83.
13. Carter G, Milner A, McGill K, Pirkis J, Kapur N, Spittal MJ. Predicting suicidal behaviours using clinical instruments: systematic review and meta-analysis of positive predictive values for risk scales. Br J Psychiatry. 2017;210(6):387–95.
14. Runeson B, Odeberg J, Pettersson A, Edbom T, Jildevik Adamsson I, Waern M. Instruments for the assessment of suicide risk: a systematic review evaluating the certainty of the evidence. PLoS One. 2017;12(7):e0180292.
15. Posner K, Brown GK, Stanley B, Brent DA, Yershova KV, Oquendo MA, Currier GW, Melvin GA, Greenhill L, Shen S, et al. The Columbia-suicide

severity rating scale: initial validity and internal consistency findings from three multisite studies with adolescents and adults. Am J Psychiatry. 2011;168(12):1266–77.
16. Posner K, Oquendo MA, Gould M, Stanley B, Davies M. Columbia classification algorithm of suicide assessment (C-CASA): classification of suicidal events in the FDA's pediatric suicidal risk analysis of antidepressants. Am J Psychiatry. 2007;164(7):1035–43.
17. Horwitz AG, Czyz EK, King CA. Predicting future suicide attempts among adolescent and emerging adult psychiatric emergency patients. J Clin Child Adolesc Psychol. 2014:1–11.
18. Greist JH, Mundt JC, Gwaltney CJ, Jefferson JW, Posner K. Predictive value of baseline electronic Columbia-suicide severity rating scale (eC-SSRS) assessments for identifying risk of prospective reports of suicidal behavior during research participation. Innov Clin Neurosci. 2014;11(9–10):23–31.
19. Madan A, Frueh BC, Allen JG, Ellis TE, Rufino KA, Oldham JM, Fowler JC. Psychometric reevaluation of the Columbia-suicide severity rating scale: findings from a prospective, inpatient cohort of severely mentally ill adults. J Clin Psychiatry. 2016;77(7):e867–73.
20. Conway PM, Erlangsen A, Teasdale TW, Jakobsen IS, Larsen KJ. Predictive validity of the Columbia-suicide severity rating scale for short-term suicidal behavior: a Danish study of adolescents at a high risk of suicide. Arch Suicide Res. 2016:1–15.
21. Gipson PY, Agarwala P, Opperman KJ, Horwitz A, King CA. Columbia-suicide severity rating scale: predictive validity with adolescent psychiatric emergency patients. Pediatr Emerg Care. 2014.
22. Youngstrom EA, Hameed A, Mitchell MA, Van Meter AR, Freeman AJ, Algorta GP, White AM, Clayton PJ, Gelenberg AJ, Meyer RE. Direct comparison of the psychometric properties of multiple interview and patient-rated assessments of suicidal ideation and behavior in an adult psychiatric inpatient sample. J Clin Psychiatry. 2015;76(12):1676–82.
23. Al-Halabi S, Saiz PA, Buron P, Garrido M, Benabarre A, Jimenez E, Cervilla J, Navarrete MI, Diaz-Mesa EM, Garcia-Alvarez L, et al. Validation of a Spanish version of the Columbia-suicide severity rating scale (C-SSRS). Rev Psiquiatr Salud Ment. 2016;9(3):134–42.
24. Hawton K, Fagg J. Suicide, and other causes of death, following attempted suicide. Br J Psychiatry. 1988;152:359–66.
25. Bolton JM. Suicide risk assessment in the emergency department: out of the darkness. Depress Anxiety. 2015;32(2):73–5.
26. Bolton JM, Gunnell D, Turecki G. Suicide risk assessment and intervention in people with mental illness. BMJ. 2015;351:h4978.
27. Glenn CR, Nock MK: Improving the short-term prediction of suicidal behavior. Am J Prev Med 2014, 47(3 Suppl 2):S176–S180.
28. Turecki G, Brent DA. Suicide and suicidal behaviour. Lancet. 2016; 387(10024):1227–39.
29. Large M, Sharma S, Cannon E, Ryan C, Nielssen O. Risk factors for suicide within a year of discharge from psychiatric hospital: a systematic meta-analysis. Aust N Z J Psychiatry. 2011;45(8):619–28.
30. O'Carroll PW, Berman AL, Maris RW, Moscicki EK, Tanney BL, Silverman MM. Beyond the tower of babel: a nomenclature for suicidology. Suicide Life Threat Behav. 1996;26(3):237–52.
31. Nock MK, Holmberg EB, Photos VI, Michel BD. Self-injurious thoughts and behaviors interview: development, reliability, and validity in an adolescent sample. Psychol Assess. 2007;19(3):309–17.
32. Ludvigsson JF, Almqvist C, Bonamy AK, Ljung R, Michaelsson K, Neovius M, Stephansson O, Ye W. Registers of the Swedish total population and their use in medical research. Eur J Epidemiol. 2016;31(2):125–36.
33. Krajniak M, Miranda R, Wheeler A. Rumination and pessimistic certainty as mediators of the relation between lifetime suicide attempt history and future suicidal ideation. Arch Suicide Res. 2013;17(3):196–211.
34. Polanco-Roman L, Jurska J, Quinones V, Miranda R. Brooding, reflection, and distraction: relation to non-suicidal self-injury versus suicide attempts. Arch Suicide Res. 2015;19(3):350–65.
35. Rogers ML, Joiner TE. Rumination, suicidal ideation, and suicide attempts: a meta-analytic review. Rev Gen Psychol. 2017;21(2):132–42.
36. Large M, Galletly C, Myles N, Ryan CJ, Myles H. Known unknowns and unknown unknowns in suicide risk assessment: evidence from meta-analyses of aleatory and epistemic uncertainty. BJPsych Bull. 2017;41(3):160–3.
37. Quinlivan L, Cooper J, Davies L, Hawton K, Gunnell D, Kapur N. Which are the most useful scales for predicting repeat self-harm? A systematic review evaluating risk scales using measures of diagnostic accuracy. BMJ Open. 2016;6(2):e009297.

38. De Leo D, Burgis S, Bertolote JM, Kerkhof AJ, Bille-Brahe U. Definitions of suicidal behavior: lessons learned from the WHo/EURO multicentre study. Crisis. 2006;27(1):4–15.

39. Silverman MM, Berman AL, Sanddal ND, O'Carroll PW, Joiner TE. Rebuilding the tower of babel: a revised nomenclature for the study of suicide and suicidal behaviors. Part 1: background, rationale, and methodology. Suicide Life Threat Behav. 2007;37(3):248–63.

40. Giddens JM, Sheehan KH, Sheehan DV. The Columbia-suicide severity rating scale (C-SSRS): has the "gold standard" become a liability? Innov Clin Neurosci. 2014;11(9–10):66–80.

41. Carroll R, Metcalfe C, Gunnell D. Hospital management of self-harm patients and risk of repetition: systematic review and meta-analysis. J Affect Disord. 2014;168:476–83.

14

Factors influencing early withdrawal from a drug and alcohol treatment program and client perceptions of successful recovery and employment: a qualitative study

Tarran Prangley[1], Sabrina Winona Pit[2,3]* (iD), Trent Rees[4] and Jessica Nealon[5]

Abstract

Background: Substance use disorders are a major contributor to the economic and healthcare burden in Australia. Therapeutic communities (TCs) are utilised treatment methods globally, though low program completion rates continue to represent a major obstacle in effective and sustainable drug and alcohol treatment. The aim of this study was to explore reasons for early withdrawal from TC programs and perceptions of successful recovery. This study also aimed to explore how employment and volunteering related to early exit and perceptions of successful recovery.

Methods: Semi-structured qualitative interviews were conducted with 13 ex-residents from a long-term TC program at a community-based rehab organisation in regional Australia.

Results: Thematic analysis revealed a complex interplay of factors contributing to early TC withdrawal, and perceptions of successful recovery from a lived experience perspective and how this was shaped by employment and volunteering. Eleven themes were identified. Three relating to reasons for joining the program, which connected with ultimate withdrawal from the program: Pre-program existing relationships, pre-program employment situation and needing a 'circuit breaker' in their life. Three relating to reasons for early withdrawal: TC program characteristics, relationships during the program and planning future employment. Five relating to perceptions of successful recovery: Improved understanding of their addiction, reduced substance use, improved physical and psychological health, relationship success and employment success.

Conclusions: Reasons for leaving treatment early are multi-faceted and revolve around relationships, planning future employment and program characteristics. The influence that each plays on their decision to leave early is varied and determined by the value they assign it. Perceived success extends far beyond achieving and maintaining abstinence to encompass improved relationships, psychological and physical wellbeing, understanding of addiction and employment, studying or volunteering. Self-worth and feeling able to contribute to society through employment, study and volunteering were perceived to be essential elements of successful recovery. Clinicians, policy makers and program developers should use the extended definition of successful recovery from the ex-clients perspective when determining the clinical and economic effectiveness of TC programs.

Keywords: Therapeutic community, Substance use disorders, Addiction, Early exit, Recovery, Employment

* Correspondence: s.pit@westernsydney.edu.au; sabrinapit@gmail.com
[2]School of Medicine, University Centre for Rural Health, Western Sydney University, 61 Uralba Street, Lismore, NSW 2480, Australia
[3]Sydney Medical School, University of Sydney, 61 Uralba Street, Lismore, NSW 2480, Australia
Full list of author information is available at the end of the article

Background

Substance use disorders are a major contributor to the economic and healthcare burden in Australia; costing $55 billion annually through crime, road accidents, workplace productivity losses and healthcare costs [1]. The National Drug Strategy [2] identified alcohol, cannabis and methamphetamine use as priority areas. Improvements in Drug and Alcohol (DA) treatment services help to address these issues, particularly by targeting demand reduction, peer-education networks, social competence training and increasing community engagement.

Therapeutic communities (TCs) are drug-free residential rehabilitation programs where clients live together in a hierarchal-based supportive environment with increasing levels of social and personal responsibility [3]. This treatment model is utilised in DA rehabilitation with the aim to socially rehabilitate drug users through personal change and skills training [4].

Success of these programs has been evaluated through a literature review of 16 controlled TC studies [5]. TC residents had superior employment outcomes and improved relationships and psychological functioning compared to controls. Length of stay in treatment and participation in subsequent aftercare were found to be consistent predictors of recovery. Contrary to these findings, a systematic review of residential treatment studies did not show superior employment outcomes in TC residents [4]. However, only one of the 11 studies included in the latter study measured employment as an outcome variable, and this study did find higher employment in the TC group at follow-up [4]. Improvements in other outcome measures included substance use, criminal activity, mental health and social engagement.

Low program completion rates, ranging from 9 to 56%, continue to represent a major obstacle in effective and sustainable DA treatment [3, 6]. Length of stay in treatment is associated with higher levels of abstinence, reduced crime and unemployment, and improved quality of life [3, 7]. Predictors of early withdrawal have therefore been explored to identify clients who may be at increased risk of dropout and enable more appropriate referral to TC services for clients who are most likely to benefit from the program.

Three quantitative studies investigated predictors of TC completion [8, 9]. Disadvantageous decision making, lower perception of likeliness to complete the program, recent prison release, aggression, self-harm or suicidality, relationships, amphetamine use and younger and older age, were all found to be predictors of early withdrawal. However, some discrepancies exist in the literature. Harley et al. found amphetamine use to be a negative predictor of program completion (Harley M, Pit SW, Rees T, Thomas S: Completion rates and psychosocial intervention effectiveness in an Australian substance abuse therapeutic community, submitted.), contrary to Darke et al. [9] who found no association with primary drug use. The relationship between disadvantageous decision making and residential treatment drop-out investigated by Stevens et al. [8] may have been mediated by potential confounders not investigated, including psychiatric comorbidities and motivation for treatment. Additionally, although the study concerned a residential treatment population, the treatment facilities did not apply the 'community as a method' approach typical for TCs. Issues with generalisability beyond cocaine dependent individuals also limits Stevens et al.'s [8] research.

A qualitative approach enables exploration of the complex relationships between client variables, treatment retention, and re-integration into society from the clients' perspective. Despite the benefit, there is a deficit of qualitative research exploring reasons for early withdrawal from adult TCs. Two qualitative studies investigating adolescent TC populations identified negative relationships with staff as major contributors to early withdrawal [10, 11]. Landrum et al. [10] investigated reasons for early withdrawal through five focus groups among judicially referred adolescents, parents and treatment staff. Five main domains affected retention: relationships, responsibility, emotional regulation, thinking and self-efficacy. The importance of motivation for treatment success was also noted.

Chen et al. [11] used semi-structured interviews to investigate the experiences of 11 adolescents who dropped out of an Orthodox Jewish TC, focusing on reasons for early TC withdrawal and recovery. Chen et al. [11] found antagonistic staff and adolescent interactions, lack of motivation and program dissatisfaction, and a desire to make positive changes in various aspects of their life. However, like Landrum et al. [10] the narrow focus on Orthodox Jewish adolescents and judicially referred adolescents limits its generalisability to other populations.

Most TC research focuses on abstinence as a surrogate for program success, however little research has investigated what recovery success looks like for clients. Aslan [12] aimed to address the question 'when is "unsuccessful" successful?' through semi-structured interviews with 13 service users who withdrew early from three TCs in the United Kingdom. Recovery success was found to manifest in various ways including improvements in psychological well-being, relationships, accommodation and employment, as well as reductions in relapse and reoffending. Eighty-five percent of participants reported using their time in positive ways such as voluntary and paid employment, college and spending time with friends or at support services. Most participants were also actively involved in further treatment after discharge.

Aslan [12] highlights an important question about redefining recovery 'success' to better reflect the clients' perspective. Similarly, Laudet [13] investigated what recovery success looks like from a lived-experience perspective through interviews with 354 individuals with resolved substance use disorders, not specifically individuals who left residential rehabilitation early. Abstinence was identified as necessary for recovery, though recovery goals extended well beyond abstinence. Recovery was seen by most as a process of growth through which the individual achieved improved financial and living conditions, social networks and physical and/or mental health.

There is a considerable lack of qualitative research, and, to our knowledge, none in an Australian context, exploring both reasons for early exit and successful recovery from a lived-experience perspective. The current study aimed to gain a better understanding of the reasons for early withdrawal from TC programs and perceptions of successful recovery. A secondary aim was to explore how employment and volunteering related to early exit and perceptions of successful recovery.

Method

Participants

Participants comprised ex-residents from a long-term TC program at a community-based rehab organisation located in regional Australia. All participants left the TC program early, either voluntarily or involuntarily, and had given consent to be contacted for future research.

Recruitment

Participants were informed about the project via email from the organisation, and given the opportunity to advise if they did not wish to be contacted by the researchers. Recruitment was targeted to ensure demographic diversity. In particular, a varied sample of age groups, gender and voluntary or involuntary withdrawal from the program was sought.

Data collection

Participants were contacted by author TP via telephone or email and provided an information sheet with the goals of the research. No prior relationship was established prior to study commencement between the participants and TP. Prior to the interview, participants were asked to sign a consent form or give verbal consent over the telephone. Participants were also provided with resources to contact should any distress arise from the interview.

The semi-structured interview schedule was developed from the literature and in consultation with the staff. Questions were designed to explore factors related to reasons for early withdrawal, substance use and treatment history, employment, social supports and perceptions of recovery. The interview schedule was pre-tested for clarity and appropriate question ordering, and further refined where necessary.

The interviews were conducted by TP via telephone from October 2017 to December 2017. TP has a bachelor degree in psychology and has received training in interviewing techniques as part of a psychology and medical degree. Author TR provided content expertise through explaining the

context of the programs. Further guidance in qualitative data analyses was provided by author SWP. Telephone interviews were conducted as the majority of participants now lived inter-state, making face-to-face interviews unfeasible. Data saturation was achieved and no new themes emerged in the final two interviews.

Analysis

Reflective notes were kept during the interview process to guide analyses. Interviews were audio-recorded, transcribed verbatim and analysed thematically [14]. Microsoft® Word was used throughout the data analyses process. The first transcript was read and analysed by TP and SWP and preliminary codes were generated after discussion. The code book was independently trialled by TP and SWP on two interviews, followed by an in-depth discussion to reach a consensus on coding. The coding tree was broadly defined into life prior to joining the drug rehabilitation program, time during the program, perceived success and factors influencing perceived success. TP coded the remaining transcripts. Coded data extracts were then collated together and emerging themes identified. Themes were discussed initially between TP and SWP, and then refined to ensure they captured the meaning of the data.. The themes were then fed back to TR to further aid in data interpretation and potential theme refinement. Data saturation was discussed between TP and SP and it was felt that data saturation was achieved after eleven interviews but two more interviews were conducted to confirm. Transcripts were not returned to participants for comment and/or correction. Quotes have been used in discussion of each topic.

Ethics

Ethics approval for this project was granted by Western Sydney University Human Research Ethics Committee (HREC No: H11353) and the University of Wollongong Human Research Ethics Committee (Ethics Number 2017/404).

Results

Thirty-five residents who left the TC program early were contacted. Reasons for non-participation were: inability to contact due to a disconnected or incorrect telephone number or email address ($n = 7$), no reply to telephone or email contact ($n = 13$), not wishing to partake (n = 1) and unable to be contacted after initial positive contact (n = 1). Thirteen interviews were conducted (7 male and 6 female). The age range was 31–61 years, mean age 44 years. The interviews varied in length, ranging from 15 to 39 min (average 27 min). Participant demographics are listed in Table 1.

The main themes and their complex relationships are depicted in Fig. 1. Figure 1 demonstrates that pre-existing relationships and participant's employment situation prior to program entry were linked with participant's need for a 'circuit breaker' in their life. The themes needing a 'circuit

Table 1 Demographics of participants

		Males	Females	Total number of participants (%)
Participants		7	6	13 (100%)
Age	31–34	0	3	3 (23%)
	35–39	0	2	2 (15%)
	40–44	2	0	2 (15%)
	45–49	2	0	2 (15%)
	50–54	1	1	2 (15%)
	55–61	2	0	2 (15%)
Reason for early exit from TC program	Voluntary	3	5	8 (62%)
	Involuntary[a]	4	1	5 (38%)
Primary dependence prior to admission[b]	Alcohol	6	0	6 (46%)
	Drug	1	3	4 (31%)
	Polysubstance	0	3	3 (23%)
Length of stay	< 2 weeks	1	0	1 (8%)
	2–4 weeks	0	2	2 (15%)
	5–8 weeks	1	3	4 (31%)
	9–12 weeks	1	1	2 (15%)
	13–16 weeks	0	0	0 (0%)
	> 16 weeks	1	3	4 (31%)

[a]The reasons for involuntary withdrawal included breaking the rules, such as bringing or purchasing illicit substances, contacting family outside of the program, having a relationship with another resident, and arguments with staff
[b]Substances included heroin, ice, cocaine, cannabis and alcohol. Prescription medication use included benzodiazepines and codeine

breaker' in life, pre-existing relationships and pre-program employment situation reflected the reasons for entry into the program, which was connected with ultimate withdrawal from the program. Furthermore, Fig. 1 shows that reasons for early withdrawal centred around three major themes: TC program characteristics, relationships during the program and planning for future employment. Finally, five themes emerged that participants perceived to be part of a successful recovery: improved understanding of their addiction, reduced substance use, improved physical and psychological health, positive relationships with others and employment success. Both relationships and employment were themes that played a major part before, during and after entering the TC program and influenced participant's reasons for withdrawing early and their perceptions of successful recovery.

Reasons for joining the program
Both existing relationships, and pre-program employment situations were linked with the need for a circuit breaker in life and formed the basis for participants' perceived need to enter the TC program.

Pre-program existing relationships
Support networks prior to the TC program were varied. Whilst some reported positive relationships with family

and friends, they also felt that their supports did not understand their journey. Others described a strong sense of isolation in the later stages of their addiction and whilst some may have had support around them at this time, it was not recognised.

'...when I was in the end of my addiction I didn't really speak to anyone...my family begrudgingly communicated with me. But I didn't really have proper conversations with anyone.'

For others, craving an emotional connection of any form resulted in maintaining destructive relationships, such as other substance users, which negatively influenced their addiction.

'......<family member> and I used a lot of ecstasy... smoked heroin once together. This is just completely what you don't do with your <family member>, ever.'

Pre-program employment situation
The influence of employment on substance abuse is complex. For most, periods of employment were interspersed with long periods of unemployment and lack of

Pre-program existing relationships

- The impact of substance use on positive relationships
- The impact of negative relationships on substance use

Pre-program employment situation

- The impact of substance use on ability to work
- The impact of employment on substance use

Needing a "circuit breaker" in life

- Early childhood trauma
- Legal issues
- Last resort
- Poor mental health
- Positive feedback about the program

Reasons for early withdrawal

TC Program characteristics

- Initial misunderstanding of the TC program
- Own reflection
- Intensity of the program
- No contact with outside world

Relationships during the program

- Missing family/ friends
- Difficulty living & communicating with others
- Unreciprocated feelings
- Misunderstanding counsellors

Planning future employment

- Work commitments
- Feeling ready to start work

Perceptions of successful recovery

Improved understanding of their addiction

- Trigger recognition
- Recovery as a journey
- Engaging in further treatment

Reduced substance use

Improved physical and psychological health

Relationship success

- Forming close relationships with new people
- Re-build existing relationships
- Being a support for others

Employment success

- Working
- Studying to gain work
- Volunteering
- Being productive: no time to use drugs

They grey areas answer the secondary aim: the relationship between employment with reasons for early withdrawal and perceptions of successful recovery

Fig. 1 Themes

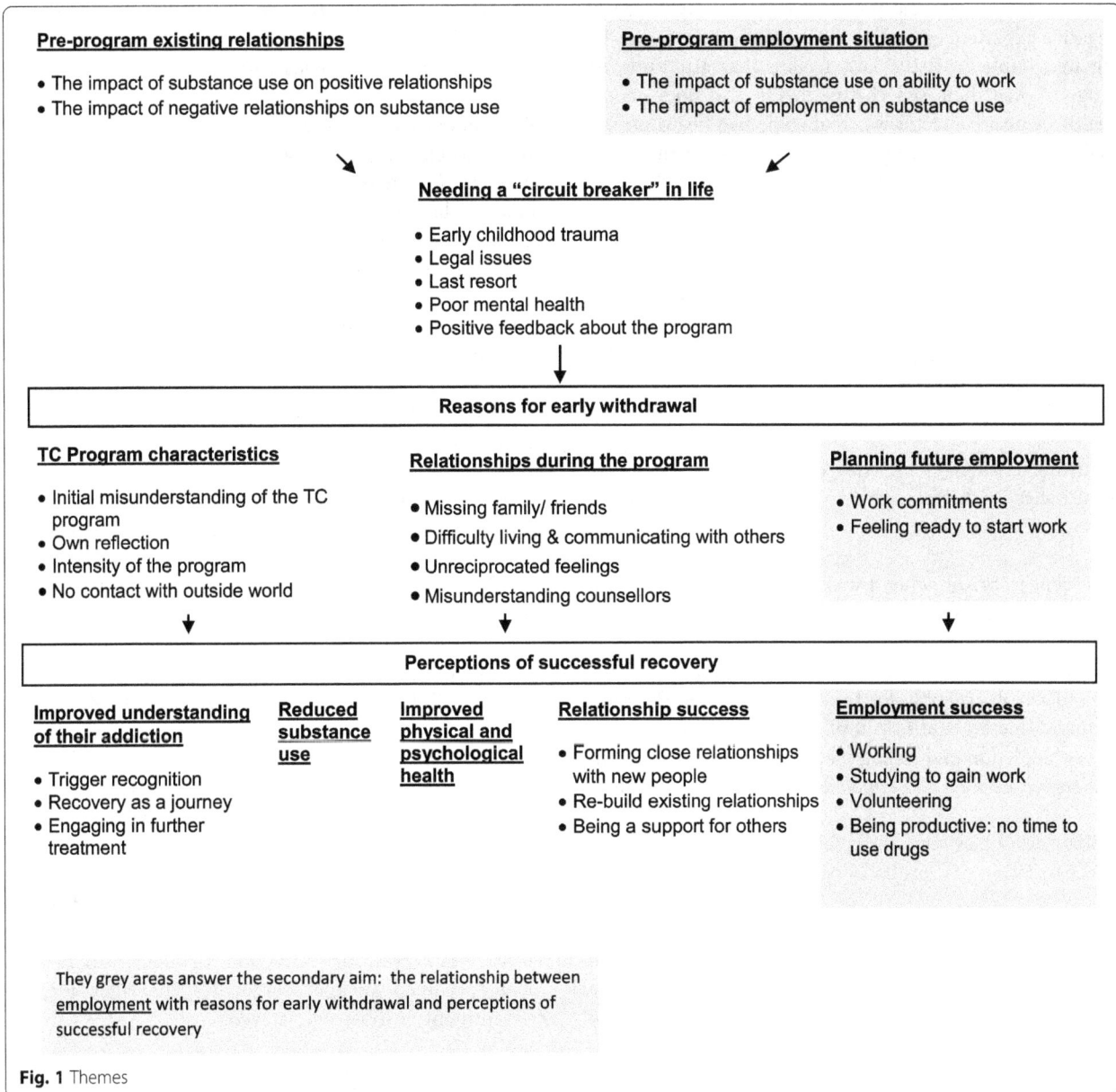

stability. For one participant, her work played such an integral part in her identity that its' loss directly influenced her to relapse. Others reported poor decision-making and lacked the skills to maintain jobs.

'...I was really good at getting jobs and really shithouse at keeping them.'

For twelve participants, employment allowed access and means to maintain their addiction, such as working in a drug and alcohol environment like clubs and pubs, or working in high paying jobs like law and finance. For others, working alone or in remote and rural locations with no oversight allowed for their addiction to continue unnoticed at work.

'I ran nightclubs for a long time ... I was given a lot of free cocaine. Um and a lot of free everything...'

Needing a 'circuit breaker' in life
Participants talked about several factors leading to them joining the program. The reasons for joining the program set the scene for being able to talk about their life in relation to the program itself, their reasons for leaving and their subsequent perceptions of successful recovery.

Reasons for joining the program were mainly based on negative experiences such as early childhood trauma, being in trouble with the law, feeling that attending the program was their last chance in life and poor mental health. A positive factor was that some had heard positive feedback about the program. Eleven participants had a history of life-long challenges. Most participants described early life challenges such as childhood trauma and substance use, isolation and complex mental health issues. For most, their substance use began in middle childhood or early adolescence as a means of escaping reality.

> '… anything you'd put in front of me that would change the way I felt and make me feel a bit better I'd take it.'

Further challenges included drug-related offences and legal issues, with three participants having spent time in prison.

> 'I went to prison when I was 23 as a result of my drug using behaviours.'

Twelve participants described a turning point that led to their decision to apply for the program. Some described feeling desperate and fearful of the consequences of continued addiction and feeling that their life was on the line. Others felt isolated and crippled by poor mental health.

> 'If I hadn't had gone through the <rehab organisation> I'd probably be dead to be honest.'

For others, decisions to attend the rehab organisation were influenced by hearing positive things about the programs from previous residents, or being referred by other treatment facilities because of their long addiction history.

Reasons for early withdrawal

Reasons for withdrawal revealed three major themes: the TC program characteristics, relationships and planning for future employment. Firstly, TC characteristics that led to participants leaving early varied, including a misunderstanding of the program and different expectations of the program when they joined. Some had time during the program to reflect on their life and substance use and mentioned they were able to come to the conclusion that the program was not for them or they felt they had learnt enough during the program and were ready to leave early. Some participants did not cope with the intensity of the program and relationships with others within the program such as being with others 24/7. On the contrary, other participants reported feeling very isolated from the outside world such as friends and family and therefore left the program early. The intensity of the program and the rule of no contact with the outside world during the program has a clear link with participants' relationships with others and their reasons for leaving early.

TC program characteristics

Four participants reported an initial misunderstanding about the TC program rules or duration. This misunderstanding had positive consequences for some whom otherwise may not have attended the program had they fully comprehended the rules.

> 'I was very naïve um about what I was getting myself in for, but that was good in a way.'

For others, a better understanding of the program duration may have allowed arrangements to be made to stay longer.

Some participants found the intensity of the TC program to be very challenging and confronting. Some described the therapy as "tiring and relentless", and found it difficult to be open about their feelings and deal with past traumas.

> '… the program's very tiring… necessary but it's work… it's therapy all day, all night it's relentless…. it's 24/7.'

Others felt uncomfortable openly confronting other residents about disagreements. One participant described a 'shame and blame' environment. Another attributed their decision to leave the program early to the 'informant culture'. Some disagreed with the program rules, and one participant described the program as 'cultish'. However, on reflection of their experiences, most developed an appreciation for the rules and the commitment of those who stayed.

> 'There were rules that I found really odd. Um but now I understand how the program works.'

For others, the decision to leave early was self-guided. Some felt they were adequately equipped and were ready to leave. Others had just had enough and expressed feelings of guilt for leaving the program early.

All participants discussed feeling isolated from the outside world. Whilst this isolation was challenging, it was also recognised as necessary. For some, isolation provided a safe environment away from violent relationships and temptations.

> ' … I needed to be taken totally out of my environment … out of the people, places and things that I was associated with, and dropped into a therapeutic community where I could recover…'

For others, isolation from their support network outside of the TC program constituted a major reason for leaving early.

Relationships during the program

For some, missing family and friends influenced their decision to leave early. Relationships formed with staff and residents within the program were challenging. In particular, some reported difficulties living and communicating with other people. Two participants developed feelings for others that were not reciprocated and one participant was asked to leave after breaching a program rule; starting a relationship with another resident. Some felt that the counsellors could have been more understanding and others felt like the counsellors weren't supportive. However, despite these difficulties, on reflection most participants recognised the necessity of the isolation and relationships within the program.

'...everyone's their brother's keeper and everyone's brother's policeman.'

Conversely, for others the support of family and friends served as a motivating factor to stay in the program, as did the support of program staff and residents. Several reported the therapeutic value of staff also being recovering addicts and seeing them as a positive role model. Living and interacting with people who had faced similar challenges to them helped to foster a sense of belonging within the community, and some reported feeling accountable to the therapeutic community.

'... I just felt for the first time that I had love around ... and I had a massive amount of support.'

Planning future employment

Work commitments outside the program also influenced the decision to leave the program early. For some this was having a job to go back to and for others this was feeling ready to find a job and start working.

'...my employer in <city> had given me time off.'

Perceptions of successful recovery

Participants discussed their life after leaving the TC program and several themes emerged that demonstrated a variety of important elements of successful recovery which will be discussed below.

Improved understanding of their addiction

Ten participants reported gaining a better understanding of their addiction triggers and barriers to ongoing recovery.

'... I didn't really want to give up that <living-place> but I understand that it was part of my recovery you know because it was a trigger with everyone using in that house ...'

Six participants learnt that 'recovery is a journey'. For some this involved sharing their own and other people's stories, whereas others felt isolated in their journey.

As part of 'recovery as a journey', most participants recognised the importance of ongoing treatment. All participants had engaged in further drug and alcohol treatments since leaving the program. The treatment varied from NA and AA support groups, counselling and doctors, medications and alternative therapies such as yoga and meditation. Most participants had engaged in a multi-faceted treatment approach.

'I've done a little bit of work with a psychologist. I've worked the steps. I've done you know I've explored meditation, acupuncture, I do Bikram Yoga.'

For some, ongoing recovery involved incorporating the TC program's morning routine into their lives. One participant attributed the core of their addiction problems to this lack of stability and routine.

'I would just get up and do my morning program which was brisk walk, some exercise, come home and eat, basically. Which would set me up you know um for the day...'

Reduced substance use

Ten participants were abstinent at the time of the interview. Five had remained abstinent since leaving the program, ranging from one to four years. For many, the achievement they are most proud of was the accomplishment and maintenance of abstinence. Most attributed their abstinence in some way to the program, in addition to external sources such as social supports, ongoing DA treatments and employment.

'... I haven't touched a drink or drugs since leaving the <rehab organisation>.'

For some, abstinence was interrupted by lapses or relapse but overall these were much shorter than previous relapses. These shorter periods were seen as success because participants reported using skills learnt at the program to better recognise the early signs and halt the progression of the lapse before losing control.

'I often use the knowledge that I gained while I was in the <rehab organisation>, like daily...'

Improved physical and psychological health

Ten participants reported an improvement in physical health, rating it as good or excellent. Two participants rated their physical health as fair or poor because of the desire to lose weight or increase fitness. Many reported improvements in psychological health and outlook on life. Some felt they had gained the ability to listen and be honest with themselves and others.

'... I was just happy that my life looked like it was going to start going in a different direction.'

Relationship success

Most participants reported the positive influence of relationships after leaving the program. They began to form close relationships with new people and rebuild existing relationships. Some participants became a source of support for others.

'...the ability to be able to listen and be honest with myself ... and be able to share other people's stories and listen to them to be a support.'

However, initial re-integration into the family model was quite challenging for one participant.

'...you know just because I'm clean, not everyone's jumping for joy and patting me on the back about that. There's a lot of damage that's done in active addiction. So dealing with some of the family members um distain, for lack of better words, of my behaviour while I was using that's been hard.'

One participant turned to helping others as a way of ignoring their own trauma.

'I tried to make my situation that I was helping other people so that I didn't have to look at my own stuff.'

Employment success

Participants recognised the positive role that the program had played in developing the skills necessary to obtain and maintain employment or study after leaving the program.

'...I wouldn't have been able to get this job without having gone through the <TC program>.'

'They may have lost me for 6 months but they've actually got a better employee.'

Eight participants reported volunteering after leaving the program, particularly in drug rehabilitation. Participants found helping and supporting others rewarding. Of the remaining five who were not volunteering, one was exploring options, two were gainfully employed and one was medically retired. For five participants, working in a volunteer position subsequently allowed them to attain paid employment.

'...from volunteer work I ended up getting a job in drug and alcohol rehab, working with women and children in a residential environment.'

For some, employment has also helped to maintain abstinence.

'... If I'm busy and being productive I'm not likely to smoke pot...'

Discussion

The current study revealed a complex interplay of factors contributing to early TC withdrawal, and the perceptions of successful recovery from a lived experience perspective and how this was shaped by employment and volunteering. Eleven main themes were identified. Three relating to reasons for joining the program, which connected with ultimate withdrawal from the program: Pre-program existing relationships, pre-program employment situation and needing a 'circuit breaker' in their life. Three relating to reasons for early withdrawal: TC program characteristics, relationships during the program and planning future employment. Five relating to perceptions of successful recovery: Improved understanding of their addiction, reduced substance use, improved physical and psychological health, relationship success and employment success.

Reasons for early withdrawal
To understand the reasons for early withdrawal, it was necessary to understand the reasons for entering the TC program.

Backgrounds of childhood trauma, abuse, isolation and an early age of first substance use were common amongst participants. Years of addiction culminated in the recognition of the need for an 'extreme' measure such as a long-term TC program, which was also influenced by pre-existing relationships and employment situation. The suffering associated with hitting rock bottom is a strong motivator for addiction recovery as individuals are forced to reassess their life and seek help [15]. The decision to leave treatment early is also heavily influenced by motivation to make positive changes in one's life [10, 15]. Similarly, lower perceived likeliness of completing the program at intake was associated with lower completion rates, whilst having fewer stressful life events was a positive predictor of completion [9]. Indeed, our participants had left treatment early and most described significant life stressors.

The reasons for early withdrawal were varied. Many participants described aspects of the TC program as challenging, such as feeling confronted by the intensity of the program, disagreement with the program rules or struggling with the isolation. Others described a misunderstanding of the program or feeling ready to leave. Relationships and work commitments were also contributory factors. These findings are consistent with Chen et al.'s [11] who found program dissatisfaction and antagonistic staff and adolescent interactions core reasons for early exit. However, the current study found that relationships can have both positive and negative effects on program retention. The role of relationships are complex and their influence changes overtime. Prior to the TC program, relationships played an important role in both maintaining addiction and the decision to seek treatment. During the program, relationships with staff and fellow residents, as well as family outside the treatment environment, were particularly important drivers in the decision to stay or leave. Consistent with Landrum et al. [10], relationships can both positively and negatively affect treatment retention. Apart from Landrum et al. [10], other research has not shown this dichotomy, though this other research has focused on predictors or reasons for early withdrawal, not protective retention factors [11].

Perceptions of successful recovery

Consistent with Aslan's [12] conclusion that *"unsuccessful" can be successful*, the current study results show that individuals who leave the TC program early can still experience recovery success, regardless of whether they left voluntarily or were asked to leave involuntarily. Participants in the current study reported improvements in relationships, psychological and physical health, stability, employment and volunteering, mirroring findings that recovery success extends beyond abstinence [4, 5, 7, 12, 13].

In line with previous research [12, 13], abstinence played an important role in perceptions of successful recovery. Whilst some participants experienced lapses, many reported using the skills learnt from the TC program to better recognise early warning signs and break the cycle before losing control and falling back into active addiction. Lapses are part of unlearning chronically habitual behaviour and should be used as a learning experience [16].

Participants reported improved trigger recognition and understanding of recovery as a journey, as described by Best [17] "recovery is a process rather than an event and it is often characterised as a journey". TC programs are structured to encourage reflective practice and this is

shown in the current results, as the understanding of recovery as a journey was not fully appreciated until reflecting on the TC program and implementing these skills into their life outside the program. Laudet [13] also found that recovery is a process of growth, leading to improved financial and living conditions, physical and/or mental health and social networks.

All participants had engaged in further treatment, compared to Aslan's [12] 85%. The strong theme of an improved understanding of recovery as a journey in the current study may account for these differences. The types of treatment were very similar, with the most commonly reported being support groups such as AA and NA used in conjunction with other treatment.

Positive relationships defined perceptions of successful recovery after leaving the program. Skills learnt from the program helped to rebuild emotional connections, which continue to positively influence their recovery. Results of the current study parallel what is shown through TC study outcomes reviews [4, 5]. However, it should be noted that some people continued to struggle after leaving the program and reported difficulties reconnecting with family and putting others above their own needs so they don't have to deal with their own traumas.

The link between employment, early withdrawal and recovery

The secondary aim was to explore how employment and volunteering related to early exit and perceptions of successful recovery. Employment, like relationships, showed varying influence across different time-points. Prior to the TC program, many reported difficulty attaining and maintaining jobs due to substance use. On the contrary, for some work was an enabler for substance use due to working in remote areas leading to social isolation, working in pubs and clubs or having the finances to afford buying substances. Commitments and motivation to find work because they felt ready to work again were reasons for leaving the program early. After leaving the program, participants reported improved self-worth and feeling able to contribute to society through study, volunteer work and paid employment, which was heavily represented in perceptions of successful recovery. These results are consistent with Vanderplasschen et al.'s [5] review of TC study outcomes and Aslan [12], who found TC residents were actively engaging in volunteering and paid employment after leaving the program.

Strengths and limitations

A qualitative approach allowed for richer data on individual reasons and challenges. Telephone interviews were used for feasibility. Given the sensitive nature of the topic this approach may have afforded more honest data. One participant discussed feeling more comfortable speaking honestly when not face-to-face, which may reflect the view of many because of associated stigma. No studies have previously looked at the extended definition of what success looks like from ex-clients point of view in an Australian context.

Recollection bias and accurate recall may have been difficult for individuals who left the program four years ago compared to one year ago, however similar themes emerged regardless of time since leaving. Similarly, selection bias was an initial concern of the researchers, that only individuals who were abstinent and doing well would be willing to take part, however this was not the case. There was a reasonable spread of participants that dropped out of the program early and those that stayed. About 50% of participants stayed less than eight weeks. We had one participant that stayed less than two weeks, two that stayed between two and four weeks and four that stayed between five and eight weeks. Seven men and six women participated in the study. This was similar to the male-female ratio of those that have taken part in the residential programs at the residential rehabilitation service provider from which our participants were sampled. This may be different compared to other organisations and readers should take this into account when interpreting the results in the light of their own organisations client base. The validity of self-report data may be threatened by social desirability bias, though telephone interviews potentially countered this. Self-report among substance users has been investigated previously and found to have acceptable levels of validity and reliability [18–21]. Additionally, research has demonstrated that telephone interviews compared to face-to-face interviews can be used reliably among people with mental health disorders [22].

Implications and recommendations

The current research illustrates the beneficial impact of the interpersonal skills training implemented in TC programs. It supports the program's role in addressing recommendations of the National Drug Strategy [2], improvements in social competence training and increased community activity engagement. The study also shows TCs to be an effective DA treatment option for individuals who partially completed the program. This may be due to a shift in the way people view recovery, away from being defined solely by abstinence towards a more holistic view. This may include supporting residents to not only focus on abstinence but also to identify how they can actively contribute to the community, through studying, volunteering or finding employment. Although care should be taken, that this happens in a supportive and safe environment. Future research could utilise a mixed-method approach to clarify the relationships between predictors of and reasons for early

withdrawal, outcome measures and perspectives of recovery success.

Many participants in the current study reported their substance use began at a young age. Future policy may look to target education around addiction at children. This education may draw parallels from other chronic conditions with a relapsing course or the anti-smoking campaigns; 'never give up giving up' [23].

Conclusion

In conclusion, reasons for leaving treatment early are multi-faceted and revolve around positive and negative relationships, planning future employment, and program characteristics. The influence that each plays on their decision to leave early is varied and determined by the value they assign it. Perceived success extends far beyond achieving and maintaining abstinence to encompass improved relationships, psychological and physical wellbeing, understanding of addiction and employment, studying and volunteering. Self-worth and feeling able to contribute to society through employment, studying and volunteering were perceived to be essential elements of successful recovery. For many, it was only after leaving the TC program that they began to understand and appreciate the skills they had learnt and recognised the importance of ongoing DA treatment. Clinicians, policy makers and program developers should use the extended definition of successful recovery from the ex-clients perspective when determining the clinical and economic effectiveness of TC programs.

Abbreviations
AA: Alcoholics Anonymous; DA: Drug and Alcohol; NA: Narcotics Anonymous; TC: Therapeutic communities

Acknowledgements
We would like to acknowledge and thank all the participants involved.

Funding
This project was partially funded by the John Shaw Warnock Research Grant provided through the Buttery. Data analyses was conducted independently from Mr. Rees, who is employed by the Buttery but his input was sought at thematic analyses stage.

Authors' contributions
SWP, TP and TR designed the study. TP conducted the interviews. TP analysed the data with input from SWP and TR. TP drafted the manuscript. SWP, TR and JN provided overall methodological and content expertise guidance. SWP led the study. All authors contributed to revising of the manuscript and have read and approved the final manuscript.

Consent for publication

Not applicable.

Competing interests

Mr. Rees is Program Manager at the Buttery, Australia. Data analyses was conducted independently from Mr. Rees but his input was sought at thematic analyses stage. No further conflict of interest is declared.

Author details

[1]School of Medicine, University of Wollongong, Wollongong, Australia. [2]School of Medicine, University Centre for Rural Health, Western Sydney University, 61 Uralba Street, Lismore, NSW 2480, Australia. [3]Sydney Medical School, University of Sydney, 61 Uralba Street, Lismore, NSW 2480, Australia. [4]The Buttery, Bangalow, Australia. [5]Faculty of Science, Medicine and Health, School of Medicine, University of Wollongong, Wollongong, Australia.

References

1. Collins, DJ & Lapsley, HM 2008, The costs of tobacco, alcohol and illicit drug abuse to Australian society in 2004/05, Commonwealth of Australia, Canberra, Australia, viewed 1 September 2017, <https://www.health.gov.au/internet/drugstrategy/publishing.nsf/Content/34F55AF632F67B70CA2573F60005D42B/$File/mono64.pdf>.

2. Department of Health 2017, National Drug Strategy 2017–2026, Department of Health, Canberra, viewed 20 October 2017, <http://www.health.gov.au/internet/main/publishing.nsf/Content/55E4796388E9EDE5CA25808F00035035/$File/National-Drug-Strategy-2017-2026.pdf>.

3. Malivert M, Fatseas M, Denis C, Langlois E, Auriacombe M. Effectiveness of therapeutic communities: a systemic review. Eur Addict Res. 2012;18:1–11.

4. Magor-Blatch L, Bhullar N, Thomson B, Thorsteinsson E. A systematic review of studies examining effectiveness of therapeutic communities. Therapeutic Communities: The International Journal of Therapeutic Communities. 2014; 35(4):168–84.

5. Vanderplasschen W, Colpaert K, Autrique M, Rapp RC, Pearce S, Broekaert E, Vandevelde S. Therapeutic communities for addictions: a review of their effectiveness from a recovery-oriented perspective. Sci World J. 2013;2013: 1–22.

6. Simpson DD, Joe GW, Broome KM, Hiller ML, Kevin K, Rowan-Szal GA. Program diversity and treatment retention rates in the drug abuse treatment outcome study (DATOS). Psychology of Addictive Behaviours. 1997;11(4):279–93.

7. Hubbard RL, Craddock SG, Anderson J. Overview of 5-year follow-up outcomes in the drug abuse treatment outcome studies (DATOS). J Subst Abus Treat. 2003;25:125–34.

8. Stevens L, Betanzos-Espinosa P, Crunelle CL, Vergara-Moragues E, Roeyers H, Lozano O, Dom G, Gonzalez-Saiz F, Vanderplasschen W, Verdejo-Garcia A, Perez-Garcia M. Disadvantageous decision-making as a predictor of dropout among cocaine-dependent individuals in long-term residential treatment. Frontiers in Psychiatry. 2013;4(149):1–9.

9. Darke S, Campbell S, Popple G. Retention, early dropout and treatment completion among therapeutic community admissions. Drug and Alcohol Review. 2012;30:64–71.

10. Landrum B, Knight D, Becan J, Flynn P. To stay or not to stay: adolescent client, parent, and counselor perspectives on leaving substance abuse treatment early. Journal of Child and Adolescent Substance Abuse. 2015; 24(6):344–54.

11. Chen G, Elisha E, Timor U, Ronel N. Why do adolescents drop out of a therapeutic community for people with drug addiction? J Child Adolescent Substance Abuse. 2016;25(1):65–77.

12. Aslan L. Dropping out of therapeutic community treatment; when is "unsuccessful", successful? Therapeutic Communities: The International Journal of Therapeutic Communities. 2015;36(2):74–88.

13. Laudet AB. What does recovery mean to you? Lessons from the recovery experience for research and practice. J Subst Abus Treat. 2007;33:243–56.

14. Braun V, Clarke V. Using thematic analysis in psychology. Qual Res Psychol. 2006;3(2):77–101.

15. Chen G. The meaning of suffering in drug addiction and recovery from the perspective of existentialism, Buddhism and the 12-step program. J Psychoactive Drugs. 2010;42(3):363–75.

16. Saunders B, Houghton M. Relapse revisited: a critique of current concepts and clinical practice in the management of alcohol problems. Addictive Behaviours. 1996;21(6):843–55.

17. Best, D 2012, Addiction recovery: a movement for social change and personal growth in the UK, Pavilion Publishing, Brighton.

18. Day C, Collins L, Degenhardt L, Thetford C, Maher L. Reliability of heroin users' reports of drug use behaviour using a 24 month timeline follow-back technique to assess the impact of the Australian heroin shortage. Addict Res Theory. 2004;(5):433–43.

19. Jackson CT, Covell NH, Frisman LK, Essock SM. Validity of self-reported drug use among people with co-occurring mental health and substance use disorders. J Dual Diagnosis. 2004;1:49–63.

20. Johnson ME, Fisher DG, Montoya I, Booth R, Rhodes F, Andersen M, Zhuo Z, Williams M. Reliability and validity of not-in-treatment drug users' follow-up self-reports. AIDS Behav. 2000;4(4):373–80.

21. Napper LE, Fisher DG, Johnson ME, Wood MM. The reliability and validity of drug users' self-reports of amphetamine use among primarily heroin and cocaine users. Addictive Behaviours. 2010;35(4):350.

22. Rohde P, Lewinsohn PM, Seeley JR. Comparability of telephone and face-to-face interviews in assessing axis I and II disorders. Am J Psychiatr. 1997; 154(11):1593–8.

23. Cancer Institute NSW 2018, Never Give Up Giving Up Anti-smoking Campaign, Cancer Institute NSW, viewed 20 March 2018, < https://www.cancerinstitute.org.au/how-we-help/cancer-prevention/stopping-smoking/quit-smoking-campaigns/never-give-up-giving-up-anti-smoking-campaign>.

15

Effectiveness of eLearning and blended modes of delivery of Mental Health First Aid training in the workplace

Nicola J. Reavley[1]* ⓘ, Amy J. Morgan[1], Julie-Anne Fischer[1], Betty Kitchener[2], Nataly Bovopoulos[2] and Anthony F. Jorm[1]

Abstract

Background: The aim of the WorkplaceAid study was to compare the effects of eLearning or blended (eLearning plus face-to-face course delivery) Mental Health First Aid (MHFA) courses on public servants' knowledge, stigmatising attitudes, confidence in providing support and intentions to provide support to a person with depression or post-traumatic stress disorder (PTSD).

Methods: A randomized controlled trial was carried out with 608 Australian public servants. Participants were randomly assigned to complete an eLearning MHFA course, a blended MHFA course or Red Cross eLearning Provide First Aid (PFA) (the control). The effects of the interventions were evaluated using online questionnaires pre- and post-training. The questionnaires centred around vignettes describing a person meeting the criteria for depression or PTSD. Primary outcomes were mental health first aid knowledge and desire for social distance. Secondary outcomes were recognition of mental health problems, beliefs about treatment, helping intentions and confidence and personal stigma. Feedback on the usefulness of the courses was also collected.

Results: Both the eLearning MHFA and blended MHFA courses had positive effects compared to PFA eLearning on mental health first aid knowledge, desire for social distance, beliefs about professional treatments, intentions and confidence in helping a person and personal stigma towards a person with depression or PTSD. There were very small non-significant differences between the eLearning MHFA and blended MHFA courses on these outcome measures. However, users were more likely to highly rate the blended MHFA course in terms of usefulness, amount learned and intentions to recommend the course to others.

Conclusions: The blended MHFA course was only minimally more effective than eLearning MHFA in improving knowledge and attitudes. However, course satisfaction ratings were higher from participants in the blended MHFA course, potentially leading to greater benefits in the future. Longer-term follow-up is needed to explore this.

* Correspondence: nreavley@unimelb.edu.au
[1]Centre for Mental Health, Melbourne School of Population and Global Health, University of Melbourne, 207 Bouverie Street, Carlton, VIC 3010, Australia
Full list of author information is available at the end of the article

Introduction

Because of the high prevalence of mental disorders, members of the public are very likely to have contact with people with mental health problems (which includes those with diagnosed disorders or subclinical symptoms) and can play a valuable role in providing support [1, 2]. It can therefore be argued that the public need knowledge and skills to provide help to people with mental health problems. This help, also known as 'mental health first aid', can be defined as the help provided to a person developing a mental health problem, experiencing a worsening of a mental health problems or in a mental health crisis (e.g. at immediate risk of suicide) [3]. The first aid is given until appropriate professional treatment is received or until the crisis resolves. The Mental Health First Aid (MHFA) training course teaching these skills was developed in Australia in 2000 [4]. It involves 12 hours of face-to-face instruction and gives an overview of the most common and disabling mental health problems, introduces a five-component action plan and then applies these actions to help people with problems of depression, anxiety disorders, psychosis and substance use disorder as well as crisis situations including suicidal behaviours, panic attacks, traumatic events, aggressive behaviour, and drug overdose [5].

Since its inception, MHFA training has expanded rapidly; there are now 1500 accredited MHFA instructors in Australia who have trained over 500,000 adults. It operates in over 20 countries and 2 million people have been trained globally [6]. Evaluation studies were first carried out in Australia and have now been undertaken in other countries. A recent meta-analysis conducted by Morgan et al. [7] included 18 randomised controlled trials that evaluated the effectiveness of MHFA in a range of settings. MHFA training led to improved mental health first aid knowledge with effects persisting up to 12 months after training. There were also moderate improvements in recognition of mental disorders and beliefs about effective treatments and and small reductions in stigmatising attitudes (ds 0.08–0.15). Perceived confidence in helping a person with a mental health problem and intentions to provide first aid were also seen post-training and persisted for up to 6 months later. There were small improvements in the amount of help provided to a person with a mental health problem at follow-up (d = 0.23) although impact of MHFA on the quality of help offered was not clear.

Eight of the studies included in the meta-analysis mentioned above were conducted in workplace settings, which is increasingly seen as an important setting for mental health education and training, not only to address mental health problems caused by work, but also to address mental health problems that arise as a result of other factors but that may become apparent in the workplace or be exacerbated by poor working conditions [8, 9]. Growing evidence suggests that workplace interventions may produce improvements in mental health literacy [10] and depression and anxiety symptoms [9, 11] as well as reductions in stigma [10].

In the context of the growing popularity of eLearning, an electronic version of MHFA was developed and evaluated in a randomised controlled trial (RCT) conducted in 2009 involving 262 members of the public, who were randomly assigned to complete the eLearning course, read a printed MHFA manual or be in a wait-list control group [12]. Participants were sent weekly emails for four weeks to prompt them to continue participating. The impact of the interventions was evaluated using online questionnaires administered at baseline, post-training and at 6-months follow-up. Both eLearning and the printed manual were superior to wait list in increasing knowledge, reducing stigmatising attitudes and increasing confidence. eLearning showed greater effects than wait-list or manual in reducing stigmatising attitudes to a person with schizophrenia and also in improving first-aid actions taken.

As with other intervention settings, recent years have seen an increase in online interventions in the workplace. eLearning may be particularly appropriate to workplace settings, where it is not always easy to roster staff to attend training simultaneously, particularly for longer courses such as face-to-face MHFA training which is 12 hours long and requires four sessions of three hours each. Other groups of people for whom attendance is difficult, are those living in remote areas or who are distant from where courses are offered, shift workers, and people who have family commitments which make it difficult to attend for this length of time. However, one of the disadvantages of the eLearning format is that it lacks the group interaction, discussion and questions that are part of a face-to-face course.

One approach to training that aims to maximise the convenience of eLearning with the interactivity of face-to-face learning, is that of blended learning. Common in the field of health professional education, blended learning has been shown to be more effective or at least as effective as non-blended instruction for knowledge acquisition [13]. However, authors of a recent meta-analysis that included 56 studies found large heterogeneity across studies and noted that their conclusions should be treated with caution [13]. Another meta-analysis of eLearning trials covered 96 studies of 168 training courses [14] and focused on comparisons between face-to-face instruction and blended learning or eLearning. Results showed that, for declarative knowledge (memory of facts and principles taught), effects were larger for blended learning (Cohen's d = 0.35 (95% CI 0.29–0.39)) than eLearning only (d = 0.15 (95% CI

0.11–0.19)). The findings were similar for procedural knowledge (information about how to perform a task or action): d = 0.53 (95% CI 0.34–0.70) vs d = – 0.07 (95% CI -0.20-0.06). This meta-analysis also looked at learner satisfaction with the mode of instruction and found a very small effect in favour of online compared to blended learning. However, the studies included in these reviews focussed specifically on its effectiveness with adults acquiring knowledge directly relevant to their current or future employment. There has been very little research into the effectiveness of mode of instruction for interventions targeted to the general public where the content does not relate to employment. Furthermore, a review of anti-stigma interventions found no difference in effects between studies with internet or non-internet delivery of content, but head-to-head comparisons of delivery mode are rare [15]. No prior studies have compared the effectiveness of MHFA training when delivered in an eLearning versus blended mode.

The principal aim of this study was to compare the effects of eLearning or blended (eLearning plus face-to-face course delivery) MHFA training on knowledge, stigmatising attitudes, confidence in providing support and intentions to provide support to a person with depression or PTSD. Participants were members of the public service in Victoria and the Australian Capital Territory (ACT), Australia.

Study hypotheses were as follows:

1. Compared to eLearning Provide First Aid (PFA) training (the control), MHFA training, whether delivered in eLearning or blended modes, will result in higher mental health first aid knowledge, lower stigmatizing attitudes, and greater confidence in providing support to a person developing a mental health problem or in a mental health crisis.
2. Compared to eLearning MHFA training, blended MHFA training will result in higher mental health first aid knowledge, lower stigmatizing attitudes, and greater confidence in providing support to a person developing a mental health problem or in a mental health crisis.
3. Compared to eLearning MHFA training, blended MHFA training will be rated higher on satisfaction than eLearning MHFA training.

Methods
Study design
The WorkplaceAid study was a parallel group RCT with participants randomized to eLearning MHFA, blended MHFA or PFA eLearning in a 1:1:1 ratio. The trial was registered with the Australian and New Zealand Clinical Trials Registry (ACTRN12614000623695, registered on 13 June 2014). PFA eLearning was chosen as a control

intervention as it deals with health problems that may occur in the workplace, uses a similar mode of administration to the eLearning MHFA training and involves a similar time commitment.

Participants
Australian public servants who were aged 18 and over and did not hold a current certificate in either MHFA or PFA were eligible for the study. Initially, state government employees in the state of Victoria, Australia, were eligible to participate. In 2016, recruitment was opened to Commonwealth government employees in the ACT in order to counteract a slow-down in recruitment in the Victorian public service after the 2014 state election and subsequent department restructure. Participants were informed about the study through flyers put up in offices, articles in newsfeed items on the staff intranet and at staff wellbeing events. Potential participants were asked to register online by going to a trial website, which contained a Participant Information Sheet, an 'I accept' checkbox and a link to the baseline Survey-Monkey questionnaire. After completion of this questionnaire, participants were randomized to one of the three groups listed above and given instructions on how to access the relevant course. Participants were advised that they could complete the training during work hours, with their manager's approval, avoiding busy times at work.

Randomization
Randomization was carried out by a random integer generator programmed on the trial website to give values of 1 = eLearning MHFA; 2 = Blended MHFA and 3 = PFA eLearning (see http://php.net/manual/en/function.-rand.php). Allocation was concealed as randomization was computer generated. Blinding was not possible due to the nature of the interventions.

Interventions
eLearning MHFA
This intervention was a 6-hour eLearning MHFA course accessed via the MHFA Australia online portal. The course teaches a 5-component action plan for responding to developing mental health problems such as depression, anxiety problems, psychosis and substance use problems, and crises including suicidal thoughts and behaviours, non-suicidal self-injury, panic attacks, traumatic events, severe psychotic states, severe effects from alcohol misuse, severe effects from drug misuse, and aggressive behaviours. The eLearning MHFA course comprised 5 modules which needed to be completed in sequence, with a quiz at the end of each: Introduction to mental health; Depression; Anxiety Problems; Psychosis and Substance Use Problems. Each module included

interactive content on case studies (click on a picture or table to answer). The course also includes audio and video content depicting stories of lived experience and demonstrating how to provide mental health first aid, following by questions or other activities.

The online content was tailored to incorporate information on resources and help-seeking pathways of specific relevance to the relevant public service (e.g. Employee Assistance Program (EAP) providers). An accompanying hard copy MHFA manual (which was regularly referred to in the eLearning course) was posted to participants when they registered for the course [5]. Participants received weekly automated emails for 6 weeks to pace them through the material. Monthly reports were extracted to monitor course progress. On course completion, an automatic email was sent to the trial manager to flag completion and another was sent to the participant containing a link to the post-course questionnaire.

Blended MHFA

This intervention included the 6-hour eLearning course described above plus a 4-hour face-to-face session, which reviewed the contents of the online course through quizzes and discussion. It also included case studies and role plays to give participants more experience in applying the MHFA Action Plan in different situations and settings. Group training was completed within 3 months of online course completion. In Melbourne and Ballarat, Victoria, two MHFA Instructors ran 16 courses individually, while one Instructor delivered 9 courses in Canberra. Courses were held in locations close to participants' workplaces.

Provide first aid

This intervention was a 4-hour eLearning PFA course delivered via the Australian Red Cross online portal. The course teaches the fundamental principles, knowledge and skills to provide emergency care for injuries and illnesses in the home or the workplace. Participants received weekly emails for 6 weeks to pace them through the material. Reports from Red Cross were obtained to monitor course progress and flag course completers.

Following online completion, participants in each course were awarded an online 'Certificate of Completion'. For the MHFA courses, participants could undertake an exam (within 3 months of course completion) to become an 'Accredited Mental Health First Aider', valid for 3 years. Staff who completed the eLearning PFA course were offered an option to attend a 1-day assessment (in their own time) to obtain a 'Statement of Attainment' for the Health Training Package, HLTAID003 – Provide First Aid, also valid for 3 years.

Outcomes

Data were collected at baseline, post training (participants were given 2 months to complete the assessment after they had completed the course), one-year follow-up and two-year follow-up. Only outcomes assessed at baseline and post training are reported here. Data from the one and two- year follow-up questionnaires will be reported in a future publication as data collection is ongoing. Participants were invited to complete an online questionnaire via SurveyMonkey after they had completed the eLearning course, or had attended the face-to-face course. The median length of time between baseline and post training assessment was 85 days.

Initial questions covered sociodemographic information (age, gender, email, daytime telephone number, employment time fraction, marital status, postcode, country of birth, language spoken at home, level of education, Aboriginal and Torres Strait Islander status and whether the respondents managed staff). Subsequent questions centred around a vignette of a person 'John' meeting the DSM criteria for major depression with suicidal thoughts and 'Paula' meeting the DSM criteria for PTSD (previously validated vignettes of two mental disorders which have high prevalence rates and are therefore relatively likely to be encountered in the workplace) [2, 16].

Primary outcomes

These were as follows:

Mental health first aid knowledge This was measured using a 16-item true/false quiz based on the content of the Mental Health First Aid Manual [5]. Respondents were presented with the statements given in Table 1 and asked whether they agreed, disagreed or did not know. The number of correct responses was converted into a percentage. A Pearson correlation coefficient was used to assess test-retest reliability in the control group, which was 0.61 (95% CI 0.44–0.73).

Desire for social distance This was measured by the Social Distance Scale [17] in relation to the vignettes described above. This scale is widely used, and many studies have shown that it has a single factor structure [18, 19]. Respondents were asked: Would you be happy to: 1) To move next door to John/Paula? 2) To spend an evening socializing with John/Paula? 3) To make friends with John/Paula? 4) To work closely with John/Paula on a project at work? 5) To have John/Paula marry into your family? Responses were scored as follows: 1 = Yes definitely (low social distance) to 4 = Definitely not (high social distance). The internal consistency of the scales in this sample (omega total) was 0.88 for depression and 0.91 for PTSD. Scores were dichotomised at the median of pre- and post-scores.

Table 1 Mental health first aid knowledge

1) Half of all people who experience a mental illness have their first episode by age 18

2) Depressive disorders are the most prevalent mental illness in the Australian population

3) If a person who is depressed does not want to seek professional help, it is important to force them to if you can

4) Exercise can help relieve depression

5) Recovery from anxiety disorders requires facing situations which are anxiety provoking

6) Antidepressant medications can be an effective treatment for most anxiety disorders

7) When interacting with a person with psychosis, it is best not to offer them choices of how you can help them because it could add to their confusion

8) A person with a psychotic illness is less likely to relapse if they have a good relationship with their family

9) A good way to help a person with a drug or alcohol problem is to let them know that you strongly disapprove of their substance use

10) People with mental illnesses are much more likely to be smokers

11) It is not a good idea to ask someone if they are feeling suicidal in case you put the idea in their head

12) It is best to get someone having a panic attack to breathe into a paper bag

13) If someone has a traumatic experience, it is best to make them talk about it as soon as possible

14) It is best not to try to reason with a person having delusions

15) If a person is intoxicated with alcohol, it is not possible to make them sober up more quickly by giving them strong coffee, a cold shower or taking them for a walk

16) If a person becomes unconscious after taking drugs, it is best to lie them on their side rather than on their back

Secondary outcomes

Recognition of mental health problems In order to assess recognition of the problems in the vignettes, participants were asked an open-ended question, "What, if anything do you think is wrong with John/Paula?" For the depression vignette, participants were assessed as having correctly recognised the problem if they mentioned 'depressed' or 'depression' in their response. For the PTSD vignette, responses with any mention of PTSD, post-traumatic stress, or post-traumatic stress disorder were assessed as correct. Pearson correlation coefficients were used to assess test-retest reliability in the control group, which were 0.56 (95% CI 0.39–0.70) for depression and 0.65 (95% CI 0.50–0.77) for PTSD.

Beliefs about treatment These were assessed using a 16-item scale based on the 2011 National Survey of Mental Health Literacy and Stigma [20] and a consensus between Australian clinical psychologists, psychiatrists,

and GPs established by a national survey [21]. Respondents were presented with sources of potential help for depression and PTSD. For the depression vignette, participants scored 1 point for 'Helpful' responses to each of the following: a typical family GP or doctor; a psychiatrist; a psychologist; becoming more physically active; reading about people with similar problems and how they have dealt with them; psychotherapy; cognitive behaviour therapy; cutting out alcohol altogether; and antidepressants. They also scored 1 point for rating 'dealing with the problem alone' as harmful. For the PTSD vignette, participants scored 1 point for 'Helpful' responses to each of the following: a typical family GP or doctor; a psychiatrist; a psychologist; becoming more physically active; reading about people with similar problems and how they have dealt with them; courses on relaxation, stress management, meditation or yoga; psychotherapy; cognitive behaviour therapy; and receiving information about his problem from a health educator. Depression treatment beliefs ranged from 0 to 10 and PTSD treatment beliefs from 0 to 9. Pearson correlation coefficients were used to assess test-retest reliability in the control group, which were 0.58 (95% CI 0.40–0.71) for depression and 0.57 (95% CI 0.40–0.70) for PTSD.

Helping intentions and confidence Intentions to provide help to the person in the vignette were assessed by asking respondents: If John/Paula was a co-worker, I would help him/her. This was scored using a 7-point scale ranging from 1 = Strongly Disagree to 7 = Strongly Agree. Responses were coded into two categories: strongly agree/agree vs other. Spearman correlation coefficients were used to assess test-retest reliability in the control group, which were 0.45 (0.25–0.61) for depression and 0.43 (0.23–0.60) for PTSD. This was followed with, "Describe all the things you would do to help John/Paula." (open-ended response). Scoring was based on the MHFA Action Plan [22] with quality of intended support ranging from 0 to 12. Open-ended responses were scored blinded to allocation or occasion. A random sample of 50 responses were double-coded for each vignette, and inter-rater reliability (ICC) was 0.88 for depression and 0.94 for PTSD. Pearson correlation coefficients were used to assess test-retest reliability in the control group, which were 0.18 (95% CI -0.04, 0.39) for depression and 0.42 (95% CI 0.21–0.59) for PTSD.

Confidence in providing help to someone at work with depression and PTSD was assessed by asking participants, "How confident do you feel in helping someone at work with a problem like John/Paula?" Confidence was rated using a 5- point scale used in previous studies, 1 = Not at all to 5 = Extremely [4]. Pearson correlation coefficients were used to assess test-retest reliability in the control group, which were 0.64 (0.49–0.76) for depression and 0.50 (0.32–0.65) for PTSD.

Personal stigma The Personal Stigma Scale was used to measure participants' stigmatising attitudes to the person described in the vignette [23]. Exploratory Structural Equation Modelling has shown this scale to have factors measuring belief that a person with a mental health problem is weak not sick, and belief that they are dangerous or unpredictable [19]. This scale includes the following 9 items: 1) (John/Paula) could snap out of it if they wanted; 2) (John/Paula)'s problem is a sign of personal weakness; 3) (John/Paula)'s problem is not a real medical illness; 4) (John/Paula) is dangerous; 5) It is best to avoid (John/Paula)'s so that you don't develop this problem yourself; 6) (John/Paula)'s problem makes him/her unpredictable; 7) You would not tell anyone if you had a problem like (John/Paula)'s; 8) I would not employ someone if I knew they had a problem like (John/Paula)'s; 9) I would not vote for a politician if I knew they had suffered a problem like (John/Paula)'s. Scoring ranged from 1 = Strongly Agree to 5 = Strongly Disagree. The Omega coefficient in this sample for' Weak not sick' stigma was 0.83 for depression and 0.82 for PTSD. For Dangerous/unpredictable stigma, the Omega coefficient was 0.70 for depression and 0.72 for PTSD. 'Weak not sick' scores showed substantial negative skew so were dichotomised at the median, which was the highest possible score (5) for both depression and PTSD vignettes.

Course satisfaction Course satisfaction was assessed using the following questions: 1) How much of the training did you complete? (1 = none of it, 2 = part of it, 3 = most of it, 4 = all of it); 2) How easy was the material to understand? (1 = very easy, 2 = easy, 3 = neither easy nor difficult, 4 = difficult, 5 = very difficult);

3) How much did you learn from the course? (1 = a great deal, 2 = a fair bit, 3 = not very much, 4 = almost nothing); 4) How useful was the course? (1 = very useful, 2 = useful, 3 = not very useful, 4 = not at all useful); 5) Do you think you will use the training material in the future? (1 = yes, 2 = no, 3 = not sure); 6) Would you recommend the course to others? (1 = yes definitely, 2 = probably, 3 = probably not, 4 = definitely not); 7) What did you like about the training materials? 8) What did you dislike about the training materials? These questions were asked post-course only.

Sample size estimation

In order to calculate the required sample size, we considered the main hypothesis of interest to be the following: that blended MHFA training would be superior to MHFA eLearning in achieving improvements in MHFA knowledge and reductions in desire for social distance. The sample size required to detect differences between these two modes of training was larger than that

required to detect differences between these modes and PFA training. Consequently, we chose a small effect size to evaluate the difference between the two modes of MHFA training, as an effect size smaller than this may not be meaningful in terms of participant outcomes. According to Stata Release 12, 165 participants were required per group. For a repeated measures design, with 1 pre-training measure and 3 post-training measures, using the change method of sample size calculation and assuming a conservative 0.70 correlation between pre- and post-measurements (based on [24]), to detect an effect size of Cohen's $d = 0.20$ (or $h = 0.20$), with a power = 0.80 and an alpha = 0.05, Increasing the sample size by 20% to account for attrition, the total sample size required was estimated to be 594 (198 participants per group).

Adverse events

In the event that a participant felt distressed during survey completion or while undertaking the training, a list of contacts was included at the end of each online survey. This included phone numbers for Lifeline, Suicideline (Victoria only), SANE, Emergency Services (000) and relevant EAP providers. Lifeline's Online Crisis Chat link was also included. Participants were encouraged to contact the trial manager to report any adverse events. None were reported.

Ethics

The study was approved by the University of Melbourne Human Ethics Sub-Committee (Ethics ID 1341345.2).

Statistical analysis

An intention-to-treat approach was used, with all participants included in the analyses. Data were analysed using mixed-effects models for continuous and binary outcome variables, with group-by-measurement occasion interactions. This method takes into account the hierarchical structure of the data in the analysis of differences between the groups, i.e. the correlation of measurement occasions within participants. It can produce unbiased estimates when a proportion of the participants withdraw before the completion of the study, based on the reasonable assumption that these data are missing at random [25]. As tertiary-educated participants were somewhat more likely to have data at post (OR = 1.39, 95% CI 0.99–1.95, $p = .057$), education was included as a fixed effect in order to help meet the missing at random assumption. For outcome measures with no substantial baseline imbalance, effect sizes (Cohen's d) were calculated by dividing the difference between the two group means at post-training by their pooled standard deviation. With baseline imbalances, Cohen's d was calculated by dividing the mean change in each condition by the pooled standard deviation post-training. Analyses were performed in Stata 14 and RStudio and the significance level was set at $p < .05$.

Results

Participant flow and numbers analysed

The CONSORT flow diagram of the number of participants at each stage of the trial is given in Fig. 1. All the participants included in the analyses completed the first questionnaire and 319 (52.5%) participants did not complete the post-test questionnaire. The sole predictor of having data at post-test was assignment to the PFA group (OR = 0.59, 95% CI 0.39–0.87, $p = 0.008$). The three groups were similar in baseline sociodemographic characteristics, indicating that randomisation resulted in comparable groups (see Table 2).

Participants' characteristics

The mean age of participants was 41.2 years (SD =10.9), 74.1% were female, 87.1% spoke English at home, 66.1% were tertiary educated, 1.2% were Aboriginal or Torres Strait Islander, 65.4% were married or in de facto relationships and 31.2% managed staff (See Table 2).

Program use

In the MHFA eLearning group, 68.8% attempted the online course compared to 73.4% of those in the blended MHFA group and 73.3% of those in the PFA eLearning group. In the MHFA eLearning group, 55.3% completed the course compared to 64.8% of those in the blended MHFA group and 43.3% of those in the PFA eLearning group, the only difference that reached statistical significance ($p < 0.001$). The MHFA course website automatically captured when each module was completed. The mean number of modules completed (among those who attempted the course) was 4.19 (SD = 1.75) for MHFA eLearning and 4.53 (SD = 1.38) for the blended group. Among all participants these means were 2.88 (SD = 2.42) and 3.32 (SD = 2.33) respectively. In the blended group, 59.8% attended face-to-face training and 58.8% attended this and also completed all five modules. The website captured first and last access of the online courses with timestamps. Among participants in the two MHFA groups, 29.2% spent less than one hour on the course, 21.4% spent 1–2 h, 16.3% spent 2–8 h and 33.1% spent more than 8 h.

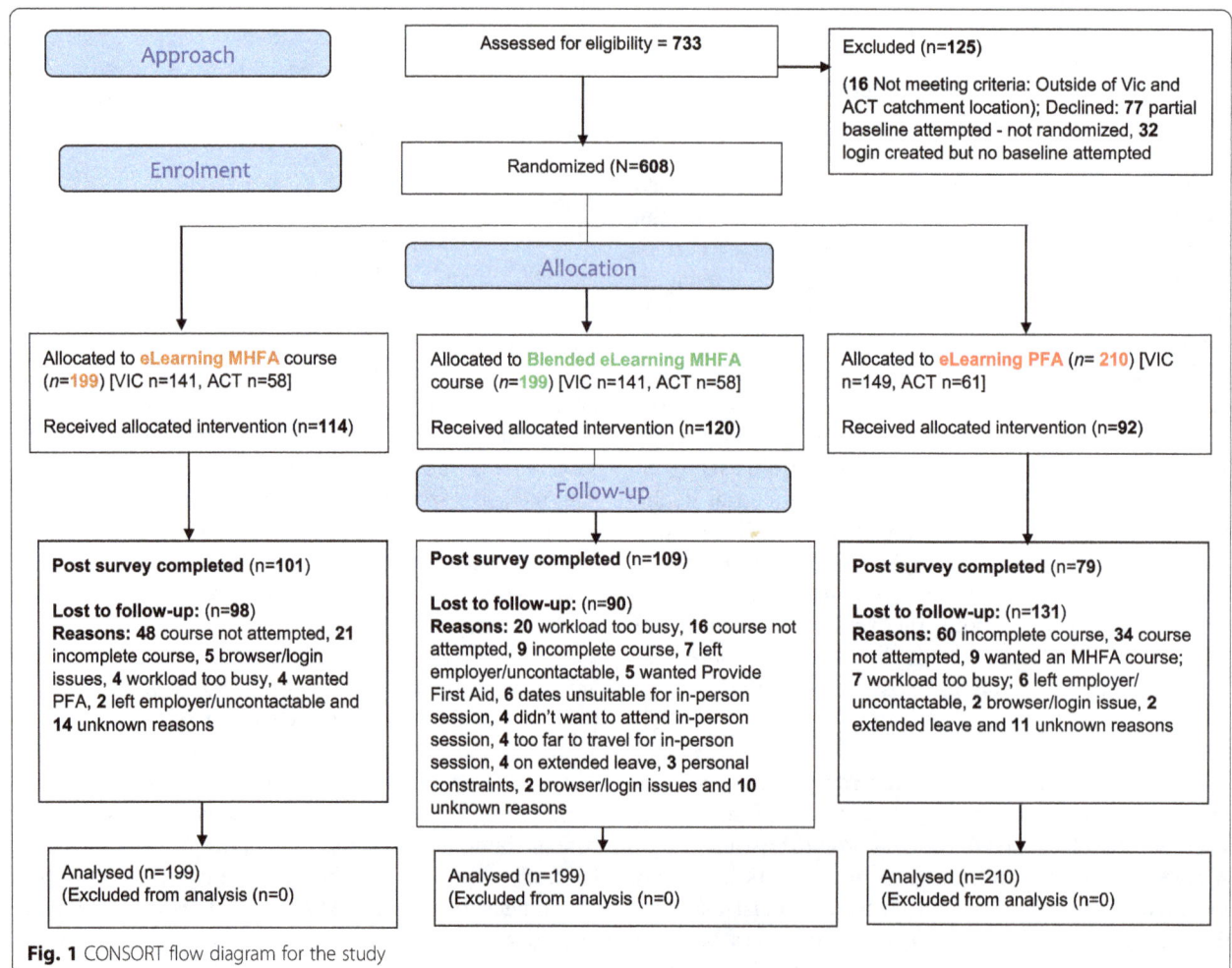

Fig. 1 CONSORT flow diagram for the study

Table 2 Baseline characteristics of participants in intervention and control groups

			Group allocation				
			MHFA eLearning	Blended MHFA	PFA elearning	Total	chi2	p
Gender							1.46	0.481
Female	N		148	140	160	448		
	%		74.8	71.1	76.2	74.1		
Male	N		50	57	50	157		
	%		25.3	28.9	23.8	26.0		
Total	N		198	197	210	605		
Only English spoken at home							4.76	0.093
Yes	N		169	180	178	527		
	%		85.4	91.4	84.8	87.1		
Total	N		198	197	210	605		
Tertiary education							1.78	0.410
Yes	N		126	127	146	399		
	%		63.6	64.8	69.5	66.1		
Total	N		198	196	210	604		
Aboriginal or Torres Strait Islander status							0.34	0.842
Yes	N		2	3	2	7		
	%		1.0	1.5	1.0	1.2		
Total	N		198	197	210	605		
Married/Defacto vs Other							2.46	0.292
Yes	N		121	131	143	395		
	%		61.1	66.8	68.1	65.4		
Total	N		198	196	210	604		
Do you manage staff							0.78	0.676
Yes	N		63	65	61	189		
	%		31.8	33.0	29.1	31.2		
Total	N		198	197	210	605		
							F	p
Age							0.3	0.737
	M		40.89	41.71	41.08	41.23		
	SD		11.30	10.93	10.60	10.93		
	N		198	196	210	604		

Primary outcomes

Baseline and post scores on all outcome measures are presented in Table 3, which also presents the results from the planned contrasts, estimating the mean difference in change over time between groups.

There were significantly greater improvements in knowledge in both MHFA eLearning and blended MHFA groups compared to PFA eLearning. These differences were greater than large in size (d = 1.35 and d = 1.55 respectively). The difference between MHFA eLearning and blended MHFA was not significant.

Those in the eLearning MHFA group were significantly more likely to show a reduced desire for social

distance from a person with depression or PTSD than those in the PFA eLearning group. The reduction in social distance in the blended group was not significantly greater than the PFA eLearning group. There were no significant differences between the MHFA eLearning and blended courses.

Secondary outcomes

Recognition of mental disorders

For the depression vignette, correct recognition was high at baseline and there was no difference in change in recognition between MHFA eLearning and PFA eLearning. There were significantly greater improvements in the

Table 3 Observed means (and standard deviations) and estimated mean differences in change over time between intervention and control groups for all outcome measures

Observed scores									Mean change over time		
Outcome	Assessment	eLearning MHFA		blended MHFA		eLearning PFA			MHFA eLearning vs PFA eLearning 95% CI	Blended MHFA vs PFA eLearning 95% CI	MHFA blended vs eLearning 95% CI
		M	SD	M	SD	M	SD				
Knowledge											
Knowledge of MHFA (% correct)	baseline	46.9	15.3	44.6	14.6	44.9	15.3	Mean diff	21.31*** 16.77–25.90	25.04*** 20.51–29.57	3.70 -0.57 – 7.98
	post	71.5	15.0	73.1	12.7	49.4	18.1	Cohen's d	1.35 1.02–1.67	1.55 1.22–1.89	0.11 -0.16 - 0.38
Beliefs about treatment - depression	baseline	5.92	2.32	5.79	2.08	5.77	2.28	Mean diff	1.80*** 1.19–2.41	2.01*** 1.40–2.61	0.20 -0.36 - 0.77
	post	7.79	1.90	7.76	1.80	5.90	2.54	Cohen's d	0.86 0.55–1.17	0.87 0.56–1.18	0.15# -0.12 - 0.43
Beliefs about treatment - PTSD	baseline	4.87	1.96	4.70	1.92	4.78	1.96	Mean diff	1.54*** 0.98–2.11	1.59*** 1.03–2.15	0.05 -0.48 - 0.58
	post	7.17	1.81	7.08	1.65	5.74	2.48	Cohen's d	0.67 0.37–0.98	0.66 0.36–0.96	-0.01# -0.26 - 0.28
		N	%	N	%	N	%				
Correct recognition of depression	baseline	190	95.5	176	88.4	190	90.5	Odds ratio	1.05 0.17–6.42	11.11* 1.60–77.28	10.57* 1.47–76.22
	post	94	93.1	103	96.3	69	88.5				
Correct recognition of PTSD	baseline	142	71.4	150	75.4	160	76.2	Odds ratio	1.28 0.38–4.32	3.61 0.96–13.57	2.83 0.84–9.55
	post	78	77.2	94	88.7	61	79.2				
Confidence		M	SD	M	SD	M	SD				
Confidence - depression	baseline	2.87	1.06	2.84	1.09	2.88	1.06	Mean diff	0.43** 0.16–0.69	0.56*** 0.29–0.82	0.13 -0.12 - 0.38
	post	3.55	0.90	3.63	0.75	3.15	1.06	Cohen's d	0.41 0.11–0.71	0.53 0.23–0.83	0.09 -0.19 - 0.36
Confidence - PTSD	baseline	2.88	1.10	2.83	1.09	2.87	1.15	Mean diff	0.58*** 0.28–0.87	0.65*** 0.36–0.94	0.07 -0.20 - 0.35
	post	3.74	0.90	3.78	0.81	3.22	1.11	Cohen's d	0.52 0.22–0.82	0.59 0.29–0.89	0.04 -0.23 - 0.32
MHFA intentions quality		M	SD	M	SD	M	SD				
Intentions - depression	baseline	3.91	1.73	3.62	1.62	3.60	1.61	Mean diff	2.06*** 1.45–2.66	3.00*** 2.41–3.60	0.95** 0.38–1.52
	post	5.67	2.35	6.35	2.45	3.31	1.55	Cohen's d	1.16	1.43	0.28

Table 3 Observed means (and standard deviations) and estimated mean differences in change over time between intervention and control groups for all outcome measures (Continued)

Outcome	Assessment	eLearning MHFA M	SD	blended MHFA M	SD	eLearning PFA M	SD		MHFA eLearning vs PFA eLearning 95% CI	Blended MHFA vs PFA eLearning 95% CI	MHFA blended vs eLearning 95% CI
									0.84–1.48	1.11–1.76	0.01–0.55
Intentions - PTSD	baseline	3.06	1.45	2.98	1.52	3.03	1.45	Mean diff	2.30*** 1.76–2.85	2.47*** 1.93–3.01	0.17 -0.35 - 0.68
	post	5.25	2.33	5.40	2.14	2.94	1.37	Cohen's d	1.17 0.85–1.49	1.33 1.00–1.65	0.07 -0.21 - 0.34
MHFA intentions – Would help		N	%	N	%	N	%				
Depression - Agree or strongly agree	baseline	156	78.4	149	74.9	158	75.2	Odds ratio	3.33* 1.06–10.44	4.26* 1.39–13.07	1.28 0.42–3.94
	post	87	86.1	93	86.9	56	71.8				
PTSD - Agree or strongly agree	baseline	150	75.4	148	74.4	160	76.2	Odds ratio	22.37*** 4.82–103.91	7.33** 2.11–25.50	0.33 0.08–1.35
	post	95	94.1	94	88.7	54	70.1				
Social distance - depression	baseline	N	%	N	%	N	%				
% scoring at or below the median. Lower scores mean less social distance	baseline	141	70.9	137	68.8	148	70.5	Odds ratio	5.30* 1.26–22.37	2.96 0.82–10.63	0.56 0.15–2.09
	post	87	86.1	88	83.0	59	76.6				
Social distance - PTSD	baseline	N	%	N	%	N	%				
% scoring at or below the median. Lower scores mean less social distance	baseline	95	47.7	102	51.3	108	51.4	Odds ratio	4.99* 1.37–18.25	2.45 0.74–8.13	0.49 0.15–1.59
	post	60	59.4	67	63.2	41	53.3				
Weak not sick – depression	baseline	N	%	N	%	N	%				
% scoring at or above the median	baseline	112	56.3	115	57.8	108	51.4	Odds ratio	1.53 0.56–4.16	1.64 0.60–4.46	1.07 0.41–2.80
	post	75	74.3	80	75.5	50	64.9				
Weak not sick – PTSD											
% scoring at or above the median	baseline	119	59.8	120	60.3	116	55.2	Odds ratio	1.20 0.42–3.42	1.89 0.63–5.61	1.58 0.56–4.43

Table 3 Observed means (and standard deviations) and estimated mean differences in change over time between intervention and control groups for all outcome measures (*Continued*)

Observed scores		eLearning MHFA		blended MHFA		eLearning PFA			Mean change over time		
									MHFA eLearning vs PFA eLearning	Blended MHFA vs PFA eLearning	MHFA blended vs eLearning
Outcome	Assessment	M	SD	M	SD	M	SD		95% CI	95% CI	95% CI
	post	76	75.3	87	82.1	55	71.4				
	baseline	M	SD	M	SD	M	SD				
Dangerous/unpredictable - depression											
	post	4.02	0.56	4.02	0.55	4.01	0.56	Mean diff	0.28*** 0.13–0.43	0.28*** 0.13–0.43	0.00 −0.14 - 0.14
	post	4.26	0.54	4.30	0.52	4.02	0.65	Cohen's d	0.42 0.12–0.72	0.50 0.20–0.80	0.08 − 0.19 −0.36
Dangerous/unpredictable - PTSD											
	baseline	4.27	0.50	4.25	0.55	4.24	0.53	Mean diff	0.27*** 0.13–0.42	0.28*** 0.14–0.43	0.01 −0.13 - 0.15
	post	4.46	0.55	4.48	0.47	4.20	0.64	Cohen's d	0.44 0.14–0.74	0.52 0.22–0.82	0.04 −0.23 - 0.32

* $p < .05$, ** $p < .01$, *** $p < .001$
# d calculated on change, rather than post due to baseline imbalances

blended MHFA vs PFA eLearning groups and in the blended MHFA vs MHFA eLearning groups. For PTSD, changes were not significantly different between groups.

Beliefs about treatment

Beliefs about treatment for depression and PTSD moved closer to those of health professionals in both the MHFA eLearning and blended MHFA groups compared to PFA eLearning. These differences were large in size for depression (d = 0.86 and d = 0.87 respectively) and medium in size for PTSD (d = 0.67 and d = 0.66 respectively). The differences between MHFA eLearning and blended MHFA were not significant.

Quality of helping intentions and confidence

There were greater increases in agreement with intentions to help a person with depression and PTSD in both the MHFA eLearning and blended MHFA groups compared to PFA eLearning. The differences between MHFA eLearning and blended MHFA were not significant.

There were greater improvements in quality of helping intentions for depression and PTSD in both the MHFA eLearning and blended MHFA groups compared to PFA eLearning. These differences were large in size for depression (d = 1.16 and d = 1.43 respectively) and PTSD (d = 1.17 and d = 1.33 respectively). There were also significantly greater improvements (of small effect size) in the blended MHFA group than in the eLearning MHFA group for depression (d = 0.28), although not for PTSD.

There were greater improvements in confidence for depression and PTSD in both the MHFA eLearning and blended MHFA groups compared to PFA eLearning. These differences were medium in size for depression (d = 0.41 and d = 0.53 respectively) and PTSD (d = 0.52 and d = 0.59 respectively). The differences between MHFA eLearning and blended MHFA were not significant.

Personal stigma

Belief that people with depression or PTSD are 'weak not sick' was low at baseline, with no significant differences in improvement between courses. For beliefs in dangerousness/unpredictability, those in the blended and eLearning MHFA groups were significantly more likely to show reduced stigma towards people with depression and PTSD than those in the PFA eLearning group. There were no significant differences between the MHFA eLearning and blended courses.

Course satisfaction

Over 90% of participants in all groups reported completing all the course and over 75% of participants in all groups reported finding the material very easy or easy to understand. However, it is interesting to note that the self-reported data differs from the objective data captured from the website, which suggested lower completion rates. Differences between groups did not reach statistical significance. When asked how much they had learnt from the course, 61.5% of participants in blended MHFA reported learning a great deal, compared to 36.6% in the eLearning course and 30.4% in the PFA course. Similarly, 72.5% of participants in the blended course reported finding it very useful, compared to 57.4% in the MHFA eLearning group and 44.3% in the PFA group. When asked if they would use the training material in future, 89.1% of those in the eLearning group, 89.0% of those in the blended MHFA group and 73.4% of those in the PFA group reported that they would. When asked if they would recommend the course to others, 72.3% of those in the eLearning group, 83.5% of those in the blended MHFA group and 62% of those in the PFA group reported that they definitely would. Differences between groups on these last four questions all reached statistical significance at $p < 0.05$ level or lower.

Discussion

Both the eLearning MHFA and blended MHFA courses had positive effects compared to PFA eLearning on the primary outcome of mental health first aid knowledge and the secondary outcomes of beliefs about professional treatments, quality of helping intentions and confidence in helping and personal stigma (related to dangerousness and unpredictability) towards a person with depression or PTSD. Thus, the first hypothesis was mostly supported. These findings are consistent with the growing number of studies demonstrating the effectiveness of MHFA courses [7], including two RCTs, one of which was conducted in Australian employees [12] and the other, more recently, in UK medical students [26].

In this study, the effects were similar for the eLearning and blended modes of MHFA courses, with most outcomes showing very small non-significant differences between the modes. There were some signs of blended MHFA being superior to eLearning MHFA, with significantly greater improvements in recognition of depression and quality of intentions to help a person with depression, although not for PTSD. Thus, the second hypothesis was mostly not supported.

This study makes a valuable contribution to the literature on the impact of modes of learning, which until now, has largely focused on students enrolled in formal education, who may be expected to have higher levels of motivation for attending and completing online courses [13, 14]. Poor retention rates in online studies are common and a key aim of the trial was to explore whether the addition of a face-to-face component was worthwhile in terms of learner outcomes in the MHFA course. It is notable that participants in the blended MHFA group were significantly more likely to complete the online course (64.8% vs 55.3%) and there were also trends towards a higher number of completed modules and more time spent on the course overall among participants in that group. Participants were also more likely to rate the blended MHFA course highly in terms of usefulness, amount learned and intentions to recommend to others, thus partly supporting the third hypothesis. It is therefore possible that blended MHFA may lead to improved behavioural changes in the longer term, such as a greater likelihood of participants providing more appropriate help to a person who develops a mental health problem. Data being collected at 1- and 2-year follow-up may shed more light on this, potentially adding to a sparse literature in the area of longer-term impacts of such training.

Additionally, one third of participants spent less than two hours online in total, despite being given permission to do the training in work time and the convenience of being able to log in as often as they wished and on more than one computer. Several factors may have contributed to the lower than expected usage, including a Victorian state government election, a department restructure (which led to email address changes) and the fact that the department-supplied internet browser was not optimal for the eLearning program. Such implementation difficulties are often seen in workplace-based interventions and complicate efforts to evaluate programs and to more widely disseminate those that are effective [27, 28].

Greater increases in depression recognition and helping intentions in the blended MHFA group may have arisen due to the in-depth discussion and mental health first aid skills practice that took place in the face-to-face component of the blended MHFA course. For example, in the blended MHFA course, there were three additional case studies, and a role play where participants practiced implementing the MHFA action plan and could then debrief with other participants and their instructor.

Strengths of the study include the use of a control intervention closely matched to the MHFA courses in time commitment and mode of delivery, while limitations include the larger than expected attrition and consequent lack of power to assess differences between the two modes of MHFA delivery. Furthermore, the majority of participants missing at post-test were those who did not complete their assigned course. An additional limitation is the fact that intentions may not translate into actual behaviours, although there is some evidence that mental health first aid intentions at baseline are associated with actual behaviour at follow-up [29, 30]. As part of the current study, data on actual behaviours will be collected at 1- and 2-year follow-up. Future studies could incorporate role plays using simulated situations to evaluate the impact of MHFA training on participant skills, although such methods may be better suited to training of health professionals than members of the public [31].

Conclusions

Both blended and eLearning MHFA courses are more effective in improving knowledge, attitudes and behavioural intentions than a control intervention. However, the blended MHFA course was minimally more effective than the eLearning MHFA course in improving recognition of depression and quality of intentions to help a person with depression Course satisfaction ratings were higher in those in the blended course, potentially leading to greater benefits in the future. Longer-term follow-up is needed to explore this.

Abbreviations
ACT: Australian Capital Territory; EAP: Employee Assistance Program; MHFA: Mental Health First Aid; OR: Odds ratio; PFA: Provide First Aid; PTSD: Post-traumatic stress disorder; RCT: Randomised controlled trial; SD: Standard deviation; VIC: Victoria

Acknowledgements
We would like to thank Anna Ross for assistance with coding open-ended responses and Stefan Cvetkovski for his assistance with the original analysis plan.

Funding
The trial was funded by the National Health and Medical Research Council (APP1061636), which played no role in the design of the study, data collection, analysis, interpretation of data or writing of the manuscript. AFJ and NJR are supported by National Health and Medical Research Council Fellowships.

Authors' contributions
AFJ, NJR, BK and JF contributed to the development and management of the project. BK and NB delivered MHFA face-to-face training. AJM carried out the data analysis. NJR drafted the manuscript and all other authors suggested improvements. All authors read and approved the final manuscript.

Consent for publication
Not applicable.

Competing interests
AFJ and BK are the co-founders of MHFA training and Chair of the Board of MHFA International. NB is the current CEO of MHFA International. NJR and JF has no competing interests. AJM is currently acting as an Associate Editor for BMC Psychiatry.

Author details

[1]Centre for Mental Health, Melbourne School of Population and Global Health, University of Melbourne, 207 Bouverie Street, Carlton, VIC 3010, Australia. [2]Mental Health First Aid Australia, 369 Royal Parade, Parkville, VIC 3052, Australia.

References

1. Reavley NJ, Jorm AF. Willingness to disclose a mental disorder and knowledge of disorders in others: changes in Australia over 16 years. Aust N Z J Psychiatry. 2014;48(2):162–8.
2. Slade T, Johnston A, Oakley Browne MA, Andrews G, Whiteford H. 2007 National Survey of mental health and wellbeing: methods and key findings. Aust N Z J Psychiatry. 2009;43(7):594–605.
3. Kitchener BA, Jorm AF, Kelly CM. mental health first aid international manual. Melbourne: Mental Health First Aid International; 2015.
4. Kitchener BA, Jorm AF. Mental health first aid training for the public: evaluation of effects on knowledge, attitudes and helping behavior. BMC Psychiatry. 2002;2:10.
5. Kitchener B, Jorm AF, Kelly C. Mental health first aid manual. 4th ed. Mental Health First Aid Australia: Melbourne; 2017.
6. Jorm AF, Kitchener BA: The truth about mental health first aid training. Psychiatr Serv 2018, 169(4):492.
7. Morgan AJ, Ross AM, Reavley NJ. Systematic review and meta-analysis of mental health first aid training: effects on knowledge, stigma, and helping behaviour. under review. 2018.
8. Sanders D, Crowe S. Overview of health promotion in the workplace. In: Scriven A, Orme J, editors. Health Professional Perspectives. London: Macmillan; 1996. p. 199–209.
9. Martin A, Sanderson K, Cocker F. Meta-analysis of the effects of health promotion intervention in the workplace on depression and anxiety symptoms. Scand J Work Environ Health. 2009;35(1):7 18.
10. Kitchener BA, Jorm AF. Mental health first aid training in a workplace setting: a randomized controlled trial [ISRCTN13249129]. BMC Psychiatry. 2004;4:23.
11. Wan Mohd Yunus WMA, Musiat P, Brown JSL. Systematic review of universal and targeted workplace interventions for depression. Occup Environ Med. 2018;75(1):66–75.
12. Jorm AF, Kitchener BA, Fischer JA, Cvetkovski S. Mental health first aid training by e-learning: a randomized controlled trial. Aust N Z J Psychiatry. 2010;44(12):1072–81.
13. Liu Q, Peng W, Zhang F, Hu R, Li Y, Yan W. The effectiveness of blended learning in health professions: systematic review and meta-analysis. J Med Internet Res. 2016;18(1):e2.
14. Sitzmann T, Kraiger K, Stewart DB, Wisher R. The comparative effectiveness of web-based and classroom instruction: a meta-analysis. Pers Psychol. 2006; 59:623–64.
15. Griffiths KM, Carron-Arthur B, Parsons A, Reid R. Effectiveness of programs for reducing the stigma associated with mental disorders. A meta-analysis of randomized controlled trials. World Psychiatry. 2014;13(2):161–75.
16. Reavley NJ, Jorm AF. Stigmatizing attitudes towards people with mental disorders: findings from an Australian National Survey of mental health literacy and stigma. Aust N Z J Psychiatry. 2011;48(12):1086–93.
17. Link BG, Phelan JC, Bresnahan M, Stueve A, Pescosolido BA. Public conceptions of mental illness: labels, causes, dangerousness, and social distance. Am J Public Health. 1999;89(9):1328–33.
18. Jorm AF, Oh E. Desire for social distance from people with mental disorders. Aust N Z J Psychiatry. 2009;43(3):183–200.
19. Yap MBH, Mackinnon AJ, Reavley NJ, Jorm AF. The measurement properties of stigmatising attitudes towards mental disorders: results from two community surveys. Int J Methods Psychiatr Res. 2014;23(1):49–61.
20. Reavley NJ, Morgan AJ, Jorm AF. Development of scales to assess mental health literacy relating to recognition of and interventions for depression, anxiety disorders and schizophrenia/psychosis. Aust N Z J Psychiatry. 2014; 48(1):61–9.
21. Morgan AJ, Jorm AF, Reavley NJ. Beliefs of Australian health professionals about the helpfulness of interventions for mental disorders: differences between professions and change over time. Aust N Z J Psychiatry. 2013; 47(9):840–8.
22. Rossetto A, Jorm AF, Reavley NJ. Quality of helping behaviours of members of the public towards a person with a mental illness: a descriptive analysis of data from an Australian national survey. Ann General Psychiatry. 2014;13(1):2.
23. Griffiths KM, Christensen H, Jorm AF, Evans K, Groves C. Effect of web-based depression literacy and cognitive-behavioural therapy interventions on stigmatising attitudes to depression: randomised controlled trial. Br J Psychiatry. 2004;185:342–9.
24. Means B, Toyama Y, Murphy R, Baki M. The Effectiveness of Online and Blended Learning: A Meta-Analysis of the Empirical Literature. Teach Coll Rec. 2010;115(030303).
25. Rabe-Hesketh S, Skrondal A. Classical latent variable models for medical research. Stat Methods Med Res. 2008;17(1):5–32.
26. Davies EB, Beever E, Glazebrook C. A pilot randomised controlled study of the mental health first aid eLearning course with UK medical students. BMC Med Educ. 2018;18(1):45.
27. Montano D, Hoven H, Siegrist J. Effects of organisational-level interventions at work on employees' health: a systematic review. BMC Public Health. 2014;14:135.
28. Olsen O, Albertsen K, Nielsen ML, Poulsen KB, Gron SM, Brunnberg HL. Workplace restructurings in intervention studies - a challenge for design, analysis and interpretation. BMC Med Res Methodol. 2008;8:39.
29. Yap MBH, Jorm AF. Young people's mental health first aid intentions and beliefs prospectively predict their actions: findings from an Australian National Survey of youth. Psychiatry Res. 2012;196(2–3):315–9.
30. Rossetto A, Jorm AF, Reavley NJ. Predictors of adults' helping intentions and behaviours towards a person with a mental illness: a six-month follow-up study. Psychiatry Res. 2016;240:170–6.
31. Boukouvalas EA, El-Den S, Chen TF, Moles R, Saini B, Bell A, O'Reilly CL. Confidence and attitudes of pharmacy students towards suicidal crises: patient simulation using people with a lived experience. Soc Psychiatry Psychiatr Epidemiol. 2018.

16

The survivability of dialectical behaviour therapy programmes: a mixed methods analysis of barriers and facilitators to implementation within UK healthcare settings

Joanne C. King[1*], Richard Hibbs[3], Christopher W. N. Saville[1] and Michaela A. Swales[1,2*] (iD)

Abstract

Background: Dialectical Behaviour Therapy (DBT) is an evidence-based intervention that has been included in the National Institute of Health and Care Excellence guidelines as a recommended treatment for Borderline Personality Disorder in the UK. However, implementing and sustaining evidence-based treatments in routine practice can be difficult to achieve. This study compared the survival of early and late adopters of DBT as well as teams trained via different training modes (on-site versus off-site), and explored factors that aided or hindered implementation of DBT into routine healthcare settings.

Methods: A mixed-method approach was used. Kaplan-Meier survival analyses were conducted to quantify and compare survivability as a measure of sustainability between early and late implementers and those trained on- and off-site. An online questionnaire based on the Consolidated Framework for Implementation Research was used to explore barriers and facilitators in implementation. A quantitative content analysis of survey responses was carried out.

Results: Early implementers were significantly less likely to survive than late implementers, although, the effect size was small. DBT teams trained off-site were significantly more likely to survive. The effect size for this difference was large. An unequal amount of censored data between groups in both analyses means that findings should be considered tentative. Practitioner turnover and financing were the most frequently cited barriers to implementation. Individual characteristics of practitioners and quality of the evidence base were the most commonly reported facilitators to implementation.

Conclusions: A number of common barriers and facilitators to successful implementation of DBT were found among DBT programmes. Location of DBT training may mediate programme survival.

Keywords: Implementation, DBT, CFIR, Kaplan-Meier, Sustainability

* Correspondence: joanne.king@belfasttrust.hscni.net; m.swales@bangor.ac.uk
[1]School of Psychology, Bangor University, Bangor, Gwynedd, UK
Full list of author information is available at the end of the article

Background

Dialectical Behaviour Therapy (DBT) [1] is a comprehensive cognitive-behavioural treatment originally developed for adult women who meet criteria for Borderline Personality Disorder (BPD), particularly those who engage in suicidal or non-suicidal self-injury. Traditionally, this client group has been perceived as "treatment resistant" and considered unsuitable candidates for psychotherapeutic intervention [2]. DBT was the first psychological therapy to challenge the culture of therapeutic rejection for individuals with BPD and has become one of the best evidenced treatments for this client group.

Numerous DBT efficacy trials [3–11] have demonstrated reductions in suicide attempts, intentional self-injury, anger, depression, hopelessness, and improvements in global functioning [12]. Recent meta-analyses have found moderate to large effect sizes indicating a beneficial effect of DBT when compared to treatment as usual on outcomes such as anger, parasuicidality, and mental health [13, 14]. Furthermore, several randomised controlled trials (RCTs) have examined the application of DBT with other client groups such as older adults with major depressive disorder, eating disorders, and forensic populations [15–19]. Thus, the data on DBT clearly indicate its efficacy for the treatment of BPD and holds promise for a host of other disorders.

In 2009, DBT was included in the National Institute of Health and Care Excellence (NICE) guidelines as a recommended treatment for females with a diagnosis of BPD and a history of repetitive self-harm [20]. Since then, a number of healthcare providers within the United Kingdom (UK) have included the provision of DBT as a quality improvement indicator in an effort to meet national targets in health outcomes for individuals with serious mental illness [21]. Preliminary efficiency research also suggests that DBT has the potential to be a cost-effective treatment for individuals presenting with parasuicidal behaviour [22, 23]. Indeed, it appears that the potential benefits DBT has to offer is gaining traction within routine healthcare settings.

Notwithstanding NICE recommendations, demonstrable treatment efficacy, and potential cost efficiencies, concerns have been raised about the sustainability of DBT programmes within the UK National Health Service (NHS) [24]. Diffusion of Innovations Theory [25] suggests that innovations must be widely adopted in order to self-sustain. Widespread adoption of a new practice depends initially on innovators and early adopters and how quickly the subsequent late majority can be persuaded to shift. Furthermore, it is proposed that ideas not sustained by early adopters are unlikely to spread elsewhere [26]. Thus, effective implementation is relevant not only to long-term sustainability but also subsequent spread of an innovation.

Other factors that can impact sustainability are those directly related to the innovation itself, such as the ease with which it can be implemented and how well treatment effects observed in efficacy trials will generalise to routine healthcare settings. The DBT model entails a comprehensive programme that structures the treatment environment across different modalities to enhance client's capabilities (skills training groups), improve their motivation (individual therapy), aid generalisation of new skills (telephone skills coaching), and supervise DBT therapists (a consultation team model) [27]. All of the treatment modalities are informed by a coherent theoretical model with associated therapeutic strategies based on cognitive behavioural principles and mindfulness [1, 28]. The programme is delivered by a team of mental health professionals all trained within the DBT model and the rationale for doing so is to alleviate the stress and anxiety of working with a high risk client group in which change is often slow [27]. Nevertheless, the requirement of a specialist trained team usually involves significant reorganisation of existing services and an ongoing commitment to delivering an intensive specialist intervention. This is likely to have an impact on how well DBT is implemented or, indeed, whether it is even considered viable for adoption within a service.

Deciding to implement a new practice is not a discrete event but a set of interactive dynamic processes. The difficulties of translating evidence-based research into real-world settings is widely acknowledged [29], which has led to a growing body of literature examining the various factors involved in the implementation and sustainability of evidence-based practices (EBPs) [30–32]. Historically, more attention has been paid to the efficacy of interventions. Whilst such information might help a consumer or agency to select a particular type of intervention, evidence of efficacy alone does not lead to more successful implementation [29], in the same way that simply training practitioners in a new approach does not sufficiently ensure behaviour change [33]. Thus, transfer of innovation needs to be considered within organisational and wider system contexts to ensure that desired change is disseminated, implemented and sustained [34]. However, because organisational restructuring requires changes in service provider behaviour and transformation of systems, translating an EBP into routine practice remains an unquestionably complex and often daunting task.

A number of conceptual frameworks have been developed to aid the process of implementation [29, 31, 35–37]. Whilst these frameworks differ somewhat on areas of emphasis and terminology, influences on implementation generally relate to the context (outer and inner), the innovation itself (fit, training, efficacy), implementation processes (planning, selection, evaluation), individual characteristics (motivation, skill), and sustainability factors (fidelity monitoring, penetration, outcomes etc.). These components are considered to be interrelated and a change in one may result in change to others. Therefore, due to the dynamic nature of healthcare systems and their external contexts, a given programme or practice may require more or less of each component at any one time in order to be successfully implemented. This represents a challenge for the implementation and sustainability of innovations, as the relative contribution of each component to overall outcome can change, resulting in the need for ongoing monitoring of processes. Such tasks can be greatly supported by the application of a guiding theoretical framework. Only recently have distinct models for sustainability of evidence-based programmes been produced [38, 39], however, most of the elements of these models (Inner and Outer Contextual Factors, Characteristics of the Interventionists and of the Intervention) are incorporated already in conceptual frameworks of implementation [32, 36].

Considering the above, implementing a comprehensive DBT programme in routine healthcare settings is unlikely to be a straightforward endeavour. Preliminary research into the sustainability of UK DBT programmes that underwent an intensive training programme between 1995 and 2007 confirmed that some teams had difficulty surviving [27]. Highest failure rates were found shortly after training ended (i.e. the second year of the programme) and again in the fifth year. Participants identified a number of challenges associated with implementing DBT in their service, which were generally characterised by an absence of organisational support. Conversely, for teams that had implemented successfully and managed to sustain, the presence of organisational support was identified as a facilitating factor.

In an effort to increase organisational support and promote effective implementation strategies, British Isles DBT (biDBT) have begun to offer an alternative training modality. Typically, training involves teams of practitioners participating in two five-day DBT intensive training events that are delivered off-site, which is known as the 'open-enrolment route'. Each training event is separated by 8 months during which teams commence the process of setting up and starting a DBT programme. With the new mode, the content and structure of the training is the same; however organisations wishing to deliver DBT programmes are encouraged to host intensive training on-site. This requires a greater financial investment and consideration of how to adapt staff roles in order to successfully deliver treatment, with the idea that greater organisational investment will have a positive influence on the implementation process. This change in training delivery warrants further investigation to examine whether it improves implementation of programmes.

The aims of the present study are threefold: 1) to investigate whether early and late adopters of DBT have differential sustainability, 2) to investigate whether change in training method delivery impacts the sustainability of DBT programmes, and 3) to examine factors that act as a barrier or facilitator to implementation by using a theoretical implementation framework to guide assessment.

Method

Participants

All biDBT programmes that underwent Intensive Training™ between January 1995 and February 2016 were eligible for this study. During this period, whether at on-site or off-site trainings, both the structure and content of the DBT Intensive Training™ remained constant, with only minor modifications to the order of topics taught. All trainings were delivered by two or three members of a six person team who had all been trained to a consistent standard of training, all of whom were adherent DBT therapists. For the sustainability analyses, the unit of analysis was DBT teams. For the survey arm of this study, only one team member from each DBT programme was invited to participate in the study. In the first instance, all DBT team leaders were invited to participate. If a team leader was unavailable, another current team member of an active team, or any former member of inactive teams, was invited to participate.

Design & Procedure

A concurrent mixed-methods approach was employed [40]. Sustainability of DBT programmes was quantified using Kaplan Meier (K-M) [41] survival analysis. biDBT maintain a database to systematically record data on programme start date, activity status (i.e. active or inactive programme), cessation date, and site of training delivery. During the period of the study all programmes were contacted by telephone to establish if they were still active i.e. delivering a DBT programme to clients, consistent with one of Scheirer's [42] definitions of sustainability. These data were used to analyse survival rates as a proxy for sustainability.

Survival data were triangulated with responses from an online survey to identify factors that may aid or hinder implementation of DBT in routine settings. Initial contact to participate in the survey was made via email to all DBT team leaders registered on the biDBT training database. If an email was returned as undeliverable, an alternative team member was contacted. Participants were provided with information on the purpose of the study and were offered the opportunity to be entered into a prize draw following completion of the survey. A link to the online survey was contained within the body of the initial email.

Measures

A 70-item online questionnaire (Additional file 1) was designed to elicit information regarding DBT teams' experiences of implementing DBT in their service. The questionnaire consisted of three types of questions (closed, free response, and rating scales) and was conceptually divided into six separate domains. The first domain relates to factors considered to be relevant to practice sustainability and is adapted from Swain and colleagues' [43] study on the sustainability of EBPs in routine mental health agencies. The remaining five domains are based on Damschroder and colleagues' [36] Consolidated Framework for Implementation Research (CFIR). The CFIR is an overarching theoretical framework that incorporates common constructs from a range of published theories on implementation and is comprised of five major domains: *Intervention Characteristics; Inner Setting; Outer Setting; Individual Characteristics*; and *Implementation Processes*. Each domain includes a constellation of interactive constructs that are purported to influence the implementation process, for a detailed discussion see [36]. Demographic information was also collected.

Analysis

Kaplan-Meier (K-M) [41] survival analyses were carried out to estimate the cumulative survival rates of DBT programmes. Based on the biDBT database teams were ascertained as either *active or inactive*. Teams that could not be contacted were considered lost to follow-up. Whilst including teams lost to follow-up as censored data is standard practice in K-M analysis, the analysis makes no distinctions within the censored data between teams that cannot be contacted (i.e. lost to follow up) and those that are still functioning. Including teams lost to follow-up as censored (i.e. assuming they are still alive) may make the survival estimate unreliable, we therefore excluded them from the survival analyses.

Study aim 1

To investigate whether there were differences in sustainability between early and late adopters, a K-M analysis comparing survival rates of teams trained between January 1995 and March 2007 (12 years) with teams trained between April 2007 and February 2016 (9 years) was carried out ($N = 468$). Programme start and cessation dates were used to calculate survival rate. To reduce the potential for unequal amounts of censored data between groups due to differences in duration of cohort timeframes (12 versus 9 years), only the first seven years of a programme within these time frames were analysed. Programmes that survived for at least 2555 days were censored regardless of whether they later became inactive. Teams active at the time of analysis (or active for

at least 2555 days) were categorised as censored data. A chi-squared test was used to check for differences in the amount of censored data between groups. A log-rank test was used to test whether the rate of programme closure varied between groups. A Cox regression model was also fitted to estimate a hazard ratio between groups, as log-rank analyses do not yield effect sizes.

Study aim 2

To examine whether training method delivery influenced the sustainability of DBT programmes, a K-M analysis comparing teams trained on-site with teams trained via open-enrolment was carried out. Teams were allocated to their respective study group based on site of training delivery. This information was extracted from biDBT database. Survival rates were calculated using programme start and cessation date. Programmes active at the time of analysis were categorised as censored data. Only DBT programmes that commenced training from January 2009, the date at which the off-site training model was introduced were included in this analysis. A chi-squared test was used to check for differences in the amount of censored data between groups. A log-rank test was used to test whether the rate of programme closure varied between training methods. A Cox regression model was also fitted to estimate a hazard ratio between groups, as log-rank analyses do not yield effect sizes.

Study aim 3

A descriptive content analysis of survey data was carried out by the first author to investigate the frequency with which individual implementation and sustainability constructs were identified as an aid or barrier to a programme's ability to successfully implement and sustain.

Results

Survival analyses

Study aim 1: Early versus late cohort comparison

A total of 468 teams were included for analysis. Of these, 160 teams were from the pre-April 2007 cohort (inactive $n = 55$, active $n = 46$) and 308 teams (inactive $n = 157$, active $n = 55$) were from the post-April 2007 cohort. A chi-squared test indicated significant differences in the distribution of active, and inactive teams between the pre and post April 2007 groups ($\chi^2 = .23.164$, df $= 1$, p-value $= 1.488e-06$), in that the post-April 2007 group had more censored and less inactive data than the pre-April 2007 group. K-M survival curves (Fig. 1) and log-rank test indicated that the pre-April 2007 group had a faster rate of closure than the post-April 2007 group ($\chi^2 = 6.819$, $p = .009$). Cox regression indicated that the hazard ratio was 0.607 (95% CI $= 0.416-0.886$, reference category $=$ pre-April 2007 group) with a Cohen's d approximation $= -.389$. Highest programme

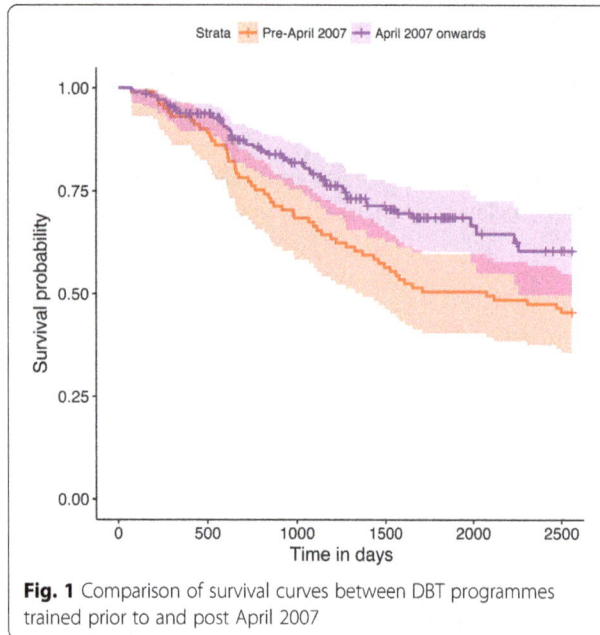

Fig. 1 Comparison of survival curves between DBT programmes trained prior to and post April 2007

failure rates were found in the second year for both cohorts.

Study aim 2: Training method comparison

A total of 266 teams were included for analysis. Fifty-two teams (active $n = 35$, inactive $n = 17$) were trained on-site and 214 teams (active $n = 187$, inactive $n = 27$) were trained off-site. A chi-squared test indicated greater levels of censored data in the on-site group ($\chi^2 = 10.802$, $p = .001$). K-M survival curves (Fig. 2) and log rank test showed that teams trained off-site had a significantly higher probability of

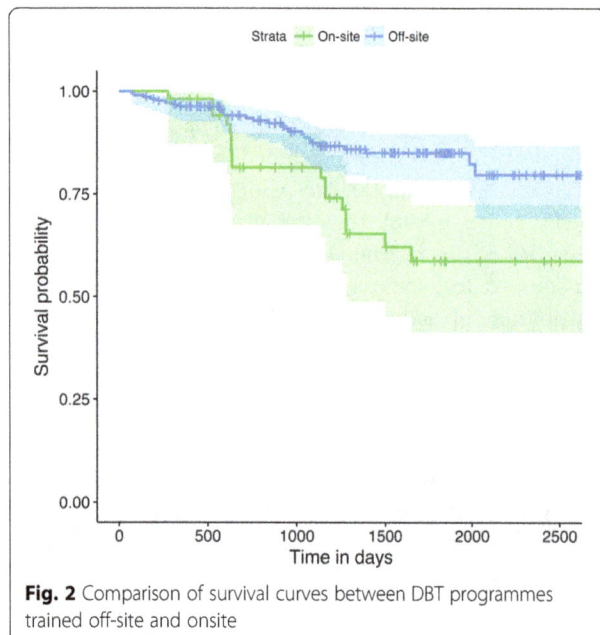

Fig. 2 Comparison of survival curves between DBT programmes trained off-site and onsite

survival than teams trained on-site ($\chi^2 = 9.801$, $p = .002$). Cox regression indicated that the hazard ratio was 2.554 (95% CI = 1.392–4.688, reference category = off-site) with a Cohen's d approximation = 0.731). Highest failure rates were found in the second year for teams that trained on-site, compared to the third year for teams trained via open-enrolment.

Barriers and facilitators to implementation
Study aim 3

The online questionnaire was completed by 68 respondents. Sixty-two (91%) were from active teams and 6 (9%) were inactive. Of the active teams, the majority of respondents were located in England ($n = 38$, 61%) and the remainder were located in Wales ($n = 8$, 13%), Scotland ($n = 2$, 3%), and Ireland ($n = 8$, 13%). The proportion of teams containing the following professions were: clinical psychologists ($n = 56$, 83%), nurses ($n = 52$, 77%), social workers ($n = 22$, 33%), psychological therapists ($n = 22$, 33%), and occupational therapists ($n = 13$, 21%). The most frequently reported number of DBT trained clinicians within a service was between 4 and 5 ($n = 23$, 37%), with a range of 2 to 12 trained clinicians. Twenty-nine (46%) respondents worked within community adult mental health services, 12 (19%) within child and adolescent mental health services (CAMHS), and the remainder across a range of learning disability ($n = 3$, 5%), eating disorders ($n = 2$, 3%), forensic ($n = 7$, 10%), youth mental health ($n = 1$, 2%), personality disorder ($n = 1$, 2%) and inpatient settings ($n = 9$, 13%). Fifty-three (85%) active teams fell within the statutory service sector and 9 (15%) within the private sector.

Of the six inactive teams who completed the online survey, the median survival time was 2015 days (5.5 years), range 635–4405 days. All respondents from inactive teams were asked to provide three reasons why they thought their DBT programme discontinued. The most frequently cited reason for programme failure was lack of management support ($n = 5$, 83%) either due to lack of understanding of how DBT works, insufficient time allocated to deliver DBT, or priority given to competing service demands. Lack of funding ($n = 3$, 50%), lack of colleague support ($n = 3$, 50%), and staff turnover ($n = 2$, 33%) were other reasons reported for programme failure. One respondent also cited high dropout rates as a reason for their programme ending but reflected that this may have been as a result of "overly rigid referral criteria".

Content analysis

Response frequencies and percentages for each implementation construct were counted for the total online survey sample. Respondents were also invited to leave comments to further elaborate their responses within each implementation domain. All comments were analysed by the lead author and grouped according to the implementation category referred. Due to the small response rate from inactive teams, comparative analyses of response differences between active and inactive programmes could not be carried out.

Barriers to implementation

The most frequently endorsed barrier to implementing DBT was practitioner turnover ($n = 40$, 59%) followed closely by financing ($n = 35$, 52%). Other common barriers were availability of resources ($n = 28$, 41%), the perceived difficulty of implementing DBT ($n = 27$, 40%), and external change events ($n = 23$, 34%). No constructs within the *Individual Characteristics* or *Outer Setting* domains were strongly endorsed as barriers to implementation. Table 1 provides illustrative comments to the most commonly reported barriers to implementing DBT.

Aids to implementation

There were a number of constructs strongly endorsed as aiding the implementation process, the most common being the quality of the DBT evidence base ($n = 60$, 88%). Other frequently endorsed constructs were practitioner skills ($n = 56$, 82%), acceptability of DBT by clients ($n = 54$, 79%), the perceived advantage to implementing DBT into practice ($n = 53$, 78%), practitioner attitudes ($n = 53$, 78%), DBT training ($n = 52$, 77%), practitioner readiness ($n = 51$, 75%), and shared willingness among DBT clinicians to implement the programme ($n = 51$, 75%). All constructs within the *Individual Characteristics* domain were strongly endorsed as aiding the implementation process. Illustrative comments are provided in Table 2.

Sustainability

Frequency and percentage data were collected on a number of factors considered to be related to sustainability of interventions such as collection of client outcome data, extent of programme penetration, ongoing training and consultation, and treatment fidelity. Of the active teams, 51 (82%) collected client outcome data, which was mainly used for tracking client progress and auditing the effectiveness of the programme. Seven (11%) respondents indicated that they were serving considerably fewer clients than when they initially commenced DBT training. Twenty-nine teams reported that they were serving approximately the same (47%) and 26 (42%) said they were serving a lot more clients since initial training. Thirty-seven (60%) respondents had received external consultation. However, only 24 (39%) reported accessing DBT expert supervision. The majority of teams, 43 (69%), carried out new team member training and 34 (55%) had received booster training. With regards to treatment modalities, 61 teams (98%) offered skills training and individual therapy, 60 (96%) ran a consultation group, and 48 (77%) offered telephone support. Finally, 41 teams (66%) had made adaptations to the DBT model and of these, 20 (32%) reported making changes during the initial training phase.

All six inactive teams collected outcome data. Four teams used the data (67%) to demonstrate clinical outcomes and cost effectiveness. One respondent (17%) indicated that they had served considerably fewer clients post initial training phase, with the remaining respondents either having served the same amount ($n = 2$, 33%) or a lot more clients ($n = 3$, 50%). Only two teams (33%) did booster training and no teams carried out new team member training. Five teams (83%) had offered all four DBT treatment modalities: individual therapy, group skills training, therapist's consultation group, and 24-h

Table 1 Barriers to Implementing DBT

Implementation domain	Construct	N	%	Example
Intervention characteristics	Financing Perceived difficulty of implementing DBT	35 29	52 40	"Cost of DBT training can be prohibitive...concern about this in future in current economic climate - despite evidence base for longer term money saving - trusts often view things in short term when lots monies need to be saved" "All DBT staff have had a long break since last running the programme and so it is harder for us to re-start the programme"
Inner setting	Practitioner turnover Available resources	40 28	59 41	"Until very recently we had no practitioner turnover this really helped with the initial establishment of DBT and refining it. We have recently had someone leave and one person is on mat leave...The people who have left are our least psychologically experienced team members and so these people delivered the groups whilst others did more primary therapy. At the moment existing team members are now doing both and this is not sustainable long term." "Failure to provide funding for a second laptop for second consecutive group and time in lieu for out-of-hours telephone consult hindered implementation."
Implementation process	External change events	23	34	–

Note. - indicates no elaborative comments provided for implementation construct

Table 2 Aids to Implementing DBT

Implementation domain	Construct	n	%	Example
Intervention characteristics	Quality of DBT evidence base	60	88	"Evidence on efficacy and cost savings also had a significant impact in securing Trust manager's interest and support"
	Perceived advantage of implementing DBT	53	78	"Business plan presented to commissioners comparing costs of often unsuccessful inpatient programmes, allegedly DBT informed, with adherent programme."
	DBT training	52	77	"The training we had from the British Isles team was excellent and central to our success. We make reference to it frequently in consult meetings."
Outer setting	Acceptability of DBT by clients	54	79	"In the past, when DBT was at risk of cuts due to financial pressures, we were able to arrange for ex-clients and current clients to talk to the senior management and explain the impact and benefits DBT had had on their lives."
Inner setting	Shared willingness to implement DBT	51	75	"We regularly meet for CPD opportunities (every 6 months) on DBT adherence and how we are implementing DBT. We use recordings/triadic observation of the 1:1 session to evaluate therapist behaviours and try to stay focused on the Consultation Supervision group agreements."
	Leadership engagement	49	72	"…so there is senior management support to find a solution quickly. Including to find resource to train a considerable number of new staff and ensure that their roles in relation to DBT are made clear going forward."
Individual characteristics	Practitioner skills	56	82	"Clinicians highly skilled and experienced so take great pleasure in learning and adhering to effective but also very creative model."
	Practitioner attitudes	53	78	"We have a team of highly motivated DBT therapists and the service has developed a good and growing reputation with referrers to the service."
	Practitioner readiness	51	75	-
Implementation process	Appointment of DBT team leader	42	62	"…but the DBT lead worked to gain this [management buy-in] and the success of the programme has led to this over time."
	Execution of implementation plan	42	62	-

Note. - indicates no elaborative comments provided for implementation construct

telephone access. One team (17%) did not offer telephone consultation. Only two teams (33%) reported modifying the DBT model to suit their service needs and of these, one team made modifications during the initial training period whilst the other implemented one full round of DBT before making adaptations.

Discussion

Consistent with earlier data [27], the highest failure rate for DBT programmes was observed in the second year post-training. Despite this early high failure rate the survivability of DBT programmes compares well with other evidence-based programmes reported in the literature. Cooper and colleagues [44] reported that 69% of delinquency and violence prevention programmes in a state-wide implementation sustained at two to four years post-initial seed-funding. Whilst the National Implementing Evidence Based Practices project reported that 80% of sites sustained at two years post implementation [45] and 47% at six years, although, in the six year data, sustainability rates varied between the five interventions studied from 25 to 69%. DBT compares favourably with these figures with survivability rates of 88% at two years and 69% at eight years.

Differences in the survival rates between the early and late implementers is not particularly surprising, although the different rates of censored data between the cohorts means that the result should be interpreted with caution.

Several factors might account for this difference. Early adopters are known to be psychologically different from their peers and often in influential positions [46]. Whilst they may have adopted DBT early they may also have been keen to move on to the next innovation. Secondly, DBTs place as an evidence-based intervention within the UK became more solid with the publication of the NICE guidance in 2009 [20]. The advocacy for DBT within the guideline may have provided an 'outer context' support to teams training post-2007, just as publication of the guidance also boosted training in DBT [47].

Traditionally, the translation from science to practice has been a passive process that has usually only involved diffusion and dissemination of EBP information, with the hope that this is sufficient to change practitioner behaviour. There is a current shift towards a more active approach whereby outside experts work alongside organisations to help achieve implementation success and assure benefits to consumers [48]. Results from the present study found that on-site training did not increase the probability of survival. Survival curve comparison of training delivery methods indicated programmes trained off-site had a significantly higher probability of surviving. This is a surprising finding, given that on-site training was designed to increase organisational investment in DBT implementation. However, this finding must be interpreted with caution, as the amount of censored data between the comparison groups was found to be significantly different, limiting conclusions that can be drawn about differences between groups. Notwithstanding this caveat, a possible explanation for the differences may be that those attending off-site training have engaged in a substantial amount of pre-planning and assessment of organisational readiness, and in efforts to obtain management buy-in, have identified an explicit need for implementing DBT in their service setting. In doing so, they are possibly more likely to have actively considered how an implementation plan may be executed. Addressing organizational funding and resources and aligning the innovation with organizational goals are factors known to be associated with sustainability [39, 43, 45, 49]. Teams attending off-site training have typically had to actively pursue funding and gain agreements from their organisation to attend. This may indicate that individuals in teams pursuing this route may possess particular leadership skills that may also relate to sustainability [49, 50]. Attending off-site training provides greater opportunities to network with other teams, allowing for the sharing of experiences and ideas, which prove beneficial to implementation and sustainability. During the second week of training teams present their initial implementation efforts for consultation and feedback from trainers and fellow trainees. In off-site trainings trainees are exposed to a wider range of systems and witness trainers applying the components of the model to these different systems. This more expansive experience may increase knowledge of the core components and principles of DBT. Cooper and colleagues [44] similarly highlighted that greater knowledge of a progammes' logic model increased the likelihood of sustainability.

Practitioner turnover and financing were the most commonly identified barriers to implementing DBT programmes. This is consistent with findings from other studies [43, 45, 50]. Indeed, these constructs may interact, as difficulty financing new team members was one of the main problems identified when practitioner turnover was high. Financing initial training was identified as a key barrier for some programmes. Although, a few overcame this difficulty by securing initial funding from external sources and then using evaluation and outcome data to secure ongoing funding from their organisations. Other programmes identified difficulties with ongoing financing, whether it was for training new team members, booster training, or accessing expert supervision or consultation. Whilst securing financing is a common theme both in this study and in others [43, 45, 50] consideration is rarely given to the costs of de-implementation and, in the case of DBT, failing to provide an intervention that may produce cost-savings [22]. Developing models that highlight the costs of failing to sustain may prove useful to influence leaders both in the inner and outer context or organisations to continue to support an evidence-based intervention.

A number of facilitators to implementation were identified. Most notably, all constructs within the *Individual Characteristics* domain were strongly endorsed as aiding the implementation process. A number of respondents reported highly motivated or skilled practitioners, effective leadership of the DBT team, or the presence of a DBT champion as key to overcoming barriers encountered to implementation and sustainability of programmes. This finding highlights how a strength in one or more areas can compensate for weaknesses in others [29]. Nevertheless, overreliance on an individual(s) to ensure effective implementation and sustainability leaves a programme particularly vulnerable to practitioner or leadership turnover. Organisations are dynamic and so the relative contribution of implementation constructs can inevitably wax and wane. This poses a difficulty for organisations because changes in one construct requires adjustments in others. Thus, successfully managing such changes will require effective monitoring and feedback systems to keep a programme on track [48], as well as ongoing availability of resources to do so.

Characteristics of the intervention, a feature in many implementation and sustainability models [31, 36, 38, 39] in particular the quality of the evidence base for DBT, was strongly endorsed as aiding the implementation process. Whilst efficacy data alone maybe insufficient for changing practice, findings from this study indicated that for some programmes research data played a crucial role in securing management commitment to delivering DBT. The quality of the evidence base may be of particular relevance during pre-planning and preparation stages, allowing for organisations to weigh up the suitability of DBT for their service and make as assessment of perceived benefits and 'fit' with the context [38]. For populations where the evidence base for DBT is not as extensive or robust, the lack of efficacy data may present a barrier to implementation. In this instance, the opportunity to trial a DBT programme and collect effectiveness data may prove beneficial.

Over half of survey respondents indicated that their programme engaged in practices which are considered pertinent to sustainability, with the exception of receiving supervision from a DBT expert. This is an encouraging finding and suggests that teams are aware of the need for continuous monitoring and collection of outcome data as an aid to sustainability [43]. Given that the highest failure rates for programmes are found within the active implementation stage (i.e. first two years), programmes should also consider identifying and monitoring implementation outcomes, distinct from service and treatment outcomes. Evaluation of implementation outcomes will provide an indicator of implementation success and yield an index of implementation processes. Also, because treatment effectiveness requires successful implementation, monitoring implementation outcomes is a necessary intermediate step to obtaining desired clinical and service outcomes [51].

There are a number of limitations to the study. The first being the small number of survey respondents from inactive teams, which prevented comparative analyses, and limits the conclusions that can be drawn from the findings. Second, the method of data collection prevented exploration of research participants' interpretation of questions or the opportunity to clarify responses. Although a summary question was included at the end of each survey domain, not all respondents chose to elaborate their responses, limiting the amount of qualitative data collected. Lastly, the retrospective accounts from individual team leaders/members must be interpreted with caution due to problems inherent with self-report, such as post-hoc rationalisation. Future research should endeavour to recruit multiple respondents from programmes to reduce the likelihood of methodological bias, as well as recruit greater numbers of inactive teams to ensure a representative sample of respondents.

Despite these limitations, the present study possessed a number of strengths. There are few studies in the literature studying sustainability beyond the early stages of implementation (post-two years) and none, to our knowledge, that allow the comparison of two different types of training delivery that may have implications for sustainability. In addition, the use of a concurrent mixed-methods approach allowed quantitative findings to be complimented with qualitative information providing greater insight into the complexities of implementation and sustainability processes. The existing implementation literature utilizes a wide range of definitions and terminologies rendering extrapolation of constructs across settings difficult. By using the CFIR as a scoping tool to guide assessment of the barriers and facilitators to DBT, a number of constructs salient to implementing DBT in routine healthcare settings were identified, allowing for refinement of more relevant assessment tools for future research.

Conclusions

Successful implementation and sustainability of healthcare innovations into routine settings poses a challenge; DBT is no exception. However, since the onset of biDBT intensive training in 1995, the sustainability of DBT programmes has remained stable and similar to the rates of other innovations, and higher than others. Given the ever-changing landscape and finite resources of healthcare systems, this is an encouraging finding. Nevertheless, a number of programmes struggle to effectively implement and sustain DBT within their organisation.

The particular adaptation to the location of training trialed here did not improve the probability of programme survival. Further augmenting on-site training with additional interventions for both inner and outer-context leadership [49, 50] could potentially improve the outcome of such training . A number of factors hindering or facilitating implementation of DBT were reported. Whilst these factors can vary between and within organisations, comparison with previous research suggests that the main barriers or aids to implementation have remained fairly consistent. Future research should include evaluation of predictive models that allow for testing the relative contribution of each implementation component, in order to identify what works in which contexts.

Abbreviations
biDBT: British Isles Dialectical Behaviour Therapy training team; BPD: Borderline Personality Disorder; CAMHS: Child and Adolescent Mental Health Service; CFIR: Consolidated Framework for Implementation Research; DBT: Dialectical Behaviour Therapy; EBP: Evidence Based Practice; K-M: Kaplan Meier survival analysis; NHS: National Health Service; NICE: National Institute for Health and Care Excellence; RCT: Randomised Controlled Trial; UK: United Kingdom

Acknowledgements
We are grateful to all the teams who participated in the study for providing information on their experience of implementation.

Funding
This research was funded by NWCPP. Survey incentives were funded by biDBT Training.

Authors' contributions
JCK is the principle researcher and was responsible for the design of the study, data collection and analyses. MAS supervised the study. RH and CWNS provided support with statistical analysis of data. JCK drafted the initial manuscript. All other authors (MAS, RH, CWNS) read and contributed to modified drafts. All authors have approved the final manuscript.

Consent for publication
Not applicable.

Competing interests
M. A. Swales is the Director of the British Isles DBT Training Team that trains practitioners in DBT with a licensed training programme. R. A. Hibbs is the Managing Director of Integral Business Support Ltd. that delivers licensed training in DBT. M. A. Swales and R. A. Hibbs are married.

Author details
[1]School of Psychology, Bangor University, Bangor, Gwynedd, UK. [2]Besti Cadwaladr University Health Board, Bangor, Gwynedd, UK. [3]Integral Business Support Ltd, Wrexham, UK.

References
1.	Linehan M. Cognitive-behavioral treatment of borderline personality disorder: Guilford press; 1993.
2.	Fonagy P, Bateman A. Progress in the treatment of borderline personality disorder. Br J Psychiatry. 2006;188(1):1–3.
3.	Clarkin JF, Levy KN, Lenzenweger MF, Kernberg OF. Evaluating three treatments for borderline personality disorder: a multiwave study. Am J Psychiatr. 2007;
4.	Koons CR, Robins CJ, Tweed JL, Lynch TR, Gonzalez AM, Morse JQ, Bishop GK, Bastian LA. Efficacy of dialectical behavior therapy in women veterans with borderline personality disorder. Behav Ther. 2001;32(2):371–90.
5.	Linehan MM, Armstrong HE, Suarez A, Allmon D, Heard HL. Cognitive-behavioral treatment of chronically parasuicidal borderline patients. Arch Gen Psychiatry. 1991;48(12):1060–4.
6.	Linehan MM, Schmidt H, Dimeff LA, Craft JC, Kanter J, Comtois KA. Dialectical behavior therapy for patients with borderline personality disorder and drug-dependence. Am J Addict. 1999;8(4):279–92.
7.	Linehan MM, Dimeff LA, Reynolds SK, Comtois KA, Welch SS, Heagerty P, Kivlahan DR. Dialectical behavior therapy versus comprehensive validation therapy plus 12-step for the treatment of opioid dependent women meeting criteria for borderline personality disorder. Drug Alcohol Depend. 2002;67(1):13–26.
8.	Linehan MM, Comtois KA, Murray AM, Brown MZ, Gallop RJ, Heard HL, Korslund KE, Tutek DA, Reynolds SK, Lindenboim N. Two-year randomized controlled trial and follow-up of dialectical behavior therapy vs therapy by experts for suicidal behaviors and borderline personality disorder. Arch Gen Psychiatry. 2006;63(7):757–66.
9.	McMain SF, Links PS, Gnam WH, Guimond T, Cardish RJ, Korman L, Streiner DL. A randomized trial of dialectical behavior therapy versus general psychiatric management for borderline personality disorder. Am J Psychiatr. 2009;166:1365–1374.
10.	Turner RM. Naturalistic evaluation of dialectical behavior therapy-oriented treatment for borderline personality disorder. Cogn Behav Pract. 2000;7(4):413–9.
11.	Verheul R, van den Bosch LM, Koeter MW, De Ridder MA, Stijnen T, Van Den Brink W. Dialectical behaviour therapy for women with borderline personality disorder. Br J Psychiatry. 2003;182(2):135–40.
12.	Lynch TR, Trost WT, Salsman N, Linehan MM. Dialectical behavior therapy for borderline personality disorder. Annu Rev Clin Psychol. 2007;3:181–205.
13.	Kliem S, Kröger C, Kosfelder J. Dialectical behavior therapy for borderline personality disorder: a meta-analysis using mixed-effects modeling. J Consult Clin Psychol. 2010;78(6):936.
14.	Stoffers JM, Völlm BA, Rücker G, Timmer A, Huband N, Lieb K. Psychological therapies for people with borderline personality disorder. Cochrane Database Syst Rev. 2012;(8):Art. No.: CD005652. https://doi.org/10.1002/14651858.CD005652.pub2.
15.	Lynch TR, Morse JQ, Mendelson T, Robins CJ. Dialectical behavior therapy for depressed older adults: a randomized pilot study. Am J Geriatr Psychiatry. 2003;11(1):33–45.
16.	Lynch TR, Cheavens JS, Cukrowicz KC, Thorp SR, Bronner L, Beyer J. Treatment of older adults with co-morbid personality disorder and depression: a dialectical behavior therapy approach. Int J Geriatr Psychiatry. 2007;22(2):131–43.
17.	Masson, P. C., von Ranson, K. M., Wallace, L. M., & Safer, D. L. (2013). A randomized wait-list controlled pilot study of dialectical behaviour therapy guided self-help for binge eating disorder. Behav Res Ther, 51(11), 723–728.
18.	Robinson AH, Safer DL. Moderators of dialectical behavior therapy for binge eating disorder: results from a randomized controlled trial. Int J Eat Disord. 2012;45(4):597–602.
19.	Shelton D, Sampl S, Kesten KL, Zhang W, Trestman RL. Treatment of impulsive aggression in correctional settings. Behav Sci Law. 2009;27(5):787–800.
20.	National Institute for Health and Clinical Excellence. Borderline personality disorder: recognition and management. [CG78]. London: National Institute for Health and Care Excellence; 2009.
21.	Services registered for CQUIN mental health. (n.d.). https://www.rcpsych.ac.uk/workinpsychiatry/qualityimprovement/cquin/cquinfaq.aspx. Accessed 14 Sept 2018.
22.	Brazier JE, Tumur I, Holmes M, Ferriter M, Parry G, Dent-Brown K, Paisley S. Psychological therapies including dialectical behaviour therapy for borderline personality disorder: a systematic review and preliminary economic evaluation. Health Technol Assess. 2006;10(35):23–48.
23.	Priebe S, Bhatti N, Barnicot K, Bremner S, Gaglia A, Katsakou C, Molosankwe I, McCrone P, Zinkler M. Effectiveness and cost-effectiveness of dialectical behaviour therapy for self-harming patients with personality disorder: a pragmatic randomised controlled trial. Psychother Psychosom. 2012;81(6):356–65.
24.	Pitman A, Tyrer P. Implementing clinical guidelines for self harm – highlighting key issues arising from the NICE guideline for self-harm. Psychol Psychother Theory Res Pract. 2008;81(4):377–97.
25.	Rogers, E. M. (2003). Diffusion of innovations (5th Ed.). https://books.google.co.uk/books?id=9U1K5LjUOwEC&printsec=frontcover&dq=editions:XNqTTc9h0ngC&hl=en&sa=X&ved=0ahUKEwjq0uWRu4HNAhVJDMAKHfKdC_MQ6wEIHTAA#v=onepage&q&f=false. Accessed 30 May 2016.
26.	Buchanan DA, Fitzgerald L, Ketley D. The sustainability and spread of organizational change: modernizing healthcare. Routledge: 2006.
27.	Swales MA, Taylor B, Hibbs RA. Implementing dialectical behaviour therapy: Programme survival in routine healthcare settings. J Ment Health. 2012;21(6):548–55.
28.	Linehan MM. Skills training manual for treating borderline personality disorder: Guilford Press; 2015.
29.	Fixsen, D. L., Naoom, S. F., Blase, K. A., & Friedman, R. M., & Wallace, F. (2005). Implementation research: a synthesis of the literature. Tampa, FL: the National Implementation Research Network, Louis de la parte Florida mental health institute, University of South Florida.
30.	Greenhalgh T, Robert G, Macfarlane F, Bate P, Kyriakidou O. Diffusion of innovations in service organizations: systematic review and recommendations. Milbank Q. 2004;82(4):581–629.
31.	Rycroft-Malone J. The PARIHS framework—a framework for guiding the implementation of evidence-based practice. J Nurs Care Qual. 2004;19(4):297–304.
32.	Stirman SW, Kimberly J, Cook N, Calloway A, Castro F, Charns M. The sustainability of new programs and innovations: a review of the empirical literature and recommendations for future research. Implement Sci. 2012;7(1):17.
33.	Swales MA. Implementing dialectical behaviour therapy: organizational pre-treatment. Cogn Behav Ther. 2010;3(04):145–57.
34.	Amodeo M, Storti SA, Larson MJ. Moving empirically supported practices to addiction treatment programs: recruiting supervisors to help in technology transfer. Subst Use Misuse. 2010;45(6):968–82.
35.	Aarons GA, Hurlburt M, Horwitz SM. Advancing a conceptual model of evidence-based practice implementation in public service sectors. Adm Policy Ment Health Ment Health Serv Res. 2011;38(1):4–23.
36.	Damschroder LJ, Aron DC, Keith RE, Kirsh SR, Alexander JA, Lowery JC. Fostering implementation of health services research findings into practice: a consolidated framework for advancing implementation science. Implement Sci. 2009;4(1):50.
37.	Glisson C, Schoenwald SK. The ARC organizational and community intervention strategy for implementing evidence-based children's mental health treatments. Ment Health Serv Res. 2005;7(4):243–59.
38.	Chambers DA, Glasgow RE, Stange KC. The dynamic sustainability framework: addressing the paradox of sustainment amid ongoing change. Implement Sci. 2013;8:117–27.

39. Shelton RC, Cooper BR, Stirman SW. The sustainability of evidence-based interventions and practices in public health and health care. Annu Rev Public Health. 2018;39:55–76.

40. Johnson RB, Onwuegbuzie AJ, Turner LA. Toward a definition of mixed methods research. J Mixed Methods Res. 2007;1(2):112–33.

41. Kaplan EL, Meier P. Nonparametric estimation from incomplete observations. J Am Stat Assoc. 1958;53(282):457–81.

42. Scheirer MA. Is sustainability possible? A review and commentary on empirical studies of program sustainability. Am J Eval. 2005;26(3):320–47.

43. Swain K, Whitley R, McHugo GJ, Drake RE. The sustainability of evidence-based practices in routine mental health agencies. Community Ment Health J. 2010;46(2):119–29.

44. Cooper BR, Bumbarger BK, Moore JE. Sustaining evidence-based prevention programs: correlates in a large-scale dissemination initiative. Prev Sci. 2015;16(1):145–57.

45. Bond GR, Drake RE, McHugo GJ, Peterson AE, Jones AM, Williams J. Long-term sustainability of evidence-based practices in community mental health agencies. Adm Policy Mental Health. 2014;41:228–36.

46. Gallo KP, Barlow DH. Factors involved in clinician adoption and nonadoption of evidence-based interventions in mental health. Clin Psychol: Scie Prac. 2012;19:93–106.

47. Swales MA, Hibbs RAB. (2014). DBT in the UK: updated dissemination and implementation data. 3rd international congress on borderline personality disorder & allied disorders. Rome. 2014:16–8.

48. Fixsen DL, Blase KA, Naoom SF, Wallace F. Core implementation components. Res Soc Work Pract. 2009;19(5):531–40.

49. Aarons GA, Green AE, Trott E, Willging CE, Torres EM, Ehrhart MG, Roesch SC. The roles of system and organizational leadership in system-wide evidence-based intervention sustainment: a mixed method study. Adm Policy Mental Health. 2016;43(6):991–1008.

50. Aarons GA, Wells RS, Zagursky K, Fettes DL, Palinkas LA. Implementing evidence-based practice in community mental health agencies: a multiple stakeholder analysis. Am J Public Health. 2009;99(11):2087–95.

51. Proctor E, Silmere H, Raghavan R, Hovmand P, Aarons G, Bunger A, Griffey R, Hensley M. Outcomes for implementation research: conceptual distinctions, measurement challenges, and research agenda. Adm Policy Ment Health Ment Health Serv Res. 2011;38(2):65–76.

17

Medication review plus person-centred care: a feasibility study of a pharmacy-health psychology dual intervention to improve care for people living with dementia

Ian D Maidment[1]*⬤, Sarah Damery[2], Niyah Campbell[1], Nichola Seare[3], Chris Fox[4], Steve Iliffe[5], Andrea Hilton[6], Graeme Brown[7], Nigel Barnes[7], Jane Wilcock[5], Emma Randle[8], Sarah Gillespie[9], Garry Barton[10] and Rachel Shaw[1]

Abstract

Background: "Behaviour that Challenges" is common in people living with dementia, resident in care homes and historically has been treated with anti-psychotics. However, such usage is associated with 1800 potentially avoidable deaths annually in the UK. This study investigated the feasibility of a full clinical trial of a specialist dementia care pharmacist medication review combined with a health psychology intervention for care staff to limit the use of psychotropics.

This paper focuses on feasibility; including recruitment and retention, implementation of medication change recommendations and the experiences and expectations of care staff.

Methods: West Midlands care homes and individuals meeting the inclusion criteria (dementia diagnosis; medication for behaviour that challenges), or their personal consultee, were approached for consent.

A specialist pharmacist reviewed medication. Care home staff received an educational behaviour change intervention in a three-hour session promoting person-centred care. Primary healthcare staff received a modified version of the training.

The primary outcome measure was the Neuropsychiatric Inventory-Nursing Home version at 3 months. Other outcomes included quality of life, cognition, health economics and prescribed medication. A qualitative evaluation explored expectations and experiences of care staff.

Results: Five care homes and 34 of 108 eligible residents (31.5%) were recruited, against an original target of 45 residents across 6 care homes. Medication reviews were conducted for 29 study participants (85.3%) and the pharmacist recommended stopping or reviewing medication in 21 cases (72.4%). Of the recommendations made, 57.1% (12 of 21) were implemented, and implementation (discontinuation) took a mean of 98.4 days. In total, 164 care staff received training and 21 were interviewed.

Care staff reported a positive experience of the intervention and post intervention adopting a more holistic patient-centred approach.

Conclusions: The intervention contained two elements; staff training and medication review. It was feasible to implement the staff training, and the training appeared to increase the ability and confidence of care staff to manage behaviour that challenges without the need for medication. The medication review would require significant modification for full trial partly related to the relatively limited uptake of the recommendations made, and delay in implementation.

Keywords: Dementia, Primary care, Care homes, Pharmacy, Medication review, Behaviour that challenges

* Correspondence: i.maidment@aston.ac.uk
[1]School of Life and Health Sciences, Aston University, Birmingham B4 7ET, UK
Full list of author information is available at the end of the article

Background

Dementia is an international healthcare priority [1, 2]. One of the key challenges within dementia care is the management of the behavioural and psychological symptoms of dementia (BPSD) [3]. Behavioural symptoms include aggression, agitation, depression and hallucinations [4]. BPSD is also referred to as behaviour that challenges, which is defined as 'any behaviour considered antisocial within the care environment or deemed dangerous to the person with dementia, their fellow residents, and staff' [5]. These two terms are used interchangeably in this paper.

Antipsychotics are frequently prescribed for people living with dementia for behaviour that challenges [3]. The usage of antipsychotics for people with BPSD is implicated in the death of 1800 people every year and two-thirds of such usage may be inappropriate [4]. The Banerjee Report found antipsychotics were often used as a first solution, yet behaviour that challenges can often be safely managed with the use of non-pharmacological approaches [2, 4]. Senior staff in care homes should be skilled in appropriate non-pharmacological techniques and be able to train other staff in these techniques [2, 4].

A recent Cochrane review concluded that antipsychotics could be successfully discontinued in older people with dementia and BPSD, but the evidence was low quality and further research was required [6]. Furthermore, solely focussing on the prescription of antipsychotics may simply drive prescribing to equally problematic alternative psychotropics (such as anti-depressants and benzodiazepines) and research should test interventions to limit the use of all psychotropics [6, 7]. Secondary care specialist dementia care pharmacists could have a vital role in ensuring the appropriate use of psychotropics for BPSD [4, 8].

This feasibility study was designed to provide key information on study processes and outcomes, so that the challenges in implementing and evaluating a pharmacy-health psychology dual intervention could be understood [9]. Incorporating learning from a feasibility study can enhance the rigour and deliverability of any subsequent full clinical trial [10, 11]. A feasibility study was needed to assess implementation of the protocol and estimate key parameters, such as recruitment, consent and follow-up rates, and the time taken to conduct the study, to inform the design of the main trial [9, 12]. It was also conducted to refine the battery of outcome measures, and understand any challenges associated with joint working between care homes, general practitioners (GPs) and pharmacists.

Aim

To determine whether it is feasible to implement and measure the effectiveness of a dual purpose pharmacy-health psychology intervention incorporating medication review and staff training to limit the prescription of psychotropics to manage BPSD in care home residents.

Method

Study design

An open label (non-blinded), mixed methods feasibility study, set within the Medical Research Council (MRC) framework for developing a complex intervention, aimed to recruit six care homes and 45 residents [13]. The study received ethical approval from National Research Ethics Services (15/EM/0314); specifically the Nottingham 1 Committee. For detailed methods refer to the published study protocol [7].

Setting

Care homes in the West Midlands, UK. Study conducted from January 2015 until December 2017.

Study participants

Residents in care homes recruited were eligible if inclusion criteria were met (see Table 1 for full details).

Study procedures

Identification and recruitment of care homes

The sampling frame was care homes (both nursing and residential) in the West Midlands (within 6 miles of

---

Table 1 Participant Inclusion and Exclusion Criteria

Participant Inclusion Criteria

1. Receiving medication (including but not limited to medicines in British National Formulary [BNF 68] sections 4.1/4.2/4.3/4.11 to treat behaviour that challenges.

2. Resident within a long-term care facility.

3. Registered with a West Midlands GP (who has also agreed to participate).

4. Dementia confirmed (dementia register, documentation of relevant read codes, confirmation of diagnosis via communication from old age psychiatry, memory clinic or clinical psychologist).

5. Patient, or personal consultee, willing to provide consent/assent.

6. A proxy informant (key worker or staff member with close working relationship) who can clearly communicate in English available.

Participant Exclusion Criteria

1. Patient, or personal consultee unable or unwilling to provide consent or lacks necessary English-language skills.

2. On palliative care register, or has pathology requiring complex specialist medication.

3. Risk of harm in line with Alzheimer's Society guidance (guidelines published in 2011, currently being updated and therefore not available).

4. Severe Mental Illness (e.g. schizophrenia) where psychotropic treatment should be continued.

Birmingham) with at least 40 residents and providing care for people living with dementia. Care Homes meeting the inclusion criteria were identified from the Care Quality Commission (CQC) and other web-sites e.g. Carehomes.co.uk including local authority sites. Eligible care homes supporting the Enabling Research in Care Homes (ENRICH; http://enrich.nihr.ac.uk/) initiative were also identified. ENRICH is an NIHR toolkit to support research in care homes. All identified care homes were invited to participate by letter with follow-up by single phone call or letter to care home manager.

Recruitment of residents

Consent for residents meeting the inclusion criteria was obtained from the resident, or their personal consultee, someone caring for them or interested in their welfare, but not acting in a professional capacity or for remuneration. Capacity was assessed using the Mental Capacity Act (2005) and local guidelines. All practical steps to maximise the individual's capacity to provide informed consent, including taking sufficient time and the use of appropriate language, were taken. If the resident lacked capacity their personal consultee was approached regarding consent to the medication review (see protocol for full description of consent; [7]). The resident's GP was then approached to consent to the medication review.

Recruitment of care staff

The care home manager allocated care staff to educational training sessions according to their shift patterns. Care home managers and care staff in each care home, and GPs who were involved in the medication review were invited to participate in qualitative interviews for the process evaluation.

Intervention

The intervention contained two elements (see Table 2 for summary of the content of both elements).

Outcome measures

The primary outcome measure was the Neuropsychiatric Inventory-Nursing Home version (NPI-NH) at 3 months [14]. This is a caregiver administered questionnaire that assesses neuropsychiatric symptoms. Other outcomes included quality of life (EQ-5D/DEMQoL) [15, 16], cognition (sMMSE) [17], health economics (modified version of Client Services Receipt Inventory [CSRI]) [18] and prescribed medication (including implementation of the review; obtained from the care home medication record). Data were collected at 8 weeks, and 3 and 6 months (findings will be reported elsewhere).

An embedded process evaluation used individual semi-structured qualitative interviews to explore the

Table 2 Description of dual-focused medication review-behavioural change intervention

Behaviour Change Intervention Overview

"Inside Out" – An interactive face-to-face three-hour educational person-centred care group based workshop, repeated twice at each home, for care staff facilitated by a researcher with health psychology training and experience of working in the social care sector. The main aim of the intervention was to provide staff with the knowledge to:
  • Understand that behaviours that challenge may be an expression of unmet need

Within this the intervention aimed to provide care home staff with the skills and resources to:
  • Investigate what the unmet need might be
  • Get to know the person with dementia as an individual to help manage their behaviour
  • Think creatively about how to prevent challenging behaviours by making sure individuals' needs are met
  • Understand that behaviours that challenge are not 'bad behaviour' and 'bad behaviour' does not equate to 'a bad person'

Training consisted of:

1. Educational elements about "behaviour that challenges", the use of antipsychotics to manage behaviour that challenges, good practice guidelines to reduce psychotropics in favour of non-pharmacological interventions.

2. Person-centred care training using the VIPS Model (V=Valuing personhood; I=Individual needs; P=Personal perspectives; S=Social environment), videos illustrating person-centred care practice and practical exercises [39].

3. Information and discussion points emphasising the importance of self-care and good communication among care staff

Primary healthcare staff received modified training primarily focussing on the treatment of BPSD.

Summary of Medication Review (based on type 3 full clinical review)

Medication reviews were conducted by two experienced clinical pharmacists (one who is a specialist dementia care pharmacist and has significant experience in the clinical area) and one, who acted as back-up and also has specialist experience in this area.

1. The primary focus is to review psychotropics used to treat behaviours that challenge; the pharmacist will also review all other medication as per routine care.

2. Establish therapeutic alliance with the person living with dementia and/or their personal consultee.

3. Collect information from clinical records, care staff, GP and any personal consultee about the patient including prescribed treatment of BPSD, medication used to treat psychotropic induced adverse events and any other medication.

4. Review medication, focussing on treatments for BPSD.

5. The GP was informed of the recommendations in writing; an individualised clinical letter from the pharmacist based on a standard proforma. The letter detailed the recommendations and the rationale for the recommendations. This was followed up with a phone call.

expectations and experiences of GPs and care home staff, including managers, both pre- and post-intervention. In addition, the chief investigator collected reflective comments from members of the team and participants ($n = 9$) to inform the potential design of the full trial. These accounts were collected during a short (up to 15 min) phone interview, which covered was the review helpful, and barriers and facilitators to participation in the study and implementation of the intervention.

All care home staff who received the behaviour change intervention were asked to complete two questionnaires. First, the Approaches to Dementia Questionnaire, which was administered pre-intervention, immediately after the training, and 3 months post-intervention; second, the Maslach Burnout Inventory – Human Services Survey which was administered pre- and 3 months post-intervention (findings will be reported elsewhere).

Results
Recruitment of care homes
Recruitment took far longer than expected. Recruiting six care homes was planned to take six months; it took 14 months to recruit five care homes. Despite two six-month extensions to the study period, it was not possible to recruit a planned sixth care home in the time available. Our original intention was to search the CQC web-site electronically, using the inclusion criteria, to identify eligible care homes. Due to the complexity of the database this did not prove possible, and it was necessary to look at each home individually on the website. Local authority and commercial websites (e.g. www.carehomes.co.uk) were searched using the same approach.

Our revised search strategy identified 82 eligible care homes. Three of these homes were recruited (conversion rate = 3.7%). Subsequently the support available from ENRICH was used; three ENRICH homes expressed an interest and one of these was recruited [19]. One care home was recruited by personal contacts – this home did not respond to the initial letter and follow-up.

At individual care home level, the decision regarding participation was largely driven by the care home manager, and personal contact between the research team and care home managers in following up initial invitations to participate was effective in securing care home sign up. The care homes recruited to the study were diverse (see Table 3 for further details).

Time to recruit care homes
The time to recruitment for care homes was calculated according to the number of days between the initial approach from the research team to the care home manager, and the receipt of local ethical approval permitting recruitment of residents to begin in that care home. The mean number of days taken to recruit care homes was 236.6 (SD 127.2). This was partly because of the time taken to recruit the final two care homes: the care home recruited via ENRICH took 314 days to recruit, and the care home recruited via the personal contacts took 421 days. The first three care homes, which were recruited following an initial letter to the care home manager took a mean of 149 days (SD 31).

Number/proportion of eligible residents in each care home and resident recruitment
Across the five participating care homes, 295 potential participants were available for eligibility screening (see Table 4). Of these, 108 (36.6%) met the inclusion criteria. The proportion of eligible residents varied from 29.2 to 58.1% across care homes.

Overall, 34 of the 108 residents were recruited to the study (conversion rate = 31.5%). Recruitment rates from individual care homes ranged from 16.7% ($n = 3/18$) in care home 005 to 58.8% ($n = 10/17$) in care home 001. Recruiting 34 individuals in total equates to a mean of 6.8 residents at each care home (range 3 to 10; Standard Deviation [SD] = 3.11). The number of individuals recruited to the study represented 75.6% of the original target ($n = 45$). Several additional potential participants were identified in the last care home recruited, but there was not enough time remaining in the study period to complete follow-up so these residents were not recruited.

Time to recruitment for study participants
Time to recruit study participants was calculated from the number of days between ethical approval being granted for recruitment to begin in each care home, and the point at which the last participant at that care home was recruited to the study. Time to complete participant recruitment ranged from 117 to 349 days (mean = 219.6; SD = 84.2).

Table 3 Characteristics of participating care homes

ID	Type	Organisation	Specialty	Number of beds
001	Nursing home	Local charity with small number (< 5) of care/nursing homes	Adults over 65	52
002	Residential home	Medium sized care home chain (50 to 100 care homes) across England	Adults over 65; Dementia	64
003	Nursing home	Small care home chain (< 5)	Adults over 65; Dementia	76
004	Nursing home	Single ownership	Adults over 65; Dementia	72
005	Nursing home	Single ownership	Adults over 65; Dementia	31 dementia (45 total)

Table 4 Eligible residents in participating care homes and recruitment rate

Care Home ID	Number eligible / number screened	Proportion eligible (%)	Number recruited	Proportion of eligible residents recruited (%)
001	17/52	32.7	10/17	58.8
002	26/64	40.6	10/26	38.5
003	24/76	31.6	6/24	25.0
004	21/72	29.2	5/21	23.8
005	18/31	58.1	3/18	16.7
ALL	108/295	36.6	34/108	31.5

Recruitment of GP practices

Consent from each participant's GP was required for the medication review. Obtaining consent was straightforward in homes predominantly supported by a single general practice with strong links between the practice and the home (care homes 001, 003, 005). It was considerably more challenging in care homes supported by multiple practices (care home 002 supported by 4 practices and 004 by 2 practices).

In care home 002 it took over 3.5 months to obtain GP consent for every resident and required a strategic and time-consuming approach to primary care engagement. This approach included working closely with the Clinical Comissioning Group (CCG), Practice-based Pharmacists (PBP) and NIHR Clinical Research Network (CRN) primary care leads, a newsletter about the study specifically written for local GPs, an article in a local NIHR "Connect" Magazine, presentation at a GP Local CRN event on Dementia and attendance at a GP practice meeting. In care home 004, it was impossible to obtain GP consent for 2 recruited participants, for whom the personal consultees had assented, despite the earlier strategic approach.

Retention rates of care homes and participants

None of the five care homes withdrew from the study. Five study withdrawals (14.7%) occurred before the medication review could be undertaken. Further participants were withdrawn at 8 week ($n = 5$; NB: one of these 5 subsequently provided data at 3 and 6 months), 3 month ($n = 8$) and 6 month ($n = 8$) follow-up. Attrition rates by care home ranged from 67 to 83.3%. Figure 1 shows participant attrition and the reasons for loss to follow-up at each data collection point.

Medication reviews: Recommendations and implementation

Medication reviews were conducted by specialist pharmacists for 29/34 study participants (85.3%) (Fig. 2). A written recommendation to stop or review medication was made for 21/29 participants (72.4%). The recommendations were implemented by the participants' GP in 12 of the 21 medication reviews (57.1%). There was

substantial variability in implementation of recommendations by care home, ranging from 0 to 100%. It took a mean of 98.4 days (range 33 to 138; SD = 42.5) to implement the recommendations. The protocol was amended so that the participant baseline assessment was repeated if the recommendation was not implemented within eight weeks of the medication review.

Behavioural change intervention

One hundred and forty-two care staff attended the person-centred care workshop and received the Behavourial Change Intervention across the five homes (mean = 28.4; range 25 to 38; SD = 5.41). For further details of participation rates, see Table 5.

In addition, 22 primary care clinical staff, including GPs ($n = 14$), GP trainees ($n = 4$), Practice Nurses ($n = 3$) and PBP ($n = 1$) across nine practices received the modified training primarily focussing on the treatment of BPSD. Four GPs were trained on the phone (one per training session); whereas 18 staff received training in five face-to-face sessions (mean of 3.6 per session).

Qualitative evaluation of expectations and experiences of care staff

Face-to-face, semi-structured interviews were conducted [by NC] with 21 participants (Care Home Managers [CHM] = 5; GPs = 3; Care Staff [CS] = 13). This paper reports expectations and experiences of the feasibility study. Participants' understanding of current guidance, person-centred care and details of changes in perceptions of people with dementia will be fully reported in a subsequent paper.

Participants found both the training and the medication review aspects of the feasibility study beneficial:

"Very useful exercise...being provided the information it helps (to) make us sure that we're prescribing appropriately." (GP1, post-intervention).

"I did ask random staff after the training and they were all really positive, said they found it really interesting, really helpful and I've actually run it past

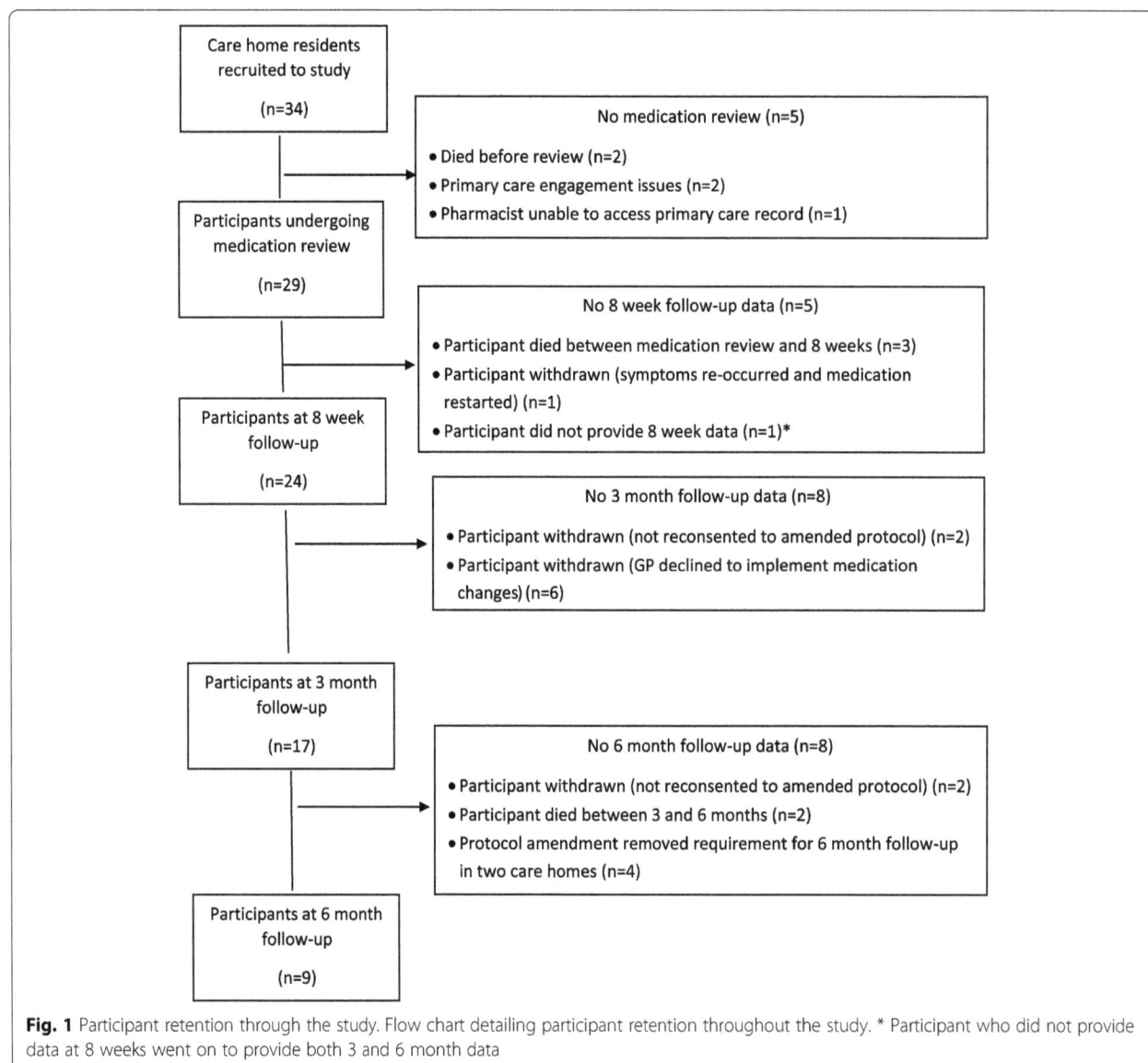

Fig. 1 Participant retention through the study. Flow chart detailing participant retention throughout the study. * Participant who did not provide data at 8 weeks went on to provide both 3 and 6 month data

my Learning and Development Partner who deals with my training in my area and they've actually sanctioned it being just as good as the (care home company) training." (CHM2, post-intervention).

Participants identified that after the training they were more likely to adopt a holistic approach with less reliance on medication:

"I think staff now discuss and think slightly different from what they did before. Before it would be 'go to the nurse', it would be 'what meds can we give?' That's still there with some but overwhelmingly it's 'what can we do different?'" (CHM5, postintervention).

"I think there's been very little (medication) put back. You know sometimes when you stop things, somebody immediately just worries about it and it just goes straight back on but I don't think that's happened." (GP2, post-intervention).

The practical training approach promoted adoption of patient-centred care, which underpinned this more holistic approach to care:

"People don't realise, a lot of time, their actions have a reaction and having– just examples and bringing it to the forefront of the mind, which is what the training does...they start thinking about things a little bit differently and I noticed that after the training the team

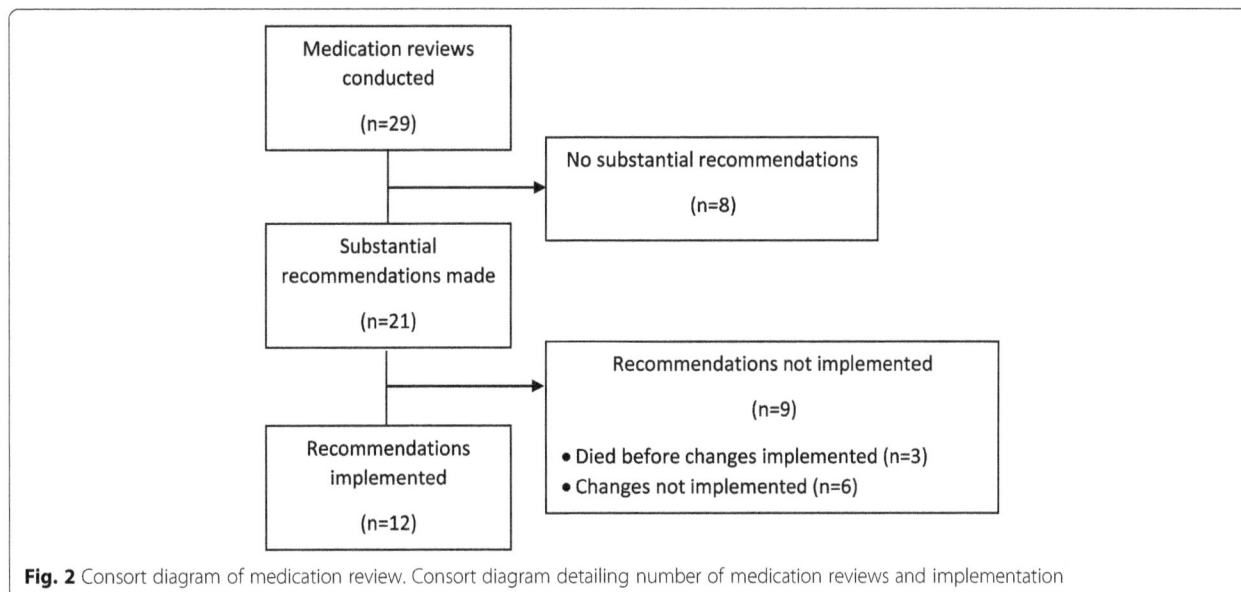

Fig. 2 Consort diagram of medication review. Consort diagram detailing number of medication reviews and implementation

did start actually trying to find what was working and what wasn't working." (CS13, post-intervention).

The holistic approach, to the medication review, with the focus on quality and safety, rather than cost also promoted adoption of the intervention:

"At the same time...a CCG pharmacist (was) going into the home to do sort of medication reviews...more of the point-of-view of reducing costs. Different approach from the MEDREV pharmacist...very much geared around using the evidence to increase the quality of care...doing it for...quality and safety rather than cost prioritisation." (GP2, post-intervention).

GPs identified that participation placed little burden on them, although some GPs identified barriers including time taken to implement the medication review:

"The study was already set up to be as easy as it can be on GP time." (GP1, post-intervention).

"That was just broadly because of timing and me not being able to...do it because of lots of things that happen in surgery." (GP3, post-intervention).

Overall, providing care staff with additional tools and skills to address behaviours that challenge appeared to have a positive impact on the attitudes and practices of care home staff:

"The care home staff have been reassured by the training...sometimes when I've done medication reviews in the past they've been a little bit cautious. "Oh, I don't think their family will like that". "Oh, this person's been on it for ages"...we've had a little bit of resistance and that's gone a little bit." (GP2, post-intervention).

"...the way that the training's done it's all about the VIPS and it's making people really think...about the individual, what might be wrong with them, how to minimise those challenging behaviours...it's giving people more tools to do their job better." (CHM2, post-intervention).

Table 5 Number of staff at each home participating in training and total number of staff

Care Home ID	Number of participating in training	Completion rate	Total number of staff in care home	Proportion of staff receiving training (%)
001	26	100%	72 (includes staff in non-caring roles)	36.1%[a]
002	25	100%	Approximately 50 carers	50%
003	26	100%	34	76.5%
004	27	100%	Approximately 63 staff in caring roles	42.9%
005	38	100%	Approximately 148 staff	25.7%[a]

[a]these figures include staff in a non-caring roles

Discussion

Increasing care home research is a key priority, and to the best of our knowledge this is the first study to report in detail the feasibility of a dual-purpose care home study involving staff training and medication review. Overall, recruitment was challenging and time-consuming, securing GP engagement was difficult, drop-out rates were high and, where substantial recommendations in relation to medication were made, these took a long time to implement, if implemented at all.

Like other care home research, recruitment was challenging [20-23]. The CQC database, as a search engine, had limited utility, confirming earlier findings (Personal Communication, Analisa Smythe, 18th October, 2017). It took 14 months rather than six months to recruit five care homes; and like other studies, the protocol was continually adapted as the team learnt from earlier experience [21]. This resulted in the need for five substantial ethical amendments during the study, which contributed to delays. Amendments included expanding the recruitment area, introducing the re-baseline procedure to account for the delay in implementation and in the final two care homes removing the six month follow-up (due to time limitations).

Our initial response rate of 3.7% is low compared to other studies that offered training to care homes; another study had a 10% response rate [21]. This was possibly because care home managers, the key decision makers, welcomed the offer of cost-free training, but were less likely to welcome a medication review, which could potentially lead to discontinuation of medication for behaviour that challenges. Informal feedback, obtained as reflective comments, from the managers and evidence from another study confirms this viewpoint; one observational/interview study on current practice for the treatment of behaviours that challenge had a similar response rate [20]. Like other studies we found that developing local relationships and using ENRICH were successful techniques [21].

It took a mean of 236.6 days to recruit homes. Like other researchers, recruiting GPs from multiple practices who provide care to participants living in a single care home was particularly challenging [22]. Our strategic approach to GP engagement was only partially successful and should be developed further for any larger trial.

At least 30% of residents were expected to meet the inclusion criteria with at least 18 potential participants per home and 7 to 8 recruited. The actual figures were 36.6% of residents with 21.6 potential participants per home and on average 6.8 recruited. On reflection, recruitment might have been improved by organising further meetings with relatives and greater involvement of care home staff in recruitment, although further training may be required for the care home staff.

Recent NICE guidance recommend that care providers should provide face-to-face training and mentoring to staff who deliver care and support to people living with dementia [24]. This training should include the management of behaviours that challenge including the appropriate use of medication [24]. MEDREV successfully developed and evaluated an acceptable and feasible training package, which was well received. A large number of staff (n = 164) received training about delivering person-centred care, and the use of psychotropics and reasons for reducing them. Furthermore, by combining staff training with a specialist medication review, the use of psychotropics was reduced [25].

The qualitative research and the reflective comments, obtained from GPs were very supportive of both the training and medication review. Staff were positive about both elements. The Behavioural Change Intervention appeared to train the care staff in person-centred care so that they would understand why reducing psychotropics is beneficial and support implementation of the recommendations from the medication review. The pharmacists who trained the GPs also reported good interaction particularly in face-to-face training, which encouraged greater participant engagement and reached more GPs.

Nearly 43% of the recommendations (n = 9/21) were not implemented. Other similar studies have found similar rates; for example one study found that 58.1% of recommendations by a clinical pharmacist were implemented [26]. The reasons for this, in our study, were not entirely clear although given the range in implementation rates between care homes, local context, and in particular the GP/care home/pharmacist relationship was likely an important factor. Informal feedback, obtained in the reflective comments, identified a perceived lack of integration with other secondary care medication reviews. The likelihood and speed of implementation may have increased with direct communication between the pharmacist and GP either by phone or face-to-face. Another possible avenue to explore is utilising the model of a practice-based pharmacist as a liaison between the specialist pharmacists conducting the medication reviews and the GP.

Other studies have found that GPs were broadly supportive of pharmacist medication reviews for BPSD and the implementation rate is similar to other studies involving clinicians implementing recommendations from a pharmacist [27, 28]. The relatively low uptake could be due to the additional time and effort needed to amend the prescription. Other studies suggest that GPs believe reducing anti-psychotic prescribing for BPSD could be achieved by increased availability of non-pharmacological approaches and staffing levels [28].

Even when supported, the medication review recommendations took on average 98.4 days to implement.

This may have clinical and medico-legal implications. It also creates methodological problems for future studies: because it was impossible to know when the recommendation was likely to be implemented, collecting outcome data was challenging. One possible reason for the delay was the use of pre-prepared medication administration packs, which are prepared every month, for care homes. Care home staff also attributed the delay in implementation of recommendations to a general low priority for healthcare for older people; this needs further exploration in future research.

Whilst problems relating to medication optimisation in care homes and in people living with dementia are widely acknowledged, there is very little research on interventions to optimise medication in care home residents [29-31]. One trial has investigated a PCT/CCG-led medication review [32]. The homes in our study already received regular medication reviews from CCG pharmacists; suggesting that CCG pharmacists may lack expertise to review psychotropics. Furthermore, the GPs, in our study, appreciated the clinical and quality focus of the medication reviews.

Limitations

This study was conducted in a single region in the UK and had a limited number of participants. However, we recruited and retained a range of care homes with differing characteristics (type of home, sociodemographic characteristics of local area). The original aim was to recruit a representative sample of staff from each home. However, only three members of staff were recruited from the final two homes, due to the difficulty and subsequent delay in recruiting these homes. Only three GPs were recruited despite efforts to recruit more. No pharmacists were interviewed; however the feasibility issues in relation to the medication review were captured in the interviews with care staff and GPs, and the reflective comments received.

Policy implications

Healthcare policy must continue to focus on optimising medication usage in care homes, including the appropriate treatment of BPSD. MEDREV developed an acceptable and feasible training programme which included the appropriate use of medication, in line with NICE guidance, suggesting that this may be a promising policy approach [24]. Since this study, NHS England has invested in pharmacy to support medication optimisation in care home [33]. This research suggests, that to successfully optimise medication, these pharmacy staff need to develop robust ways of working across organisational boundaries linking primary, secondary and social care.

There are also implications for research policy makers. Recruiting the care homes and people with living dementia was time-consuming and difficult, confirming other studies. The NIHR and other funders have prioritised high quality research both in care homes, and on medication optimisation in older people [31, 34]. Yet despite this, there is limited research on medication optimisation in care homes [35] perhaps because care home research involving medication optimisation is uniquely challenging, as we found. This suggests that research into medication optimisation in care homes needs to be a specific priority.

Future research

One of the key challenges in this study was the delay in implementation of recommendations. Whilst our solution, of repeating the baseline measurements, might work for a single location feasibility study, when the chief investigator is able to work closely with the Clinical Study Officers, it is less likely to work for a larger multiple centre study. Expert recommendations on medication optimisation did not appear to be implemented in a significant minority of residents; this needs further investigation. From the care home point of view, it may be a question of who has the greater authority, the GP or the pharmacist and established relationships.

GP engagement could be improved by holding an initial event very early in the study. This event should carry Continuing Professional Development accreditation from the appropriate Royal College and include education from expert speakers, ideally with international reputations, in addition to information on the study.

Specialist pharmacists may not have had time to build a good relationship with the GP and without good communication and trust implementation of the recommendations may be challenging as we found. Since this study began, there has been significant investment in primary care clinical pharmacy including within care homes [36-38]. These practice-based pharmacists (PBP) are perhaps ideally placed to deliver the medication review; they have access to records and the autonomy to change the repeat template particularly if an independent prescriber. Involving such PBPs in the delivery of the medication review could address some of the feasibility issues identified and is a hypothesis for a future trial. Yet this area may be outside the scope of their practice and competency. Future research should explore the best way for pharmacy staff to deliver this specialist medication review and the training requirements.

Conclusion

The feasibility study contained two linked elements; staff training and medication review. We found it feasible to develop, deliver and evaluate a well-received staff training programme both in the care home and the GP surgery. The dual intervention appeared to increase the ability of care staff to manage BPSD appropriately with less reliance on medication. Although we found a clear need for specialist medication review of psychotropics for care home residents with dementia, the medication review would require significant modification for full trial.

Abbreviations

BPSD: Behavioural and Psychological Symptoms of Dementia; CHM: Care Home Manager; CRN: Clinical Research Network, an NIHR Research Network Coordinating Centre for UK clinical research studies in the NHS; CS: Care Staff; ENRICH: Enabling Research in Care Homes an NIHR research ready initiative for care homes in the UK; GP: General Practitioner; MRC: Medical Research Council; PBP: Practice Based Pharmacist; SD: Standard Deviation; VIPS: Valuing personhood; Individual needs; Personal perspectives; Social environment

Acknowledgements

We acknowledge the support from all the care homes, residents, next of kin and healthcare professionals involved in the study. The study was supported by the West Midlands Clinical Research Network including Mary Tooley (ENRICH Care Home Research Facilitator) and Louise Jones, Carly Craddock, Di Baines, Nadezda Starkova and Liz Bates. Naveed Iqbal – Aston University – also provided support liaising with primary care. Jo Deekes in addition to GBr (Pharmacy, Birmingham and Solihull Mental Health NHS Foundation Trust) conducted the medication reviews and along with IM delivered the GP training.

Funding

This paper presents independent research funded by the National Institute for Health Research (NIHR) under its Research for Patient Benefit (RfPB) Programme (Grant Reference Number PB-PG-0613-31071). The views expressed are those of the author(s) and not necessarily those of the NHS, the NIHR or the Department of Health. Sarah Damery is supported by the National Institute for Health Research (NIHR) Collaboration for Leadership in Applied Health Research and Care West Midlands (CLAHRC WM).

Authors' contributions

IM was the chief investigator and led the research. RS led the health psychology aspects with support from NC, who delivered the training and conducted the interviews. SD led the quantitative analysis. NS provided project management support. SG led the Public Patient Involvement and ER co-ordinated and led quantitative data collection. NB, SI, AH and CF gave clinical advice and input throughout the project. SI and JW gave advice on care home recruitment. All authors were members of the steering group, gave general advice on study design and conduct, read and approved the final manuscript.

Consent for publication

Not applicable.

Competing interests

The authors declare that they have no competing interests.

Author details

¹School of Life and Health Sciences, Aston University, Birmingham B4 7ET, UK. ²Institute of Applied Health Research, College of Medical and Dental Sciences, University of Birmingham, Edgbaston, Birmingham B15 2TT, UK. ³Aston Health Research Innovation Cluster, Aston University, Birmingham B4 7ET, UK. ⁴Norwich Medical School, University of East Anglia, Earlham Road, Norwich, Norfolk NR4 7TJ, UK. ⁵Research Department of Primary Care & Population Health, University College London, Royal Free Campus, Rowland Hill St, London NW3 2PF, UK. ⁶Faculty of Health Science, University of Hull, Hull HU6 7RX, UK. ⁷Birmingham and Solihull Mental Health NHS Foundation Trust, Unit 1, B1, 50 Summer Hill Road, Birmingham B1 3RB, UK. ⁸National Centre for Mental Health, Research and Innovation Department, The Barberry, 25 Vincent Drive, Birmingham B15 2FG, UK. ⁹Department of Clinical Healthcare, Faculty of Health and Life Sciences, Oxford Brookes University, Gipsy Lane Campus, Headington, Oxford OX3 0FL, UK. ¹⁰Norwich Clinical Trials Unit, University of East Anglia, Earlham Road, Norwich, Norfolk NR4 7TJ, UK.

References

1. Department of Health. Prime Minister's challenge on dementia 2020; 2015. p. 49. Available from: https://www.gov.uk/government/uploads/system/uploads/attachment_data/file/406076/Dementia_vision.pdf. Accessed 30 Aug 2018

2. World Health Organization and Alzheimer's Disease International. Dementia: a public health priority; 2012. p. 112. Available from: http://www.who.int/mental_health/publications/dementia_report_2012/en/. Accessed 30 Aug 2018

3. Ballard C, Lana MM, Theodoulou M, Douglas S, McShane R, Jacoby R, et al. A randomised, blinded, placebo-controlled trial in dementia patients continuing or stopping neuroleptics (the DART-AD trial). PLoS Med. 2008;5: 0587–99.

4. Banerjee S. The use of antipsychotic medication for people with dementia: Time for action: Department of Health; 2009. p. 60. Available from: http://webarchive.nationalarchives.gov.uk/20130107105354/http://www.dh.gov.uk/prod_consum_dh/groups/dh_digitalassets/documents/digitalasset/dh_108302.pdf. Accessed 30 Aug 2018

5. Andrews GJ. Managing challenging behaviour in dementia. BMJ. 2006;332: 741 Available from: http://www.bmj.com/content/332/7544/741.abstract. Accessed 30 Aug 2018.

6. Van Leeuwen E, Petrovic M, van Driel M, De Sutter A, Vander Stichele R, Declercq T. Withdrawal versus continuation of long-term antipsychotic drug use for behavioural and psychological symptoms in older people with dementia. Cochrane Database Syst Rev. 2018;2018:CD007726 Available from: https://www.cochranelibrary.com/cdsr/doi/10.1002/14651858.CD007726.pub3/information. Accessed 2 Aug 2018.

7. Maidment ID, Shaw RL, Killick K, Damery S, Hilton A, Wilcock J, et al. Improving the management of behaviour that challenges associated with dementia in care homes: protocol for pharmacy–health psychology intervention feasibility study. BMJ Open. 2016;6 Available from: http://bmjopen.bmj.com/content/6/3/e010279.abstract. Accessed 30 Aug 2018.

8. Dementia Action Alliance. The Right Prescription : a call to action on the use of antipsychotic drugs for people with dementia; 2009. p. 1–32. Available from: http://www.institute.nhs.uk/qipp/calls_to_action/dementia_and_antipsychotic_drugs.html. Accessed 30 Aug 2018

9. Leblanc A, Légaré F, Labrecque M, Godin G, Thivierge R, Laurier C, et al. Feasibility of a randomised trial of a continuing medical education program in shared decision-making on the use of antibiotics for acute respiratory infections in primary care: the DECISION+ pilot trial. Implement Sci. 2011;6:5 Available from: https://implementationscience.biomedcentral.com/articles/10.1186/1748-5908-6-5. Accessed 30 Aug 2018.

10. McCluskey A, Middleton S. Increasing delivery of an outdoor journey intervention to people with stroke: A feasibility study involving five community rehabilitation teams. Implement Sci. 2010;5:59 Available from: http://www.implementationscience.com/content/5/1/59%5Cn. Accessed 30 Aug 2018.

11. Arain M, Campbell MJ, Cooper CL, Lancaster GA. What is a pilot or feasibility study? A review of current practice and editorial policy. BMC Med Res Methodol. 2010;10:1–7. Available from: https://doi.org/10.1186/1471-2288-10-67. Accessed 30 Aug 2018.

12. NIHR. NIHR Glossary of Terms. Available from: https://www.nihr.ac.uk/glossary. Accessed 30 Aug 2018.

13. MRC. Developing and evaluating complex interventions: new guidance. MRC. 2008; Available from: https://www.mrc.ac.uk/documents/pdf/complex-interventions-guidance/. Accessed 28 Oct 2016.

14. Cummings J, Mega M, Gray K, Rosenberg-Thompson S, Carusi D, Gornbein J. The neuropsychiatric inventory: comprehensive assessment of psychopathology in dementia. Neurology. 1994;44:2308–14.

15. Herdman M, Gudex C, Lloyd A, Janssen M, Kind P, Parkin D, et al. Development and preliminary testing of the new five-level version of EQ-5D (EQ-5D-5L). Qual Life Res. 2011;20:1727–36.

16. Smith SC, Lamping DL, Banerjee S, Harwood R, Foley B, Smith P, et al. Measurement of health-related quality of life for people with dementia. Heal Technol Assess. 2005;9:1–93.

17. Molloy D, Alemeyehu E, Roberts R. Reliability of a Standardized Mini-Mental State Examination compared with the traditional Mini-Mental State Examination. Am J Psychiatry. American Psychiatric Publishing. 1991;148: 102–5 Available from: https://doi.org/10.1176/ajp.148.1.102. Accessed 30 Aug 2018.

18. Beecham J, Knapp M. Costing psychiatric interventions. In: Thornicroft G, editor. Meas Ment heal needs. 2nd ed. London: Royal College of Psychiatrists; 2001.

19. NIHR. ENRICH (Enabling Research in Care Homes). 2018. Available from: https://enrich.nihr.ac.uk/pages/care-home-staff. Accessed 30 Aug 2018.

20. Mallon CM. Managing behaviours that challenge within English care homes: an exploration of current practices; 2015. p. 336. Available from: https://kar.kent.ac.uk/54752/ PhD Thesis.pdf. Accessed 30 Aug 2018

21. Jenkins C, Smythe A, Galant-Miecznikowska M, Bentham P, Oyebode J. Overcoming challenges of conducting research in nursing homes. Nurs Older People. 2016;28:16–23.

22. Shepherd V, Nuttall J, Hood K, Butler CC. Setting up a clinical trial in care homes: challenges encountered and recommendations for future research practice. BMC Res Notes. BioMed Central. 2015;8:306 Available from: http://www.biomedcentral.com/1756-0500/8/306. Accessed 30 Aug 2018.

23. Hall S, Longhurst S, Higginson IJ. Challenges to conducting research with older people living in nursing homes. BMC Geriatr. 2009;9.38 Available from: http://bmcgeriatr.biomedcentral.com/articles/10.1186/1471-2318-9-38. Accessed 30 Aug 2018.

24. NICE. Dementia - assessment, management and support for people living with dementia and their carers. NICE Guideline 97 (NG97). 2018. Available from: https://www.nice.org.uk/guidance/NG97. Accessed 30 Aug 2018).

25. Ballard C, Corbett A, Orrell M, Williams G, Moniz-Cook E, Romeo R, et al. Impact of person-centred care training and person-centred activities on quality of life, agitation, and antipsychotic use in people with dementia living in nursing homes: A cluster-randomised controlled trial. PLOS Med. 2018;15:e1002500 Available from: http://dx.plos.org/10.1371/journal.pmed. 1002500. Accessed 30 Aug 2018.

26. Nishtala PS, McLachlan AJ, Bell JS, Chen TF. A retrospective study of drug-related problems in Australian aged care homes: medication reviews involving pharmacists and general practitioners. J Eval Clin Pract. 2011;17:97–103.

27. Ravn-Nielsen LV, Duckert M-L, Lund ML, Henriksen JP, Nielsen ML, Eriksen CS, et al. Effect of an In-Hospital Multifaceted Clinical Pharmacist Intervention on the Risk of Readmission. JAMA Intern Med. 2018:1–8 Available from: https://jamanetwork.com/journals/jamainternalmedicine/article-abstract/2670037. Accessed 30 Aug 2018.

28. Cousins JM, Bereznicki LR, Cooling NB, Peterson GM. Prescribing of psychotropic medication for nursing home residents with dementia: a general practitioner survey. Clin Interv Aging. 2017;12:1573–8 Available from: https://www.dovepress.com/prescribing-of-psychotropic-medication-for-nursing-home-residents-with-peer-reviewed-article-CIA. Accessed 30 Aug 2018.

29. Barber ND, Alldred DP, Raynor DK, Dickinson R, Garfield S, Jesson B, et al. Care homes' use of medicines study: prevalence, causes and potential harm of medication errors in care homes for older people. Qual Saf Heal Care. 2009;18:341–6 Available from: http://qualitysafety.bmj.com/lookup/doi/10.1136/qshc.2009.034231. Accessed 30 Aug 2018.

30. Maidment I. Medication -related adverse events in older people with dementia causes and possible solutions. 2013. Available from: http://eprints.aston.ac.uk/21396/1/Studentthesis-2013.pdf. Accessed 8 Nov 2016.

31. NIHR. Dissemination Centre. Themed Review. Advancing Care. Research with Care Homes. 2017; Available from: http://www.dc.nihr.ac.uk/themed-reviews/advancing-care-themed-review.pdf. Accessed 30 Aug 2018.

32. Desborough J, Houghton J, Wood J, Wright D, Holland R, Sach T, et al. Multi-professional clinical medication reviews in care homes for the elderly: study protocol for a randomised controlled trial with cost effectiveness analysis. Trials. 2011;12:218 Available from: http://trialsjournal.biomedcentral.com/articles/10.1186/1745-6215-12-218. Accessed 30 Aug 2018.

33. NHS-England. Care home pharmacists to help cut overmedication and unnecessary hospital stays for frail older patients. 2018 [cited 2018 Mar 19]. Available from: https://www.england.nhs.uk/2018/03/care-home-pharmacists-to-help-cut-over-medication-and-unnecessary-hospital-stays-for-frail-older-patients/. Accessed 30 Aug 2018.

34. NIHR. NIHR Themed Calls. 2017. Available from: https://www.nihr.ac.uk/funding-and-support/themed-calls/index-old.htm. Accessed 30 Aug 2018.

35. Millar AN, Daffu-O'Reilly A, Hughes CM, Alldred DP, Barton G, Bond CM, et al. Development of a core outcome set for effectiveness trials aimed at optimising prescribing in older adults in care homes. Trials. 2017;18:1–12.

36. Robinson J. Integration fund to pay for pharmacist medicine optimisation posts in care homes. Pharm J. 2018; Available from: https://www.pharmaceutical-journal.com/news-and-analysis/news/integration-fund-to-pay-for-pharmacist-medicine-optimisation-posts-in-care-homes/20204365.article. Accessed 30 Aug 2018.

37. NHS-England. General Practice Forward View (GPFV) Clinical Pharmacists in General Practice Phase 2 Guidance for applicants. 2017. Available from: https://www.england.nhs.uk/wp-content/uploads/2017/07/clinical-pharmacists-phase-2-guidance-application.pdf. Accessed 4th Oct 2017.

38. Deeks LS, Naunton M, Kosari S. Pharmacists' perceptions of their emerging general practice roles in UK primary care: a qualitative interview study. Br J Gen Pract. 2017:67, 396.1–39396 Available from: http://bjgp.org/lookup/doi/10.3399/bjgp17X692237. Accessed 30 Aug 2018.

39. Brooker D. What is person-centred care in dementia? Rev Clin Gerontol. 2004;13:215–22.

18

Diagnosis of somatoform disorders in primary care: diagnostic agreement, predictors, and comaprisons with depression and anxiety

Katharina Piontek[1,2]* (iD), Meike C. Shedden-Mora[2], Maria Gladigau[2], Amina Kuby[2] and Bernd Löwe[2]

Abstract

Background: To investigate (a) the diagnostic agreement between diagnoses of somatoform disorders, depressive and anxiety disorders obtained from a structured clinical interview and diagnoses reported from primary care physicians (PCPs) and (b) to identify patient and PCP-related predictors for the diagnostic agreement regarding the presence of a somatoform disorder.

Methods: Data from a cross-sectional study comprising 112 primary care patients at high risk for somatoform disorders were analyzed. Diagnoses according to International Classification of Diseases, 10th revision (ICD-10) for somatoform, depressive and anxiety disorders were obtained from the Composite International Diagnostic Interview (CIDI) and compared with the diagnoses of the patients' PCPs documented in their medical records. Using multiple regression analyses, predictors for the PCPs' diagnosis of a somatoform disorder were analyzed.

Results: The agreement between PCP diagnoses and CIDI diagnoses was 32.3% for somatoform disorders, 48.0% for depressive disorders and 25.0% for anxiety disorders. Multiple regression analyses revealed the likelihood of being diagnosed with a somatoform disorder by PCP increased with somatic symptom severity (OR = 1.22, 95% CI 1.03–1.44). Regarding PCP-related characteristics, a specialization in internal medicine (OR = 5.95, 95% CI 1.70–20.80) and working in a solo practice (OR = 2.92, 95% CI 1.02–8.38) increased the likelihood that patients were diagnosed with a somatoform disorder.

Conclusions: The present results indicate that the process of diagnosing somatoform disorders in primary care needs to be improved. Findings further underline the necessity to implement appropriate strategies to improve early detection of patients.

Keywords: Somatoform disorders, Depressive disorder, Anxiety disorder, Primary care Diagnostic agreement, Detection rate, Structured clinical interview

* Correspondence: katharina.piontek@uni-greifswald.de
[1]Institute for Medical Psychology, University Medicine Greifswald, Greifswald, Germany
[2]Department of Psychosomatic Medicine and Psychotherapy, University Medical Center Hamburg-Eppendorf, Hamburg, Germany

Background

The burden of disease due to non-specific, functional and somatoform disorders is high and the presence of recurrent or persistent medically unexplained symptoms is associated with impaired physical and mental quality of life, increased utilization of healthcare services and the development of comorbidities like depressive and anxiety disorders [1, 2]. Available data regarding the prevalence of somatoform disorders are inconsistent and vary considerably in dependence on the underlying study population and the diagnostic criteria applied in the single studies (e.g. [3–6]). A recent meta-analysis of 32 studies investigated the prevalence of somatoform disorders and medically unexplained symptoms in primary care patients using both strict diagnostic criteria according to clinical assessments (*International Classification of Diseases; ICD* [7], *Diagnostic and Statistical Manual of Mental Disorders; DSM* [8]) and standardized questionnaires [9]. That study revealed a high heterogeneity of the primary studies and substantial differences in the prevalence rates in the diagnoses of somatoform disorders according to ICD or DSM criteria with prevalence rates of 34.8% and 26.2%, respectively. Further, in 40% to 49% of the primary care patients, at least one medically unexplained symptom was detected using questionnaires. These numbers underline that somatoform disorders pose a highly relevant public health problem, but existing literature suggests that the process of diagnosing somatoform disorders is challenging and that the different diagnostic criteria may have a substantial impact on the detection rate. The low detection rate in primary care is one key problem in the management of somatoform disorders [6]. It has been demonstrated that only 33% to 60% of the patients are correctly diagnosed by their primary care physician (PCP) and referred to a specialist for further treatment [4]. This is particularly alarming as the primary care practice serves as the patient's first point of entry into the health care system and access to mental health services. Furthermore, according to current guidelines for non-specific, functional, and somatoform bodily complaints [1], management of somatoform disorders is recommended within a stepped care model according to the course of disease, in collaboration with other physicians and therapists and coordinated by the PCP, thereby emphasizing the high responsibility of the PCP in the diagnostic and therapeutic procedure [10].

Several barriers have been identified with respect to the diagnosis of somatoform disorders in primary care settings [11]. Present data indicate that a lack of specific training, a lack of experience and a lack of reliable diagnostic tools may hinder the diagnosis of somatoform disorders [11]. It has been further demonstrated that the application of the diagnostic criteria seem to be problematic for many PCPs and existing classification systems have been described as being difficult to use,

impractical, not distinct, overlapping or too restrictive [11]. Besides these conceptual barriers, both patient and PCP-related characteristics might contribute to a correct diagnosis, and it is of importance to identify relevant predictors of a correct PCP diagnosis of a somatoform disorder to improve early detection of the disease.

The aims of the present study are, first, to investigate the level of agreement between diagnoses of somatoform disorders and its comorbidities depression and anxiety disorder obtained from a structured clinical interview and diagnoses reported from PCPs and, second, to identify patient and PCP-related predictors of PCPs' diagnoses of a somatoform disorder.

Methods

Sample recruitment

Data were collected within the project "Network Somatoform and Functional disorders" (*Sofu-Net*), a sub-project of the Hamburg Network for Mental Health *psychenet* [12, 13]. The study is registered at ISRCTN (ISRCTN55870770). *Sofu-Net* aimed to improve early detection of patients with somatoform disorders in primary care and to refer patients more quickly into effective treatment [14].

Between September and December 2012, all patients at least 18 years old attending the participating primary care practices were asked to take part in a screening regarding bodily complaints and well-being. Patients with severe physical illness, cognitive impairment or insufficient German language skills were excluded from the study. Patients with a positive screening result were asked to participate in a telephone interview within 4 weeks after the screening. All patients gave informed written consent. The study protocol is consistent with the principles of the Declaration of Helsinki and was approved by the ethics committee Medical Chamber Hamburg, Germany.

Measures

The self-administered screening questionnaire included data on the patients' age, gender, marital status, and school education. The Patient-Health-Questionnaire (PHQ) [15] was used to screen for somatoform disorders (PHQ-15), depression (PHQ-9) and anxiety (Generalized Anxiety Disorder Assessment; GAD-7) [16]. The PHQ-15 comprises of 15 items assessing somatic symptoms and their severity within the last 4 weeks. The 3-point Likert scale ranges from *not bothered* (0) to *bothered a lot* (2). The PHQ-9 comprises nine items assessing depressive symptoms and their severity within the last 2 weeks. The 3-Point Likert Scale ranges from *not at all* (0) to *nearly every day* (2). The GAD-7 comprises of seven items assessing anxiety-related symptoms within the last 2 weeks. The 3-Point Likert Scale ranges from *not at all* (0) to *nearly every day* (2). On all three scales, cutoff-values of 5, 10 and 15 represent mild, moderate and severe symptom levels, respectively [15]. Patients were considered screening positive if one the following conditions was fulfilled: (a) PHQ-15 ≥ 15, (b) PHQ-15 ≥ 10 and GAD-7 or PHQ-9 ≥ 10. Further, patients were asked how often they talk about psychosocial complaints and private problems with their PCP using the following question: 'Do you talk about psychological complaints and private problems with your primary care physician?' Patients responded on a 6-point Likert Scale ranging from *never* (1) to *always* (6).

The telephone interview encompassed the sections for somatoform disorders, depressive and anxiety disorders of the Composite International Interview (CIDI) [17]. The CIDI assesses mental disorders according to the criteria of the *International Classification of Diseases, 10th revision* (ICD-10) [7] and the criteria of the *DSM-IV Diagnostic and Statistical Manual of Mental Disorders, 4th edition* (DSM-IV) [8]. For the present analyses, diagnostic codes according to ICD-10 were analyzed. ICD-10 diagnoses obtained from the CIDI were considered as reference standard. CIDI interviews were conducted by research assistants who were extensively trained and supervised. Patients fulfilling the diagnostic criteria within the last 6 months were classified as having a current somatoform disorder, depressive or anxiety disorder. The category of somatoform disorders included somatization disorder (F45.0), undifferentiated somatoform disorder (F45.1), and persistent pain disorder (F45.4). Within a decision tree, it was assessed for each reported complaint whether it was medically unexplained. Mild, moderate and severe depressive episodes as well as dysthymia were summarized in the category depressive disorders (F32-F34). Anxiety disorders included agoraphobia, social phobia, specific phobias (e.g. animal phobias), phobic anxiety disorder, panic disorder, and generalized anxiety disorder (F40-F41).

PCP data form
The PCPs completed a form assessing their patients' medical history based on the data in their medical records. This form consisted of 6 sections encompassing the following topics: (1) reason for the patients' consultation (using ICD-10 codes), (2) present somatic diseases (list of 26 diseases and an additional open question, e.g. cardiovascular, endocrine, neurological, lung and autoimmune diseases), (3) present mental disorders (list of 13 disorders and an additional open question, e.g. dementia, alcohol, drug and medication dependence, schizophrenia, depression, anxiety disorder, somatoform disorder), (4) somatic explanation of the patients' bodily symptoms from the PCPs' perspective, (5) recommendation of psychological treatment by PCP, and (6) intake of medication (antidepressants, analgesics, benzodiazepines, and antipsychotic drugs). The form was

completed by PCPs for all screening-positive patients when the screening procedure had been finished.

Data from treating physicians
Using a questionnaire, the following characteristics of the participating PCPs were assessed: age, gender, specialization, training in psychosomatic basic care, years in general practice, and type of practice.

Data analyses
Data are reported as means (standard deviation) for continuous variables and as numbers (percentages) for categorical variables. Group comparisons were performed using t-tests (mean) for continuous variables and Pearson χ^2-tests for categorical variables. Tests were considered statistically significant at a two-sided p-value < 0.05. Kappa-statistics were calculated to determine the diagnostic agreement between diagnoses of somatoform disorders, depressive and anxiety disorders obtained from the CIDI and diagnoses obtained from PCPs. The following agreement levels were considered: discrete (0–0.20), regular (0.21–0.40), moderate (0.41–0.60), substantial (0.61–0.80), almost perfect (0.81–1.00) [18].

Two multiple logistic regression analyses were conducted to identify predictors for a PCP diagnosis of a somatoform disorder. The diagnoses obtained from CIDI were used as reference standard. The first model included the following patient-related predictors: age, gender, marital status, school education, comorbid depressive disorder, comorbid anxiety disorder, discussion of psychosocial problems with PCP, somatic symptom severity, and the number of PCP visits within the last 6 months. The second model included the following PCP-related predictors: age, gender, specialization, years in general practice, training in psychosomatic basic care, and type of practice.

Data analyses were conducted using STATA 13.0 (Stata Corporation, College Station, TX, USA).

Results
Characteristics of the study population
From 1826 screening participants, 283 (15.5%) were screened positive for somatoform disorders, depression and anxiety. From those screening positive, 137 (48.4%) patients participated in the telephone interview. After the exclusion of patients with incomplete interviews and missing data, 112 cases were available for the present analyses (Fig. 1).

Among the study population, the majority of patients was female. Data showed that patients with and without somatoform disorders did not differ in their sociodemographic and clinical characteristics (Table 1).

Within the study population, 65 (58.0%) patients were diagnosed with a current somatoform disorder according to CIDI and 29 (25.9%) patients were diagnosed with a current somatoform disorder according to their PCP.

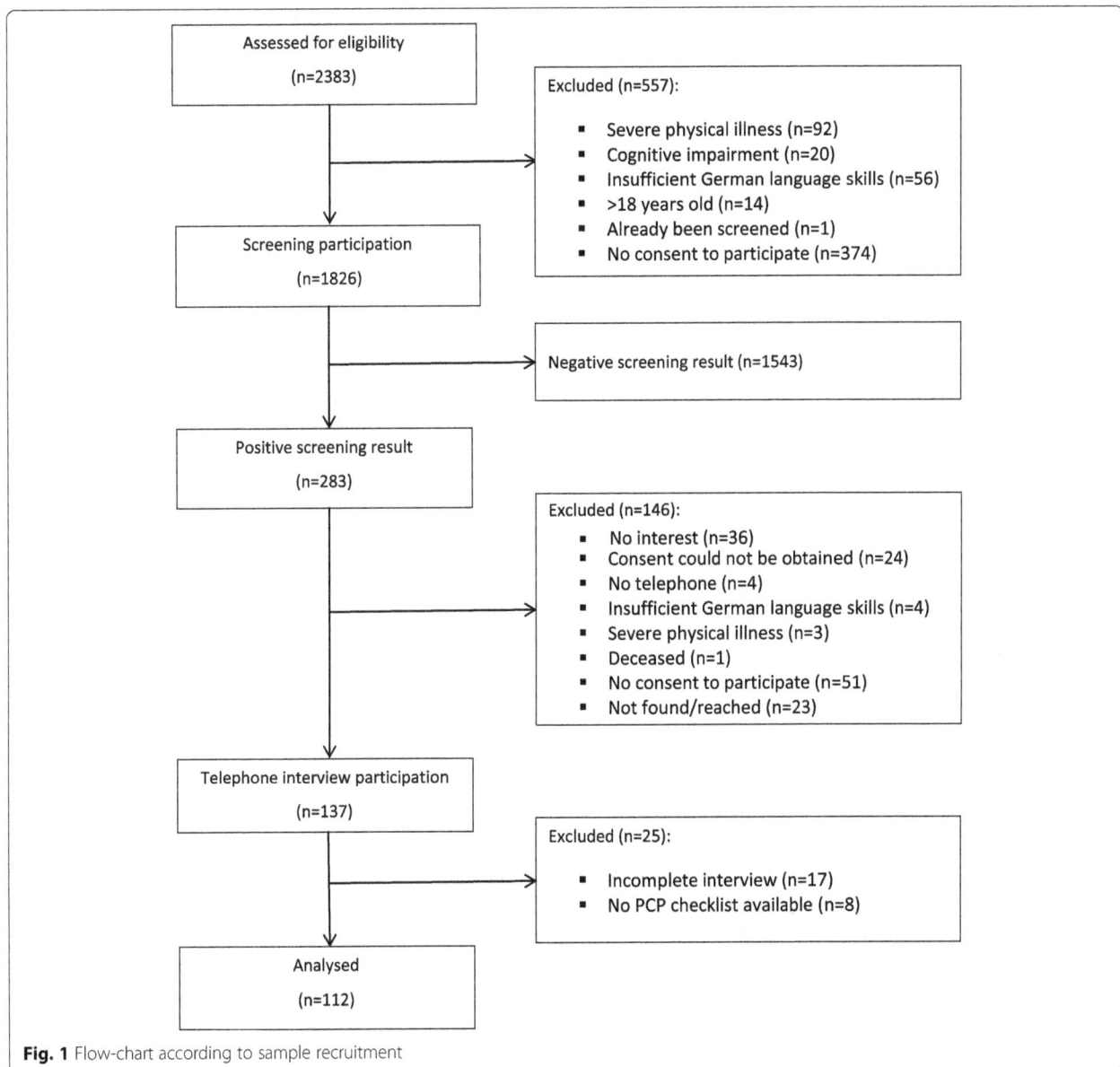

Fig. 1 Flow-chart according to sample recruitment

The rates of comorbidity with current depressive or anxiety disorders according to CIDI were 43.1 and 47.7%, respectively, while 26.6% of the patients presented both disorders (data not shown).

Characteristics of the participating PCPs

The characteristics of the participating PCPs are illustrated in Table 2. PCPs were on average 49.3 years old, and 53.7% were female. Most PCPs had a specialization in general medicine (58.5%) and 85.4% had completed training in psychosomatic basic care. Most frequently, PCPs worked in a group practice (75.6%) and had worked in general practice for on average 10.5 years.

Diagnostic agreement

The results of the analyses regarding the diagnostic agreement are displayed in Table 3. Using the CIDI diagnosis as gold standard, data analyses revealed that PCPs diagnosed 21 (32.3%) patients with a somatoform disorder, while they did not reach agreement with the CIDI diagnosis in 44 (67.7%) patients. PCPs classified 8 (17.0%) patients as having a somatoform disorder although a negative result was obtained using CIDI. Diagnostic agreement of not having a somatoform disorder according to CIDI or PCPs was found for 39 (83.0%) patients. Kappa value was 0.14 ($P < .05$), indicating a significant discrete diagnostic agreement.

Table 1 Characteristics of the study population according to the presence of a somatoform disorder as diagnosed using CIDI

	Total	With somatoform disorder	Without somatoform disorder
	$n = 112$	$n = 97$ (86.0%)	$n = 15$ (14.0%)
Female sex, n (%)	88 (78.6%)	79 (81.4%)	9 (60.0%)
Age (years), M (SD)	47.1 (15.9)	45.5 (15.2)	57.5 (17.1)
School education, n (%)			
< 10 years	28 (25.5)	25 (26.0)	3 (21.4)
10 years	35 (31.8)	29 (30.2)	6 (42.9)
> 10 years	47 (42.7)	42 (43.8)	5 (35.7)
Marital status, n (%)			
Married	42 (37.8)	35 (36.5)	7 (46.7)
Unmarried	38 (34.2)	35 (36.5)	3 (20.0)
Separated, divorced, widowed	31 (27.9)	26 (27.1)	5 (33.3)
PHQ-15 score, M (SD)	14.6 (3.3)	14.9 (3.4)	13.2 (2.6)
Age (years) at the onset of somatoform symptoms, M (SD)	19.3 (13.7)	19.3 (13.7)	n/a
Comorbid depressive disorder (CIDI) within the last 6 months, n (%)	50 (44.6)	43 (44.3)	7 (46.7)
Comorbid anxiety disorder (CIDI) within the last 6 months, n (%)	48 (42.9)	43 (44.3)	5 (33.3)
Currently in psychotherapy, n (%)	24 (22.0)	21 (22.3)	3 (20.0)
PCP visits within the past 6 months, M (SD)	6.1 (4.8)	6.0 (4.4)	6.6 (6.7)
Discussion of psychosocial distress with PCP, n (%)			
Never, seldom/rarely, sometimes	69 (61.6)	59 (60.8)	10 (66.7)
Often, very often, always	43 (38.4)	38 (39.2)	5 (33.3)

CIDI Composite International diagnostic interview
PHQ-15 Patient Health Questionnaire
PCP Primary care physician

Regarding depressive disorders, PCPs diagnosed 24 (48.0%) patients, while they did not reach agreement with the CIDI diagnosis in 26 (52.0%) patients. In contrast, PCPs classified 14 (22.6%) patients as having a depressive disorder although a negative result was obtained using CIDI. Diagnostic agreement of not having a depressive disorder according to CIDI or PCPs was found

for 48 (77.4%) patients. Kappa value was 0.26 ($P < 0.01$), indicating a significant regular diagnostic agreement.

Regarding anxiety disorders, PCPs diagnosed 12 (25.0%) of patients, while they did not reach agreement with the CIDI diagnosis in 36 (75.0%) patients. In contrast, PCPs classified 5 (7.8%) patients as having an anxiety disorder

Table 2 Characteristics of PCPs ($n = 41$)

Age (years), M (SD)	49.3 (7.7)
Female sex, n (%)	22 (53.7)
Specialization, n (%)	
General medicine	24 (58.5)
Internal medicine	12 (29.3)
Other specialization	5 (12.2)
Training in psychosomatic basic care, n (%)	35 (85.4)
Type of practice, n (%)	
Solo practice	10 (24.4)
Group practice	31 (75.6)
Years in general practice, M (SD)	10.5 (5.6)

Table 3 Diagnostic agreement between PCP ratings and CIDI results ($n = 112$)

		CIDI	
		n (%) yes	n (%) no
Somatoform disorder			
PCP rating	n (%) yes	21 (32.3)	8 (17.0)
	n (%) no	44 (67.7)	39 (83.0)
Depressive disorder			
PCP rating	n (%) yes	24 (48.0)	14 (22.6)
	n (%) no	26 (52.0)	48 (77.4)
Anxiety disorder			
PCP rating	n (%) yes	12 (25.0)	5 (7.8)
	n (%) no	36 (75.0)	59 (92.2)

although a negative result was obtained using CIDI. Diagnostic agreement of not having an anxiety disorder according to CIDI or PCPs was found for 59 (92.2%) patients. Kappa value was 0.19 ($P < 0.01$), indicating a significant discrete diagnostic agreement.

Patient and PCP-related predictors for the diagnosis of a somatoform disorder by PCPs

Regarding patient-related characteristics, multiple regression analysis revealed that with every point increase in PHQ-15 mean score, the chance of being diagnosed with a somatoform disorder increased by 1.2 (OR = 1.22; 95% CI 1.03–1.44) (Table 4).

Regarding PCP-related characteristics, multiple regression analysis revealed that a specialization in internal medicine was associated with a 6-fold higher chance that patients were diagnosed with a somatoform disorder by their PCP (OR = 5.95; 95% CI 1.70–20.80) (Table 5). Further, working in a solo practice was associated with a 3-fold higher chance of patients being diagnosed with a somatoform disorder (OR = 2.92; 95% CI 1.02–8.38). With respect to the PCPs' age, younger age was associated with a higher chance of patients being correctly diagnosed with a somatoform disorder (OR = 0.90; 95% CI 0.81–1.00). This effect was borderline significant ($p = 0.06$). In the single models, all predictors explained 11.8 and 17.2% of the model variance, respectively.

Discussion

In the present population of primary care patients at high risk for somatoform disorders, the diagnostic agreement between PCPs' diagnoses and diagnoses obtained from a structured clinical interview was highest for depressive disorders, followed by somatoform disorders and anxiety disorders. Our analyses further revealed that somatic symptom severity was a relevant patient-related predictor for PCPs' diagnosis of a somatoform disorder,

Table 4 Patient-related predictors for PCPs' diagnosis of a somatoform disorder ($n = 85$)

Patient-related characteristics	OR (95% CI)	P-value
Age	1.00 (0.97; 1.05)	0.75
Female gender	0.42 (0.10; 1.67)	0.22
Marital status, married	1.52 (0.75; 3.10)	0.25
At least 10 years of schooling	1.45 (0.71;2.96)	0.31
Comorbid depressive disorder	1.70 (0.52; 5.55)	0.38
Comorbid anxiety disorder	0.92 (0.20; 4.32)	0.92
Discussion of psychosocial distress	1.90 (0.60; 6.00)	0.27
Somatic symptom severity (PHQ-15)	1.22 (1.03; 1.44)	0.04
Number of PCP visits within the last 6 months	0.94 (0.80; 1.10)	0.44

Results of multiple logistic regression analysis
PHQ-15 Patient Health Questionnaire
PCP Primary care physician

Table 5 Physician-related predictors for PCPs' diagnosis of a somatoform disorder ($n = 99$)

Physician-related characteristics	OR (95% CI)	P-value
Age	0.90 (0.81; 1.00)	0.06
Female sex	2.26(0.74; 6.85)	0.15
Specialization internal medicine	5.95 (1.70; 20.80)	<.01
Years in general practice	1.06 (0.93; 1.21)	0.38
Training in psychosomatic basic care	0.58 (0.15; 2.96)	0.51
Solo practice	2.92 (1.02; 8.38)	<.05

Results of multiple logistic regression analysis

while a specialization in internal medicine and working in a solo practice were relevant physician-related predictors for PCPs' diagnosis of a somatoform disorder.

We showed that PCPs identified 32.3% of the patients with a somatoform disorder using the CIDI diagnosis as reference. This finding is in line with data from previous studies which revealed agreement rates ranging from 18% to 56%, depending on the investigated populations and the methods applied in the single studies [19–22]. This variety may reflect the difficulties in the terminology and conceptualization of somatoform type disorders which have often been discussed in previous research [11]. Regarding conceptual barriers in the process of diagnosing somatoform disorders, existing classification systems have been described by PCPs as being difficult to use, as providing little information about the illness, or as too restrictive [11].

In the present study, all PCPs participating in *Sofu-Net* had attended network meetings and quality circles which were an inherent part of the network providing information about diagnostic approaches and management of somatoform disorders. Moreover, participating PCPs were prompted to use the PHQ as screening tool for early detection and contemporary referral to psychotherapeutic co-treatment. We therefore suppose that participation in *Sofu-Net* has promoted the PCPs' awareness for patients with somatoform complaints and their diagnostic knowledge and skills. Further, among the participating PCPs, 85% had a training in psychosomatic basis care, suggesting that these PCPs may be particular interested in the field of psychosomatic care which might has enhanced the detection of patients with somatoform complaints. In addition, PCPs were aware of the patients' positive screening result, giving advice that somatoform complaints were present in their patients. Nevertheless, using CIDI as reference, a large part of the patients with somatoform as disorders remained unrecognized by their PCPs. However, it is of importance to note that among all patients who had been "overlooked" by their PCPs (67.7%), PCPs stated for 54.6% of these patients that they do not consider the patients' complaints as medically explained and therefore suspect the presence of a somatoform disorder. This finding suggests that PCPs were aware of somatization in their patients, although not having labelled their patients as having a somatoform disorder. A recent qualitative study by our group among PCPs investigated the process of coding somatoform disorders in primary care [23]. In that study, PCPs reported that coding is done for reimbursement purposes, that they use other information in their personal documentation, for example about the patients' psychosocial background or potential causes about the presented symptoms, and that they do not necessarily need to document a confirmed diagnosis for treatment. Moreover, PCPs reported that they restrain their coding to protect patients from stigma trough certain diagnoses or other negative consequences. Inaccurate coding was further described to arise from uncertainties regarding the diagnostic criteria and that finding the definite diagnosis is seen as the responsibilities of psychiatric specialists [23]. Although we have not investigated these processes in the present study, it might be assumed that the described factors were of relevance among the PCPs in the present study and have contributed to the relatively low detection rate.

In the present study, the diagnostic agreement was highest for depressive disorders (48%). It has been argued that PCPs are better acquainted with depression than with other mental disorders and may therefore have a greater ability to detect depressive disorders [24]. Regarding the presence of an anxiety disorder, the diagnostic agreement was only 25.0%. When interpreting this result, it needs to be considered that the diagnostic classification of anxiety disorders in the present study encompassed conditions of differential severity (i.e. panic disorder, animal phobia). It is possible that PCPs did not to diagnose light cases, given that symptoms might not have been apparent or might not have been associated with severe impairments. In turn, patients might have not disclosed their symptoms when feeling only slightly impaired.

We demonstrated that somatic symptom severity was a relevant predictor for a diagnosis of a somatoform disorder by PCPs, while the patient's sociodemographic characteristics had no impact on the detection rate. Possibly, an increasing symptom severity presumably has prompted patients to describe their bodily complaints more often and striking to their PCPs, thereby facilitating the detection of a somatoform disorder.

We further showed that a specialization in internal medicine and working in a solo practice were relevant physician-related predictors for a diagnosis of a somatoform disorder. This result is in line with findings from a study demonstrating that physicians who saw themselves as more effective in dealing with somatoform symptoms were more likely to be working in a solo practice [25]. Data from that study further showed that PCPs working in solo practices and those who were in the same practice

for 5 years felt most comfortable in dealing with patients with somatoform disorders. It might be assumed that these PCPs had a better chance to establish a close relationship with their patients and had more time to explore their patients' complaints and psychosocial background facilitating the diagnostic process. With regard to the PCPs' education, we found that PCPs with training in internal medicine were more successful in diagnosing somatoform disorders compared to PCPs with training in general medicine, suggesting that training in internal medicine encompasses knowledge and skills facilitating the process of diagnosing somatoform disorders. It might be further possible that training in internal medicine makes PCPs more confident of declaring symptoms as medically explained, and thus diagnosing somatoform disorders. Taken together, the present findings underline that structural circumstances are essential for improving early detection and care for patients with somatoform disorders.

Strengths of the present study encompass the well characterized population of primary care patients at high risk for somatoform disorders as identified using established screening instruments and the structured diagnostic procedure using CIDI interviews. Our analyses are further based on different data sources including patient self-report, diagnoses obtained from CIDI interviews, and a PCP questionnaire, thereby integrating different perspectives on somatoform disorders diagnoses. Limitations may arise from the low response rate in the telephone interview, which potentially has introduced a selection bias. However, screening-positive patients who participated in the telephone interview did not differ from those who dropped out with regard to age, gender and PHQ-scores. Another weakness of the present study is the lack of data from screening-negative patients, which may has led to a misclassification bias underrepresenting the rate of patients with somatization. On the other hand, the PHQ has been demonstrated to be a well-validated measure for detecting and monitoring somatization, depression, and anxiety [15]. Nevertheless, as data on screening-negative patients are lacking, no data are available regarding PCPs diagnostic assessment of these patients.

Conclusions

Our data demonstrate that the process of diagnosing somatoform disorders in primary care remains challenging. We showed that the diagnostic agreement between diagnoses obtained from CIDI and diagnoses obtained from PCPs was low, but there is reason to assume that PCPs were aware of somatization in their patients without labelling them as having a somatoform disorder. Even with the release of the DSM-5, conceptual and practical problems of the previous classification remain unresolved. However, our data indicate that structural circumstances are crucial in the diagnostic process, as

PCPs training in internal medicine and working in a solo practice were associated with a higher chance of detecting a somatoform disorder. As structural circumstances are changeable, more research is necessary to assess and overcome situational barriers. Our data further suggest that there might be particular knowledge and skills taught during the education in internal medicine helping PCPs to detect patients with somatoform disorders. Likewise demonstrated in previous studies, the restricted time during consultations may hinder PCPs to build a strong doctor-patient relationship and to explore the psychosocial background of their patients, thereby impeding the correct diagnosis. Thus, continuity of care, as provided potentially stronger in solo practices, might facilitate the diagnosis of somatoform disorders in primary care. Furthermore, collaborative networks of PCPs and psychotherapists like *Sofu-Net* may contribute to the improvement of care in somatoform type disorders.

Abbreviations
CI: Confidence interval; CIDI: Composite International Interview; DSM: Diagnostic and Statistical Manual of Mental Disorders; GAD: Generalized Anxiety Disorder Assessment; ICD: International Classification of Diseases; OR: Odds Ratio; PCP: Primary care physician; PHQ: Patient-Health-Questionnaire

Acknowledgments
The authors would like to thank all patients for participating in the study and all network partners for their work.

Funding
The study was funded by the German Federal Ministry of Education and Research (BMBF) as part of *psychenet - Hamburg Network for Mental Health*, a large health services research study in the Hamburg Metropolitan Area (sub-project somatoform disorders; principal investigator: Bernd Löwe, grant number 01KQ1002B). The sponsor of the study was not involved in the design of the study, data collection, data analysis, data interpretation and writing the manuscript.

Authors' contributions
KP analyzed and interpreted the data and wrote the manuscript. MSM, MG, AK contributed to writing the manuscript. BL designed the study and was a major contributor in writing the manuscript. All authors read and approved the final manuscript.

Authors' information
Not applicable.

Consent for publication
Not applicable.

Competing interests
The authors declare that they have no competing interests.

References
1. Schaefert R, Hausteiner-Wiehle C, Hauser W, Ronel J, Herrmann M, Henningsen P. Non-specific, functional, and somatoform bodily complaints. Dtsch Arztebl Int. 2012;109(47):803–13.
2. Shedden-Mora M, Lau K, Kuby A, Gross B, Gladigau M, Fabisch A, Loewe B. Improving health Care for Patients with somatoform and functional disorders: a collaborative stepped care network (Sofu-net). Psychiatr Prax. 2015;42(Suppl 1):S60–4.
3. Loewe B, Spitzer RL, Williams JB, Mussell M, Schellberg D, Kroenke K. Depression, anxiety and somatization in primary care: syndrome overlap and functional impairment. Gen Hosp Psychiatry. 2008;30(3):191–9.
4. Steinbrecher N, Koerber S, Frieser D, Hiller W. The prevalence of medically unexplained symptoms in primary care. Psychosomatics. 2011;52(3):263–71.
5. de Waal MW, Arnold IA, Eekhof JA, van Hemert AM. Somatoform disorders in general practice: prevalence, functional impairment and comorbidity with anxiety and depressive disorders. Br J Psychiatry. 2004;184:470–6.
6. Fink P, Sorensen L, Engberg M, Holm M, Munk-Jorgensen P. Somatization in primary care. Prevalence, health care utilization, and general practitioner recognition. Psychosomatics. 1999;40(4):330–8.
7. World Health Organization. The ICD-10 classification of mental and behavioural disorders: clinical description and diagnostic guidelines. Geneva: World Health Organization; 1992.
8. American Psychiatric Association. Diagnostic and statistical manual of mental disorders (4th ed., text rev.). Washington, DC: American Psychiatric Publishing; 2000.
9. Haller H, Cramer H, Lauche R, Gobos G. Somatoform disorders and medically unexplained symptoms in primary care-a systematic review and meta-analysis of prevalence. Dtsch Arztebl Int. 2015;112:279–98.
10. Hanel G, Henningsen P, Herzog W, Sauer N, Schaefert R, Szecsenyi J, Lowe B. Depression, anxiety, and somatoform dirsorders: vague or distinct categories in primary care? Results from a large cross-sectional study. J Psychosom Res. 2009;67:189–97.
11. Murray AM, Toussaint A, Althaus A, Lowe B. The challenge of diagnosing non-specific, functional, and somatoform disorders: a systematic review of barriers to diagnosis in primary care. J Psychosom Res. 2016;80:1–10.
12. Haerter M, Brandes A, Hillebrandt B, Lambert M. psychenet - Das Hamburger Netz psychische Gesundheit [psychenet - The Hamburg Network for Mental Health]. Psychiatr Prax. 2015;42(Suppl 1):S4–8.
13. Shedden-Mora MC, Gross B, Lau K, Gumz A, Wegscheider K, Loewe B. Collaborative stepped care for somatoform disorders: a pre-post-intervention study in primary care. J Psychosom Res. 2016;80:23–30.
14. Loewe B, Piontek K, Daubmann A, Harter M, Wegscheider K, Koenig HH, Shedden-Mora M. Effectiveness of a stepped, collaborative, and coordinated health care network for somatoform disorders (Sofu-net): a controlled cluster cohort study. Psychosom Med. 2017;79(9):1016–24.
15. Kroenke K, Spitzer RL, Williams JB, Loewe B. The patient health questionnaire somatic, anxiety, and depressive symptom scales: a systematic review. Gen Hosp Psychiatry. 2010;32(4):345–59.
16. Spitzer RL, Kroenke K, Williams JB, Loewe B. A brief measure for assessing generalized anxiety disorder: the GAD-7. Arch Intern Med. 2006;166(10):1092–7.
17. Kessler RC, Ustun TB. The world mental health (WMH) survey initiative version of the World Health Organization (WHO) composite international diagnostic interview (CIDI). Int J Methods Psychiatr Res. 2004;13(2):93–121.
18. Landis JR, Koch GG. The measurement of observer agreement for categorical data. Biometrics. 1977;33(1):159–74.
19. Pols RG, Battersby MW. Coordinated care in the management of patients with unexplained physical symptoms: depression is a key issue. Med J Aust. 2008;188(12 Suppl):S133–7.
20. Norton J, de Roquefeuil G, David M, Boulenger JP, Ritchie K, Mann A. Prevalence of psychiatric disorders in French general practice using the patient health questionnaire: comparison with GP case-recognition and psychotropic medication prescription. Encéphale. 2009;35(6):560–9.
21. Pilowsky I. Dimensions of hypochondriasis. Br J Psychiatry. 1967;113(494):89–93.

22. H G, Henningsen P, Herzog W, Sauer N, Schaefert R, Szecsenyi J, Lowe B. Depression, anxiety, and somatoform disorders: vague or distinct categories in primary care? Results from a large cross-sectional study. J Psychosom Res. 2009;67(3):189–97.

23. Pohontsch NJ, Zimmermann T, Jonas C, Lehmann M, Lowe B, Scherer M. Coding of medically unexplained symptoms and somatoform disorders by general practitioners - an exploratory focus group study. BMC Fam Pract. 2018;19(1):129.

24. Nuyen J, Volkers AC, Verhaak PF, Schellevis FG, Groenewegen PP, van den Bos GA. Accuracy of diagnosing depression in primary care: the impact of chronic somatic and psychiatric co-morbidity. Psychol Med. 2005;35(8):1185–95.

25. Hartz AJ, Noyes R, Bentler SE, Damiano PC, Willard JC, Momany ET. Unexplained symptoms in primary care: perspectives of doctors and patients. Gen Hosp Psychiatry. 2000;22(3):144–52.

19

Humanistic outcomes in treatment resistant depression: a secondary analysis of the STAR*D study

Allitia DiBernardo[1], Xiwu Lin[1], Qiaoyi Zhang[1], Jim Xiang[1], Lang Lu[1], Carol Jamieson[1], Carmela Benson[2], Kwan Lee[1], Robert Bodén[3,4], Lena Brandt[4], Philip Brenner[4], Johan Reutfors[4] and Gang Li[1,5*]

Abstract

Background: In the Sequenced Treatment Alternatives to Relieve Depression (STAR*D) study, a third of patients did not achieve remission or adequate response after two treatment trials, fulfilling requirements for treatment resistant depression (TRD). The present study is a secondary analysis of the STAR*D data conducted to compare the humanistic outcomes in patients with TRD and non-TRD MDD.

Methods: Patients with major depressive disorder who entered level 3 of the STAR*D were included in the TRD group, while patients who responded to treatment and entered follow-up from level 1 or 2 were included in the non-TRD group. The first visit in level 1 was used for baseline assessments. The time-point of assessments for comparison was the first visit in level 3 for TRD patients (median day: 141), and the visit closest to 141 ± 60 days from baseline for non-TRD patients. Outcomes were assessed by the 12-item Short Form Health Survey (SF12), 16-item Quality of Life Enjoyment and Satisfaction Questionnaire (Q-LES-Q), Work and Social Adjustment Scale (WSAS), and Work Productivity and Activity Impairment scale (WPAI). Scores were compared in a linear model with adjustment for covariates including age, gender, and depression severity measured by the 17-item Hamilton Rating Scale for Depression (HDRS17) and Quick Inventory of Depressive Symptomatology (QIDS).

Results: A total of 2467 (TRD: 377; non-TRD: 2090) patients were studied. TRD patients were slightly older (mean age 44 vs 42 years), had a higher proportion of men (49% vs 37%, $p < .0001$), and baseline depression severity (HDRS17: 24.4 vs 22.0, p < .0001) vs non-TRD patients. During follow-up, TRD patients had lower health-related quality of life (HRQOL) scores on mental (30 vs 45.7) and physical components (47.7 vs 48.9) of the SF12, and lower Q-LES-Q scores (43.6 vs 63.7), greater functional and work impairments and productivity loss vs non-TRD patients (all $p < 0.05$).

Conclusion: Patients with TRD had worse HRQOL, work productivity, and social functioning than the non-TRD patients.

Keywords: Health-related quality of life, Humanistic outcomes, Social functioning, Star*d, Treatment resistant depression

* Correspondence: gli@its.jnj.com
[1] Janssen Research & Development, LLC, Titusville, NJ, USA
[5] Real World Evidence, Statistics & Decision Sciences, Janssen R&D US, 920 US Highway 202 S, Raritan, NJ 08869, USA
Full list of author information is available at the end of the article

Background

According to the World Health Organization, more than 300 million people worldwide suffer from depression. Depression is a leading cause of disability and a major contributor to global disease burden [1]. By 2020, major depressive disorder (MDD) is expected to be the second global leading cause of disability. MDD exhibits more debilitating effects on physical, social, and emotional functioning compared to any other chronic medical illness [2]. Although, several therapeutic options have proven efficacious in the treatment of MDD, [3] about 30% of patients with MDD fail to respond to antidepressant therapy, a condition referred to as treatment resistant depression (TRD) [4–7]. Factors such as fewer interpersonal or economic resources, minority status, lower function and quality of life, poor social and family support, and treatment non-compliance contribute to TRD [8–10].

The National Institute of Mental Health (NIMH)-- sponsored Sequenced Treatment Alternatives to Relieve Depression (STAR*D) is the largest and most comprehensive clinical trial conducted in real-world settings of psychiatry and primary care to date, and included patients with nonpsychotic MDD [11]. In STAR*D study, patients were treated sequentially with a series of antidepressants or psychotherapy trials and the resistance was found to be increasing at Level 3 (failure of 2 therapies). Therefore, Conway et al. recently proposed an operational definition of TRD i.e., the failure of 2 adequate dose-duration antidepressants from different classes and/or psychotherapeutic treatments (either in combination or succession) in the current episode [5]. We have used a similar definition for TRD and used data from STAR*D study.

Humanistic outcomes as measured by health-related quality of life (HRQOL), functional and work productivity instruments, characterize the patient's experience with the medical care. HRQOL equals perceived physical and mental health over time, and incorporates domains related to physical, mental and emotional, and social functioning. In addition to conventional clinical measures of health, HRQOL is increasingly used for assessing the quality of care in outcomes research [12].

It is well-known that depression has a debilitating effect on HRQOL [2, 13]. Symptoms of depression are associated with significant interference with functioning including absence from work, productivity loss, and lower job retention, resulting in an increased indirect cost [14, 15]. Patients with TRD have greater healthcare resource utilization and experience more difficulties in social and occupational function and a larger decline in physical health compared with other MDD patients [16]. The repeated and continuous symptoms of depression and associated distress experienced by TRD patients, and the associated social morbidity and chronic suffering, can infer vast socio-economic implications [17, 18].

Only a few studies have assessed the HRQOL in patients with TRD, [19–21] however, to our knowledge, none of the studies has compared the humanistic outcomes in TRD and non-TRD patients using a larger cohort from a real-world setting. Therefore, this study was conducted to evaluate various HRQOL and work productivity domains in patients with TRD versus those with non-TRD MDD using the STAR*D database.

Methods

Data source and study population

In the STAR*D study, outpatients from mental health and primary care practices, aged between 18 to 75 years, who met the Diagnostic & Statistical Manual Disorders (DSM-IV) criteria and had a 17-item Hamilton Rating Scale for Depression (HDRS17) [22] score ≥ 14 for nonpsychotic MDD were enrolled. Patients with bipolar or psychotic disorders, primary diagnosis of obsessive-compulsive disorder or an eating disorder, general medical conditions that contraindicated protocol medications in the first two treatment steps, substance dependence that required inpatient detoxification, and suicidal patients who required immediate hospitalization were excluded [23].

All patients provided written informed consent at study entry, at entry into each level, and the follow-up phase. For the present analysis, the study team obtained the limited access STAR*D dataset, following the NIMH procedure for obtaining and analyzing the research data [24]. As this was a retrospective analysis, so the institutional review board approval and informed consent were not required. Patient identifiers are not disclosed and only summary data are presented.

STAR*D study design

A detailed description of STAR*D study design has been presented elsewhere [23]. The STAR*D was a prospective, pragmatic clinical trial conducted at multiple sites in the United States that evaluated the relative efficacy and tolerability of various antidepressants in outpatients with nonpsychotic MDD [25, 26]. All patients started with a single selective serotonin reuptake inhibitor (SSRI) (citalopram) and followed an algorithm-based acute phase treatment over a 12-week period. Patients who did not have remission after the initial treatment, participated in a sequence of up to three randomized trials (Levels). Patients who achieved remission or a response with an adequate benefit according to clinician's judgment after any of the treatment levels could enter the 12-month naturalistic follow-up phase. Patients were allowed to choose among acceptable treatment options reflecting the clinical practice. Patients could switch to bupropion, venlafaxine, sertraline, cognitive therapy (Level 2), mirtazapine, nortriptyline (Level 3), tranylcypromine, mirtazapine+venlafaxine (Level 4) or augment the current treatment with bupropion, buspirone, cognitive therapy (Level 2), lithium, T3 thyroid hormone (Level 3). There were no meaningful clinical differences due to pharmacological differences between treatment options and probability of remission was not clearly dependent on choice of medication [25] (Table 1).

The present study is a secondary analysis based on data collected in the STAR*D. For the present study, TRD and non-TRD MDD patients were compared. Patients who entered level 3 of the STAR*D trial (i.e. failed to remit or achieve adequate response after two antidepressant trials) were included in the TRD group, while patients who entered follow-up after level 1 or level 2 (or 2A) and were included in the non-TRD group. The first visit in level 1 was used for baseline assessments. Comparison of outcome measures between TRD and non-TRD groups was made at primary visits which for TRD patients was the first visit in level 3. The median day of the primary visit for TRD patients was 141, therefore, the visit closest to 141 days from baseline with a deviation ±60 days was considered the primary visit for a non-TRD patient. Treatment response of patients in both the cohorts was also observed at a longer duration including at 12-month, considering a window period of 365 ± 60 days. However, due to low number of patients in both the cohorts (TRD: 28; non-TRD: 16), no analysis was performed.

Assessments

Demographics and baseline clinical characteristic
Demographics and baseline clinical characteristics were assessed at the first visit of level 1 using HDRS17, [22] the 14-item Cumulative Illness Rating Scale (CIRS),

[27] and the 16-item Quick Inventory of Depressive Symptomatology (QIDS) Self-Reported (QIDS-SR16) and Clinician-rated (QIDS-C) versions [28]. To equate HDRS17 total scores indicating no depression (score = 0–7), mild depression (score = 8–13), moderate depression (score = 14–19), severe depression (score = 20–25), and very severe depression (score = 26+) with QIDS-SR16 total scores, a conversion table was used to provide equivalent QIDS-SR16 ratings (no depression: score = 0–5; mild: score = 6–10; moderate: score = 11–15; severe: score = 16–20; very severe: score = 21+).

Outcome assessments at primary visit
The HRQOL was measured using the Short Form Health Survey (SF-12) and the Quality of Life Enjoyment and Satisfaction Questionnaire (Q-LES-Q). The SF-12 is a 12 item, self-report instrument that assesses mental and physical health status [29], while the 16-item short version of Q-LES-Q, a self-report instrument, was used that measures the degree of enjoyment and satisfaction experienced by patients in several domains of functioning (e.g., physical health, feelings, work, household duties, school/house work) [30].

Functioning was measured using the Work and Social Adjustment Scale (WSAS), and the Work Productivity and Activity Impairment scale (WPAI). The WSAS is a 5 item self-reported instrument that measures functional impairment (the ability to work, manage home, social and personal leisure activities, and the ability to form and maintain close relationships) and the WPAI is a six-item self-report questionnaire that measures the number of work hours missed or the number of hours worked in the past 7 days, and impairment resulting from health conditions while working or performing usual daily activities other than work.

Table 1 STAR*D study design and categorization of patients (TRD vs non-TRD)

	Non-TRD			TRD	
	Non-TRD 1	Non-TRD 2		TRD1	TRD2
	Patients Entered Follow-up after	Patients Entered Follow-up after	Patients Entered Follow-up after	Patients Entered	Patients Entered
	Level 1	Level 2	Level 2A	Level 3	Level 4
Level 1 Baseline	X	X	X	X	X
Level 2		X	X	X	X
Level 2A			X	X	X
Level 3				X	X
Level 4					X
Follow-up	X	X	X	X	X

TRD treatment resistant depression
A detailed description of STAR*D study design and different levels of treatment has been presented elsewhere: Rush AJ, Fava M, Wisniewski SR et al. Sequenced treatment alternatives to relieve depression (STAR*D): rationale and design. Control Clin Trials 2004; 25: 119–42

Statistical analysis

The sample size of this study was not calculated based on any statistical consideration, however all patients with measurements available at both baseline and primary visits were included in the analysis. Demographics and baseline clinical characteristics were summarized descriptively in each group using mean and standard deviations (SD) for continuous variables and frequencies for categorical variables. Association of baseline clinical characteristics with TRD was investigated by t-test or logistic regression models. Humanistic outcomes were compared between TRD and non-TRD patients using a linear model adjusting for the covariates that could potentially affect the outcome such as baseline of the variable, age category, gender, and baseline values of total severity score of comorbidity, Depression severity by HDRS17, and Depression severity by QIDS. Missing values were not imputed, as the exact reason for missing data in the STAR*D study was not clear.

Results

Demographics and baseline clinical characteristic

Out of 3671 patients who entered level 1, 2467 (67%) patients with both baseline and first visit assessments at level 3 (or around 141 days) were included in the analysis. The remaining 1204 patients were lost to follow up. Of the 2467 patients included in the analysis, 377 entered level 3 (TRD group), while 2090 entered follow-up from levels 1 and 2 (non-TRD group). (Table 1).

The TRD patients were slightly older than the non-TRD patients (mean [SD] age 44 [11.97] vs 42 [13.26] years, $p = .0005$). The TRD group had a higher proportion of men compared with the non-TRD group (49% vs 37%, $p < .0001$). Patients with TRD had higher scores of HDRS17 (24.4 vs 22.0, p < .0001) and QIDS-SR16 (17.0 vs 14.7, p < .0001) compared with the non-TRD patients. More patients in the TRD group than in non-TRD group had a very severe depression as measured by HDRS17 (40% vs 22%) and QIDS-SR16 (20% vs 10%). In general, TRD patients were observed with either

Table 2 Demographics and baseline clinical characteristics of TRD and non-TRD patients

Variable	N	TRD	N	Non-TRD	P-Value
Age at entry to study; mean years (SD)	377	44.3 (11.97)	2090	41.8 (13.26)	0.0005
Age, years; (%)					0.0004
18–34	98	26	734	35.1	
35–49	145	38.5	744	35.6	
50–64	122	32.4	512	24.5	
65+	12	3.2	100	4.8	
Gender; n (%)					<.0001
Female	193	51.2	1322	63.2	
Male	184	48.8	769	36.8	
HDRS17 current score (transcribed); mean (SD)	377	24.4 (5.10)	2089	22.0 (4.80)	<.0001
Depression severity by HDRS17; (%)					<.0001
Mild (score: 8–13)	0	0	3	0.1	
Moderate (score:14–19)	63	16.7	703	33.7	
Severe (score: 20–25)	164	43.5	920	44	
Very severe (score:26+)	150	39.8	463	22.2	
QIDS-C current score (transcribed); mean (SD)	377	17.5 (3.19)	2089	15.8 (3.27)	<.0001
Depression severity by QIDS-SR16; (%)					<.0001
No Depression (score:0–5)	0	0	25	1.2	
Mild (score:6–10)	18	4.8	308	14.8	
Moderate (score:11–15)	115	30.6	861	41.3	
Severe (score:16–20)	168	44.7	693	33.3	
Very severe (score:21+)	75	19.9	197	9.5	
QIDS-SR current score (transcribed); mean (SD)	376	17 (3.86)	2084	14.7 (4.25)	<.0001
Total severity score of comorbid condition; mean (SD)	377	5.6 (4.43)	2091	4.3 (3.66)	<.0001

HDRS17 The Hamilton Rating Scale for Depression, *QIDS-C* Quick inventory of depressive symptomatology (clinician-rated), *QIDS-SR* Quick inventory of depressive symptomatology (self-rated), *SD* Standard deviation, *TRD* Treatment resistant depression

comparable or worse depression scores compared to non-TRD patients at baseline (Table 2).

Humanistic outcomes

HRQOL

The number of patients observed at the primary visit for all the outcome measures varied from those at baseline, as not all data were collected at every visit for all patients. Majority of the patients (n = 316) with both baseline and primary visit values were observed for outcome based on SF12 measurement. The median and mean (standard deviation) day of primary visit was 133 and 136 (37.9) for non-TRD patients, respectively. Patients with TRD had significantly lower scores on the mental component (p < .0001) and physical component (p = 0.0126) of the SF-12 scale compared with non-TRD patients being at the same time window. The TRD patients also reported lower Q-LES-Q global scores compared with non-TRD patients (p < .0001) (Table 3).

Work and social functional impairment

At the time of meeting the TRD criteria, patients in the TRD group reported greater functional impairments in work and social functioning compared with the non-TRD group. TRD patients had higher scores at WSAS and all scales of WPAI compared with the non-TRD group (p < .0001) (Table 3), indicating greater functional and work impairments, and higher productivity loss due to health.

Discussion

This study shows that patients meeting the TRD criteria in the STAR*D had worse HRQOL scores, work productivity, and greater functional impairments compared to non-TRD patients. At baseline, the TRD patients exhibited greater depression severity, however the quality of life and functional parameters were equal in both the cohorts. The difference in humanistic outcomes several months later suggests a decrease in quality of life and functioning, over time in patients with depression that is not alleviated in comparison to those effectively treated. To our knowledge, the present study is the first to compare the humanistic outcomes in TRD with non-TRD patients using a large dataset and a working definition of TRD [5].

In the present study, patients with TRD had poorer HRQOL scores compared with non-TRD patients, as measured by the SF-12. A few studies have evaluated the screening performance of the mental health component of SF-12 and suggested a cutoff value of 42 [31] or 45.6 as the best screening cutoff for depression [32]. In the present study, patients with TRD had lesser mental health component scores (30) than these cutoffs. However, the scores in non-TRD patients (45.7) were almost equal to at least one of the suggested cutoffs. The physical health component scores in both TRD and non-TRD groups were comparable suggesting a greater impairment in mental health of TRD patients compared to physical health impairment.

Table 3 Quality of life and functional impairment at Primary Visit[a] for TRD and non-TRD patients

Endpoint	TRD	Non-TRD	Mean Difference TRD vs non-TRD	95% CI	P-value
Quality of Life, mean					
Short form (SF-12) scores[c]					
Mental component	30.0	45.7	−15.7	−17, −14.4	<.0001
Physical component	47.7	48.9	−1.2	−2.1, −0.3	0.0126
Q-LES-Q General activities index	43.6	63.7	−20.1	−22.2, −18.1	<.0001
Functional impairment					
WSAS score	23.4	11.3	12.0	10.9, 13.2	<.0001
WPAI, %[b]					
Activity impairment	54.5	30.5	24.0	20.8, 27.2	<.0001
Percent hours missed	19.6	9.5	10.1	6.4, 13.8	<.0001
Work impairment	43.0	19.2	23.8	19.7, 27.9	<.0001
Overall work impairment	52.9	24.9	28.0	23, 33	<.0001

[a] The primary visit is the first visit in level 3 for TRD patients and the visit closest to 141 days from baseline visit and with a deviation ≤60 days for non-TRD patients

Least square means, 95% CIs, and p-values were obtained from a linear model adjusted for baseline of the variable, age category, gender, and baseline values of total severity score of comorbidity, Depression severity by HDRS17, and Depression severity by QIDS-SR16

[b]WPAI scores are based on 7-day recall period

SFHS Short form health survey, Q-LES-Q Quality of life enjoyment and satisfaction, WSAS Work and social adjustment scale, WPAI Work productivity and activity impairment, TRD Treatment resistant depression, CI Confidence interval

[c]Range of SF-12 scores reported: Mental Component 13.8 to 67.9; Physical Component 7.4 to 70.5. Lower score indicates poorer mental or physical health-related function and wellbeing

A previously published study used STAR*D data to assess the HRQOL of patients with MDD using Q-LES-Q. In that study, it was found that patients who did not remit or achieve adequate response to first line selective serotonin reuptake inhibitor treatment had poor Q-LES-Q scores which, while improved after second line therapy, however still failed to achieve normal scores [33]. The Q-LES-Q scores observed in the present study also indicate a generally poor HRQOL status in both TRD and non-TRD patients. However, the scores were significantly worse in TRD patients compared with non-TRD patients.

In the present study, it was found that patients with TRD had significantly greater functional impairments compared with non-TRD patients as measured by WSAS and WPAI scores. This finding is in agreement with a Canadian study [21] of outpatients with various depressive conditions, which found that patients with TRD had greater functional impairments when compared to patients with treatment responsive depression. Another study [20] showed that patients with primary unipolar major depression who achieved remission with residual symptoms had a longer period of impairment in occupational functioning, with worse overall scores on the Social Adaptation Scale and the Global Assessment of Functioning, compared to those who had remission without residual symptoms.

Generally, in the assessment of mental disorders, more importance has been given to management of symptoms rather than functional impairment [34]. The traditional HRQOL scales were based on symptomatic assessments made by a single respondent (either patient or physician). However, an emerging consensus has been developed in considering the patient's perspective related to functional impairment as an important aspect in monitoring and evaluating HRQOL outcomes [34, 35]. Thus, an increasing importance in the assessment of patient's perspective on impairments in addition to symptoms is needed.

We used patient-reported outcome (PRO) data from the STAR*D study to compare various aspects of humanistic burden in TRD and non-TRD patients. The STAR*D study was the first major study that investigated the effectiveness of treatments in outpatients with nonpsychotic MDD who did not achieve an adequate response after an initial antidepressant trial. The STAR*D study was designed to achieve more generalizability by including a more representative population, using minimal exclusion criteria and keeping the treatments unblinded [23]. Therefore, the results of the present study may be generalizable to the overall humanistic burden in TRD and non-TRD patients.

The use of STAR*D data may have limitations. As the STAR*D study was completed in 2006, the results do not fully reflect current medical practice and healthcare policies. It has been reported that TRD patients in the STAR*D study had higher rates of psychiatric comorbidities, [10] and the status of comorbidities or the association of comorbidities with clinical severity, HRQOL, and functional impairment was not addressed in our study. Also, since this is a secondary analysis of the STAR*D and based on a subgroup of patients (patients who entered level 3 of the STAR*D), there may be some selection bias.

Severity of illness, age at onset of MDD, ethnicity, marital status, employment status, educational level, and a number of other sociodemographic factors have been found to be associated with several domains of HRQOL in patients with depression [17, 36]. For instance, increased comorbidities, fewer years of education, unemployment, or belonging to a minority group were associated with worse physical and mental functions on the HRQOL domains [17, 36]. Since the baseline characteristics in our study were not balanced due to lack of randomization, it could have been a source of potential confounding. However, we adjusted the estimates for demographic and clinical characteristics including age, gender, the CIRS, HDRS17 and the QIDS-SR16. Additionally, as we did not assess any causal association, we can consider both the possibilities that it is the humanistic outcomes that interfered with the treatment effect or lack of effective treatment worsened humanistic outcomes.

Conclusion

The findings of the present study expand the evidence that patients with TRD experience greater humanistic burden measured as HRQOL, work and social functioning and work productivity compared with non-TRD patients. This highlights the humanistic burden of TRD, and its potential impact on the individual patient as well as on societal burden and costs. Further measures should be taken to limit the humanistic as well as the clinical and economic consequences of TRD.

Abbreviations

HRQOL: Health-related Quality of Life; MCS: Mental Component Summary; MDD: Major depressive disorder; NIMH: National Institute of Mental Health; PCS: Physical Component Summary; PRO: Patient-reported outcome; QIDS: Quick Inventory of Depressive Symptomatology; TRD: Treatment Resistant Depression; WPAI: Work Productivity and Activity Impairment; WSAS: Work and Social Adjustment Scale

Acknowledgements

The authors thank Dr. Rishabh Pandey (SIRO Clinpharm Pvt. Ltd.) for writing assistance and Dr. Ellen Baum (Janssen Research & Development, LLC) for additional editorial assistance.

Funding

This study was sponsored by Janssen Research & Development, LLC, and through the public-private real world evidence collaboration between Karolinska Institutet and Janssen Pharmaceuticals (contract: 5-63/2015). Authors designed the study and data collection, and performed analysis and interpretation of data. All authors fully met ICMJE authorship requirements. Janssen provided funding for medical writing support.
RB received funding from the Swedish Research Council (grant 2016-02362).

Authors' contribution

Conception and design: GL, LB, RB, JR, AD. Collection and assembly of data: N/A. Data analysis and interpretation: GL, XL, JX, LL, LB, PB, RB, JR, AD. Manuscript writing: All authors read and approved the final manuscript.

Consent for publication

Not applicable.

Competing interests

AD, XL, QZ, JX, LL, CJ, CB, KL, GL are employees of Janssen Research & Development, LLC and hold stocks in the company. LB, PB, RB, and JR are in research collaboration with Janssen for which grant support has been received by Karolinska Institutet. JR has been a speaker for Eli Lilly, received unrestricted grant support from Schering-Plough, and has conducted research in collaboration with AstraZeneca, and Pfizer, for which grant/research support has been received by Karolinska Institutet.

Author details

[1]Janssen Research & Development, LLC, Titusville, NJ, USA. [2]Janssen Scientific Affairs, LLC, Titusville, NJ, USA. [3]Department of Neuroscience, Psychiatry, Uppsala University, Uppsala, Sweden. [4]Centre for Pharmacoepidemiology, Clinical Epidemiology, Department of Medicine Solna, Karolinska Institutet, Karolinska University Hospital, Stockholm, Sweden. [5]Real World Evidence, Statistics & Decision Sciences, Janssen R&D US, 920 US Highway 202 S, Raritan, NJ 08869, USA.

References

1. The World Health Organization. Depression. http://www.who.int/mediacentre/factsheets/fs369/en/. Accessed 12 May 2017.
2. Papakostas GI, Petersen T, Mahal Y, Mischoulon D, Nierenberg AA, Fava M. Quality of life assessments in major depressive disorder: a review of the literature. Gen Hosp Psychiatry. 2004;26(1):13-7.
3. Gartlehner G, Wagner G, Matyas N, Titscher V, Greimel J, Lux L, Gaynes BN, Viswanathan M, Patel S, Lohr KN. Pharmacological and non-pharmacological treatments for major depressive disorder: review of systematic reviews. BMJ Open. 2017;7(6):e014912.
4. Al-Harbi KS. Treatment-resistant depression: therapeutic trends, challenges, and future directions. Patient Prefer Adherence. 2012;6:369-88.
5. Conway CR, George MS, Sackeim HA. Toward an evidence-based, operational definition of treatment-resistant depression: when enough is enough. JAMA Psychiatry. 2017;74(1):9-10.
6. Amos TB, Tandon N, Lefebvre P, Pilon D, Kamstra RL, Pivneva I, Greenberg PE. Direct and Indirect Cost Burden and Change of Employment Status in Treatment-Resistant Depression: a Matched-Cohort Study using a U.S. Commercial Claims Database. J Clin Psychiatry. 2018;79(2).
7. Olfson M, Amos T, Benson C, McRae J, Marcus S. Prospective service use and health care costs of Medicaid beneficiaries with treatment-resistant depression. J Managed Care Pharm. 2018;24(3):226-36.
8. Thase ME. Treatment-resistant depression: prevalence, risk factors, and treatment strategies. J Clin Psychiatry. 2011;72(5):e18.
9. Amital D, Fostick L, Silberman A, Beckman M, Spivak B. Serious life events among resistant and non-resistant MDD patients. J Affect Disord. 2008;110(3):260-4.
10. Rush AJ, Warden D, Wisniewski SR, Fava M, Trivedi MH, Gaynes BN, Nierenberg AA. STAR*D: revising conventional wisdom. CNS drugs. 2009;23(8):627-47.
11. Rush AJ, Trivedi MH, Wisniewski SR, Nierenberg AA, Stewart JW, Warden D, Niederehe G, Thase ME, Lavori PW, Lebowitz BD, et al. Acute and longer-term outcomes in depressed outpatients requiring one or several treatment steps: a STAR*D report. Am J Psychiatry. 2006;163(11):1905-17.
12. Bungay KM. Methods to assess the humanistic outcomes of clinical pharmacy services. Pharmacotherapy. 2000;20(10 Pt 2):253S-8S.
13. Barge-Schaapveld DQ, Nicolson NA, Berkhof J, de Vries MW. Quality of life in depression: daily life determinants and variability. Psychiatry Res. 1999;88(3):173-89.
14. Beck SL, Falkson G. Prevalence and management of cancer pain in South Africa. Pain. 2001;94(1):75-84.
15. Woo JH, Park HS, Kim SC, Kim YH. The effect of lumbar sympathetic ganglion block on gynecologic cancer-related lymphedema. Pain Physician. 2013;16(4):345-52.
16. Corey-Lisle PK, Birnbaum HG, Greenberg PE, Marynchenko MB, Claxton AJ. Identification of a claims data "signature" and economic consequences for treatment-resistant depression. J Clin Psychiatry. 2002;63(8):717-26.
17. Trivedi MH, Corey-Lisle PK, Guo Z, Lennox RD, Pikalov A, Kim E. Remission, response without remission, and nonresponse in major depressive disorder: impact on functioning. Int Clin Psychopharmacol. 2009;24(3):133-8.
18. Greenberg P, Corey-Lisle PK, Birnbaum H, Marynchenko M, Claxton A. Economic implications of treatment-resistant depression among employees. PharmacoEconomics. 2004;22(6):363-73.
19. Dunner DL, Rush AJ, Russell JM, Burke M, Woodard S, Wingard P, Allen J. Prospective, long-term, multicenter study of the naturalistic outcomes of patients with treatment-resistant depression. J Clin Psychiatry. 2006;67(5):688-95.
20. Kennedy N, Paykel ES. Residual symptoms at remission from depression: impact on long-term outcome. J Affect Disord. 2004;80(2-3):135-44.
21. Ravindran AV, Matheson K, Griffiths J, Merali Z, Anisman H. Stress, coping, uplifts, and quality of life in subtypes of depression: a conceptual frame and emerging data. J Affect Disord. 2002;71(1-3):121-30.
22. Hamilton M. A rating scale for depression. J Neurol Neurosurg Psychiatry. 1960;23:56-62.
23. Rush AJ, Fava M, Wisniewski SR, Lavori PW, Trivedi MH, Sackeim HA, Thase ME, Nierenberg AA, Quitkin FM, Kashner TM, et al. Sequenced treatment alternatives to relieve depression (STAR*D): rationale and design. Control Clin Trials. 2004;25(1):119-42.
24. National Institute of Mental Health (NIMH). NIMH Data Archive Data Use Certification. https://data-archive.nimh.nih.gov/s/sharedcontent/about/policy. Accessed 9 Oct 2018.
25. Gaynes BN, Warden D, Trivedi MH, Wisniewski SR, Fava M, Rush AJ. What did STAR*D teach us? Results from a large-scale, practical, clinical trial for patients with depression. Psychiatr Serv. 2009;60(11):1439-45.
26. Lavori PW, Rush AJ, Wisniewski SR, Alpert J, Fava M, Kupfer DJ, Nierenberg A, Quitkin FM, Sackeim HA, Thase ME, et al. Strengthening clinical effectiveness trials: equipoise-stratified randomization. Biol Psychiatry. 2001;50(10):792-801.
27. Linn BS, Linn MW, Gurel L. Cumulative illness rating scale. J Am Geriatr Soc. 1968;16(5):622-6.
28. Rush AJ, Trivedi MH, Ibrahim HM, Carmody TJ, Arnow B, Klein DN, Markowitz JC, Ninan PT, Kornstein S, Manber R, et al. The 16-item quick inventory of depressive symptomatology (QIDS), clinician rating (QIDS-C), and self-report (QIDS-SR): a psychometric evaluation in patients with chronic major depression. Biol Psychiatry. 2003;54(5):573-83.
29. Salyers MP, Bosworth HB, Swanson JW, Lamb-Pagone J, Osher FC. Reliability and validity of the SF-12 health survey among people with severe mental illness. Med Care. 2000;38(11):1141-50.
30. Wyrwich KW, Harnam N, Revicki DA, Locklear JC, Svedsater H, Endicott J. Assessment of quality of life enjoyment and satisfaction questionnaire-short form responder thresholds in generalized anxiety disorder and bipolar disorder studies. Int Clin Psychopharmacol. 2011;26(3):121-9.

31. Gill SC, Butterworth P, Rodgers B, Mackinnon A. Validity of the mental health component scale of the 12-item short-form health survey (MCS-12) as measure of common mental disorders in the general population. Psychiatry Res. 2007;152(1):63–71.

32. Vilagut G, Forero CG, Pinto-Meza A, Haro JM, de Graaf R, Bruffaerts R, Kovess V, de Girolamo G, Matschinger H, Ferrer M, et al. The mental component of the short-form 12 health survey (SF-12) as a measure of depressive disorders in the general population: results with three alternative scoring methods. Value Health. 2013;16(4):564–73.

33. IsHak WW, Mirocha J, Pi S, Tobia G, Becker B, Peselow ED, Cohen RM. Patient-reported outcomes before and after treatment of major depressive disorder. Dialogues Clin Neurosci. 2014;16(2):171–83.

34. Mundt JC, Marks IM, Shear MK, Greist JH. The work and social adjustment scale: a simple measure of impairment in functioning. Br J Psychiatry. 2002; 180:461–4.

35. Sainfort F, Becker M, Diamond R. Judgments of quality of life of individuals with severe mental disorders: patient self-report versus provider perspectives. Am J Psychiatry. 1996;153(4):497–502.

36. Daly EJ, Trivedi MH, Wisniewski SR, Nierenberg AA, Gaynes BN, Warden D, Morris DW, Luther JF, Farabaugh A, Cook I, et al. Health-related quality of life in depression: a STAR*D report. Ann Clin Psychiatry. 2010;22(1):43–55.

20

A qualitative analysis of suicidal psychiatric inpatients views and expectations of psychological therapy to counter suicidal thoughts, acts and deaths

Yvonne F Awenat[1,2,4*] [iD], Sarah Peters[1,2,3], Patricia A Gooding[1,2,3], Daniel Pratt[1,2,4], Emma Shaw-Núñez[1,4], Kamelia Harris[1] and Gillian Haddock[1,2,4]

Abstract

Background: Suicide is a global problem and suicidal behavior is common in acute psychiatric wards. Inpatient suicides regularly occur with 10.4/100,000 such deaths recorded in the UK in 2016. Inpatient suicides are potentially the most avoidable of all suicides as inpatients have 24-h staff contact. Current inpatient treatment prioritizes maintenance of physical safety by observation, medication and general supportive measures, however efficacious and effective specific treatments are lacking. Psychological treatments have a growing evidence base for suicide prevention yet provision of inpatient therapy is uncommon. The present qualitative study aimed to understand the patient acceptability issues by investigating suicidal inpatients views and expectations of a novel suicide-focussed cognitive behavioural psychological therapy which was nested alongside a pilot clinical trial of the intervention.

Methods: Thematic analysis of semi-structured individual qualitative interviews with twenty suicidal psychiatric inpatients to investigate their views and expectations about ward-based suicide-focused psychological treatment.

Results: Two main themes were identified. The first, 'A therapy that works', revealed inpatients' views of the necessary components for effective ward-based suicide-focused psychological therapy. The second, 'Concerns about in-patient suicide-focused therapy', depicted their fears about engaging in this treatment. Results suggested that suicide-focused psychological therapy was cautiously welcomed by inpatients' whose narratives expressed their needs, priorities and concerns. Further data analysis enabled formation of a user-informed model of suicide-focussed psychological therapy which offers guidance for researchers and clinicians.

Conclusions: We conclude that hospitalization of suicidal individuals offers a critical opportunity to intervene with effective treatment to preserve life and that suicide-focussed psychological therapy is likely to be well received by suicidal inpatients warranting further testing with a sufficiently powered definitive trial. It is important that provision of ward-based psychological therapy for suicidal inpatients addresses the considerable context-specific challenges inherent in this setting.

Keywords: Suicide prevention, Psychiatric inpatients, Psychological therapy, Qualitative, User-views, Implementation

* Correspondence: Yvonne.awenat@manchester.ac.uk
[1]Division of Psychology and Mental Health, School of Health Sciences, University of Manchester, Zochonis Building, Brunswick St, Manchester M13 9PL, UK
[2]Manchester Academic Health Science Centre, MAHSC, Manchester, UK
Full list of author information is available at the end of the article

Background

Suicide is a global problem equating to one death and 20 attempted suicides every 40 s [1]. Internationally suicide rates vary, with 13.4/100,000 population suicide deaths recorded for 2016 in USA [2] and 10.91/100,000 population suicides recorded across Europe [3] during 2015. UK data for 2016 indicates 13.4/100,000 suicide deaths of which 28% were by mental health patients, 9% of which are attributed to inpatients [4]. Morbidity from repetitious suicidal behaviour is common in UK psychiatric wards where individuals at high risk of suicide are frequently admitted [5]. Psychiatric in-patient treatment prioritizes maintenance of physical safety by observation, medication and general supportive measures, yet despite 24-h staff presence, in-patient suicides persist, with 1443 suicides recorded during 2005–2015 [4, 5].

International health reforms driven by greater focus on community based treatment and economic pressures have resulted in reduced psychiatric bed availability in the USA [6], Europe [7], Israel [8] and in the UK, where 42% of psychiatric beds were closed during 2000–2012 [9]. Consequently, pressure on remaining beds has resulted in shorter hospitalization episodes, with those lasting less than one week being linked to post-discharge suicide [4]. In-patient suicides are particularly preventable as the 24-h staff contact offers a unique opportunity to intervene [10], yet effective suicide prevention interventions for in-patients remain elusive.

Psychological therapy has a growing evidence base for suicide prevention, for example: dialectical behavioural therapy (DBT) [11], psychodynamic-interpersonal therapy [12], suicide-focused counselling [13], and cognitive behaviour therapy (CBT) [14–18]. A systematic review and meta-analysis [18] of several forms of psychological therapy found CBT to demonstrate superior outcomes for repetition of self-harm at 12 months follow-up (OR 0.80, 95%; CI 0.65–0.98; 10 trials; n = 2232), which accords with the results of an earlier systematic review [14] which also found CBT to be most efficacious. The UK National Institute for Health and Care Excellence (NICE) [16]. recommends CBT for suicidal patients in any treatment setting. However, despite international recognition of the value of psychological treatment for suicidal in-patients (e.g., South Africa [19], USA [20]; UK [16], Sri Lanka [21], India [22]), provision remains inconsistent. Within UK psychiatric hospitals suicidal in-patients rarely receive psychological therapy as usual practice favours post-discharge referral for psychological treatment [23]. Consequently, publications of studies about adult in-patients' experiences of psychological suicide-prevention treatments are scarce. Several studies of community-dwelling patients' evaluations of suicide-focused psychological interventions exist [24–26], all reporting generally positive experiences and satisfaction

of participants. Most participants continued to experience suicidal ideation but perceived that therapy had equipped them with skills to avert transition of thoughts to suicidal behaviour [24–26]. However congruence of views and experiences of community and in-patient populations cannot be assumed given their different clinical and contextual situations [27].

Evaluations of psychological treatments for suicide-prevention commonly report standardised measures of psychopathology, which although crucial to quantifying clinical efficacy, fail to address patient expectations and experiences which, as determinants of treatment response, also impact on clinical efficacy [28]. It is therefore important that therapy is 'efficacious' in terms of having demonstrated positive clinical outcomes for research participants under strictly controlled scientific conditions, *and* is 'effective' in terms of real-world patient acceptability [29]. Where patient experience of suicide-focussed therapy has been studied, the focus is typically on post-therapy evaluations [24–26], however, this fails to elicit the beliefs and expectations of *potential* recipients [28]. Patient's 'expectancy effects' [30] and role expectations of self and therapist influence the quality of the therapeutic alliance [31], which, as a component of efficacy [32], is essential for therapeutic change [33, 34]. Such constructs are suggested to account for 15–33% of the treatment effect [30, 35], indicating the importance of attention to such issues during treatment innovation as recommended by the UK Medical Research Council [36].

As uptake of and adherence to psychological interventions by suicidal populations is problematic [37–39], it is imperative to develop therapies that are acceptable to patients. Within health behaviour theory [40] Janz's value-expectancy health belief model [41] offers guidance for improving adherence to psychological treatments by suicidal patients, purporting that an individual's willingness to enact change behaviour (i.e., uptake psychological therapy) is dependent on how likely that action is perceived to achieve their desired outcome. It is therefore important that patients comprehend and have confidence in their treatment which accords with UK National Health Service (NHS) priorities [42].

Historical literature portrays the challenges and complex interpersonal dynamics for suicidal inpatients and professional staff alike with Morgan's [43] conceptualisation of 'malignant alienation' whereby pernicious contextual psychosocial forces within inpatient wards alienate staff from inpatients and vice versa. Indeed, contemporary qualitative accounts of inpatients' experiences of psychiatric hospitalisation continue to attest to perceptions of untherapeutic regimes which fail to meet their psychological needs [19, 44, 45]. Whilst there is an urgent need for effective treatments for suicidal in-patients whose hospitalisation offers a critical opportunity to avert suicide, the psychiatric ward setting itself presents major contextual challenges [46], including the potential of exacerbation of self-harm behaviour [47] and heightened suicide risk [48]. It is important that treatments aimed at helping are acceptable to the suicidal patients as negative experiences of suicide-prevention treatments may worsen the patients' condition [49]. The qualitative study presented in this paper therefore aimed to investigate suicidal in-patients' views and expectations of a novel ward-based suicide-focussed psychological therapy intervention nested within a pilot feasibility clinical trial [50]. We believe this to be the first study of this population and topic.

Methods

Design

This qualitative study was nested within a mixed-method feasibility study involving a pilot clinical trial which was conducted from October 2013 to December 2016 across five acute adult psychiatric wards of a NHS mental health service in Northern England. Qualitative approaches have been successfully applied in previous studies of suicidal patients views [18, 25, 49, 51] and were therefore selected as suitable to investigate the plethora of 'unknowns' regarding potential therapy recipients' views, perceptions and expectations of a new suicide-focussed psychological treatment. Data collection was by face-to-face semi-structured individual interviews to provide inpatient participants' with a calm and private setting conducive to discussion of personal and potentially sensitive views [51].

Inclusion and exclusion criteria

Participants were current in-patients of a public mental health hospital in Northern England who were aged 18 years or over and had self-reported experience of suicidal thoughts or behaviour within the past three months. Participants were excluded if they lacked capacity to provide informed consent.

Recruitment

Ethical approval was granted by a statutory UK Research Ethics Committee (13/NW/0504). Recruitment for this qualitative study occurred during the consultation period during which trial procedures and therapy content were being refined [50], hence participants had real potential to influence the intervention. Purposive sampling [52, 53] was employed to recruit current inpatients who met the eligibility criteria necessary to provide data to address the aims of this research. All in-patients were informed about the study by ward staff in the first instance. Those who expressed interest in taking part were then contacted by either the first and fifth authors who provided further verbal and written information and allowed a minimum of 24 h for individuals to

consider their decision. All patients informed about the study ($N = 20$) expressed interest and subsequently provided written informed consent. Researchers involved in direct contact with participants were trained in ethical participant care including assessment of participant's capacity to provide informed consent. An 'ethics-as-process' approach [54] was taken whereby assessment of capacity was conducted during inpatients' initial meeting with researchers and then re-confirmed during the subsequent meeting prior to obtaining formal written informed consent, and again prior to and during qualitative interviewing. Recruitment continued until theoretical saturation was reached at which point sufficient data to satisfy the study aims had been collected [52].

Semi-structured interview

Given the sensitive topic and participants' vulnerability, considerable attention was invested in interviewer training to ensure participant safety [51]. A semi-structured interview schedule based on current literature with further refinement and piloting by a Service User Group (comprised of eight people with past experience of psychiatric inpatient treatment for suicidality) was developed. Interview questions were 'funnelled' to present opening questions about general experiences of ward treatments and psychological therapy prior to suicide-focused questions (e.g., views about suicide-focussed psychological therapy), finally ending with less personal topics (e.g., views of the interview process). Interviews were digitally audio-recorded and transcribed verbatim (at which point all identifying data was anonymised) following which recordings were deleted. All participants were debriefed post-interview to ensure provision of appropriate support for any distress.

Analysis

Analysis was led by the first author assisted by the second, fifth and sixth authors who contributed to initial and iterations of coding with further contributions to critical discussions of analytic interpretations from the third, fourth and seventh authors thereby enhancing trustworthiness of the final themes [55]. Inductive Thematic Analysis, recognised as a systematic method of identifying thematic patterns across the data corpus was employed utilizing Braun and Clark's [56] recommended six-phase analytical procedures. We adopted constant comparative approach whereby data generation and coding occurred in parallel to enable ongoing analysis to inform questioning in subsequent interviews [56, 57]. This was achieved by reflection on field notes taken during interviews and review of recent audio-recordings to identify topics requiring further probing or participant generated issues not listed in the core interview schedule. As such, this represented the first phase of analysis although not being a discreet entity, this was continued throughout the analytic process. First phase familiarisation with the data continued by reading each transcript several times to identify potential relevant areas of interest. Moving into the second phase of analysis involved manual line-by-line analysis to name segments of data as tentative codes, following which in the third phase codes with a common meaning were clustered together as potential themes. During the fourth and fifth phases theme names and contents were reviewed and subjected to critical interrogation by the wider research team to check their data-driven genesis. The final sixth phase comprised preparation of the manuscript involving conceptualising the explanatory narrative and selection of the most pertinent data extracts as illustrative quotes.

A reflexive stance of 'empathic neutrality' was taken by the research team who recognised the potential influence of personal beliefs and preconceptions on analytic processes yet aspired to interpret and report participants' narratives as true to their experience. The research team comprised academics (a doctoral student and junior / senior researchers) and academic / clinicians (two Clinical Psychologists' and one Registered Nurse) assisted by the Service User Reference Group comprised of eight individuals' with prior experience of psychiatric hospitalisation and suicidality. This enabled a wide range of views to be considered during research meetings where analytic interpretations were discussed.

Results

Participants

Twenty participants, comprising fourteen males, were recruited from five acute psychiatric wards in a NHS psychiatric hospital in Northern England, UK. Self-reported demographic data indicated participants' ages ranged from 22 to 65 years (median 38.1); duration of hospitalisation spanned from two to 672 days (median:21); and previous admissions during the past year ranged from none to three. Participants self-reported their reasons for admission, choosing to provide their diagnosis or perception of a precipitant event. Further details are provided in Table 1.

Overview of key findings

Analysis identified two themes (Table 2), each with three sub-themes. Theme 1 - 'A therapy that works', epitomised participants' perceptions of the influences and necessary components for effective ward-based suicide-focused psychological therapy. Theme 2 - 'Concerns about in-patient suicide-focused therapy' depicted participants' fears about engaging with therapy. Findings were further synthesized to develop a user-informed model (Table 3).

Theme 1: A therapy that 'works'

This theme reflected participants' perceptions of context-specific internal and external influences and necessary features required for a therapy that would 'work' for suicidal psychiatric in-patients.

Past experiences shaped expectations

One-fifth of participants reported they had previously received psychological therapy, although only one participant had received therapy in a psychiatric ward setting. Some participants were perplexed about the different terms used to depict psychological therapy: *"I don't know. What is psychological therapy? ... I've done CBT?" (P09).*

CBT was the most commonly experienced therapy, although participants tended to speak of 'counselling' when referring to any type of psychotherapy. Discussions about experiences of therapy invariably gravitated to whether it had *'worked'* or not.

Evaluations were judged according to perceptions of how successful therapy had been in addressing personally held goals, which for some, was eradication of particular symptoms:

"I've had CBT, I've had lots and lots of therapies in [hospital]... when it comes to the severe depression, the suicidal feelings, the attempted suicides – they went away." (P07)

Dissatisfaction with psychological therapy resulted when it failed to meet prior expectations. Some participants were unprepared to openly discuss difficult and sensitive issues from their past, attributing subsequent worsening of their condition to such talk:

"When I used to see the psychologist sometimes and started drinking heavier and heavier because I was having to talk a lot about me past and stuff... it was just all buried stuff." (P02).

For some, the therapist's passive style was incompatible with their expectations: *"I've had counselling... it was drink-related but I didn't find it helpful at all... all the guy did was just nod and it started to irritate me." (P05).* An expectation of two-way communication was common and, where lacking, could precipitate collapse of the therapeutic relationship, *"It was me doing all the talking, it was him listening with no feedback and if I don't get any feedback then I can't work with anybody." (P02).*

Suicidality-specific goals Participants described some expectations or goals for therapy that were particularly

Table 1 Participant Socio-demographic Information

Ppt.	Reason for admission	Length of stay on ward in days	Admissions in last 12 months	Diagnosis	Previous psychological therapy
1.	Hearing voices	21	1	SCZ[4]	No
2.	Overdose	21	1	U	Yes
3.	U	112	u	MDD[2]	No
4.	Sectioned	336	u	Alcoholism	No
5.	Breakdown; overdose	10	2	U	Yes
6.	Repeated overdoses	49	1	Emotionally unstable PD[1]	No
7.	Overdose (Sectioned)	u	u	Anxiety	Yes
8.	U	u	u	U	No
9.	Manic / high; overdose	38	u	Bipolar / PD[1]	Yes
10.	Hearing voices	21	1	Voices / SCZ[4]	No
11.	Suicidal	17	1	U	No
12.	U	14	1	Bipolar / PD[1]	No
13.	U	84	2	SCZ[4]	No
14.	Suicidal	21	0	Depression	No
15.	Stopped clozapine	7	0	SCZ[4]	No
16.	Suicidal	10	0	U	No
17.	Self-harm	672	u	PTSD[2] / Emotionally unstable PD[1]	No
18.	Feeling down	2	0	Depression	No
19.	Mental breakdown	7	0	U	No
20.	Hearing voices	12	3	U	No

Abbreviations: Gender *M* Male, *F* Female, *PD*[1] Personality Disorder; *PTSD*[2] Post Traumatic Stress Disorder, *MDD* Major Depression Disorder[3], *SCZ* Schizophrenia [4], *U* data unavailable

related to addressing their suicidality (i.e., their suicidal thoughts or behaviours) which invariably prioritised relief from distress:

"I'm willing to give anything a go to stop me feeling like this." (P11).

Another priority was discharge from hospital, yet participants understood that discharge was unlikely while still engaging in suicidal behaviour, making cessation of such behaviour important:

"probably any idea or whatever to try and stop self-harming or doing overdoses ... I just hope it [therapy] would help and then I can get discharged." (P06).

Table 2 Themes and Sub-themes

Theme 1: A Therapy that 'works'	Theme 2: Concerns about inpatient suicide -focused therapy
Past experiences shaped expectations	A secure therapeutic relationship
Suicidality-specific goals	Potential for harm
Mechanisms: how suicide-focussed therapy works	Ending therapy

Participants perceived that suicide-focused therapy could offer a route to understanding and making sense of their suicidal crisis. Improved self-understanding and development of self-management strategies were seen as pivotal to avoid future suicidal behaviour representing strategies that could be used beyond hospitalisation:

"Now, if you're to sit me down and say, "Well, why do you want to take your life? What's your thinking behind wanting to take your life? What's causing you to think the way you do?" . . . looking at cognition, thinking styles, patterns, trying to challenge them." (P07).

"help me to recognise when I'm going to be suicidal and perhaps be able to do something about it." (P02).

Suicide-focussed therapy was welcomed as participants' recounted few opportunities to talk about being suicidal with ward staff. Talk was perceived as an essential vehicle for self-understanding with therapy being recognised as a potentially helpful intervention.

"just talking about the suicidal thoughts... and why I've got them... talking about it would just help really 'cos there's no one to talk to about it, so it'd be best to

Table 3 User-informed conceptual model of in-patient suicide-focused psychological therapy [52]

Stage of therapy	Client's Need	Supporting data	Therapeutic approach
Immediate	Feel safe. Overcome fear of talking about suicide.	"… it might make me more suicidal. Because the question is being asked all the time and even though I have tried to take my life numerous times …And if it's prevalent, if it's there and somebody's reminding you of it, you're more likely to do it" (P02)	Explore potential barriers to therapy and if necessary defuse fears of talking about suicide.
	Development of strong therapeutic relationship.	"You can go and just relax and like express yourself with that person, with free of them judging you. .." (P19)	Create a safe environment conducive to building secure, 'containing' therapeutic relationship. Promote trust by empathic validation of client's distress and by allowing client to set the pace and depth of discussions. Demonstrate collaboration with client by negotiating acceptable levels of information sharing with ward staff.
	Catharsis / Relief from distress.	"Being able to talk about what you've done [suicidal behaviour] and someone to listen" (P06)	Facilitate client to share experiences of suicidal ideation and behaviour by demonstrating non-judgement and empathy. Normalise client's experiences to promote a sense of feeling understood. Self-soothing by relaxation/breathing practices. End of session grounding techniques during last 5–10 min.
	Tolerating intense negative emotions / suicidal thoughts and prevention of suicidal behaviour.	"I'd be worried what will happen once that barrier's been broke down to tell you the truth. Because I don't know whether I'd start crying or get angry." (P14)	Guide development and practice of distress tolerance skills / techniques to overcome emotional avoidance and emotional dysregulation. Develop attentional control, attentional broadening and switching techniques to reduce threat-based information processing biases. Promote clients' sense of agency by assisting recall of experiences of overcoming suicidal states.
Intermediate	Make sense of suicidal thoughts and behaviour.	"Trying to get rid of the suicidal thoughts, just talking about the suicidal thoughts… and why I've got them… talking about it would just help really 'cos there's no one to talk to about it, so it'd be best to just to have someone to talk to about the suicidal thoughts and what they're about." (P10)	Collaborative development of individualised formulation. Foster therapist - client's shared understanding of drivers and inhibitors of suicidality/suicidal behaviour. Identify therapeutic goals targeting suicide reduction. Reflect on experiences of helpful and unhelpful escapes from distress.
	Self-understanding and self-management of emotions and cognitions.	"Help me to recognise when I'm going to be suicidal and perhaps be able to do something about it." (P02)	Provide exit points from suicidal thoughts and cognitions by: - Identifying and challenging negative self-appraisals. - Cultivating emotional regulation skills and positive affect / self-image techniques. - Generating problem-solving strategies to manage threats associated with suicidal cognitions.
	Regain personal independence, and social confidence / functioning.	"It's more like building up my social skills a bit more and like talking to people in a group". (P19)	Behavioural activation and activity scheduling. Improve self-esteem / confidence building to develop stronger sense of personal agency. Promote positive beliefs about coping and resilience.
Longer term	Reclaim personhood and positive self-identity.	"Getting me life back. Yeah and get back in work and get back to the person I used to be."(P05).	Develop stronger recognition of own values and hopes for the future. Re-establish connecting with previous achievements.
	Re-establishment / improvement of close relationships. Harnessing support and understanding of family.	"And it would help others come to terms with the illness as well, i.e. your mum or your dad or your brother or your sisters who you live with or your partner." (P01)	Discuss possibility of information sharing with and/or involvement of family in therapy and longer-term suicide prevention plans.

Table 4 Recommendations for research and practice of suicide-focused psychological therapy

In-patients' views	Implications for suicide-focused therapy	Recommendations for therapist
Past negative experiences of therapy	Unsatisfactory previous experience of therapy may prevent uptake of suicide-focused therapy. May lead to avoidable dissatisfaction and attrition if therapist not aware of clients' expectations and preferences.	Enquire about and consider the impact of any past experiences of therapy. Provide clear information about the nature and demands of suicide-focused therapy and the potential for negative therapeutic reaction.
Confusion / lack of understanding of aims and functions of psychological therapy	Potential for disappointment if client's expectations of therapy cannot be met. Need to identify and manage realistic expectations. Need for active client engagement during and in-between sessions.	Discuss and mutually agree expectations including client's expectations of own and therapist's role, and therapist's expectations of client's role.
Concerns about trust and confidentiality of information disclosed in therapy	Lack of trust and confidence in confidentiality may impact on continued uptake and engagement. Demonstration of openness and transparency by therapist explaining own responsibility for breaking confidentiality if concerned for client's safety may serve to build trust. Therapist must inform ward team if actual or risk of harm to client or others disclosed in therapy. Need to clarify client's wishes of who non-risk information may or may not be shared with.	Allow time for trust to develop recognising the particular challenges for inpatients who may be involuntarily detained. Demonstrate consistent reliable behaviour Discuss limits of confidentiality with client. Discuss when and how any disclosures of actual or risk of harm to self or others would be managed respecting clients' preferences where possible. Agree what and with whom other information may be shared with (e.g., ward staff, family).
Fear or unwillingness to talk about suicide	Willingness to discuss suicide is essential for suicide-focused therapy. Covert fears of potential for harm may impede engagement in therapy.	Important to give full information about the need to talk about suicide to enable informed consent. Proactive discussion to elicit any client fears about perceived dangers of talking about suicide. Provide reassurance that client will retain control of the depth and pace of therapy.
Concerns about the ending of therapy	Anxiety about possibility of abrupt ending of sessions may affect ability to engage in therapy.	Involve client in discussions about preferences for ending of therapy. Offer ways of gradual spacing of session intervals, follow-up or booster sessions.

just to have someone to talk to about the suicidal thoughts and what they're about." (P10).

In expressing optimism towards the possibility of a suicide-focused psychotherapy, one participant alluded to the quintessential dilemma inherent in the suicidal crisis itself, of the ambivalence between wanting to die, and also wanting to be saved. This dilemma occurred at a time when help appeared inaccessible or unavailable suggesting that provision of a suicide-focused psychological therapy could address an important unmet need:

"if I really wanted to kill myself I wouldn't tell anybody I was going to do it I would go to a forest where no one would find me and hang myself from a tree... these people, who have had five failed suicide attempts, they are cries for help, they wanted to be found, because if you wanted to kill yourself, you're not daft you know how to do it, wouldn't you? It's because they can't get help, but now that your thing [suicide-focused therapy] will be implemented they won't have to do that, think of all of the lives you'll save." (P12).

Mechanisms: How suicide-focused therapy 'works'
Participants perceived that therapy would work by fulfilling

their need to talk about their suicidal thoughts and behaviours. They perceived this necessary to understand and make sense of their situation. The option of a suicide-focussed psychological therapy was attractive, as requests to talk with staff were frequently reported as unavailable leaving participants feeling isolated and frustrated when the only intervention offered was a pharmacological sedative.

"in hospital they just ask you have you got them [suicidal thoughts] and if you have then they just try and give you some medication for it, they don't talk about why you've got them..." (P10).

Participants alluded to a belief that in-depth reflection and discussion of their innermost fears was necessary in order to overcome these, and that therapy would enable cathartic ventilation of worries and purposeful endeavour to problem-solve underlying issues.

"Well, it's to try to get you to open up isn't it? ... And talk about things that are on your mind and your worries and all that. And I think the therapy part of it is to... help you to face your fears and your worries." (P14).

Therapy was seen as a route to recovery beyond hospitalisation during the suicidal crisis, offering individuals' support to improve social confidence and other aspects of psychological wellbeing necessary for restoration of usual lifestyle roles despite the challenges of on-going problems. For example, recovery of lost personhood and meaningful occupation were important to participants:

"Getting me life back. Yeah and get back in work and get back to the person I used to be."(P05).

"building up my social skills a bit more and like talking to people in a group." (P19).

Participants also perceived that the benefits of therapy could extend to family members:

"coming to terms with your illness is one part. And it would help others come to terms with the illness as well, i.e., your mum or your dad or your brother or your sisters who you live with or your partner." (P01).

Participants articulated clear expectations of the essential qualities necessary for an in-patient therapist, recognising the importance of a strong therapeutic relationship for successful therapy:

"empathy, having the ability to climb into someone's internal frame of reference... communicate on their wavelength. Being able to listen actively" (P07).

Theme 2: Concerns about inpatient suicide-focused therapy

The second theme illustrated participants' perceptions of contextual barriers for ward-based suicide-focused therapy specific to the therapeutic relationship and therapy process.

A secure therapeutic relationship The primacy of a safe therapeutic relationship built on trust and confidentiality was universal among participants; *"If you don't establish trust or the chemistry is wrong between the therapist and the client, it won't work." (P07).* However, there were concerns that trust could be particularly challenging for suicidal in-patients: *"I don't know how you convince people to trust you when they're finding it hard to trust people anyway?" (P14).*

Participants' related past negative experiences of broken trust where disclosure of suicidal thoughts and covert suicidal acts to staff had resulted in undesirable consequences; *"I've opened up to people in the past and they've used it against me" (P14).* However, mistrust was not global and fellow in-patients sometimes became trusted confidantes; *"last night I wanted to [ligature]... I can talk to my friend in here, not the staff" (P06).*

Similar concerns were held about confidentiality of therapy sessions: *"They [inpatients] can be very suspicious with therapies... they don't trust the information they give will be confidential, even though they [therapists] say it will be..." (P07).* Tension existed between participants' need to talk about suicide during therapy knowing that the therapist would have to inform ward staff should there be concerns of imminent risk of self-harm which could threaten willingness to engage in therapy and divulge suicidal thoughts:

"If I told you I'm going to hang myself tonight, you'd have to tell the nurses, wouldn't you?" (P13).

Others were more comfortable with the therapist sharing risk information with ward staff, but would wish to impose restrictions and exercise control over the destiny of particularly personal information:

"Well with me, it [sharing information] wouldn't bother me. It just depends what they're going to do with that information... How far is it allowed to go? ... In my case, there'd be one or two things where I wouldn't be comfortable with staff knowing." (P14).

There were greater concerns about sharing information with relatives and some participants would refuse permission for the therapist to discuss matters with family:

"The family, I think, would, that's on a need-to-know basis. You don't want to upset family members for no reason." (P11).

"No, I wouldn't want it shared with family and friends 'cause it's supposed to be a private session." (P10).

Potential for harm Emotional avoidance was evident with one participant alluding to a protective 'barrier' behind which intense and potentially overwhelming emotions were contained, being fearful of negative consequences if required to talk about sensitive matters; *"I'd be worried what will happen once that barrier's been broke down to tell you the truth. Because I don't know whether I'd start crying or get angry." (P14).* Others feared that talking about being suicidal might make them more suicidal: *"... it might make me more suicidal...and if it's prevalent, if it's there and somebody's reminding you of it, you're more likely to do it" (P02).*

Ending therapy There were concerns that abrupt ending of therapy could result in 'unfinished business' leaving individuals vulnerable and unsupported with suggestions for provision of post-discharge community therapy:

"If you give therapy and it's not completed, they may have issues, very sensitive, emotionally driven issues, that have been touched upon, which made it worse and it's not been treated effectively. You can end up being worse off. Whereas, to give them the continuous care therapy in the community, if they do get discharged... that would be a very good thing" (P07).

A therapy that 'works': User-informed conceptual model of in-patient suicide-focused psychological therapy

Further analysis enabled creation of a framework linking user-informed acceptability prerequisites with tenets of suicide-focused psychological therapy [52] expressed as a tentative conceptual model (see Table 3). This offers information to assist future researchers and clinicians in delivering 'psychologically-informed' suicide prevention interventions and provides a benchmark for further testing and hypothesis development. A collective of participant's expressed needs and valued outcomes have been aligned with temporal stages of suggested therapeutic techniques based on a cognitive behavioural suicide prevention therapy manual [52]. Flexibility and individualisation for particular clients is required. In the immediacy of suicidal crisis, individual's needs for catharsis and relief of psychological distress by therapeutic talk within a safe, secure and trusting therapeutic relationship are prioritised. Following this, the need for self-understanding to enable proactive self-care and avert future suicidal behaviour is suggested. Quality of life and functional outcomes were also seen as important to support and sustain maintenance of improved psychological health.

Discussion
Main findings
This is the first study to investigate suicidal in-patients views and expectations of suicide-focused psychological therapy and offers important insights of the 'real-world' contextual needs and challenges around provision of psychological therapy for suicidal in-patients.

Incompatibility of service objectives and in-patient needs
Dominating the findings was in-patients' needs for therapeutic talk to process, make sense of, and address their suicidality which does not accord with prevailing models of psychiatric treatment for suicidal in-patients, which prioritize physical safety by observation and containment [58]. Insufficient opportunity to explore the emotional impact of being suicidal and to find solutions to the problems that precipitated admission creates the potential for reinforcement and entrenchment of the in-patients' status quo. Despite the existence of scientific knowledge of the modifiable psychological factors which have been shown to be associated with suicidality (i.e., hopelessness, defeat and entrapment [59]), we found that suicidal inpatient participants' reported no opportunities to receive any psychological treatment. Such lack of attention to the psychological architecture of suicidality along with the associated negative experiences of in-patient treatment may be contributory factors to the persistently high 'revolving-door' readmission rates and post-discharge escalations of suicide rates [4, 48, 60].

Participants described how attempts to discuss suicidal thoughts with staff were thwarted by rebuffs or offers of sedative medication to the detriment of addressing their needs for therapeutic talk. Whilst sedation offers temporary relief from intense emotional distress, it is not an appropriate substitute for substantive treatment of suicidality, and used in this manner may impose a state of emotional avoidance likely to perpetuate psychological morbidity [61–64]. This exposes a major conflict between the aims and priorities of staff and in-patients. In reality, staff have limited access to nonpharmacological interventions and psychiatric wards are busy, unpredictable and impose vast personal demands on staff caring for suicidal in-patients [5, 46, 58]. A recent study of ward staff experiences of working with suicidal in-patients identified a culture where risk aversive avoidance of suicide-talk dominated their practice highlighting the need for staff training [65]. Indeed the results from this study of suicidal inpatients' experiences confirm this and demonstrate the impasse between the needs and fears of suicidal in-patients and those of ward staff adding further support of the need for ward staff training.

Barriers to suicide-focussed therapy
Past negative experiences
Some participants held negative views of psychological therapy based on past unsatisfactory experiences, for example, discussion of sensitive matters during therapy was perceived to have worsened their condition. Past experiences are important as they impact on expectations of future therapy [28, 66] and where negative, are likely to adversely affect desire and willingness to engage in further therapy. The notion of 'negative therapeutic reaction' is recognised within psychotherapy, commonly presenting during initial therapy sessions as a transient sequel to discussion of painful and deeply suppressed issues [67]. Therefore, to avoid disengagement or withdrawal from therapy, it is important to inform recipients of the potential for a transient worsening of their condition and discuss how this would be managed. Some participants perceived therapist passivity as disengaging, indicating the need to discuss role expectations with potential clients as pre-therapy *'role induction'* is strongly

associated with reduced attrition and better clinical outcomes [68].

Fears of increased suicidality

Participants viewed relief of distress as the prime goal of therapy, yet some feared that suicide-focussed therapy might increase distress or even trigger suicidal ideation representing a potential barrier to accepting such treatment. Willingness to talk about suicide is essential for suicide-focussed psychological therapy, and indeed, has been shown to be a key aspect of effective psychological treatments for suicide [59]. However, this presented particular challenges concerning trust and confidentiality for psychiatric in-patients, as many are involuntarily detained [69]. Although participants understood the therapist's responsibility to break confidentiality by informing ward staff of heightened suicide risk [70], this did present a potential barrier to uptake and engagement in suicide-focused therapy. A paradox existed whereby inpatients wanted to talk about their distress and suicidal thoughts, yet recognised discharge as unlikely should staff become aware of their persistent suicidal ideation. This quandary may have led some in-patients to feign cessation of suicidal thoughts in order to gain discharge [71] and may also be implicated within the escalation of suicide rates during the immediate post-discharge period [4].

Strengths

The contextual challenges of conducting research in psychiatric wards are extensive [72]. However, our results offer particular insights to assist others wishing to implement psychological treatments in this setting. Participants raised many context-specific concerns which are important to consider as contextual influences within treatment settings impact on the therapeutic alliance and ultimately on the treatment effect [73, 74].

Our study researched the expectations of suicidal in-patients as part of the development of a suicide-focussed psychological intervention. Our participants were not involved in the clinical trial of this intervention but their status mirrored the eligibility requirements of trial participants thereby enabling them to represent a 'by-proxy potential participant' identity. This may help to overcome a recognised limitation with traditional approaches of participant evaluations *following* receipt of therapy which frequently report high levels of positive affirmations suggestive of social desirability bias [66]. We therefore suggest an important role for investigation of potential recipients' views and expectations as a method to enhance the ecological validity of novel psychological treatments. Patient acceptability of treatments aimed at suicidal in-patients is particularly important as their admission presents a critical opportunity to intervene and save life [10] which for some, (given that 43%

of inpatient suicides occur in the month following discharge, and of these, 47% had died in the first week prior to receiving any community follow-up [75]), may represent our last opportunity.

Further, this study demonstrates the unique role of qualitative approaches in 'giving voice' to highly sensitive, often covert, personal views of vulnerable populations [76]. Our sample comprised suicidal psychiatric inpatients from whose rich accounts a unique data-driven user-informed model for suicide-focussed psychological therapy was devised. Our model, unlike others that have relied on secondary documentary sources [77], represents contemporary 'real-world' verbatim accounts directly obtained from participants' whose precise clinical and contextual situation mirrored that of individuals who would be eligible for future ward-based suicide-focused therapy. As such this affords a high level of ecological validity.

Limitations

It is possible that individuals who volunteered to participate may have been more comfortable and interested in talking about suicide and we may not have recruited people who would be less likely to engage in a suicide-focused talking therapy. By accessing individuals outside from the therapy trial this bias is likely to be minimised. Nevertheless it is possible that findings relating to concerns about suicide-focused therapy are underestimated and the need to address these concerns may be lacking from the user-informed model of suicide-focussed psychological therapy which derived from the analysis. As only one-fifth of participants had any prior experience of psychological therapy their views should be interpreted cautiously. A further limitation is that our sample was drawn from one (albeit large) mental health trust and further study with larger samples of broader sociodemographic variability including more balanced gender composition is indicated.

Recommendation for research and clinical practice

We have demonstrated that the suicidal in-patient participants in this study would welcome ward-based suicide-focussed psychological therapy as an additional treatment choice as recommended in UK statutory guidelines [16]. Further research with a sufficiently powered sample size is required to determine efficacy and to further advance intervention development regarding effectiveness with all stakeholders. Participant generated constructs within our user-informed model of suicide-focused therapy (See Table 3) offers a basis for further research to develop a user-defined outcome measure of recovery from suicidal episodes. More generally, further research to uncover and generate workable solutions for the precise organisational and ward level cultural dynamics that perpetuate the dissonance of needs and views of suicidal inpatients and the ward staff who look after them is required.

Our approach of formal research investigation to exploring the views, expectations and priorities of individuals who would fulfil eligibility criteria for the intervention being developed may be a useful pre-randomised clinical trial phase to extend to other new treatments and populations. However, further research with longitudinal correlational design would be required to determine how this approach impacts on research participant recruitment, retention and definitive trial clinical outcomes. Recipient understanding of the nature of any treatment is essential for ethical research [70] and our findings confirm the importance of providing potential participants' with information of the key requirements of complex therapy, especially if willingness to discuss distressing topics is necessary. Table 4 contains a body of user-generated issues constituting potential avoidable barriers and associated recommendations as guidance for clinicians / research therapists pursuing the practice of suicide-focused psychological therapy.

Conclusion

Hospitalisation of suicidal individuals offers a critical opportunity to engage inpatients in effective treatment and preserve life. Provision of ward-based suicide-focused psychological therapy was cautiously welcomed by suicidal in-patients whose expressed needs, concerns and priorities have been presented and collated into a user-informed model of the key components of suicide-focussed therapy. Patients comprise the largest and potentially most influential stakeholder group in terms of ultimate uptake of health interventions and opportunities to enhance treatment acceptability by understanding their 'real-world' context offer great promise yet remain underexploited [78]. Notwithstanding the need for further research, we cautiously suggest that pre-clinical trial investigation of research participants' views of novel treatments may positively contribute to the future development of better quality treatments likely to improve participant / patient uptake whilst also optimising efficient use of public funding.

Abbreviations
CBT: Cognitive Behavioural therapy; DBT: Dialectical Behavioural Therapy; NHS: National Health Service; NICE: National Institute for Health and Care Excellence

Acknowledgements
We are grateful to members of our Service User Reference Group (INSURG) who provided advice throughout the study and also to Stockport and District Mind and the Samaritans who also provided support and consultation. We are also grateful to Isabelle Butcher for technical assistance with formatting of the tables.

Funding
This paper presents independent research funded by the National Institute for Health Research (NIHR) under its Research for Patient Benefit (RfPB) Programme (Grant Reference Number PB-PG-1111-26026). The views expressed are those of the author(s) and not necessarily those of the NHS, the NIHR or the Department of Health.

Authors' contributions
The first author YA conceived the idea for the study, YA and ESN recruited participants and conducted the interviews to collect the data. Analysis was led by YA and SP with assistance from KH, ESN and GH, PG and DP contributing to critical discussions of analytic interpretations thereby enabling trustworthiness of the final themes. All authors contributed to iterations of drafting and approval of the manuscript.

Consent for publication
Not Applicable.

Competing interests
Yvonne Awenat is a Trustee for a North-West England mental health charity affiliated to Mind. All other authors confirm that they have no competing interests.

Author details
[1]Division of Psychology and Mental Health, School of Health Sciences, University of Manchester, Zochonis Building, Brunswick St, Manchester M13 9PL, UK. [2]Manchester Academic Health Science Centre, MAHSC, Manchester, UK. [3]Manchester Centre for Health Psychology, University of Manchester, Manchester, UK. [4]Greater Manchester Mental Health NHS Trust, Manchester, UK.

References
1. WHO. World Health Organisation. Preventing Suicide: A global imperative. 2014. Geneva. WHO Available at: http://www.who.int/mental_health/suicide-prevention/world_report_2014/en/. Accessed 24 July 2018.
2. CDCP. Centre for Disease Control and Prevention. Web Based Injury Statistics Query and Reporting System (WISQARS). 2016. Atlanta, GA. National Centres for injury prevention and control. Available at: http://www.cdc.gov/injury/wisqars/leading_causes_death.html. Accessed 22 July 2018.
3. EUROSTAT. Eurostat. European commission. 2018. available at. http://ec.europa.eu/eurostat/web/health/causes-death. Accessed 22 July 2018.
4. NCISH. National confidential inquiry into suicide and homicide by people with mental illness. 2017. Annual report. UK: University of Manchester; 2017.
5. Bowers L, Banda T, Nijman H. Suicide inside: a systematic review of inpatient suicides. J Nerv Ment Dis. 2010;198(5):315–28.
6. Bastiampillai T, Sharfstein S, Allison S. Increase in US suicide rates and critical decline in psychiatric beds. JAMA. 2016;316(24):2591–2.
7. Priebe S, Frottier P, Gaddini A, Kilian R, Lauber C, Martinez-Jorgerson P, et al. Mental health care institution in nine European countries. Psychiatr Serv. 2008;59(5):570–3.
8. Abramorowitz M, Grinshpoon A, Priebe S. New institutionalization as a rebound phenomenon? The case of Israel. Isr J Psychiatry Relat Sci. 2008; 45(4):272–7.
9. OECD. Organisation for Economic Cooperation and Development. (UK) Health status. Available at: http://stats.oecd.org. Accessed 20 Nov 2017.
10. Appleby L, Shaw J, Kapur N, Windfuhr K, Ashton A, Swinson N, et al. Avoidable deaths: five-year report of the National Confidential Inquiry into suicide and homicide by people with mental illness National Confidential

Inquiry into suicide and homicide by people with mental illness (NCISH). UK: University of Manchester; 2006.

11. Linehan M, Comtois K, Murray A, Brown M, Gallop R, Heard H, et al. Two-year randomised controlled trial and follow-up of dialectical behaviour therapy vs therapy by experts for suicidal behaviors and borderline personality disorder. Arch Gen Psychiatry. 2006;63(7):757–66.

12. Guthrie E, Kapur N, Mackway-Jones K, Chew-Graham C, Moorey J, Mendel E, Francis F, Sanderson S, Turpin C. Predictors of outcome following brief psychodynamic-interpersonal therapy for deliberate self-poisoning. Aust N Z J Psychiatry. 2003;37(5):532–6.

13. Aoun S. Deliberate self-harm in rural Western Australia. Australian and New Zealand J Mental Health. 1999;8:65–73.

14. Hawton K, Witt K, Taylor Salisbury T, Arensman E, Gunnell D, Hazell P, et al. Psychosocial interventions following self-harm in adults: a systematic review and meta-analysis. Lancet. 2016;3(8):740750.

15. NICE. National Institute for Health & Care Excellence. Self-harm: the short term physical and psychological management and secondary prevention of self-harm in primary and secondary care. 2014. NICE CG 16, Available at http://www.nice.org.uk/guidance/CG16. Accessed 9 Sept 2017.

16. NICE. National Institute for Health & Care Excellence. Self-harm: Longer term management. CG133. 2011a Available at www.nice.org.uk/guidance/CG133 Accessed 9 Sept 2017.

17. Tarrier N, Taylor P, Gooding P. Cognitive-behavioral interventions to reduce suicide behaviour: a systematic review and meta-analysis. Behav Modif. 2008;32:77–108.

18. Winter D, Bradshaw S, Bunn F, Wellsted D. A systematic review of the literature on counselling and psychotherapy for the prevention of suicide: 1. Quantitative outcome and process studies. Couns Psychother Res. 2013;13(3):164–83.

19. Bantjes J, Nel A, Louw K, Frenke L, Benjamin E, Lewis I. 'This place is making me more depressed': the organisation of care for suicide attempters in a south African hospital. J Health Psychol. 2016. https://doi.org/10.1177/1359105316628744.

20. Cox G-HM, D. Greene F. Post-admission cognitive therapy: a brief intervention for psychiatric inpatients admitted after a suicide attempt. Cogn Behav Pract. 2010;19:233–44.

21. Samaraweera S, Sivayogan S, Sumathipala A, Bhugra D, Siribaddana S. RCT of cognitive Behavioural therapy in active suicidal ideation – a feasibility study in Sri Lanka. Eur J Psychiatry. 2007;21(3):175–8.

22. Raj M, Kumaraih V, Bhide V. Cognitive-behavioural intervention in deliberate self-harm. Acta Psychiatr Scand. 2001;104(5):130–5.

23. Durrant C, Clarke I, Tolland A, Wilson H. Designing a CBT service for acute inpatient settings: a pilot evaluation study. Clin Psychol Psychother. 2007;14:117–25.

24. Aoun S, Johnson L. A consumer's perspective of a suicide intervention programme. Aust N Z J Mental Health Nurs. 2001;10:97104.

25. Awenat, Y. Shaw-Nunez, E. Kelly J. Law H. Ahmed S. Welford M. Tarrier N. Gooding P. A qualitative analysis of the experiences of people with psychosis of a novel cognitive behavioural therapy targeting suicidality. Psychosis Psychol Soc Integr App. 2016. https://doi.org/10.1080/17522439.2016.1198827.

26. Perseius K, Ojehagen A, Ekdahl S, Asberg M, Samuelson M. Treatment of suicidal and deliberate self-harming patients with borderline personality disorder using dialectical behavioural therapy: the patients' and therapists' perceptions. Arch Psychiatr Nurs. 2003;17(5):218–27.

27. Bowers L. Reasons for admission and their implications for the nature of acute inpatient psychiatric nursing. J Psychiatric Mental Health Nurs. 2005; 12(2):231–6.

28. Greenberg R, Constantino M, Bruce N. Are patient expectations still relevant for psychotherapy process and outcome? Clin Psychol Rev. 2006;26:657–78.

29. Hendricks Brown C, Curran G, Palinkas L, Aarons G, Wells K, Jones L, et al. An overview of research and evaluation designs for dissemination and implementation. Ann Rev Public Health. 2017;38:1–22.

30. Lambert M. Psychotherapy outcomes research: Implications for integrative and eclectic therapists. In: Norcross J, editor. Psychotherapy relationships that work: Therapists contributions and responsiveness to patient. New York: Oxford University Press; 1992. p. 94–129.

31. Arnkoff D. Glass C. Shapiro S. Expectations and preferences. In Norcross, J. Psychotherapy relationships that work: Therapists contributions and responsiveness to patient. New York. Oxford University Press 2002 (325–346).

32. Roth A. Fonagy P. Parry G. What works for whom? A critical review of psychotherapy research. New York: Guilford Press; 2006.

33. Wolfe B, Goldfried M. Research on psychotherapy integration: Recommendations and conclusions from a NIMH workshop. J Consult Clin Psychol. 1998;56:448–51.

34. Safran J, Muran J, Samstag L, Stevens C. Repairing alliance ruptures. In: Norcross J, editor. Psychotherapy relationships that work: Therapists contributions and responsiveness to patient. New York: Oxford University Press; 2002. p. 235–254.

35. Constantino M, Arnow B, Blasey C, Agras W. The association between patient characteristics and the therapeutic alliance in cognitive-behavioral and interpersonal therapy for bulimia nervosa. J Consult Clin Psychol. 2005;73:203–11.

36. Medical Research Council. UK. MRC. Developing and evaluation complex interventions: New guidance. 2008. London. MRC. http://www.mrc.ac.uk/complexinterventionsguidance. Accessed 23 Aug 2017.

37. Brown G, Ten Have T, Henriques G, Xie S, Hollander J, Beck A. Cognitive therapy for the prevention of suicide attempts: a randomised controlled trial. J Am Med Assoc. 2005;294(5):563–70.

38. DeRubeis R, Hollon S, Amsterdam J, Shelton R, Young P, Salomon R, et al. Cognitive therapy vs medications in the treatment of moderate to severe depression. Archives of General Psychiatry. 2005;62:409–16.

39. Sokero P, Melartin T, Rytsala H, Leskela U, Lestela-Mielonen P, Isometsa E. Adequacy of, attitudes toward, and adherence to treatments by suicidal and non-suicidal depressed patients. J Nerv Ment Dis. 2008;196(3):223–9.

40. Gipson P, King C. Health behavior theories and research. Cog Behav Pract. 2012;19:209–17.

41. Janz N, Champion V, Strecher V. The health belief model. In: Glanz BRK, Lewis F, editors. Health behavior and heath education. San Francisco: Wiley; 2002.

42. National Institute for Health & Care Excellence. NICE. Service user experience in adult mental health: Improving the experience of care of people using mental health services CG136. Available at. http://www.nice.org.uk/guidance/CG133. 2011b;(Accessed 7 Sept 2017).

43. Morgan H. Death Wishes: The Understanding and Management of Deliberate Self Harm. Chichester: Wiley; 1979.

44. Gilburt H, Rose D, Slade M. The importance of relationships in mental health care: A qualitative study of service users' experiences of psychiatric hospital admission in the UK. BMC Health Serv Res. 2008;(8):92. https://doi.org/10.1186/1472-6963-8-92.

45. Wood L, Alsawy S. Patient experiences of psychiatric inpatient care: a systematic review of qualitative evidence. J Psychiatric Intensive Care. 2016. https://doi.org/10.20299/jpi.2016.001.

46. Holmes J. Acute wards: problems and solutions. Psychiatric Bull. 2002;26:383–5.

47. Bohus M, Haaf B, Stiglmayr C, Pohl Y, Bohme R, Linehan M. Evaluation of inpatient Dialectical-Behavioral Therapy for borderline personality disorder – a prospective study. Behav Res Ther. 2000;38:875–87.

48. Large M, Chung D, Davidson M, Weiser M, Ryan C. In-patient suicide: selection of people at risk, failure of protection and the possibility of causation. BJP Open. 2017;3:102–5.

49. Hunter C, Chantler K, Kapur N, Cooper J. Service user perspectives on psychosocial assessment following self-harm and its impact on further help-seeking: A qualitative study. J Affective Disord. 2013;145:315–23.

50. Haddock G, Davies L, Evans E, Emsley R, Gooding P, Heaney L, Jones S, Kelly J, Munroe A, Peters S, Pratt D, Tarrier N, Windfuhr K, Awenat Y. A study to investigate the feasibility and acceptability of a cognitive behavioural suicide prevention therapy for people in acute psychiatric wards: The rationale and design of the 'INSITE' randomised control trial. Trials. 2016;17: 79 DOI: 10.1186/s13063-016-1192-9.

51. Biddle L, Cooper J, Owen-Smith A, Klienberg E, Bennewith O, Hawton K, Kapur N, Donovan J, Gunnell D. Qualitative interviewing with vulnerable populations: Individuals' experiences of participating in suicide and self-harm based research. J Affective Disord. 2013;145:356–62.

52. Marshall M. Sampling for qualitative research. Fam Pract. 1996;13(6):522–5.

53. Ritchie J, Lewis J, McNaughton Nicholls C, Ormston R. Qualitative Research Practice. 2nd ed. London: Sage; 2013.

54. Cutcliffe R, Ramcharan P. Levelling the playing field? Exploring the merits of the ethics-as-process approach for judging qualitative research proposals. Qualitative Health Res. 2002;12(7):1000–10.

55. Peters S. Qualitative research methods in mental health. Evidence Based Mental Health. 2010;13:35–40.

56. Braun V, Clarke V. Successful Qualitative Research: a practical guide for beginners. London: Sage; 2013.

57. Charmaz K. Constructing Grounded Theory. A practical guide through qualitative analysis. London: Sage; 2006.

A qualitative analysis of suicidal psychiatric inpatients views and expectations of psychological therapy...

211

58. Bowers L, Simpson A, Eyres S, Nijman H, Hall C, Grange A, et al. Serious untoward incidents and their aftermath in acute inpatient psychiatry: The Tompkins Acute Ward Study. Int J Mental Health Nurs. 2006;15(4):226–34.

59. Tarrier N, Kelly J, Gooding P, Pratt D, Awenat Y, Maxwell J. Cognitive Behavioural Prevention of Suicide in Psychosis: A treatment manual. London: Routledge; 2013.

60. Qin P, Nordentoft M. Suicide risk in relation to psychiatric hospitalization: evidence based on longitudinal registers. Archives of General Psychiatry. 2005;62:427432.

61. Berking M, Neacsiu A, Comtois K, Linehan M. Experiential avoidance in the reduction of depression in treatment for borderline personality disorder. Behav Res Ther. 2009;47:663–70.

62. Chawla N, Ostafin B. Experiential avoidance in functional dimensional approach to psychopathology: An empirical review. J Clin Psychol. 2007;63:871–90.

63. Hayes S, Wilson K, Gifford F, Follelle V, Strosahl K. Experiential avoidance and behavioural disorders: a functional dimensional approach to diagnosis and treatment. J Consult Clin Psychol. 1996;64:1152.

64. Wells A. Emotional disorders and metacognition: Innovations in cognitive therapy. Chichester: Wiley; 2000.

65. Awenat Y, Peters S, Shaw-Nunez E, Gooding P, Pratt D, Haddock G. Staff experiences of working with in-patients who are suicidal: qualitative analysis. Br J Psychiatry. 2017. https://doi.org/10.1192/bjp.bp.116.191817.

66. Holding J, Gregg L, Haddock G. Individuals' experiences and opinions of psychological therapy for psychosis: A narrative synthesis. Clin Psychol Rev. 2016;43:142–61.

67. Seinfield J. A Primer for Handling the Negative Therapeutic Reaction. New York: Jason Aronson Inc; 2002.

68. Barrett M, Chua W, Crits-Christoph P, Gbbons M, Casiano D, Thompson D. Early withdrawal from mental health treatment. Implications for Psychother Pract. 2008;45(2):247–67.

69. NHS Digital. National Health Service Digital online. Inpatients formally detained in hospitals under the Mental Health Act 1983 and patients subject to supervised community treatment: 2015/16. Available at www.digital.nhs.uk Accessed 6 Aug 2017.

70. Mishara B, Weisstub D. Ethical and legal issues in suicide research. Int J Law Psychiatry. 2005;28(1):23–41.

71. Simon R, Gutheil T. Sudden improvement among high-risk suicidal patients; should it be trusted? Psychiatric Serv. 2009;60(5):387–9.

72. Mccann E, Bowers L. Training in cognitive behavioural interventions on acute psychiatric wards. J Psychiatric Mental Health Nurs. 2005;12:215–22.

73. Clark D. Developing new treatments: on the interplay between theories, experimental science and clinical innovation. Beha Res Ther. 2004;42:1089–104.

74. Dunn G, Bentall R. Modelling treatment-effect heterogeneity in randomized controlled trials of complex interventions (psychological treatments). Stat Med. 2017;26:4719–45.

75. Hunt I, Kapur N, Webb R, Robinson J, Burns J, Shaw J, et al. Suicide in recently discharged psychiatric patients: a case-control study. Psychol Med. 2009;39(2):443–9.

76. Hjelmeland H, Knizek B. Why we need qualitative research in suicidology research. Suicide and Life Threatening Behavior. 2010;40(1):74–80.

77. Leamy M, Bird V, Le Boutillier C, Williams J, Slade M. Conceptual framework for personal recovery in mental health: systematic review and narrative synthesis. Br J Psychiatry. 2001;199(6):445–52.

78. Waddell C. So much research evidence, so little dissemination and uptake: mixing the useful with the pleasing. Evidence Based Mental Health. 2001;4: 3–5. https://doi.org/10.1136/ebnh.4:1.3.

21

'Suicide rates in Crete, Greece during the economic crisis: the effect of age, gender, unemployment and mental health service provision'

Maria Basta[1], Alexandros Vgontzas[1*], Anastasia Kastanaki[2], Manolis Michalodimitrakis[2], Katerina Kanaki[2], Katerina Koutra[3], Maria Anastasaki[1] and Panagiotis Simos[1]

Abstract

Background: Recently, suicides in Greece have drawn national and international interest due to the current economic crisis. According to published reports, suicides in Greece have increased up to 40% and Crete has been highlighted as an area with the sharpest increase.

Aim: To investigate the suicide mortality rates in Crete between 1999 and 2013 and their association with the economic crisis.

Methods: Data on suicides were selected from the Department of Forensic Medicine files of the University of Crete.

Results: Our analysis showed that (1) Crete, has the highest suicide mortality rate in Greece, however no significant increase was observed between 1999 and 2013, (2) there were opposing trends between men and women, with women showing a decrease whereas men showed an increase in that period, (3) there was a significant increase of suicides in middle-aged men (40–64 yrs) and elderly, although the highest unemployment rates were observed in young men and women, and (4) finally, there was a regional shift of suicides with a significant decrease in Western Crete and a significant increase in Eastern Crete.

Conclusions: Although, Crete has the highest suicide mortality rates in Greece, we did not observe an overall increase during the last 15 years, including the period of economic crisis. Furthermore, there was an increase in middle-aged and elderly men, whereas young men and women showed oppositional trends during the years of austerity. This may be related to the culturally different expectations for the two genders, as well as that younger individuals may find refuge to either strong family ties or by immigrating abroad. Finally, the relative increase of suicides in Eastern Crete may be explained by factors, such as the lack of community mental health services in that area.

Keywords: Suicides, Gender, Health services, Economic crisis, Greece

* Correspondence: avgontzas@hmc.psu.edu
[1]Department of Psychiatry, University Hospital of Heraklion, Voutes,Heraklion, 71110 Crete, Greece
Full list of author information is available at the end of the article

Background

For the last several years suicides in Greece have drawn national and international interest due to the current economic crisis, which has engulfed Europe since 2008. This period coincided with the implementation of fiscal austerity, increase of unemployment rates and negative economic growth, and had severe adverse effects on various aspects of people's daily life and probably on their mental health. Studies in European Union countries conducted during the recent economic crisis period have found associations between suicide mortality rates (SMRs) and unemployment [1]. In Greece, according to published reports, SMRs have been on a remarkable upward trend up to 40% [2–4]. In 2011 a brief report in Lancet suggested a 40% rise in suicides in the first half of 2011 compared to 2010 [5]. Kontaxakis et al. reported that in the decade between 2001 and 2011 SMRs increased by 38.4%, with women showing the highest rise (69.6% as compared to 33.1% among men) [3]. In a similar vein, another recent study reported a 35% increase in suicides between 2010 and 2012, with unemployment being significantly associated with suicide mortality, especially among men of working-age, which coincided with austerity measures [4]. In another study it was suggested that fiscal austerity measures and negative economic growth were related to significantly increased male SMRs, whereas fiscal austerity affected mostly the population between 45 and 89 years of age [6]. Conversely, another long-term study from North Greece found no associations between SMRs and unemployment [7].

Based on a previous report, Crete displayed the highest suicide rate in Greece between 1999 and 2010 [8] and the lay press have designated the island of Crete as the area with the sharpest increase of suicides in Greece during the first years of the crisis. It should be noted, however, that although suicide mortality rates are known to fluctuate yearly, requiring relatively longer study periods, the aforementioned issue has not been systematically addressed using data from subsequent years (http://agonaskritis.gr/οι-αυτοκτονίες-στην-κρήτη; https://www.neakriti.gr/article/eidiseis/989417/kriti-tragiki-prwtia-stis-aytoktonies/).

The present study included data from 1999 to 2013 in order (a) to compare suicide mortality rates before and during the economic crisis, and (b) to examine short and long term effects of the crisis. Furthermore, we assessed the association between specific sociodemographic parameters (i.e. gender, age, unemployment rates and availability of mental health services in Western vs. Eastern Crete) on differences in SMRs between the two time periods. Our initial hypothesis was that suicides have increased during the crisis period, and that this increase is associated with economic indices, i.e.

unemployment, and is influenced by the availability of mental health services.

Methods
Study design

A retrospective study was undertaken reviewing all suicide cases in Crete between January 1, 1999 and December 31, 2013. Crete is the largest of the Greek islands with a population of 623,065 in the 2011 by the Hellenic Statistical Authority (ELSTAT) census. The island of Crete is divided into four prefectures, which from west to east are the following: Chania, Rethymnon, Heraklion and Lasithi. Data on the suicide fatalities in Crete were obtained from the Department of Forensic Sciences, Faculty of Medicine, University of Crete, Greece. A total of 651 cases were registered during this period. National suicide data were provided by ELSTAT, an independent, national authority in Greece that follows European and international standards of data collection and statistical analyses. The study has been approved by the IRB Committee of the University of Crete, School of Medicine.

Data analysis

Suicide mortality rates (SMRs) per 100,000 inhabitants were calculated for each calendar year as well as age-adjusted SMRs (based on the 2001 population census) with the direct method. Region-specific (i.e., Western and Eastern Crete) and gender-specific rates were also calculated. Previous research has shown that the association of suicide with socio-economic variables varies with gender and age [9]. Thus, we also stratified the sample into meaningful age-subgroups to depict those who had recently entered the labor market (< 40 years old), those who had been in the workforce longer (40–64 years old) and finally those at retirement age (> 64 years) and calculated age- by gender-specific SMRs for each subgroup. Yearly trends in SMRs were modeled using Poisson Regression. Model fit was assessed using the Wald Chi-square test at $p = 0.05$. Further the association between suicide and unemployment rates as a function of Age Group was examined using Generalized Linear Model analysis. All analyses were performed with IBM-SPSS v. 20.

Given that prior studies have raised the issue of potential misclassification of suicide as a cause of death in numerous countries, including Greece (mostly due to religious and other reasons) [10–12], more recent studies took measures to eliminate this possibility [2]. Following this suggestion and in order to investigate the potential bias of suicide misclassification in our analyses, we performed a series of sensitivity analyses including a comparison of official suicide mortality data from ELSTAT with validated coroner death certificate data for the same suicides in the island of Crete.

Results

During the 15 years examined a total of 651 suicides were recorded in Crete, 527 (80.9%) were committed by men and 124 (19.1%) by women. Standardized SMRs were nearly four times higher among men than among women (11.69 vs. 2.75 per 100.000 residents; Wald's $X^2[1] = 6.94$, $p = 0.007$).

Suicide mortality rates in Crete vs. Greece

The first significant finding of this study is that SMRs in Crete are higher compared to the SMRs in Greece (see Table 1). This finding is verified based both on ELSTAT (Hellenic Statistical Authority) and the Archives of Forensic Medicine [Forensic Medicine, University of Crete (AFM)]. Specifically, based on ELSTAT data, the mean yearly SMR between 1999 and 2013 for Crete vs. Greece was 5.2 vs. 2.4 per 100,000 for the total group (Wald's $X^2[1] = 11.43$, $p = 0.001$), 10.8 vs. 5.3 for men (Wald's $X^2[1] = 7.79$, $p = 0.005$) and 2.5 vs. 1.1 for women (Wald's $X^2[1] = 5.84$, $p = 0.0016$), respectively. The men/women ratio was similar in both groups: 4.03 in Crete vs. 4.7 in Greece. In Crete there was a significant linear rise in this ratio during the study period ($R^2 = 0.577$, $p = 0.001$).

The high SMR in Crete vs. Greece was verified by the data provided by the Archives of Forensic Medicine,

although the number of suicides per year was higher compared to the numbers given by ELSTAT throughout all years by 8.2%.

Suicide mortality rates in Crete during the period of the economic crisis: Gender effect

The second important finding of this study is that overall suicidal rates in Crete were rather stable during the 15-year study period, including the 2008–2013 interval of the financial crisis in Greece. Specifically, the Poisson regression analysis revealed that for every year during the study period there was a slight increase of 0.010 suicides per 100,000 residents, which failed to reach significance (95% CI =0.980 to 1.041, $p = 0.5$). Given that this effect was superseded by a Year by Gender interaction (Wald's $X^2[1] = 4.96$, $p = 0.05$), yearly suicide trends were assessed separately for men and women. As shown in Fig. 1, the SMR among men in Crete between 1999 and 2013 rose at an average annual rate of 0.025 instances per 100,000 residents, a trend that failed to reach significance ($p = 0.16$). Conversely, the SMR among women displayed a decreasing trend averaging 0.50 cases per year per 100,000 residents also failing to reach significance ($p = 0.15$).

Systematic differences in SMRs as a function of age were also assessed given a significant Age Group (< 40, 40–64, and > 64 years) by Year interaction among men (Wald's $X^2[1] = 12.19$, $p = 0.002$). Specifically, SMRs displayed average yearly increases of 0.48 and 0.31 suicides per year per 100,000 residents in the 40–64 year group (95% CI = 1.019 to 1.078, $p = 0.001$) and the > 64 year group, respectively (95% CI = 1.005 to 1.057, $p = 0.018$) (Table 2). In women annual trends in SMRs did not vary significantly across Age Groups (Age Group by Year interaction: $p = 0.1$).

Suicide mortality rates in Crete during the period of the economic crisis: Age effect

Another interesting finding is that SMRs in younger people of both genders were lower compared to those of middle-aged and retirement-age people. In both genders the Age Group main effect was significant (Men: Wald's $X^2[2] = 11.09$, $p = 0.004$; Women: Wald's $X^2[2] = 9.02$, $p = 0.01$) indicating significantly lower overall SMRs in the youngest age groups (6.01 in men and 1.03 suicides in women per 100,000 residents) as compared to both the 40–64 year group (17.44 in men and 4.53 suicides in women per 100,000 residents; $p < 0.007$) and to the > 64 year group (21.54 in men and 4.96 suicides in women per 100,000 residents; $p < 0.007$).

To assess the hypothesis that suicides may be associated with the economic crisis in Greece, we examined the relation between suicide and unemployment rates in Greece during 2013—i.e., the year with the highest unemployment

Table 1 Standardized annual suicide mortality rates in Crete and Greece for men and women between 1999 and 2013

Crete			Greece			
Year	Men	Women	Total	Men	Women	Total
1999	10.43	3.71	7.13	5.13	1.35	3.19
2000	14.38	5.10	9.73	5.07	1.35	3.16
2001	9.39	1.59	5.44	4.81	0.77	2.75
2002	8.89	2.42	5.68	4.22	1.00	2.56
2003	11.11	2.40	6.83	5.13	1.12	3.07
2004	6.62	2.54	4.60	4.62	1.04	2.78
2005	11.98	2.71	7.27	5.07	1.25	3.10
2006	10.36	2.56	6.50	5.09	1.11	3.05
2007	8.59	1.84	5.17	4.34	0.91	2.60
2008	11.33	2.40	6.84	4.78	0.99	2.85
2009	11.18	2.69	6.92	5.23	0.86	3.02
2010	8.78	1.14	4.94	5.17	0.62	2.86
2011	12.6	2.26	7.46	6.17	1.32	3.71
2012	13.95	1.69	7.85	7.83	1.65	4.70
2013	12.66	2.38	7.57	8.01	1.96	4.93
Mean	10.81	2.49	6.66	5.38	1.15	3.10

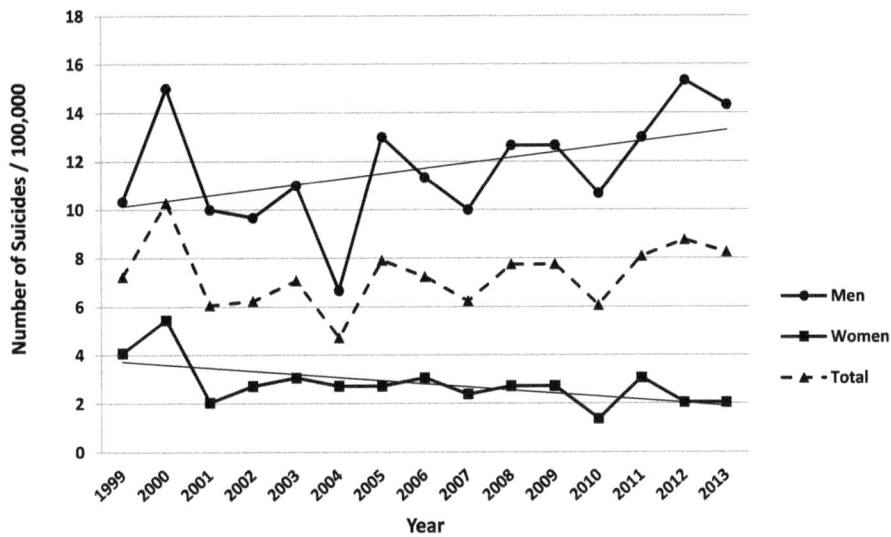

Fig. 1 Yearly trends in standardized suicide mortality rates for the entire population of Crete (dashed line), men (solid line, circles) and women (solid line, squares) between 1999 and 2013

rate and the longest, cumulative crisis impact, among the years of the crisis examined in our study—based on data given by ELSTAT (http://www.statistics.gr/en/home/) (as an indicator of the impact of the economic crisis) stratified by gender and age group (Fig. 2). In men the significant *positive* association between age and SMR (Wald's $X^2[2]$ = 13.88, p = 0.001) was paralleled by a significant *negative* association with unemployment rates (Wald's

Table 2 Standardized annual suicide mortality rates in Crete by gender and age group between 1999 and 2013

Age Group						
	Men			Women		
Year	18–39 yrs	40–64 yrs	> 64 yrs	18–39 yrs	40–64 yrs	> 64 yrs
1999	7.00	18.95	6.78	1.91	3.57	11.33
2000	12.25	13.02	29.36	3.18	10.71	3.78
2001	2.92	16.58	24.84	0.00	2.38	7.55
2002	8.17	10.66	13.55	1.27	3.57	5.66
2003	6.42	17.76	15.81	1.27	2.38	9.44
2004	5.25	8.29	9.03	3.18	1.19	3.78
2005	5.83	17.76	31.62	1.91	3.57	3.78
2006	8.17	14.21	18.07	0.64	5.95	5.66
2007	3.50	13.02	29.36	1.27	2.38	5.66
2008	4.67	21.31	27.10	0.00	7.14	3.78
2009	4.67	21.31	27.10	0.64	8.33	0.00
2010	7.00	11.84	22.59	0.00	3.57	1.89
2011	5.83	26.05	15.81	1.27	3.57	7.55
2012	5.83	28.42	27.10	1.27	3.57	1.89
2013	4.08	28.42	27.10	0.00	4.76	3.78
Mean	6.11	17.84	21.68	1.19	4.44	5.03

$X^2[2]$ = 22.75, $p < 0.0001$). In women, whereas SMR did not vary significantly with age ($p > 0.3$), unemployment rates were also negatively associated with age (Wald's $X^2[2]$ = 29.55, $p < 0.0001$). Specifically, younger men (< 40 years of age) had the highest unemployment rates (45%) and the lowest SMR (4.1 per 100,000 residents) among all age groups. Conversely, men aged 40–64 years had lower unemployment rates (20%) but presented the highest SMR among all age groups (28.42 per 100,000 residents). Similarly, younger women (aged < 40 years) had the highest unemployment rates (53%) and the lowest SMR (0 cases) among all age groups, while middle-aged women (aged 40–64 yrs) had lower unemployment rates (27%) and higher SMR (4.8 per 100,000 residents).

Suicide mortality rates in Crete during the period of the economic crisis: Region effect

Finally, SMRs were analyzed based on the region where they took place. Crete was divided into two main regions: Western Crete (Chania and Rethymno prefectures), and Eastern Crete (Heraklion and Lasithi prefectures). The division "western" and "eastern" was based on the fact that after the closure of the only psychiatric hospital, that was located in Chania (western Crete), most of the new community mental health services were created on this area of the island, whereas there was a scarcity of mental health services in the east part. As already stated, one of the objectives of the study was to assess the influence of the availability of mental health services on SMR. Poisson regression results on SMR values revealed a significant Region main effect (Wald $X^2[1]$ = 8.42, p = 0.004), indicating overall higher SMRs in Western Crete, and a Region by Year interaction (Wald's $X^2[1]$ = 5.43, $p < 0.02$). Figure 3

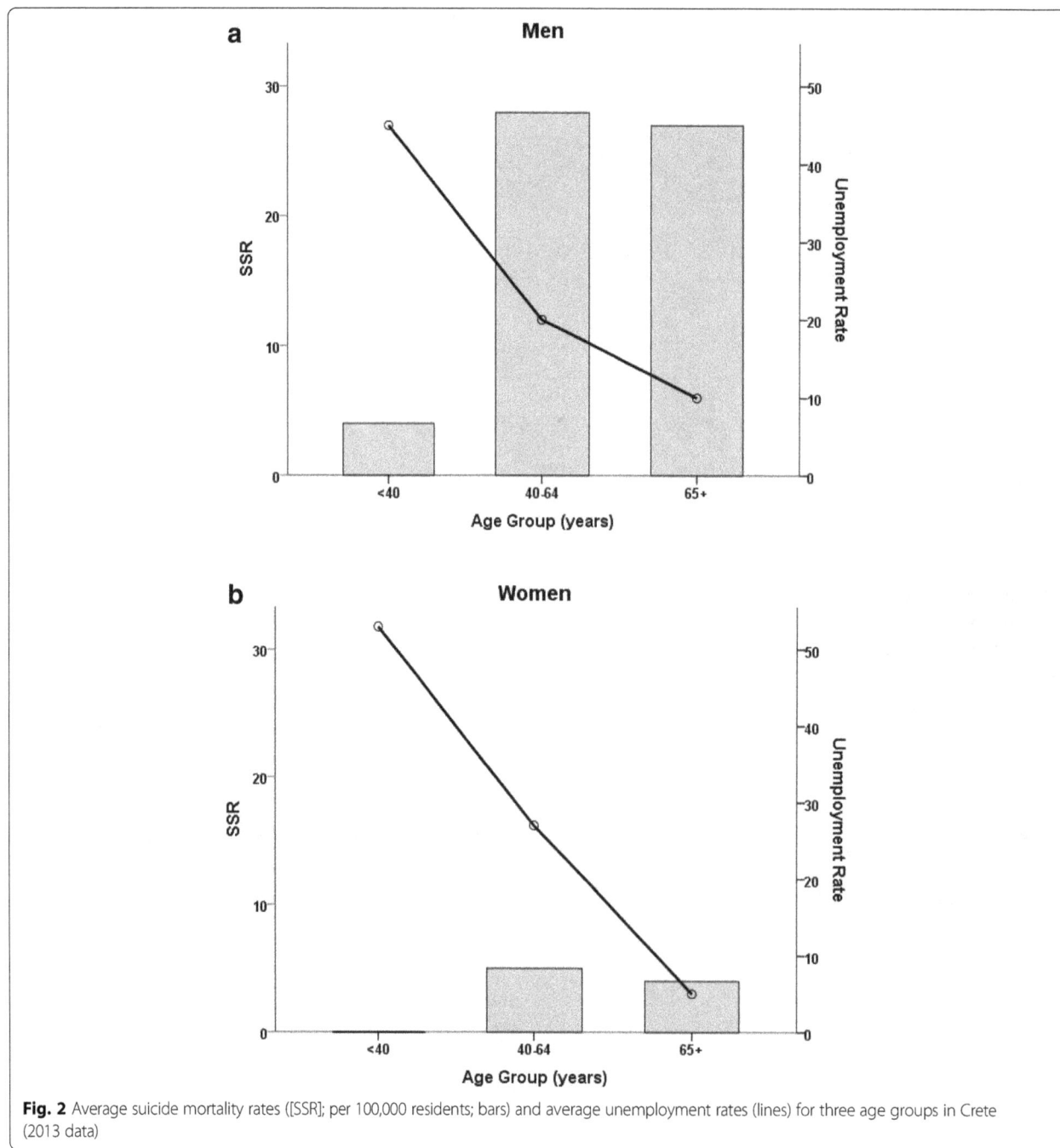

Fig. 2 Average suicide mortality rates ([SSR]; per 100,000 residents; bars) and average unemployment rates (lines) for three age groups in Crete (2013 data)

shows SMR values in Eastern and Western Crete. In Eastern Crete, the annual SMR rose significantly between 1999 and 2013 at an average rate of 0.39 suicides per 100,000 residents (95% CI = 1.014 to 1.064, $p = 0.002$). Conversely, in Western Crete there was a significant reduction in the total number of suicides at an average annual rate of 0.34 suicides per 100,000 residents during the same period (95% CI = 0.943 to 0.995, $p = 0.020$).

We should note that although the population of Western Crete (227,407) is considerably smaller compared to Eastern Crete (366,961), the availability of inpatient beds for psychiatric care in general hospitals is considerably higher in the former region than in the latter (15/100,000 vs. 9/100,000, respectively). A similar trend is noted for outpatient facilities available to support psychosocial rehabilitation (70/100,000 vs. 7/100,000, respectively) (https://www.hc-crete.gr/ψυχικη-υγεια/χαρτης-ψυχικης-υγειας).

Discussion

This is the first long-term (1999–2013) study of suicides in the island of Crete based on data from the

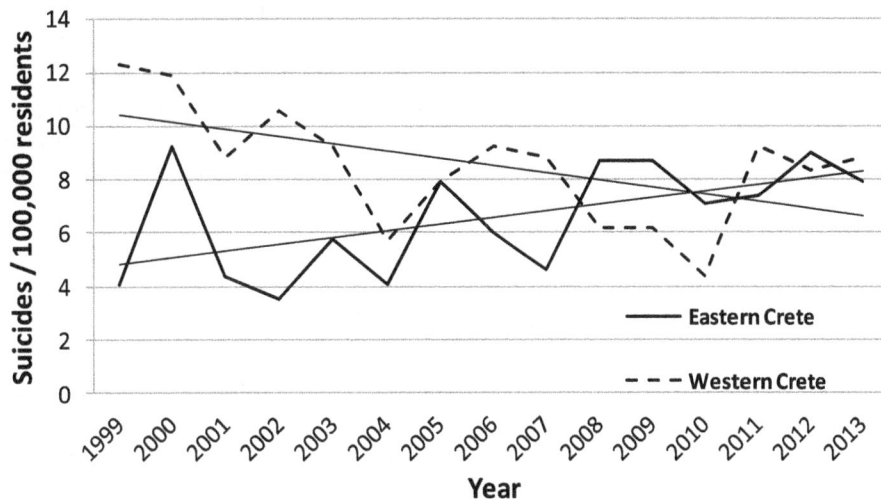

Fig. 3 Yearly trends in standardized suicide mortality rates in Eastern (solid line) and Western Crete (dashed line) between 1999 and 2013

Department of Forensic Medicine of the University of Crete. The primary findings of the study are: (1) Crete has overall and yearly, higher SMRs compared to the national SMR in Greece, (2) there is no overall increase of SMRs including the period of the economic crisis (2008–2013), (3) there were opposing trends between men and women, with women showing a decrease, whereas men displaying increased rates in that period, (4) in men, there was a significant increase in middle-aged and elderly but not in the younger persons, although the highest unemployment rates were observed in young men and women and (5) SMRs have decreased in Western Crete and increased in Eastern Crete, an area where the network of mental health services is markedly underdeveloped.

Our data clearly indicate that the island of Crete in this 15-year period has both yearly and overall higher SMRs compared both to the national average SMR, as well as to the SMR of other parts of Greece, a phenomenon that is difficult to explain [13]. There is a popular belief that Crete has higher rates of psychopathology compared to the rest of Greece, but there are no epidemiological data to support such a claim. Well-established differences in terms of culture, such as large, close-knit families, high frequency of gun ownership and limited access to mental health services due to geographical factors and scarcity of such services may explain the higher SMRs in the island of Crete.

A major finding of our study is that the overall SMRs in Crete have remained stable across 15 years including the economic crisis period. This counters popular beliefs and previous study findings claiming an increase of suicides driven by the economic crisis. In 2011, a brief report in Lancet suggested that SMRs rose by 17% between 2007 and 2009 with a further 40% rise in the first half of 2011 as compared with the same period in 2010

[5]. Following this initial report, several studies reported modest, non-significant increases [3] based on unofficial sources, such as police announcements and news coverage [6], or even a reduction in suicides in 2012 [14]. Notably these studies contrasted short periods before and during the initial period of the crisis [3, 5]. A study based on ELSTAT data reported an increase in SMRs by 18% in men during the 2009–2012 period as compared to the 2005–2008 period, with relative stable rates among women [15]. Compared to these earlier studies, our study covers a much longer time period (including nine years prior to and six years during the crisis). This feature is important in light of the well-known yearly fluctuation of SMRs. For instance, the by-far highest suicide rate in Crete during the present study period occurred in 2000, a year marked by a steady rise of both national and regional gross income. Consistent with our study, Fountoulakis et al. reported no increase in SMRs in the area of Thessaloniki in Northern Greece for the same twelve year period (2000–2012) [7].

An interesting finding of our study is the age- and gender-dependence of SMRs. There was a significant increase of SMRs in middle aged men whereas no such association was observed in younger men (< 40 years old), despite the highest unemployment rates observed in this group ($> 60\%$) (http://www.statistics.gr/en/home/). Similarly to our findings, a study in Italy reported decline of SMRs among younger men and increase among men involved in the labor force during the economic crisis compared to the period before [16]. One explanation of these findings is that a young man who is unemployed can either rely on the support of his family, a very common phenomenon in the Cretan culture indicating family members' strong adherence to the family bonds, or can choose to emigrate in search of better job opportunities. Based on national statistics it is estimated that between 2008 and 2016, 300,000 young Greeks went abroad to find better job opportunities, the so called "brain-drain" phenomenon (http://www.bankof-greece.gr/BogEkdoseis/ekthdkth2015.pdf; http://www.kath imerini.gr/865921/article/epikairothta/ellada/to-trito-me-tanasteytiko-kyma-twn-ellhnwn) [17]. In contrast, middle-aged men traditionally carry the main burden of the economic well-being of the family. Thus, losing their job or business can have a devastating effect both on the socio-economic status of their families as well as on their self-esteem. Rising SMRs among elderly men in Greece, unlike findings from Italy [16] may be related to signifi-cant reductions in already modest pensions enforced as part of the austerity measures in our country. In women we observed a decreasing trend of SMRs during the period of the economic crisis, consistent with other studies con-ducted in Greece and other southern European countries [14–16]. A possible explanation is that during stressful periods women revert to their more traditional role of sup-porting their entire family at a social and personal level.

A recent 30-year interrupted time series analysis on the influence of austerity-related and prosperity-related events on SMRs in Greece during the period 1983–2012 found a significant increase in total suicides by 36%, and male suicides by 19%, after the introduction of new austerity measures in June 2011 [2] and in women an abrupt and sustained increase by 36% following austerity-related events in May 2011. Interestingly, during one prosperity-related event, i.e. the January 2002 launch of the Euro in Greece, there was an abrupt but temporary significant decrease in male suicides [2].

An important and novel finding of our study is that regional SMRs vary systematically with the amount of available mental health services. The results from the lit-erature are mixed. One study in Greece reported a posi-tive association between mental health services and suicide mortality rates. [18] However, another recent study including 10 European countries failed to find significant associations between available psychiatric beds and SMRs, after controlling for economic variables [19]. In our study, there was a significant decrease of suicides during this 15-year period in Western Crete, whereas there was a sig-nificant increase in Eastern Crete. Traditionally and for historical reasons, both inpatient and outpatient services have been more strongly developed in the western part of the island although the population in the eastern part of the island comprises 2/3 of the total population of Crete. Notably, in 2014 all parties of the Greek parliament recog-nized that mental health services were grossly underdevel-oped in the eastern part of Crete [17] and that there is an urgent need to support and to expand these services in that region.

Strengths and limitations

There are several strengths and limitations associated with this study. This is the longest –ever period studied for SMRs in Greece covering nine years preceding and six years after the economic crisis. Also, this study is based on data from the Forensic Medicine Department of the University of Crete, whereas suicides may be underreported in official national statistics due to family or social pressures to attribute death from suicide to other causes as a result of religious and cultural beliefs [9–11]. One limitation of our study is the relatively small sample size that might have affected the statistical significance of some of our findings, such as the gender effect. A further limitation of our study is that un-employment was the only indicator used to examine the impact of the crisis on economy, while others such as Per Capita Income, Household Income, home ownership etc. were not included. Finally, in interpreting the results of this study, we should consider some cultural and eco-nomic characteristics of the island of Crete. For example, the island is well-known for the close relationships of the members of the nuclear and extended family. More-over, the burden of the economic crisis may have been contained in Crete by the fact that many residents benefit from additional sources of income (tourism and farming).

Conclusions

In conclusion, our study indicates that in the island of Crete, despite overall stable SMRs during the economic cri-sis period, it appears that middle-aged and elderly men may be more vulnerable to the burden of economic turmoil and should be specifically targeted for appropriate prevention services. For example, "crisis lines" can be of particular value in the workplace to support middle-aged men who lose their jobs are laid off, supplemented by hot lines oper-ated by "business associations". Furthermore, our study strongly supports the usefulness of mental health services in preventing suicides during the years of economic crisis. In this regard, the delay in developing these services in Eastern Crete as a result of fiscal austerity and lack of avail-able funds, can have a perpetuating and lasting effect on the observed rise of suicides in this part of the island. Finally, the decreasing trends of SMRs in younger men and in women, suggests that in this region, traditional values, such as close family and social ties, and lower social expec-tations may have a protective role against suicides in these age and gender groups. In this vein, advancing our under-standing of those aspects of family and social life that may serve as protective factors against suicide risk is critical to develop prevention strategies.

Abbreviations
ELSTAT: Hellenic statistical authority; SMR: Suicide mortality rate

Acknowledgements
Not applicable

Funding
The work presented here received *no funding* for the design of the study, collection of data, analysis and data interpretation, as well as manuscript preparation and submission.
This paper is dedicated to the memory of our colleague, M. Michalodimitrakis, Professor and Chair of the Department of Forensic Science, University of Crete who passed away in 2016.

Authors' contributions
MB contributed to the interpretation of results and writing and final revision of the manuscript, AV: participated in the design, interpretation and preparation of the manuscript, and overall supervision of the study, AK: participated in data collection and preparation of the manuscript, MM: participated in study design and collection of data, KK1 participated in the collection and preparation of data for statistical analysis and preparation of the manuscript, KK2 and MA contributed to the interpretation of the results and preparation of the manuscript, PS: contributed to data analysis, interpretation of results preparation and final revision of the manuscript. All authors read and approved the final manuscript.

Consent for publication
Not applicable.

Competing interests
The authors declare that they have no competing interests.

Author details
[1]Department of Psychiatry, University Hospital of Heraklion, Voutes,Heraklion, 71110 Crete, Greece. [2]Department of Forensic Science, School of Medicine, University of Crete, Voutes, Heraklion, 71003 Crete, Greece. [3]Department of Psychology, School of Social Sciences, University of Crete, Gallos, Rethymnon, 74100 Crete, Greece.

References
1. Stuckler D, Meissner C, Fishback P, Basu S, McKee M. The health implications of financial crisis: a review of the evidence. Ulster Med J. 2009;78:142–5.
2. Branas CC, Kastanaki AE, Michalodimitrakis M, Tsougas J, Kranioti EF, Theodorakis P, et al. The impact of economic austerity and prosperity events on suicide in Greece: a 30-year interrupted time-series analysis. BMJ Open. 2014;5:e005619.
3. Kontaxakis V, Th P, Havaki-Kontaxaki B, Tsouvelas G, Giotakos O, Papadimitriou GN. Suicide in Greece: 2001-2011. Psychiatriki. 2013;24(3):170–4.
4. Rachiotis G, Stuckler D, McKee M, Hadjichristodoulou C. What has happened to suicides during the Greek economic crisis? Findings from an ecological study of suicides and their determinants (2003-2012). BMJ Open. 2015;5:e007295.
5. Kentikelenis A, Karanikolos M, Papanicolas I, Basu S, McKee M, Stuckler D. Health effects of financial crisis: omens of a Greek tragedy. Lancet. 2011;378:1457–8.
6. Antonakakis N, Collins A. The impact of fiscal austerity on suicide: on the empirics of a modern Greek tragedy. Soc Science Med. 2014;112:39–50.
7. Fountoulakis K, Savopoulos C, Zannis P, Apostolopoulou M, Fountoukidis I, Kakaletsis N, Kanellos I, Dimellis D, Hypantis T, Tsikerdekis A, Pompili M, Hatzitolios A. Climate change but not unemployment explains the changing suicidality in Thessaloniki Greece (2000–2012). J Affective Dis. 2016;193:331–8.
8. Kastanaki A. Thesis: "Suicides in Crete during the psychiatric reform: an epidemiological and forensic medicine approach". www.didaktorika.gr/eadd/handle/10442/27862
9. Gunnell D. Time trends and geographic differences in suicide: implications for prevention. In: Hawton K, editor. Prevention and treatment of suicidal behaviour: from science to practice. New York: Oxford University Press; 2005. p. 29–52.
10. Zacharakis CA, Madianos MG, Papadimitriou GN, Stefanis CN. Suicide in Greece 1980–1995: patterns and social factors. Soc Psychiatry Psychiatr Epidemiol. 1998;33:471–6.
11. Chang S, Stuckler D, Yip P, Gunnell D. Impact of 2008 global economic crisis on suicide: time trend study in 54 countries. BMJ. 2013;17:347–62.
12. Rockett I, McKinley T. Reliability and sensitivity of suicide certification in higher-income countries. Suicide Life Threat Behav. 1999;29:141–9.
13. Fountoulakis K, Savopoulos C, Apostolopoulou M, Dampali R, Zaggelidou E, Karlafti E, et al. Rate of suicide attempts and their relationship to unemployment in Thessaloniki Greece (2000-2012). J Affect Disord. 2015;124:131–6.
14. Michas G. Suicides in Greece: a light in the end of the tunnel. BMJ. 2013; 347:f6249.
15. Vlachadis N, Vlachadi M, Iliodromiti Z, Kornarou E, Vrachnis N. Greece's economic crisis and suicide rates: overview and outlook. J Epidemiol Community Health. 2014;68(12):1–2.
16. Pompili M, Vichi M, Innamorati M, Lester D, Yang B, De Leo D, Girandi P. Suicide in Italy during a time of economic recession: some recent data related to age and gender based on a nationwide register study. Health Soc Care Community. 2014;22(4):361–7.
17. "Praktika Voulis" (Minutes of the Greek Parliament), Σύνοδος Β' Σύνοδος (07/10/2013–04/06/2014):40.
18. Giotakos O, Tsouvelas G, Kontaxakis V. Suicide rates and mental health services in Greece. Psychiatriki. 2012;23(1):29–38.
19. König D, Fellinger M, Pruckner N, Hinterbuchinger B, Dorffner G, Gleiss A, Vyssoki S, Vyssoki B. Availability and use of mental health services in European countries: influence on national rates. J Affect Disord. 2018;239:66–71.

22

Predictors of quality of care in mental health supported accommodation services in England: a multiple regression modelling study

Christian Dalton-Locke[1*†] ⓘ, Rosie Attard[1†], Helen Killaspy[1] and Sarah White[2]

Abstract

Background: Specialist mental health supported accommodation services are a key component to a graduated level of care from hospital to independently living in the community for people with complex, longer term mental health problems. However, they come at a high cost and there has been a lack of research on the quality of these services. The QuEST (Quality and Effectiveness of Supported tenancies) study, a five-year programme of research funded by the National Institute for Health Research, aimed to address this. It included the development of the first standardised quality assessment tool for supported accommodation services, the QuIRC-SA (Quality Indicator for Rehabilitative Care – Supported Accommodation). Using data collected from the QuIRC-SA, we aimed to identify potential service characteristics that were associated with quality of care.

Methods: Data collected from QuIRC-SAs with 150 individual services in England (28 residential care, 87 supported housing and 35 floating outreach) from four different sources were analysed using multiple regression modelling to investigate associations between service characteristics (local authority area index score, total beds/spaces, staffing intensity, percentage of male service users and service user ability) and areas of quality of care (Living Environment, Therapeutic Environment, Treatments and Interventions, Self-Management and Autonomy, Social Interface, Human Rights and Recovery Based Practice).

Results: The local authority area in which the service is located, the service size (number of beds/places) and the usual expected length of stay were each negatively associated with up to six of the seven QuIRC-SA domains. Staffing intensity was positively associated with two domains (Therapeutic Environment and Treatments and Interventions) and negatively associated with one (Human Rights). The percentage of male service users was positively associated with one domain (Treatments and Interventions) and service user ability was not associated with any of the domains.

Conclusions: This study identified service characteristics associated with quality of care in specialist mental health supported accommodation services that can be used in the design and specification of services.

Keywords: Mental health, Supported accommodation, Quality assessment, Quality of care, Predictors of quality, Multiple regression

* Correspondence: c.dalton-locke@ucl.ac.uk
†Christian Dalton-Locke and Rosie Attard contributed equally to this work.
[1]Division of Psychiatry, University College London, Maple House, 149 Tottenham Court Road, London W1T 7NF, UK
Full list of author information is available at the end of the article

Background

Specialist mental health supported accommodation services support an estimated 60,000 people in England [1, 2] and form an essential component of the whole-system care pathway for people with complex, longer term mental health problems [3]. They provide a graduated level of support for people discharged from hospital and are usually found in countries which have gone through a process of deinstitutionalisation i.e. the closure of asylums and development of community care.

In England, these services can be classified into three main types [4]: (1) residential care homes, which are staffed 24 h per-day, provide day-to-day necessities such as meals and medication administration, and are usually not time-limited; (2) supported housing services, which provide time-limited tenancies with shared or self-contained flats with staff on-site up to 24 h per-day; and (3) floating outreach services, which provide visiting (off-site) support to service users in permanent (not time-limited) tenancies. Most service users in residential care and supported housing have a diagnosis of psychosis compared to around half of those using floating outreach (the remainder have common mental disorders such as depression or anxiety). Service users in residential care have the highest level of needs followed by supported housing and floating outreach [3].

Despite the large number of people using mental health supported accommodation services and the associated costs, these services have been under researched. The Quality and Effectiveness of Supported Tenancies for people with mental health problems project (QuEST), a five-year research programme that commenced in 2012 funded by the National Institute for Health Research (NIHR) (Application RP-PG-0610-10,097), aimed to address this evidence gap. It included: the adaptation of a standardised quality assessment tool (the Quality Indicator for Rehabilitative Care – QuIRC) for use in supported accommodation services; a national survey of supported accommodation services and their service users across England [3]; a naturalistic, prospective cohort study investigating 30-month outcomes for service users; and a feasibility study to assess whether it is possible to carry out a large scale randomised control trial comparing two supported accommodation models (supported housing and floating outreach).

The QuIRC was developed to assess the quality of care in psychiatric and social care facilities for adults with longer term mental health problems across Europe and its development has been described elsewhere [5]. In summary, its content was derived from triangulation of the results of a systematic literature review [6], international Delphi exercise [7] and review of care standards in each of ten participating European countries. Item scores are collated to assess seven domains of care: the Living (built) Environment; the Treatments and Interventions provided; the Therapeutic Environment (culture of the unit); the promotion of Self-Management and Autonomy; the promotion of Social Interface with the community and family/friends; the protection of Human Rights; the implementation of Recovery Based Practice. Examples of questions and the domains they score on are presented in Table 1. Some questions score on more than one domain, for example, question 'Roughly what percentage of your residents/service users will be assisted to vote in the next political election?' scores for Social Interface, Human Rights and Recovery Based Practice.

The QuIRC has good inter-rater reliability [5] and the domain scores derived are positively associated with service users' experiences of care [8]. It is available as a web based application (www.quirc.eu) in the ten languages of the countries that participated in its development. Results are presented in a printable report showing the unit's performance on each domain as a percentage on a "spider web" diagram, which also shows the average performance for similar units in the same country.

The QuIRC was adapted for supported accommodation services (QuIRC-SA) through an iterative process of consultation with relevant stakeholders in England during the QuEST Study and its psychometric properties assessed [9]. Specifically, focus groups were carried out with staff from the three main types of supported accommodation service and three expert panels were consulted (two comprised individuals with lived experience of supported accommodation services and one comprised senior professionals and policy makers with expertise in supported accommodation) to suggest appropriate amendments. The adapted tool has good psychometric properties [9]. The QuIRC-SA comprises the same seven domains as the original QuIRC but floating outreach services are not assessed on the Living Environment domain as staff visit service users in their own homes (the service does not provide the building).

The QuIRC has been used in national and international studies investigating longer term mental health services [8, 10] which have found quality of services to be positively associated with geographic location (urban/rural) and smaller, mixed sex units with an expected maximum length of stay and where there is a range of disability amongst service users.

The QuIRC-SA was used in the QuEST programme during the national survey of supported accommodation carried out in 2013–14 [3]. This involved 87 services (22 residential care, 35 supported housing, 30 floating outreach) randomly selected from 14 nationally representative areas across England. Supported housing services scored higher than residential care and floating outreach on six of the seven QuIRC-SA domains and floating outreach scored highest on the human rights domain.

Table 1 QuIRC-SA domains and example questions[a]

Domain	Example question 1 [and response options/format]	Example question 2 [and response options]
Living Environment	What do you think of the general condition of the building outside? (Select one) [Very poor condition/Quite poor condition/Acceptable condition/Quite good condition/Very good condition]	What do you think of the general décor indoors? (Select one) [Very poor condition/Quite poor condition/Acceptable condition/Quite good condition/Very good condition]
Therapeutic Environment	How hopeful are you that the majority of your current residents/service users will show improvement in their general functioning over the next 2 years? [Number]	We know it is not always possible to keep staff up to date with new developments but we are interested in knowing what types of training the staff in your project/service have received. In which of the following areas have your staff received FORMAL training in the last 12 months and how many staff members received this training? [Yes / No to several areas in mental health (e.g. comunication skills, mental health awareness), and number of staff that received training]
Treatments and Interventions	How many of your residents/service users regularly take part in programmed activities in the project/service? [Number]	Do you use individual care-plans for all residents/service users? [Yes / No]
Self-Management and Autonomy	Do residents/service users who have legal capacity have full control over their finances? [Yes / No]	Is there a process for supporting service users to manage their own medication? [Yes/No]
Social Interface	How many of your residents/service users have regular contact with non-service user friends? [Number]	Roughly what percentage of your residents/service users will be assisted to vote in the next political election? [Percentage]
Human Rights	Are patient's/residents' records kept in a locked environment (e.g. locked staff office, locked cabinet, password-protected computer)? [Yes/No]	Do you have a formal complaints procedure? [Yes / No]
Recovery Based Practice	In general, how would you say your project/service mostly aims to assist residents/service users? (Select one) [To assist residents/service users to gain and regain skills to live more independently/To provide residents/service users with the care they need because of their disability / Both equally]	How often do you have meetings where staff and residents/service users discuss the running of the project/service? (Select one) [Never/Every 7 to 12 months/Every 4 to 6 months/Every 2 to 3 months/Every 2 to 6 weeks/Weekly or more than weekly]

[a]Please note that some questions score on to more than one domain

In 2016, the QuIRC-SA was also completed with four supported housing service managers during the feasibility study component of the QuEST programme, and with 80 supported housing services as part of a national survey of staff morale being undertaken by the QuEST team. It was also completed with managers of 54 supported accommodation services in the London boroughs of Camden and Islington as part of a local audit in 2016 (11 residential care, 34 supported housing, nine floating outreach).

We aimed to use these four sources of QuIRC-SA data to investigate service characteristics associated with quality of care in mental health supported accommodation services in England.

Methods

Sample

A total of 195 QuIRC-SAs were completed for 150 specialist mental health supported accommodation services across England between October 2013 and January 2017. Where a service had completed the QuIRC-SA more than once (45 services), only the most recently completed QuIRC-SA was retained for the current analysis. The final sample comprised 28 residential care, 87 supported housing and 35 floating outreach services. Table 2 shows the data sources for this study.

Data analysis

The sample of 150 services provided 80% power to estimate the association of six service characteristics with each of the seven QuIRC-SA domain scores with a small to medium effect size (of 0.35) at a significance level of 0.7% [11]. This reduced significance level accounts for the multiple hypothesis testing conducted (seven regression models, one for each domain of the QuIRC-SA).

The following six service characteristics were investigated for their association with domain scores and entered as independent variables into multiple linear regression models using Stata 14: (1) local authority area rank index score for the location of the service. This is a sampling index developed previously by Priebe and colleagues [11] used to sample the geographical regions across England from where the supported accommodation services were recruited for the national survey conducted during the QuEST study [3]. It provides a spread of scores on local authority areas on factors that influence mental health supported accommodation provision (mental health morbidity, social deprivation, degree of urbanisation, provision of community mental health care, provision of supported accommodation, mental health care spend per capita and housing demand); (2) service size (total number of service user beds/places per service); (3) staffing intensity (total full-time-equivalent (FTE) staff divided by total number of service user beds/

places); (4) usual expected length of stay; (5) service user sex ratio (total number of males divided by total number of occupied beds/places) and (6) service user ability (number of current service users 'generally able to do very little without assistance' divided by the number of service users 'generally able to do some things without assistance' plus the number of service users 'generally able to most things without assistance').

Staffing intensity withstanding, these characteristics were selected as they have previously been shown to be associated with quality of care in inpatient mental health rehabilitation services [10, 12]. We included staffing intensity as we were aware this varies considerably between different types of supported accommodation services. We used the local authority area rank index [13] score rather than the previously used urban/rural dichotomous variable [12] as it provided a more comprehensive composite score of factors relating to location, including urban/rural setting. The other five variables are descriptive items collected during the completion of the QuIRC-SA (they do not contribute to any of the domain scores). These six variables were tested for multicollinearity and found not to be highly correlated.

All seven QuIRC-SA domain scores were normally distributed and were separately analysed as dependent variables using multiple linear regression models (thus creating seven models). Parameter estimates of the linear regression models were computed using robust clustered standard errors, with service type as the cluster variable (residential care, supported housing, floating outreach). Changes in domain scores per one unit increase for service variables with continuous data and their 95% confidence intervals (estimated using bootstrapping) are presented (local authority area index score, total beds/places and expected usual length of stay). For service variables that are ratios (staffing intensity, service user sex and service user ability), we present change in the domain score for one standard deviation (SD) increase in service variable.

Results

Missing data

Having an expected usual length of stay was missing for 13 of the 150 completed QuIRC-SAs (12 residential care and 1 supported housing services). It was assumed that this was most likely to be due to the service not having an expectation of service users moving on and thus no usual expected length of stay. Therefore, these missing values were replaced with the maximum value for this variable (20 years) prior to any analysis.

Service characteristics

The total number of beds/places per service ranged from 3 to 80 with floating outreach tending to have larger

Table 2 Data sources and number of QuIRC-SAs completed and retained in the current analysis

Data source	Residential care			Supported housing			Floating outreach			All services		
	N	Services completed > one QuIRC-SA	QuIRC-SAs retained[a]	N	Services completed > one QuIRC-SA	QuIRC-SAs retained[a]	N	Services completed > one QuIRC-SA	QuIRC-SAs retained[a]	N	Services completed > one QuIRC-SA	QuIRC-SAs retained[a]
National survey	22	5	17	6	5	1	31	5	26	59	5	44
Staff morale survey	0	0	0	79	0	79	0	0	0	79	0	79
Local audit	11	0	11	4	0	4	9	0	9	24	0	24
Feasibility trial	0	0	0	3	0	3	0	0	0	3	0	3
TOTAL	33	5	28	92	5	87	40	5	35	165	5	150

[a]Where services completed more than one QuIRC-SA, only the most recently completed QuIRC-SA was retained for the regression models

services (mean 23 places) and supported housing having the fewest places per service (mean 11). Residential care services had the highest staff to client ratio (0.72), and floating outreach the lowest (0.17). The mean length of stay was longest in residential care services (mean 12.32 years) and lowest in floating outreach (2.83 years). The percentage of beds/places occupied by male service users was similar for residential care (70%) and supported housing (71%), and slightly lower for floating outreach (59%). Seven (24%) residential care and 19 (22%) supported housing services only accepted male service users. As expected, residential care services had a much higher proportion of residents able to do very little without assistance (28%), compared to supported housing (11%) and floating outreach (12%) services. Table 3 shows the service characteristics.

Service quality (QuIRC-SA domain scores)

Supported housing scored higher than residential care on all seven of the QuIRC-SA domains, and higher than floating outreach on six of the domains. Floating outreach scored 88% on the Social Interface domain, the highest domain score by service type. On average (mean), the Social Interface domain was also the highest scoring out of all the domains across the service types (81%), and Human Rights the lowest (52%). Table 4 shows the mean and standard deviation of each QuIRC-SA domain score by service type and across services.

Associations between service quality (QuIRC-SA domain scores) and service characteristics

Table 5 shows the estimated change in QuIRC-SA domain score per one unit increase in the service variable. Where the service variable is a ratio (staffing intensity, service user sex ratio and service user ability), the change in domain score per one SD increase in the service variable is also presented. Associations between service variables and domain scores with p values less than 0.05 are described below.

Living Environment

For this domain there were no ratings available for floating outreach services and therefore analysis was based on 115 rather than 150 services. The mean Living Environment domain score across all services was 78% (residential care 77%, supported housing 78%). Each one point increment in the local authority area index score was associated with a reduction in the Living Environment score of 2.3 percentage points. With each additional year of usual expected length of stay, the Living Environment domain score decreased by 0.2 percentage points (95% CI: -0.4 to – 0.0).

Therapeutic Environment

The mean Therapeutic Environment domain score across all services was 60% (residential care 57%, supported housing 61%, floating outreach 59%). Each one point increment in the local authority area index score was associated with a reduction in the Therapeutic Environment score of 1.8 percentage points. Each additional bed/place was associated with a decrease in the Therapeutic Environment domain score of 0.1 percentage points (95% CI: -0.1 to 0.0). An increase in the staff to service user ratio of 0.3 (one SD) was associated with an increase of 0.5 percentage points in the Therapeutic Environment domain score (95% CI: 0.3 to 0.7). With each additional year of usual expected length of stay, was associated with a decrease in the Therapeutic Environment domain score of 0.4 percentage points (95% CI: -0.5 to – 0.3).

Treatments and Interventions

The mean Treatments and Interventions domain score across all services was 67% (residential care 63%, supported housing 69%, floating outreach 66%). Each additional bed or place per service was associated with a reduction in this domain score of 0.1 percentage points (95% CI: -0.2 to – 0.1). Each increase in the staff to service user ratio of 0.3 (one standard deviation) was associated with an increase in the Treatments and Interventions domain score of 2.0 percentage points (95% CI: 3.9 to 8.1). With each additional year of usual expected length of stay was associated with a decrease in the Treatments and Interventions domain score of 0.1 percentage points (95% CI: -0.2 to 0.0). An increase of 0.2 (one SD) in the ratio of male service users to places was associated with an increase in the Treatments and Interventions domain score of 1.4 percentage points (95% CI: 0.2 to 2.6).

Self-Management and Autonomy

The mean Self-Management and Autonomy domain score across all services was 54% (residential care 51%, supported housing 55%, floating outreach 53%). Each additional year of usual expected length of stay was associated with a decrease in this domain score of 0.4 percentage points (95% CI -0.8 to – 0.1).

Social Interface

The mean Social Interface domain score across all services was 81% (residential care 76%, supported housing 80%, floating outreach 88%). Each additional year of usual expected length of stay was associated with a decrease in this domain score of 0.3 percentage points (95% CI: -0.4 to – 0.2).

Table 3 Descriptive statistics of service variables, by type of service

Service variable	Residential care			Supported housing			Floating outreach			All types		
	N	Range	Mean (SD)	N	Range	Mean (SD)	N	Range	Mean (SD)	N	Range	Mean (SD)
Local authority area index score	28	-0.54, 1.78	0.91 (0.83)	87	-0.76, 1.96	0.90 (0.99)	35	-0.76, 1.78	0.62 (0.92)	150	-0.76, 1.96	0.84 (0.95)
Total beds/places	28	7.00, 40.00	19.46 (7.59)	87	3.00, 28.00	11.20 (5.20)	35	5.00, 80.00	29.97 (22.90)	150	3.00, 80.00	17.12 (14.35)
Staffing intensity (total staff FTE divided by total beds/places)	28	0.34, 2.25	0.72 (0.40)	87	0.10, 1.61	0.45 (0.27)	35	0.03, 0.97	0.17 (0.17)	150	0.03, 2.25	0.43 (0.33)
Expected usual length of stay (years)	28	2.00, 20.00	12.32 (7.82)	87	1.00, 20.00	3.38 (3.43)	35	1.00, 9.00	2.83 (2.16)	150	1.00, 20.00	4.92 (5.63)
Service user sex ratio (percentage of male service users)	28	0.30, 1.00	0.70 (0.22)	87	0.00, 1.00	0.71 (0.25)	35	0.00, 0.90	0.59 (0.20)	150	0.00, 1.00	0.68 (0.24)
Service user ability (percentage 'able to do very little')	28	0.00, 1.00	0.28 (0.30)	87	0.00, 0.71	0.11 (0.18)	35	0.00, 0.50	0.12 (0.16)	150	0.00, 1.00	0.15 (0.21)

Table 4 QuIRC-SA domain scores, by service type

QuIRC-SA domain	Residential care (n = 28)		Supported housing (n = 87)		Floating outreach (n = 35)		All types (n = 150ª)	
	Range	Mean (SD)	Range	Mean (SD)	Range	Mean (SD)	Range	Mean (SD)
Living Environment %	54, 96	77 (10)	62, 96	78 (8)	–	–	54, 96	78 (8)
Therapeutic Environment %	38, 72	57 (7)	41, 77	61 (7)	45, 71	59 (5)	38, 77	60 (7)
Treatments and Interventions %	32, 80	63 (11)	54, 84	69 (7)	58, 75	66 (4)	32, 84	67 (7)
Self Management and Autonomy %	30, 67	51 (9)	28, 85	55 (12)	38, 77	53 (9)	28, 85	54 (11)
Social Interface %	55, 96	76 (10)	58, 92	80 (8)	77, 97	88 (5)	55, 97	81 (9)
Human Rights %	39, 69	53 (7)	36, 78	53 (8)	35, 62	48 (6)	35, 78	52 (8)
Recovery Based Practice %	20, 86	61 (14)	47, 87	69 (10)	50, 77	66 (7)	20, 87	67 (10)

ªFloating outreach services do not score for Living Environment, therefore 35 QuIRC-SAs are removed from the total sample of 150 for this domain

Human Rights

The mean Human Rights domain score across all services was 52% (residential care 53%, supported housing 53%, floating outreach 48%). Each one point increment in the local authority area index score was associated with a reduction in the Human Rights domain score of 2.2 percentage points. An increase in the staff to service user ratio of 0.3 (one SD) was associated with a decrease in this domain score of 2.0 percentage points (95% CI: -3.5 to − 0.6). An increase in the ratio of male service users to places of 0.2 (one SD) was associated with a reduction in the Human Rights domain score of 0.6 percentage points (95% CI: -1.2 to 0.0).

Recovery Based Practice

The mean Recovery Based Practice domain score across all services was 67% (residential care 61%, supported housing 69%, floating outreach 66%). Each one point increment in the local authority area index score was associated with a reduction in this domain score of 2.0 percentage points. Each additional bed/place per service was associated with a reduction in this domain score of 0.1 percentage points (95% CI: -0.2 to 0.0) and each additional year of usual expected length of stay was associated with a reduction of 0.7 percentage points (95% CI: -0.8 to − 0.6).

Resident ability was not associated with any of the QuIRC-SA domains.

Discussion

Supported accommodation is a key component of community mental health care for service users with more complex needs. Identification of service characteristics that are associated with better quality care is of obvious importance. The QuIRC-SA is a standardised quality assessment measure with good inter-rater reliability across a range of different service types.

Six of the seven service characteristics we investigated were associated with one or more of the QuIRC-SA domain scores; local authority area index score, service size

(number of beds/places), proportion of male service users, staffing intensity, and the expected usual length of stay. The latter variable was negatively associated with six of the seven QuIRC-SA domains. The Local Authority index had the most influence on domain scores, with a one point increment being associated with a reduction of up to 2.3% in four of the QuIRC-SA domains. This multi-dimensional index includes markers of demand (urbanicity, psychiatric morbidity and housing) and investment (spend on mental health and supply of community based services). Salisbury and colleagues recently established the association between the amount spent on mental health in a geographic area and the quality of longer term care [14]. Our results appear to corroborate this at the local level, suggesting that local investment needs to respond to local demands to ensure adequate quality of care is provided to people with longer term and more severe mental health problems living in supported accommodation.

Staffing intensity was positively associated with two domains (Therapeutic Environment, Treatments and Interventions), and negatively associated with one of the domains (Human Rights). This is consistent with findings by Sandhu and colleagues [15], where adequate staffing was considered by staff and service users to be key to facilitating recovery. The negative association we found between this variable and Human Rights could perhaps reflect services with higher staffing having a more restrictive approach to supporting service users with more complex needs. In supported housing services in Canada, authoritarian staff management structures were found to have the least positive impact on services users where a "democratic, shared decision-making style" (p.1256) of staffing was preferred [16]. Additionally, Nelson and colleagues [17] report lower levels of staffing encouraged increased engagement with service users.

Increasing service size was negatively associated with Therapeutic Environment, Treatment and Interventions and Recovery Based Practice domain scores. This finding

Table 5 Change in domain score per one unit/SD[a] increase in service variable (95% confidence intervals) and p values, for each linear regresion model (domain)

Service variable	SD for ratio service variables[a]	Living Environment (n = 115)	Therapeutic Environment (n = 150)	Treatments and Interventions (n = 150)	Self-Management and Auton. (n = 150)	Social Interface (n = 150)	Human Rights (n = 150)	Recovery Based Practice (n = 150)
Local authority area index score	—	-2.3 (-2.6, -2.0), <0.001	-1.8 (-3.2, -0.5), 0.007	-1.4 (-3.3, 0.5), 0.140	-0.4 (-1.5, 0.7), 0.512	-2.9 (-6.6, 0.7), 0.114	-2.2 (-3.8, -0.6), 0.006	-2.0 (-2.9, -1.2), <0.001
Total beds/places	—	-0.0 (-0.4, 0.4), 0.908	-0.1 (-0.1, 0.0), 0.001	-0.1 (-0.2, -0.1), 0.001	-0.1 (-0.2, 0.0), 0.072	-0.1 (-0.3, 0.0), 0.052	0.0 (-0.3, 0.3), 0.996	-0.1 (-0.2, 0.0), 0.043
Staffing intensity (total staff FTE divided by total beds/places)[a]	—	-0.4 (-1.5, 0.7), 0.474	1.5 (0.8, 2.2), <0.001	6.0 (3.9, 8.1), <0.001	1.4 (-10.6, 7.8), 0.061	-1.4 (-10.6, 7.8), 0.767	-6.1 (-10.4, -1.8), 0.006	1.3 (-3.4, 6.0), 0.598
	0.3	-0.1 (-0.5, 0.2), 0.474	0.5 (0.3, 0.7), <0.001	2.0 (1.3, 2.7), <0.001	0.5 (0.0, 0.9), 0.061	-0.5 (-3.5, 2.6), 0.767	-2.0 (-3.5, -0.6), 0.006	0.4 (-1.1, 2.0), 0.598
Expected usual length of stay (years)	—	-0.2 (-0.4, 0.0), 0.017	-0.4 (-0.5, -0.3), <0.001	-0.1 (-0.2, 0.0), 0.019	-0.4 (-0.8, -0.1), 0.019	-0.3 (-0.4, -0.2), <0.001	-0.3 (-0.6, 0.1), 0.151	-0.7 (-0.8, -0.6), <0.001
Service user sex ratio (percentage of male service users)[a]	—	-1.5 (-10.7, 7.8), 0.753	3.2 (-1.3, 7.7), 0.166	5.9 (1.0, 10.8), 0.018	3.9 (-0.7, 8.5), 0.098	5.0 (-0.2, 10.3), 0.061	-2.5 (-5.0, 0.0), 0.046	4.6 (-4.3, 13.5), 0.308
	0.2	-0.4 (-2.5, 1.8), 0.753	0.8 (-0.3, 1.8), 0.166	1.4 (0.2, 2.6), 0.018	0.9 (-0.2, 2.0), 0.098	1.2 (-0.1, 2.4), 0.061	-0.6 (-1.2, 0.0), 0.046	1.1 (-1.0, 3.2), 0.308
Service user ability (percentage 'able to do very little')[a]	—	-0.1 (-2.0, 1.9), 0.942	-1.5 (-7.0, 3.9), 0.583	1.0 (-8.3, 10.3), 0.83	-3.7 (-14.2, 6.7), 0.485	5.1 (-5.8, 16.1), 0.357	-1.4 (-8.2, 5.5), 0.691	-5.5 (-13.1, 2.2), 0.160
	0.2	0.0 (-0.4, 0.4), 0.942	-0.3 (-1.5, 0.8), 0.583	0.2 (-1.8, 2.2), 0.833	-0.8 (-3.0, 1.4), 0.485	1.1 (-1.2, 3.4), 0.357	-0.3 (-1.8, 1.2), 0.691	-1.2 (-2.8, 0.5), 0.160

[a]For service variables that are ratios (staffing intensity, service user sex ratio and service user ability), the change in domain score per one SD increase in the service variable has also been included

Predictors of quality of care in mental health supported accommodation services in England: a multiple...

229

concurs with previous research [6, 10], suggesting that larger services tend to be more institutional and less able to offer an individualised, rehabilitative approach.

Our results on the proportion of male service users per service differs somewhat from a previous study showing a negative association between the percentage of male service users in an inpatient rehabilitation unit and quality [12]. We found that having a higher proportion of male service users was negatively associated with the Human Rights domain score but positively associated with the Treatments and Interventions domain score. This could be an artefact in that many male only supported accommodation services cater for service users who have a forensic history, offering specialist treatments (such as substance misuse interventions) in an environment which is necessarily more rule bound than other services since service users are often subject to legal restrictions and conditions associated with being permitted to live in the community.

We found no association between service user ability and quality of care. This concurs with findings from a national survey of inpatient mental health rehabilitation services [12]. This is important as service user ability can sometimes be cited by staff as a reason for being unable to deliver a high quality service.

Strengths and limitations

The data analysed in this study were collected using a specialist, standardised service quality assessment tool for mental health supported accommodation services that has been shown to have good psychometric properties [9]. We used multilevel modelling for our data analysis to take account of clustering at the service type level. We agreed the variables that we would investigate for their association with quality of care prior to carrying out our analyses, choosing these on the basis of previous research. In addition, our sample size was adequate for our analyses. The sample included more supported housing services than the other two service types, in keeping with national provision [3]. However, our analyses used data collected for other purposes and not all the services were randomly selected (87 were randomly selected for the QuEST national survey). Furthermore, we only included services based in England and therefore the findings cannot be generalised to supported accommodation services in other countries.

Implications

Whilst under resourcing of supported accommodation services can only be addressed at a political level, we have identified other factors that are associated with better service quality that could be incorporated into service planning. Having a shorter expected length of stay was associated with better quality services, presumably

because it facilitates a more focused approach to individual goal setting with service users that can assist their recovery and help them gain the necessary skills to move on successfully to more independent accommodation (reflected in the Self-Management and Autonomy QuIRC-SA domain). This creates a positive and hopeful culture reflected in the Therapeutic Environment and Recovery Based Practice domains, and is not limited by general service user ability. However, adequate staffing is clearly essential to achieve this, a factor related to the size of the service. Larger service size was negatively associated with three of the seven QuIRC-SA domains. A balance therefore has to be struck between providing adequate staffing and a service size that is economically viable. Finally, services with higher male service user ratios fared better on quality, but single sex services will continue to be needed due to the challenges posed by individuals with certain types of risk.

Conclusions

This study has helped to identify general service structures and characteristics that can drive up quality of care in supported accommodation services. Services should adopt an expected usual length of stay and be of a moderate size with adequate staffing to support service users to gain and regain skills for more independent living. However, the feasibility of such changes are likely to be constrained by resources and the nature of services; an expected usual length of stay and move-on to more independent settings might be less realistic for services to implement that provide high levels of support.

Abbreviations
FTE: Full-time-equivalent; NIHR: National Institute for Health Research; QuEST: Quality and Effectiveness of Supported Tenancies for people with mental health problems; QuIRC: Quality Indicator for Rehabilitative Care; QuIRC-SA: Quality Indicator for Rehabilitative Care-Supported Accommodation; SD: Standard deviation

Acknowledgements
The authors would like to acknowledge the support of the accommodation services who completed the QuIRC-SAs in this study; the QuEST team (www.ucl.ac.uk/quest) who developed the QuIRC-SA and collected the data; and the DEMoBinc team (Development of a European Measure of Best Practice) for their development of the QuIRC.

Authors' contributions
CDL, RT, HK and SW conceived and designed the study. The data were analysed by CDL & RT under the supervision of SW. CDL and RT made the first draft of the article which was reviewed and revised by HK and SW. All authors read and approved the final manuscript.

Consent for publication
Not applicable

Competing interests
The authors declare that they have no competing interests.

Author details
[1]Division of Psychiatry, University College London, Maple House, 149 Tottenham Court Road, London W1T 7NF, UK. [2]Population Health Research Institute, St George's, University of London, Cranmer Terrace, London SW17 0RE, UK.

References
1. Department for Communities and Local Government. Research into the effectiveness of floating support services for the Supporting People programme. 2008.
2. National Statistics. Community care statistics, supported residents (adults) - England, 2007. London: NHS Digital; 2007.
3. Killaspy H, Priebe S, Bremner S, McCrone P, Dowling S, Harrison I, et al. Quality of life, autonomy, satisfaction, and costs associated with mental health supported accommodation services in England: a national survey. Lancet Psychiatry. 2016;3:1129–37.
4. Priebe S, Saidi M, Want A, Mangalore R, Knapp M. Housing services for people with mental disorders in England: patient characteristics, care provision and costs. Soc Psychiatry Psychiatr Epidemiol. 2009;44:805–14.
5. Killaspy H, White S, Wright C, Taylor TL, Turton P, Schützwohl M, et al. The development of the quality Indicator for rehabilitative care (QuIRC): a measure of best practice for facilities for people with longer term mental health problems. BMC Psychiatry. 2011;11. https://doi.org/10.1186/1471-244X-11-35.
6. Taylor TL, Killaspy H, Wright C, Turton P, White S, Kallert TW, et al. A systematic review of the international published literature relating to quality of institutional care for people with longer term mental health problems. BMC Psychiatry. 2009;9:55.
7. Turton P, Wright C, White S, Killaspy H. Promoting recovery in long-term institutional mental health care: an international Delphi study. Psychiatr Serv. 2010. https://doi.org/10.1176/ps.2010.61.3.293.
8. Killaspy H, White S, Wright C, Taylor TL, Turton P, Kallert T, et al. Quality of longer term mental health facilities in Europe: validation of the quality indicator for rehabilitative care against service users' views. PLoS One. 2012. https://doi.org/10.1371/journal.pone.0038070.
9. Killaspy H, White S, Dowling S, Krotofil J, McPherson P, Sandhu S, et al. Adaptation of the quality Indicator for rehabilitative care (QuIRC) for use in mental health supported accommodation services (QuIRC-SA). BMC Psychiatry. 2016;16. https://doi.org/10.1186/s12888-016-0799-4.
10. Killaspy H, Cardoso G, White S, Wright C, Caldas de Almeida JM, Turton P, et al. Quality of care and its determinants in longer term mental health facilities across Europe; a cross-sectional analysis. BMC Psychiatry. 2016;16. https://doi.org/10.1186/s12888-016-0737-5.
11. Dunlap WP, Xin X, Myers L. Computing aspects of power for multiple regression. Behav Res Methods, Instrum, Comput. 2004;36:695–701.
12. Killaspy H, Marston L, Omar RZ, Green N, Harrison I, Lean M, et al. Service quality and clinical outcomes: an example from mental health rehabilitation services in England. Br J Psychiatry. 2013;202:28–34. https://doi.org/10.1192/bjp.bp.112.114421.
13. Priebe S, Saidi M, Kennedy J, Glover G. How to select representative geographical areas in mental health service research: a method to combine different selection criteria. Soc Psychiatry Psychiatr Epidemiol. 2008;43:1004–7. https://doi.org/10.1007/s00127-008-0383-4.
14. Salisbury TT, Killaspy H, King M. Relationship between national mental health expenditure and quality of care in longer-term psychiatric and social care facilities in Europe: cross-sectional study. Br J Psychiatry. 2017;211:45–9. https://doi.org/10.1192/bjp.bp.116.186213.
15. Sandhu S, Priebe S, Leavey G, Harrison I, Krotofil J, McPherson P, et al. Intentions and experiences of effective practice in mental health specific supported accommodation services: a qualitative interview study. BMC Health Serv Res. 2017;17. https://doi.org/10.1186/s12913-017-2411-0.
16. McCarthy J, Nelson G. An evaluation of supportive housing for current and former psychiatric patients. Hosp Community Psychiatry. 1991;42:1254–6 https://ps.psychiatryonline.org/doi/abs/10.1176/ps.42.12.1254?journalCode=ps.
17. Nelson G, Hall GB, Walsh-Bowers R. A comparative evaluation of supportive apartments, group homes, and board-and-care homes for psychiatric consumer/survivors. J Community Psychol. 1997;25:167–88. https://doi.org/10.1002/(SICI)1520-6629(199703)25:2<167::AID-JCOP6>3.0.CO;2-V.

23

Health care utilization and cost after discharge from a mental health hospital; an RCT comparing community residential aftercare and treatment as usual

Eirik Roos[1,2]* ⓘ, Ottar Bjerkeset[3,4] and Aslak Steinsbekk[1]

Abstract

Background: Community residential aftercare (step-down) services can ease the transition after a mental health hospital stay for patients with severe mental illness (SMI).

Aims: To investigate use of community and specialised mental health care services and costs in patients with SMI the first 12 months after discharge from a mental health hospital (MHH), comparing community residential aftercare (CRA) and treatment as usual.

Methods: An open parallel group randomised controlled trial with 41 participants. Data on use of specialist services (hospital, ambulant treatment and outpatient treatment) and community services (residential stays, home help, home care nursing, mental health consultation) were collected from specialist and community registers and health records.

Results: For the primary outcome, utilisation of community mental health services, the intervention group used, on average, 29% fewer hours (mean differences − 21.6 h, 95% CI -93.1 to 44.9, p = .096) with a cost saving of 29% (mean differences − 1845 EUR, 95% CI -8267 to 4171, p = .102), but the estimates were imprecise. For the secondary outcome, the study groups had the same total number of inpatient days (66 days), but the intervention group had on average of 13.4 fewer inpatient days in the mental health hospital (95% CI -29.9 to 0.9. p = .008). The number of inpatient admissions (mean difference − 0.9 admissions, 95% CI -3.5 to 1.5, p = .224) and readmissions (− 0.8, 95% CI -2.5 to 0.9. p = .440) was lower in the intervention group. The intervention group had on average a total cost saving of 38.5% (mean differences − 23,071 EUR, 95% CI -45,450 to 3027. p = .057). A post hoc multivariable regression analysis controlling for baseline characteristics gave a reduction in total cost in favour of the intervention group of − 19,781 EUR (95% CI -44,072 to 4509, p=,107).

Conclusion: In this study, it was not possible to draw a definite conclusion about the effect, due to the small sample and imprecision of the estimates. The direction of the results and size of the point estimate, in addition to findings in other studies, indicates that transferring patients ready for discharge from mental hospital to community residential aftercare can have the potential to reduce total consumption of health services and costs without increased hospital admissions.

Keywords: Community residential aftercare, Step-down, Discharge-ready mental health patients, Severe mental illness

* Correspondence: eirik.roos@trondheim.kommune.no
[1]Department of Public Health and Nursing, Norwegian University of Science and Technology, 7491 Trondheim, Norway
[2]Health and Welfare, Trondheim, Norway
Full list of author information is available at the end of the article

Background

Most psychiatric inpatients can be discharged without comprehensive follow-up, yet patients with severe mental illness (SMI) often need long-term aftercare [1]. This is a particularly vulnerable group, as patients with SMI have a 10–25 year shorter life expectancy than the general population [2]. Furthermore, a Danish population-based cohort study found increased risk of hospitalisations and rehospitalisation within 30 days for patients with SMI compared with the general population [3].

The duration of hospital stays is a major driver for health costs [4] and most Western countries have shifted more mental health care towards community-based settings [5]. However, it is a challenge to provide timely community services for patients who are ready for discharge from mental health hospitals. A study in the UK in 2005 found that the proportion of discharges classified as "delayed" varied from 4 to 16% of all hospital beds [6]. A study from Norway in 2013 found that 7% of all patients in mental health hospitals were ready for discharge, but were still waiting for municipal services to take over, mainly to provide sheltered housing [7]. A review of 35 studies, mostly from general hospitals, on delayed discharge [8] found that the average cost of one extra day per patient was between £200 and £565.

Early psychiatric readmission serves as a negative quality of care indicator in the mental health services [9, 10]. Some studies report that short inpatient treatment stays (< 28 days) increase readmission rates [11–13]. In contrast, a Cochrane review from six randomised studies did not find evidence suggesting that short-stay hospitalisation (< 28 days), compared to long stay (> 28 days), encouraged a 'revolving door' pattern of admission to hospital [14].

Community based residential mental health services can serve as an alternative to both inpatient admissions (step-up) and aftercare (step-down). A review from 2013 [15] evaluated such services for acute [16–18] and sub-acute admissions (step-up) [19] and concluded that these step-up residential community services offered a cost-effective alternative to hospital based inpatient services. Similarly, a few studies have evaluated community-based services in the form of residential aftercare after hospital stays (step-down) [20–23]. An RCT study on inpatient treatment for substance use disorders compared the effects of two types of community-based, residential treatment programs among justice involved persons with dual diagnosis and reported significant reductions in psychiatric severity for those assigned to residential conditions [23]. An observational study found that a staffed residential step-down facility with a comprehensive program improved symptoms and functioning for persons with psychosis or mood disorder [21].

Taken together, this indicates that patients ready for discharge could be discharged as early as possible to a community residential service, without the shorter stay leading to increased risk of readmission [14], and the costs would be reduced [8]. To make this happen for in-patients with SMI, there is a need for improved collaboration and communication between service levels [24, 25] as well as services that can receive patients who need community services after their hospital stay [20].

There is, however, still a need for studies on the effect and costs of residential aftercare services in the community. One type not previously investigated, is residential aftercare services that do not offer organised in-house activities. Offering organised in-house activities may substitute for future local activities and integration in the local community. Thus, not offering in-house activities could potentially help patients use community services more actively and promote more independent living. The reason being that the patients would have to orient themselves more towards the activities in the community during the stay [26].

The aim of this RCT study was to investigate use of community and specialist mental health care services and costs in patients with severe mental illness (SMI) the first 12 months after discharge from a mental health hospital (MHH), comparing community residential aftercare (CRA) and treatment as usual.

Methods

This was an open parallel group randomised controlled trial including patients from January 2013 to April 2015. It was approved by the Committee for Medical and Health Research Ethics in Central Norway (2011/1770) and was registered in clinicaltrials.gov (NCT01719354).

Change to protocol

Fewer patients than aimed for were included due to problems with recruitment (59% of calculated sample size). It was planned to collect self-reported outcome at 1, 4 and 12 months, but it proved very difficult to get the participants to complete the questionnaires even after 1 month despite several attempts. The collection of these data was therefore stopped, meaning that only outcomes on the consumption of health care services and costs as outcomes were used.

Settings

In Norway, the health and social care services are mainly financed by and provided for in the public sector [27]. Community health and long-term care is the responsibility of the municipalities, while acute somatic and psychiatric hospitals and specialist services are run by the government. Community health and social care includes GPs, public health nurses, nursing homes, home care and mental health care (some places including residential care). Specialist health care organises acute and psychiatric specialist services into mental health hospital (MHH), community mental health centre (CMHC), mental health outpatient treatment and mental health ambulant treatment.

In central Norway, community residential aftercare units (CRA) have been established in order to improve the discharge process from hospital to independent supported living [26]. They facilitate the process of establishing community health and social services, support self-care and engagement, but do not offer organised in-house activities, to ensure community orientation and the fostering of initiatives among the patients. Both the community residential aftercare (CRA) unit and the university mental health hospital (MHH), the setting for this study, are in the City of Trondheim (190,000 inhabitants), in central Norway. The municipality of Trondheim offers a multitude of mental health services to people with mental disorders: community mental health consultation, home care nursing, home help, day centre, short-stay residential aftercare, self-referral and housing arrangement. The MHH has 81 beds, half for acute admissions and half for long-stay patients.

Eligibility criteria

All in-patients with severe mental illness (SMI) at the MHH who were assessed as discharge ready and in need of aftercare services from the municipality after discharge were eligible for this study. However, they had to have a treatment aftercare plan initiated by the time of inclusion. Furthermore, there were no requirements regarding specific diagnostic criteria, and this group mainly concerns people with a diagnosis of schizophrenia, schizoaffective disorders, bipolar disorder, major depression or personality disorders. Furthermore, the patients had to be older than 18 years and they had to sign the informed consent. The exclusion criteria were patients with impaired level of consciousness or acute confusion, those who were under involuntary observation or admission according the Norwegian mental health care act (those involuntary admitted were included if it had been converted to voluntary hospitalisation) and patients assessed by the hospital to be without need of community services after discharge.

Recruitment

All patients were recruited at the MHH in both acute and long stay departments after they were declared by the hospital to be ready for discharge. Staff in the departments identified eligible patients. The doctors in the hospital were responsible for assessing whether the patients were able to understand the consequences of participating in the study. The hospital nurses were the

ones mainly responsible for informing the patients orally about the study and giving them written information and the informed consent. The patients were given one day to decide on their participation and those who wanted to take part signed the consent and gave it to the staff who collected baseline data.

Randomisation and allocation

The randomisation was done using a web-based computer program provided by a trial service at the Norwegian University of Science and Technology. The staff at the MHH conducted the randomisation after receiving the informed consents and the baseline data, and they informed the patients about the allocation.

Intervention – The CRA

A more detailed description of the community residential aftercare unit has been published previously [26]. Briefly, the CRA was established in 2009 and has 14 rooms in total. A stay at the CRA is voluntary and the tentative length of a stay is up to 4 w, but for homeless patients the stay is longer due to the practicalities of making housing arrangements (14 homeless patients in 2016 had an average stay of 64 days) [26].

The CRA operates 24/7 and is staffed by psychiatric nurses, general nurses and nursing assistants. A general practitioner (GP) is present in the CRA one day a week and offers a consultation to all patients who have recently been admitted, and those in need of medical follow-up at the CRA.

The philosophy of the CRA involves the conscious decision not to offer any in-house activities. Instead, the patients are informed about activities in their neighbourhood and in the community. Therefore, there are no organised activities at the CRA such as meals in common, therapy options or use of exercise equipment.

The CRA staff facilitates the process of establishing community health and social services to support the transition from the hospital to independent supported living. The process is started as early as possible to establish a relationship between the patient, the responsible case handler in the municipality and the service providers offering follow-up services after discharge. During the stay, the result of the individual assessment is discussed with the patient, the case handler and it is communicated to the community Health and Welfare agency to help it to decide on the level of services provided by the municipality after discharge. Before discharge from the CRA, patients receive information about the possibility of later self-referral to a short (maximum of three days) inpatient stay at the CRA.

Control – Treatment as usual (TAU)

The TAU discharge process in the MHH for discharge ready patients in need of community follow-up typically includes one of the following: (1) The staff in the hospital contact the Health and Welfare agency in the municipality to clarify which type of follow-up services are needed from the municipality, including housing. This is settled before discharge to the home. (2) The staff in the hospital refers the patient to a community mental health centre (CMHC), which is part of the specialist services, where they continue the treatment plan initiated by the MHH before the CMHC contacts the municipality to make plans before discharge to home.

Measures

To document the implementation of the intervention, the following data were collected: (1) days in the MHH before randomisation (expected to be equal between the groups). (2) Days from randomisation to discharge (expected to be shorter in the intervention group). (3) Where they were discharged immediately after the index stay in the MHH (only the intervention group should be discharged to the CRA). (4) The length of stay at an inpatient unit or residential unit immediately after the index stay (expected to be longer in the intervention group).

Primary outcome

The primary outcome was total hours of community health services and costs for these services during a 12-month period. This included total number of hours with home help (cleaning, shopping etc.), home care nursing and community mental health consultation. The reason for having this as the primary outcome was that it was expected based on experience that patients discharged to the CRA was assessed to need less community services compared to the assessment made based on observation in a hospital setting.

Secondary outcome

The secondary outcomes were number of and cost for the total inpatient days in the MHH, CMHC and CRA, total hours with outpatient treatment including ambulant treatment and the total number of admissions and readmissions from baseline to 12 months after inclusion. Readmission was defined as acute, unplanned admissions to the MHH, CMHC or the CRA within 30 days after last discharge. As a summary measure for the secondary outcomes, total cost of all services was used.

Data collection

All data were provided by the staff in the community health and social care and specialist health care services. They collected the data from registries with data on contacts with the services ("consultations") which are registered with a very high grade of accuracy as it is both demanded by law to be registered and in the interest of the services to do so as it is connected to the use of resources and thus financing. In addition, data on patient characteristics was collected at baseline.

Calculation of cost

The cost of the different services was provided by employees in the administration of the municipality of Trondheim and the university hospital, using the cost from 2015 (Table 1). These figures included the total staff costs, rent and operating expenditures.

Sample size

As there were no publications on which to base the power calculation, it was based on historical data (one month in 2012) from the municipal health registers for 14 patients who had stayed at the CRA and 13 who had been discharged directly from MHH. The mean number of hours of community care services per week was 3.7 (SD 3.5) for CRA patients and 20.91 (SD 40.4) for MHH patients. Mean daily function (ADL) score for CRA patients on a 1–5 scale was 1.58 (SD 0.37) and it was 1.94 (SD 0.65) for MHH patients.

Including 35 patients in each group, using a two-tailed t-test with a 5% statistical significance level and power of 80% would detect these differences. The aim was to include a total sample of 140 to allow for an expected high dropout and withdrawal rate.

Blinding

There was no blinding of the patients or staff due to the nature of the intervention. The persons extracting the data from the registers were not aware of the allocation. The outcome data only included data registered as part of the patients' regular care and, therefore, could not be influenced by the study staff.

Statistical methods

The comparison between the groups was based on the intention to treat principle, where the participants were analysed according to the group they were randomised to. No per protocol test was planned or done. There were complete data on the use of all the outcomes for all participants, meaning that no measures had to be taken regarding missing. Due to the outcome data having a strong non-normal distribution and outliers, and the small sample size ($n = 41$), the comparison of the continuous variables was analysed with the non-parametric Mann-Whitney U-test [28]. The categorical data were calculated using Pearson chi square or Fisher exact test.

Table 1 Cost in 2015 per inpatient day and per hour for various mental health services, with the sector responsible for financing

Place	Cost	Financed by university hospital	Financed by municipality
Cost per inpatient day (24 h)			
Mental health hospital	1065 EUR	ⅰ X	
Community mental health centre	619 EUR	X	
Community residential aftercare[a]	270 EUR		X
Cost per hour:			
Outpatient treatment at hospital	292 EUR	X	
Ambulant treatment[b]	181 EUR	X	X
Home help	84 EUR		X
Home care nursing	84 EUR		X
Community mental health consultation	90 EUR		X

The exchange rates were €100 = 948.50 NOK, rate at the Norges Bank on 05.07. 2017 using the mid-price (the midpoint between the buying and selling price)
[a]For the community residential aftercare, all operating cost (staff cost, and all expenditures) in 2015 was 805,738 EUR excluding capital cost. The operating cost was divided by 14 beds and 365 days and gave a cost of 184 EUR per inpatient day. The capital costs used was the mean of all nursing homes and residential aftercare units in the municipality (86 EUR)
[b]For the ambulant treatment, the cost was recalculated, as the cost provided by the administration (1168 EUR per hour) seemed too high. This was due to the hour cost being higher than the cost of one day in the hospital, and those providing the cost figures could not specify this figure. The recalculation was based on the yearly budget in 2015 of 1,062,309 EUR. It was assumed that the 10-full time equivalent employees had face-to-face time contact with the services user in 1/3 (due to travel, sometimes more than one employee visiting, administrative work etc.) of their work-time. One full time equivalent equals 1750 h per year (37.5 h per week). This gives some 5800 h of face-to-face services to the approximately 100 users receiving this service. This corresponds well with the number of hours of ambulant treatment observed in the trial among those receiving such services (median 53 h)
Cost is in EUR

The outcomes in the groups is presented with both median and mean values and mean difference with 95% confidence interval (95% CI) which were calculated using t-tests with bootstrapping for the continuous data. Thus, the 95% CI (from the parametric test) does not correspond to the p-values reported (from non-parametric test). For the categorical data, the difference is presented in percentage points.

There were some differences between the characteristics of the groups at baseline. Therefore, a post hoc analysis was done using linear regression analysis with total cost as dependent variable and baseline variables as independent variables. Total cost was chosen as it best captures the overall picture of the participants' health care use. Due to the small sample, and the rule of thumb of having at least 10 observation for every variable included in a regression analysis [29], only the baseline variables with more than 20%-point differences between the groups (Table 2, Homeless, Diagnosis, Employment status, Living alone) were included in the model as independent variables in addition to group allocation.

All analyses were done with SPSS 24 for Windows (IBM Corp. Armonk, NY).

Results

Participants flow

The total number of participants assessed for eligibility was not registered. However, in the weekly meetings between the researcher and the contact nurses (one nurse from each department in the MHH), the nurses reported

that almost all participants who were introduced to the study, said that they would participate. Forty-one participants met the inclusion criteria and were randomised Fig. 1.

Baseline data

There were some differences between the groups on some variables at baseline. There were more patients living alone, being homeless and unemployed in the intervention group, with one patient with a F6 diagnosis (personality disorder). In the control group, (Table 2) more patients were involuntary admitted and had a F6 diagnosis.

Implementation of the intervention

The intervention was implemented as planned, with changes in the observed variables in the direction expected (Table 3). All patients in the intervention group were discharged to the CRA. The difference in mean length of mental hospital inpatient stay (LOS) from randomisation to discharge was 6.3 days (3.8 days in the intervention group and 10.1 days in the control group, $p = .023$).

Outcomes

There were large variation and some outliers for most of the outcomes (Fig. 2).

Primary outcome

Those randomised to the CRA had on average 29% fewer hours of community mental health services for

Table 2 Demographic variables and diagnosis for patients at baseline

	All (n = 41)	Intervention (N = 21)	Control (N = 20)	Difference in % points
Age, mean (SD)	42.9 (14.7)	42.2 (14.9)	43.8 (14.8)	0
Female	21 (51%)	9 (43%)	12 (60%)	− 17
Living alone	29 (71%)	17 (81%)	12 (60%)	21
Homeless	15 (37%)	12 (57%)	3 (15%)	42
Sheltered housing	0	0	0	0
Involuntary admitted	8 (20%)	3 (14%)	5 (25%)	− 11
Employment status				
Full-time employment	2 (5%)	1 (5%)	1 (6%)	−1
Part-time employment	2 (5%)	2 (10%)	0 (0%)	10
Unemployment	10 (24%)	8 (40%)	2 (13%)	27
Disability pension	23 (56%)	10 (48%)	13 (65%)	− 17
Student	1 (2%)	0 (0%)	1 (6%)	− 6
Highest level of education				
Compulsory school	11(31%)	7 (37%)	4 (23%)	− 14
Middle level education	20 (55%)	9 (47%)	11 (65%)	− 18
Higher education	5 (14%)	3 (16%)	2 (12%)	4
Main Diagnosis (ICD- 10 code)				
Mental and behavioral disorders (F1)	4 (10%)	2 (10%)	2 (10%)	0
Schizophrenia, schizotypal, delusional disorders (F2)	10 (24%)	5 (24%)	5 (24%)	0
Mood (affective) disorders (F3) and anxiety disorders (F4)	17 (41%)	12 (57%)	5 (24%)	33
Behavioral and personality disorders (F6)	5 (12%)	1 (5%)	4 (20%)	−15
Observation for suspected mental and behaviour disorders (Z03.2)	5 (12%)	1 (5%)	4 (20%)	−15

N varies due to missing: Employment (control: three missing). Education (intervention: two missing. Control: three missing)
Numbers are N (%) except for age which is mean (SD)

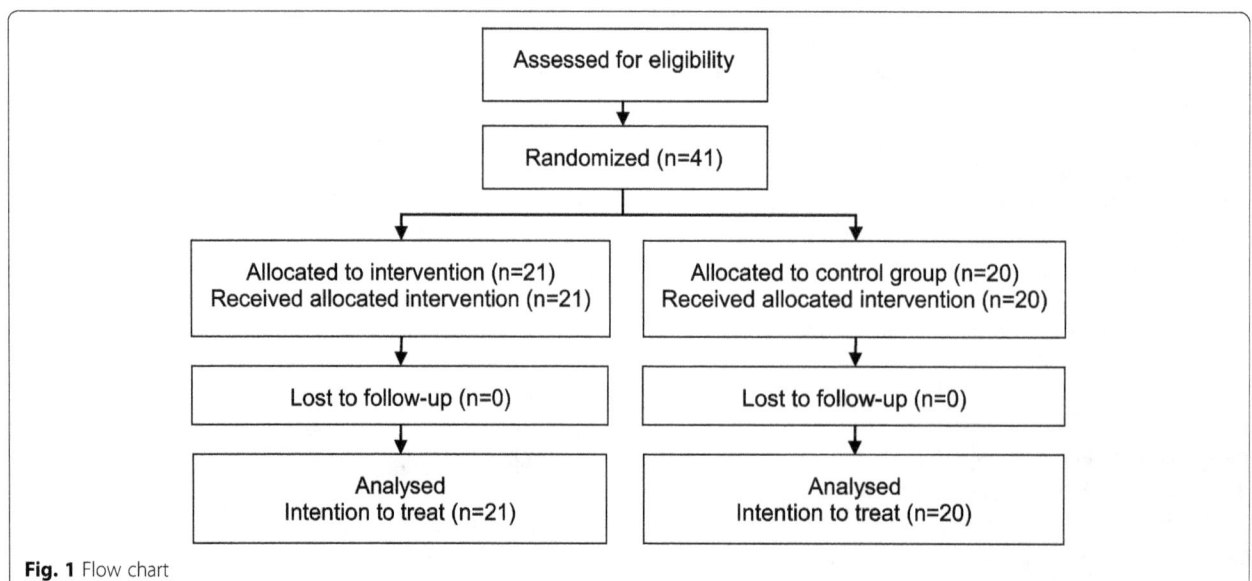

Fig. 1 Flow chart

Table 3 Implementation of the intervention

Variable	All (n = 41)	Intervention (N = 21)	Control (N = 20)	P-value
Discharged to	N (%)	N (%)	N (%)	
Home	11(27%)	0 (0%)	11 (55%)	
CMHC	9 (22%)	0 (0%)	9 (45%)	
CRA	21 (51%)	21 (100%)	0 (0%)	
Number of hospital inpatient days from index admission to discharge from MHH				
Mean (SD)	18.3 (26.9)	20.4 (30.9)	16.1 (22.5)	
Median (IQR), range	11 (5–16), 113	9 (4.3–17.5), 112.5	12.5 (6.5–16), 107	.531
Number of hospital inpatient days from index admission to date of randomisation (baseline)				
Mean (SD)	11.4 (19.9)	16,6 (26.9)	6.0 (4.1)	
Median (IQR), range	6 (3–10.5), 90	6 (2.5–13), 90	6 (3–8.5), 14	.495
Number of hospital inpatient days from date of randomisation (baseline) to discharge date				
Mean (SD)	6.9 (15.4)	3.8 (5.8)	10.1 (21.1)	
Median (IQR), range	3 (1–7), 97.5	1 (1–4), 23.5	4.5 (1.3–10), 97.0	.023
Length of stay at an institution immediately after discharge from the mental health hospital				
CMHC				
Mean (SD)	5.9 (12.8)	0 (0)	12 (16.4)	
Median (IQR), range	0 (0–0), 55	0 (0–0), 0	0 (0–23), 55	
CRA				
Mean (SD)	24.1 (35.6)	45.9 (37.6)	0 (0)	
Median (IQR), range	1.5 (0–44), 176	44 (28–58), 175	0 (0–0), 0	

MHH Mental health hospital, *CMHC* Community mental health centre, *CRA* Community residential aftercare

12 months but the precision of the estimate was low, i.e. wide confidence intervals (mean difference – 21.6 h, 95% CI -93.1 to 44.9, p = .096) (Table 4). This difference was mainly due to less use of home care nursing. The cost for the community mental health services was 29% lower with a mean difference of – 1845 EUR (95% CI -8267 to 4171, p = .102) with similar imprecision in the estimates.

Secondary outcomes
The total number of inpatients days after discharge from the initial stay to 12 months was 66 days for both groups

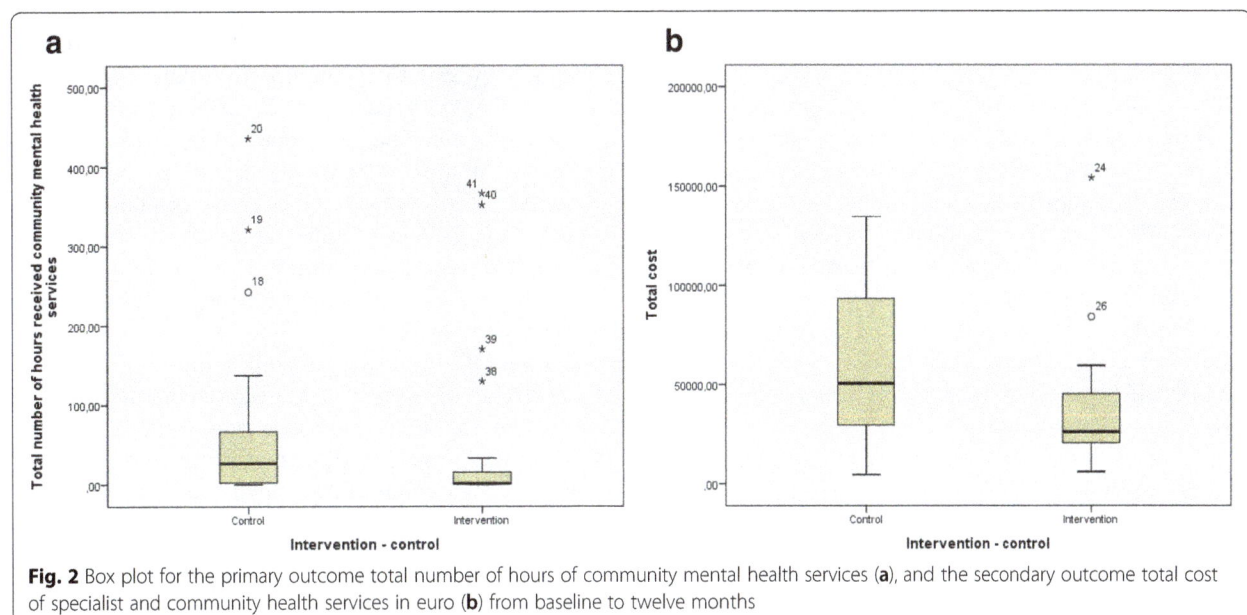

Fig. 2 Box plot for the primary outcome total number of hours of community mental health services (**a**), and the secondary outcome total cost of specialist and community health services in euro (**b**) from baseline to twelve months

Table 4 Primary outcomes: Total number of hours, number of patients and costs of community mental health services from baseline (date of randomisation) to 12 months

Variable	All (n = 41)		Intervention (N = 21)	Control (N = 20)	Between groups	P- value
Number of hours	Mean (SD)	Median (IQR), range	Mean (SD)	Mean (SD)	Mean diff (95% CI)	
Total number of hours received community mental health services	62.9 (115.1)	6.0 (0.0–54.0), 436.0	52.4 (111.4)	74 (120.8)	−21.6 (−93.1 to 44.9)	.096
Home help (cleaning, shopping etc.)	1.8 (6.6)	0 (0–0), 39.3	1.4 (3.7)	2.3 (8.8)	−0.9 (−5.5 to 2.4)	.680
Home care nursing	55.3 (106.3)	0 (0–49.4), 396.7	47.4 (111.0)	63.5 (103.4)	−16 (−85.5 to 51.2)	.023
Community mental health consultation	5.9 (20.7)	0(0–3.3), 128.6	3.6 (8.2)	8.2 (28.6)	−4.5 (− 20.9 to 4.5)	.758
Number of patients	N (%)		n (%)	n (%)	Difference in %- points	
Total number of patients with the listed services[a]	29 (71%)		13 (62%)	16 (80%)	− 18	.209
Home help (cleaning, shopping etc.)	5 (12%)		3 (14%)	2 (10%)	4	.679
Home care nursing	20 (49%)		6 (29%)	14 (70%)	− 41	.009
Community mental health consultation	14 (34%)		8 (38%)	6 (30%)	8	.589
Costs	Mean (SD)	Median (IQR), range	Mean (SD)	Mean (SD)	Mean diff (95% CI)	
Total cost of Community mental health services	5345 (9752.6)	546 (0–4587), 36,773	4444.7 (9399)	6290.5 (10,266.7)	− 1845 (−8267 to 4171)	.102
Home help (cleaning, shopping etc.)	153 (558)	0 (0–0), 3313	116 (310)	191 (743)	−74 (− 476 to 200)	.680
Home care nursing	4661 (8966)	0 (0–4165), 33,460	3999 (9359)	5357 (8721)	− 1357 (− 7124 to 4683)	.023
Community mental health consultation	530 (1864)	0 (0–300), 11,605	328 (742)	741 (2577)	− 413 (− 1784 to 457)	.758

[a]Each patient could receive more than one service

(Table 5), but patients randomised to the CRA had 54% fewer inpatient days in the MHH (mean differences – 13.4 days, 95% CI -29.9 to 0.9, p = .008). About half (6.3 days, Table 3) of the difference between the groups in MHH inpatients days (13.4 days) was due to the patients in the control group being discharged later from the MHH after the initial stay. The total number of admission to any institution after the initial stay was 3.9 times in the intervention group and 4.9 times in the control group (mean difference – 0.9 times, 95% CI -3.5 to 1.5, p = .224).

The number of and proportion of persons with admissions and readmissions was not statistically significant different between the groups, but was slightly lower in the intervention group (Table 5).

The total cost for all mental health services for 12 months was 38.5% lower for patients randomised to the CRA (mean differences – 23,071 EUR, 95% CI -45,450 to 3027, p = .057) (Table 6). This was mainly due to lower inpatients costs which had a mean difference of – 17,741 EUR (95% CI -36,824 to 4503, p = .042) in favour of the intervention.

Post hoc analysis
The post hoc analysis was done due to the observed differences in patient characteristics at baseline, using a multivariable linear regression model with total cost as the independent variable and the four baseline

characteristics with the largest %-point differences between the groups (> 20%-points, Table 2) as dependent variables. The difference between the groups in favour of the intervention group was a reduced cost of – 19,781 EUR (95% CI -44,072 to 4509, p=,107) in the best model, which included three of the four independent variables (Homeless, Diagnosis and Employment status).

Discussion
This is the first RCT study on the effect of discharge for patients with SMI to a community residential aftercare facility (CRA) with no organised in-house activities or on-site treatment. The differences in utilisation and cost during 12 months were in favour of the intervention group, but mostly with p-values above the conventional cut-off p < 0.05. The confidence intervals were wide, meaning that there was imprecision in the estimates. Thus, no final conclusion on the effect of the CRA can be made based on this study.

However, the study gives indication of a potential effect of discharging patient in need of community aftercare to the CRA. The best estimates for this potential based on the present study is that it can reduce the use of hourly based community mental health services with 29% (22 h), with a cost saving of 29% (1845 EUR) for each patient compared to usual care. The total number of inpatient days for one year was the same (66 days), but the number of inpatient days in the mental health

Table 5 Secondary outcomes. Number of mental health inpatient days, number of admissions and number of readmission < 30 days from baseline (date of randomisation) to twelve months

Variable	All (n = 41)		Intervention (N = 21)	Control (N = 20)	Between groups	P- value
	Mean (SD)	Median (IQR), range	Mean (SD)	Mean (SD)	Mean diff (95% CI)	
Total inpatient days	66.5 (61.4)	50 (34.5–77.5), 306	66.7 (55.9)	66.4 (68.1)	0.3 (−35.8 to 40.3)	.629
MHH	17.8 (25.0)	8 (3–18), 97.5	11.2 (19.8)	24.7 (28.5)	−13.4 (−29.8 to 0.9)	.008
CMHC	17.9 (31.5)	0 (0–27.5), 120	7.9 (22.3)	28.4 (36.7)	−20.4 (−38.8 to − 2.8)	.004
CRA	29.7 (50.3)	2 (0–47.5), 255	45.9 (37.6)	12.8 (57.0)[a]	33.2 (− 0.1 to 60)	.000
CRA self-referral	1.2 (2.8)	0 (0–0), 12	1.7 (2.8)	0.6 (2.7)[b]	1.1 (− 0.6 to 2.7)	.035
Total number of admission after initial stay	4.4 (4.0)	3 (1–5), 15	3.9 (3.9)	4.9 (4.1)	−0.9 (−3.5 to 1.5)	.224
MHH	2.8 (2.9)	2 (1–3.5), 12	2.6 (2.8)	3.1 (3.0)	−0.5 (−2.3 to 1.2)	.358
CMHC	1.2 (2.5)	0 (0–2), 14	0.7 (1.7)	1.8 (3.1)	−1.0 (−2.8 to 0.3)	.016
CRA	0.5 (0.5)	1 (0–1),1	1.0 (0.0)	0.05 (0.22)[a]	0.9 (0.8 to 0.9)	0.00
CRA self-referral	0.4 (0.83)	0 (0–0), 3	0.7 (1.1)	0.05(0.22)[b]	0.6 (0.2 to 1.1)	.019
Total number of readmissions after initial stay	1.5 (2.8)	0 (0–2.5), 11	1.2 (2.4)	1.9 (3.2)	−0.8 (−2.5 to 0.9)	.440
MHH	1 (1.9)	0 (0–1), 8	0.81 (1.7)	1.2 (2.2)	−0.4 (−1.7 to 0.8)	.820
CMHC	0.5 (1.9)	0 (0–0), 11	0.38 (1.2)	0.7 (2.5)	−0.3 (−1.7 to 0.7)	.396
CRA	0		0	0	0	
	N (%)		n (%)	n (%)	Difference %- points	
Number of patients admitted after initial stay	38 (93%)		21 (100%)	17 (85%)	15	.069
MHH	21 (51%)		9 (43%)	12 (60%)	− 17	
CMHC	17 (41%)		4 (19%)	13 (65%)	− 46	
CRA aftercare	22 (54%)		21 (100%)	1 (5%)	95	
CRA self-referral	8 (20%)		7 (33%)	1 (5%)	28	
Number of patient with readmission	15 (37%)		6 (29%)	9 (45%)	− 16	.281
MHH	12 (29%)		6 (29%)	6 (30%)	−1	
CMHC	6 (15%)		2 (10%)	4 (20%)	−10	
CRA	0		0	0	0	

MHH Mental Health hospital, CMHC Community mental health centre, CRA Community residential aftercare

[a]One patient in the control group, who after the initial stay at the MHH was discharged to home, later had several acute admissions to the MHH. After the last of these, the patient was discharged to the CRA from the MHH as the CMHC declined the referral of this patient from the MHH, and a solution had to be found. This patient then stayed at the CRA for 255 days

[b]One patient in the control group was admitted to a self-referral bed at the CRA from the patient's residence by a community mental health team as an emergency measure due to lack of other suitable services. The patient stayed at the CRA for 12 days

hospital was 54% (13 days) lower. Importantly, although using less services, the point estimate for the number of inpatient admissions and readmissions was respectively 18% (− 0.9 admissions) and 42% (− 0.8 readmissions) lower in the intervention group indicating at least no major worsening in the intervention group.

Considering possible mechanisms and explanations for the direction of the observed effect, it seems that the CRA is successful in facilitating independent living which, in turn, leads to less mental health service use. Even if a stay at the CRA does not reduce the total number of inpatient days during the first year, spending more time in residential aftercare service can leave room for better assessment of and subsequent alignment between the patients' actual care needs in the community and the services offered. Another explanation can be that when the hospital staff communicate the care needs of the patient to the community services, they do so based on what they have seen during the hospital stay (observer bias) [30]. This can differ from the patients' behaviour in a CRA setting where there are no in-house organised activities, and where, consequently, the staff can observe how the patient manages in a more home like setting. In addition, a stay in the CRA allows for more time in assessing and setting up the required level of services to support independent living. This is in line with the finding in an observational cohort study among six community residential alternatives compared to six standard acute wards [18], which found that patients having used the community alternative had more contact with community mental health teams, early intervention services and crisis teams.

Table 6 Cost for all inpatient and outpatient services from baseline (date of randomisation) to twelve months. Values are in euro (EUR)

Variable	All (n = 41)		Intervention (N = 21)	Control (N = 20)	Between groups	P- value
	Mean (SD)	Median (IQR), range	Mean (SD)	Mean (SD)	Mean diff (95% CI)	
Total cost	48,131 (39726)	31,232 (20813–57,209), 149,638	36,877 (32647)	59,948 (43745)	−23,071 (−45,450 to 3027)	.057
Sum inpatient service cost	38,321 (34137)	25,825 (14808–46,641), 142,643	29,667 (31543)	47,408 (35161)	−17,741 (−36,824 to 4503)	.042
MHH	18,920 (26663)	8518 (3194–19,167), 103,821	11,941 (21085)	26,248 (30304)	−14,306 (−31,754 to 912)	.008
CMHC	11,073 (19526)	8518 (3194–19,167), 74,237	4896 (13812)	17,559 (22703)	−12,663 (−23,568 to − 2632)	.004
CRA	8018 (13573)	539 (0–12,810), 68,770	12,380 (10142)	3428 (15377)	8941 (− 608 to 16,194)	.000
CRA – self-referral	309 (749)	0 (0–0), 3236	449 (764)	161 (723)	287 (− 199 to 714)	.035
Sum outpatient services cost	9809 (12934)	4916 (875–15,192), 49,443	7210 (9578)	12,539 (15501)	− 5329 (−13,216 to 2546)	.215
Mental health outpatient treatment	2678 (7128)	486 (0–2178), 43,757	2145 (3603)	3239 (9625)	− 1094 (− 6125 to 2240)	.843
Mental health ambulant treatment	1786 (4050)	0 (0–180), 15,619	620 (1920)	3010 (5250)	− 2389.7 (− 4681 to 90.6)	.160
Home help (cleaning, shopping etc.)	153 (558)	0 (0–0), 3313	116 (310)	191 (743)	−74.5 (− 412.6 to 214.5)	.680
Home care nursing	4661 (8966)	0 (0–4165), 33,460	3999 (9359)	5357 (8721)	−1357.7 (− 6520 to 4051)	.023
Community mental health consultation	530 (1864)	0 (0–300), 11,605	328 (742)	741 (2577)	−413.6 (−1773 to 411)	.758

Furthermore, the patient's own role can be important, especially what the patients can learn and do differently after a stay at a "boring hotel" [26]. This study cannot answer whether the CRA might increase the patients' contribution or abilities such as agency, responsibility, self-management, coping and empowerment. One way of looking at independence is by examining motivation and behaviour, as the CRA attempt to motivate the patients to adopt a more independent behaviour. The self-determination theory (SDT) can shed some light on this, as it claims to provide a universal framework for understanding the individual and environmental factors that shape motivation and subsequent behaviour [31]. According to SDT, motivation depends on the (lack of) support for three basic psychological needs: autonomy, competence, and relatedness. It does not seem to be fare fetched to suggest that these areas were strengthened; leading to the patients' feeling more equipped to do self-care activities such as preparing their own meals, structuring their daily routines and introducing activities in their neighbourhood.

The chosen primary outcome, use of hourly based community health and social services, was chosen based on an assumption that discharge to the CRA would help identify the best level of service for each patient, which was expected to be lower than usual care. This does not imply that less use of community health and social services was a desired outcome by itself. The aim must be to balance the level of services to the patient's needs. However, with the aim to promote independency among service users, the level of services should not be so high as to jeopardise this. To be almost self-reliant and be in command of one's own life are basic rights that most humans takes for granted. Given the direction of the results in this study, pointing towards both less use of services and fewer re-/admissions for those randomised to the CRA, there are indications that having a strong community orientation in the discharge process can result in a service level promoting independency.

Even if both step-up [15–19] and step down [20–23] community residential services exist, none of the studies investigating the effects and costs are directly comparable to this study, as they offer in-house activities or treatment. However, according to these studies, there seems to be a clear indication that community residential services can reduce costs [17, 18, 20], similar to the point estimates found in this study of around 1/3 reduction: Byford et al. [17] found 22% lower total 12-month costs (£14,952 vs. £19,288), a UK based study by Slade et al. [18] reported 61% lower 12-month inpatient costs (£3832 vs. £9850) and Thomas et al. in Australia [20] found that the cost per day per client in the step-up step-down program was 32% lower ($517 vs. $758). The explanation for reduced costs in these studies and in our

study, is chiefly due to reduced inpatient stays and use of specialist services.

We did not measure change in patients' level of symptoms and functioning, but two other studies on community residential aftercare have done this [21, 23]. An observational study from Australia [21] found improvement in patients' symptoms and functioning three months after discharge from the residential inpatient step-down unit. An RCT among justice involved persons [23] found a significant reduction in psychiatric symptom severity after two years in those who had been admitted to self-run community residential aftercare (Oxford House).

Strength and limitations

To the best of our knowledge, this is the first RCT-study to investigate a step-down model of a staffed residential aftercare not offering in-house activities or treatment therapy. The strength of this study is the use of data from health service registers covering both specialist and community mental health care utilisation, which provided complete data on all participants.

One major limitation was that the sample size was smaller than what was pre-planned, which in addition to giving imprecise estimates, also is the most likely explanation for the differences in patient characteristics at baseline. An alternative explanation of baseline difference is flaws in the randomisation and allocation process. However, the randomisation was internet based and it was not possible for anyone involved in the study processes to influence the allocation.

The recruitment was both slow and low despite a range of study activities from information meetings to encouragement from management. The main reason expressed by some of the inpatient staff in the MHH was scepticism about the level of competence at the CRA, particularly the lack of psychologists. This scepticism was surprising as the CRA had been in operation before the study and should thus be known to the hospital staff with treatment responsibility. Furthermore, it cannot be ruled out that the persons with treatment responsibility recruiting patients to the CRA previously and maybe to the study represent a sub-set, as it was not collected data on who recruited patients.

Another reason for the recruitment problem can be that the staff at the hospital did not include patients for this study to avoid them being randomised to the control group, which meant that they would get a delayed discharge compared to being discharged to the CRA. This suspicion is strengthening by the fact that some patients were discharged directly to the CRA instead being recruited to the study.

Nevertheless, it is a major limitation that the number of eligible patients was not recorded. However, it is obvious that the number of eligible patients was far higher than the 41 patients recruited, as the recruitment took place in an 81-bed unit over 26 months. Thus, caution is needed when generalising the result of this study to other settings, as the sample in this study represents a subset of hospitalised persons with SMI. The best description of this subset is that it is representative of the group of patients with SMI that were considered suitable for the CRA by personnel with treatment responsibility in the hospital who are willing to refer patients to the CRA. This assumption is strengthened by the contact nurses for the study who reported that almost all participants that were introduced to the study agreed to participate.

Conclusion

In this study, it was not possible to draw a definite conclusion about the effect, due to the small sample and imprecision of the estimates. The direction of the results and size of the point estimate, including findings in other studies, indicates that transferring patients ready for discharge from mental hospital to community residential aftercare without organized in-house activities has the potential to reduce total consumption of health services and costs without increased hospital admissions.

Abbreviations
CMHC: Community mental health centre; CRA: Community residential aftercare; MHH: Mental health hospital; RCT: Randomized controlled trial; SMI: Severe mental illness

Acknowledgements
The authors would like to thank participants that took part in the study, the staff at the mental health hospital, the staff at the community residential aftercare, city of Trondheim, Norway for ongoing support.

Funding
Part of ER salary was covered by a grant from the Norwegian directorate for health.

Authors' contributions
ER conceived of the study, participated in the design of the study, collected and led the analysis of the data and drafted the manuscript. OB participated in analysing the data and contributed to the manuscript drafts. AS participated in the design, analysing the data and contributed to the manuscript drafts. All authors read and approved the final manuscript.

Consent for publication
Not applicable.

Competing interests
The first author (ER) worked with the establishment of the CRA as an advisor to the chief officer in the municipality, but has not been involved in the day to day operation of the service. The other authors declare that they have no competing interests.

Author details
[1]Department of Public Health and Nursing, Norwegian University of Science and Technology, 7491 Trondheim, Norway. [2]Health and Welfare, Trondheim, Norway. [3]Faculty of Nursing and Health Sciences, Nord University, Levanger, Norway. [4]Department of Mental Health, Norwegian University of Science and Technology, Trondheim, Norway.

References
1. Zhang J, Harvey C, Andrew C. Factors associated with length of stay and the risk of readmission in an acute psychiatric inpatient facility: a retrospective study. Aust N Z J Psychiatry. 2011;45(7):578–85.
2. Laursen TM, Munk-Olsen T, Vestergaard M. Life expectancy and cardiovascular mortality in persons with schizophrenia. Curr Opin Psychiatry. 2012;25(2):83–8.
3. Davydow DS, Ribe AR, Pedersen HS, Fenger-Gron M, Cerimele JM, Vedsted P, Vestergaard M. Serious mental illness and risk for hospitalizations and Rehospitalizations for ambulatory care-sensitive conditions in Denmark: a Nationwide population-based cohort study. Med Care. 2016;54(1):90–7.
4. Tulloch AD, Fearon P, David AS. Length of stay of general psychiatric inpatients in the United States: systematic review. Admin Pol Ment Health. 2011;38(3):155–68.
5. Kunitoh N. From hospital to the community: the influence of deinstitutionalization on discharged long-stay psychiatric patients. Psychiatry Clin Neurosci. 2013;67(6):384–96.
6. Lewis R, Glasby J. Delayed discharge from mental health hospitals: results of an English postal survey. Health Soc Care Community. 2006;14(3):225–30.
7. Ose SO, Slettebak R. Unødvendige innleggelser, utskrivningsklare pasienter og samarbeid rundt enkeltpasienter-omfang og kjennetegn ved pasientene. SINTEF, rapport A. 2013;25247.
8. Rojas-García A, Turner S, Pizzo E, Hudson E, Thomas J, Raine R. Impact and experiences of delayed discharge: a mixed-studies systematic review. Health Expect. 2018;21(1):41-56.
9. Vigod SN, Kurdyak PA, Dennis CL, Leszcz T, Taylor VH, Blumberger DM, Seitz DP. Transitional interventions to reduce early psychiatric readmissions in adults: systematic review. Br J Psychiatry J Ment Sci. 2013;202(3):187–94.
10. Sfetcu R, Musat S, Haaramo P, Ciutan M, Scintee G, Vladescu C, Wahlbeck K, Katschnig H. Overview of post-discharge predictors for psychiatric re-hospitalisations: a systematic review of the literature. BMC Psychiatry. 2017;17(1):227.
11. Leff J, Trieman N. Long-stay patients discharged from psychiatric hospitals social and clinical outcomes after five years in the community. The TAPS Project 46. Br J Psychiatry. 2000;176(3):217–23.
12. Manuel JI, Gandy ME, Rieker D. Trends in hospital discharges and dispositions for episodes of co-occurring severe mental illness and substance use disorders. Admin Pol Ment Health. 2014;42(2):168-75.
13. Taft Parsons I. Length of stay: managed care agenda or a measure of clinical efficiency? Psychiatry (Edgmont). 2006;3(6):46.
14. Babalola O, Gormez V, Alwan NA, Johnstone P, Sampson S. Length of hospitalisation for people with severe mental illness. Cochrane Database Syst Rev. 2014;1:CD000384.
15. Thomas KA, Rickwood D. Clinical and cost-effectiveness of acute and subacute residential mental health services: a systematic review. Psychiatr Serv. 2013;64(11):1140–9.
16. Fenton WS, Hoch JS, Herrell JM, Mosher L, Dixon L. Cost and cost-effectiveness of hospital vs residential crisis care for patients who have serious mental illness. Arch Gen Psychiatry. 2002;59(4):357–64.
17. Byford S, Sharac J, Lloyd-Evans B, Gilburt H, Osborn DP, Leese M, Johnson S, Slade M. Alternatives to standard acute in-patient care in England: readmissions, service use and cost after discharge. Br J Psychiatry Suppl. 2010;53:s20–5.

18. Slade M, Byford S, Barrett B, Lloyd-Evans B, Gilburt H, Osborn DP, Skinner R, Leese M, Thornicroft G, Johnson S. Alternatives to standard acute in-patient care in England: short-term clinical outcomes and cost-effectiveness. Br J Psychiatry Suppl. 2010;53:s14–9.

19. Borge FM, Hoffart A, Sexton H, Clark DM, Markowitz JC, McManus F. Residential cognitive therapy versus residential interpersonal therapy for social phobia: a randomized clinical trial. J Anxiety Disord. 2008;22(6):991–1010.

20. Thomas K, Rickwood DJ, Bussenschutt G. Adult step-up step-down: a sub-acute short-term residential mental health service. Int J Psychosoc Rehabil. 2015;19(1):13–21.

21. Thomas KA, Rickwood DJ, Brown PM. Symptoms, functioning and quality of life after treatment in a residential sub-acute mental health service in Australia. Health Soc Care Community. 2017;25(1):243–54.

22. Zarzar T, Sheitman B, Cook A, Robbins B. Reducing length of acute inpatient hospitalization using a residential step down model for patients with serious mental illness. Community Ment Health J. 2018:54(2):180-3.

23. Majer JM, Chapman HM, Jason LA. Comparative analysis of treatment conditions upon psychiatric severity levels at two years among justice involved persons. Adv Dual Diagn. 2016;9(1):38–47.

24. Armijo J, Mendez E, Morales R, Schilling S, Castro A, Alvarado R, Rojas G. Efficacy of community treatments for schizophrenia and other psychotic disorders: a literature review. Front Psychol. 2013;4:116.

25. Craven MA, Bland R. Better practices in collaborative mental health care: an analysis of the evidence base. Can J Psychiatry. 2006;51(6 Suppl 1):7S–72S.

26. Roos E, Bjerkeset O, Svavarsdóttir MH, Steinsbekk A. Like a hotel, but boring: users' experience with short-time community-based residential aftercare. BMC Health Serv Res. 2017;17(1):832.

27. Romoren TI, Torjesen DO, Landmark B. Promoting coordination in Norwegian health care. Int J Integr Care. 2011;11(Spec 10th Anniversary Ed):e127.

28. Hollander M, Wolfe DA, Chicken E. Nonparametric statistical methods (vol. 751). Wiley; 2013.

29. Lydersen S. Statistical review: frequently given comments. Ann Rheum Dis. 2015;74(2):323–5.

30. Burghardt GM, Bartmess-LeVasseur JN, Browning SA, Morrison KE, Stec CL, Zachau CE, Freeberg TM. Perspectives–minimizing observer bias in behavioral studies: a review and recommendations. Ethology. 2012;118(6):511–7.

31. Deci EL, Ryan RM. The "what" and "why" of goal pursuits: human needs and the self-determination of behavior. Psychol Inq. 2000;11(4):227–68.

24

Residential green space quantity and quality and symptoms of psychological distress: a 15-year longitudinal study of 3897 women in postpartum

Xiaoqi Feng[1,2,3*] and Thomas Astell-Burt[1,2,3,4]

Abstract

Background: Experiments and large-scale epidemiological studies indicate the importance of green space for mental health. However, little research has been conducted to elucidate whether these mental health benefits are more dependent upon the quantity or quality of the green space.

Methods: Symptoms of psychological distress were measured in 3897 women who did not change neighbourhood up to 15 years postpartum using the Kessler 6 psychological distress scale from 2004 onwards. The percentage land-use of the neighbourhood was used to ascertain a measure of green space quantity. A Likert scale was used to measure green space quality in response to the statement *"there are good parks, playgrounds and play spaces in this neighbourhood."* Multilevel negative binomial growth curve regression models were used to examine the patterning of symptoms of psychological distress across the postpartum period in relation to green space quantity and quality, adjusting for person-level and geographical markers of confounding. The same variables were also fitted in multilevel logistic regressions to examine the odds of reporting serious mental illness (as defined by K6 scores ≥ 13 out of 24).

Results: Symptoms of psychological distress were fewer among women who agreed (rate ratio (RR) 0.95, 95%CI 0.91 to 0.98) and strongly agreed (RR 0.89, 95%CI 0.85 to 0.93) local parks were good quality. The odds of reporting serious mental illness were also lower among women who agreed (odds ratio (OR) 0.88, 95%CI 0.77 to 1.00) and strongly agreed (OR 0.74, 95%CI 0.64 to 0.86) local parks were good quality. No association was found between green space quantity and symptoms of psychological distress or the odds of reporting serious mental illness.

Conclusions: This study suggests it may be how mothers perceive green space nearby and what those spaces enable them to do, rather than simply how much there is overall, that is important for promoting mental health in the postpartum period. In conclusion, community consultation is likely to be a crucial part of strategies that maximise the health benefits of urban greening for everyone.

Keywords: Mental health, Green space quality, Green space quantity, Women, Postpartum

* Correspondence: xfeng@uow.edu.au
[1]Population Wellbeing and Environment Research Lab (PowerLab), School of Health and Society, Faculty of Social Sciences, University of Wollongong, Wollongong, NSW, Australia
[2]Menzies Centre for Health Policy, University of Sydney, Sydney, NSW, Australia
Full list of author information is available at the end of the article

Background

Urban greening and restoration of green space is widely believed to promote mental health through a range of pathways. This is supported by evidence from experiments and large-scale observational studies [1–4] which suggest contact with green spaces (e.g. parks) provides effortless restoration and opportunities for stress reduction. This includes a range of studies suggesting views of nature promote memory recall [5], relaxed wakefulness [6], altered cerebral blood flow and brain activation patterns consistent with relaxation [7, 8]. Studies have suggested that physical (and probably also social) recreation in environments containing green space also reduces the risk of minor psychiatric morbidity [9, 10] and facilitates an enhanced sense of self and connectedness with nature [11]. This in turn stimulates forward-looking, pro-social thinking and reductions in future discounting associated with depression and negative health behaviours [12]. Other pathways may include natural soundscapes that enhance stress reduction and cognitive restoration [13], phytochemicals that might have benefits for immune and central nervous systems [14], higher levels of negative ions [15] that may have value for the treatment of depression [16] and increased exposure to lactic acid bacteria and microbial genera which are ubiquitous in the natural environment and could influence depression, fatigue, and cognition [17].

Reviewing many of the epidemiological studies conducted so far on adults in Australia [9, 18, 19], New Zealand [20], the UK [21–24], the US [25, 26], the Netherlands [27–29] and Denmark [30] reveals that the majority of evidence is based upon cross-sectional data and supports interventions that focus on increasing the quantity of residential green space. This conclusion is also supported by recent systematic reviews of research on adults and children [31, 32]. This is important to help set guidelines on how much green space is needed to promote mental health, given that opportunities for coming into contact with nature worldwide are becoming rarer as parks within cities and around the urban fringe are redeveloped into new housing, commercial premises and other forms of built environment. Within this context, however, even maintaining a certain quantity of green space may be very challenging and might ultimately take a lower priority in comparison to other needs. Evidence is required on not just how much green space is needed, but also what green space is fit for purpose.

'Fit for purpose' is a concept that pushes beyond quantity to notions of quality, which given its policy relevance is a surprisingly far less researched issue in epidemiological studies of green space and health. In fact, only three studies have examined the potential mental health benefit of quality green space in adult samples. One study in Perth (Australia) found lower odds of psychological distress among participants living near moderate to high quality green spaces, but no association with green space quantity [19]. A study of four cities in the Netherlands found evidence of mental health benefits of both green space quantity and quality, but with the strongest evidence for high quality greenery [29]. A third study in Santiago (Chile) reported better mental health among people living in areas where there were more green spaces viewed as appropriately maintained [33]. Each of these studies was reliant upon cross-sectional data and could not examine how green space quantity and quality might matter as people age, which is important as many studies have already shown that mental health varies across the lifecourse (e.g. [21]).

Accordingly, our aim was to answer the question 'is green space quantity or quality more important for mental health?' using a longitudinal study. We focussed upon adult women who were followed-up biennially from 0-1y up to 15y postpartum. The purpose of focussing upon women postpartum was to recognise an under-researched yet very large population subgroup within which depression is common and a significant cause of morbidity and mortality [34, 35]. For example, recent work suggested that 14.5% of women experienced symptoms of depression at 4 years postpartum, higher than at any point in the first 12 months following childbirth [36]. It may also be that green space quality matters more than quantity during this sensitive period of the lifecourse, given the needs of the mother and that it remains common for them to be responsible for the majority of childrearing activities. For example, it is plausible that for mothers of infants a small but high quality green space nearby that affords opportunities for outdoor relaxation and socialising within a short walk of home has greater restorative potential than a large amount of green space viewed as poor quality. With evidence from prior studies suggesting that there can be a discrepancy between subjective and objective distance to the nearest green space (e.g. [37]), it may be that nearby green spaces that are perceived to be low in quality may offer very little restorative benefit. As such, this sample was considered to provide an important test of whether a focus on green space quantity is sufficient, or if green space quality also matters for protecting mothers' mental health in the postpartum period.

Methods

Data on mothers in the postpartum period was obtained from Australia's definitive birth cohort, the Longitudinal Study of Australian Children (LSAC). Permission to obtain and analyse the LSAC was granted through a formal application to The Department of Social Services of the Australian Government (the data custodian). The LSAC

Table 1 Sample counts and percentage reporting serious mental illness, as defined by scores ≥ 13 out of 24 on the Kessler 6 Psychological Distress Scale, across sample characteristics

	N	% K6 ≥ 13	Chi2 (p-value)
Total	20,407	12.4	
Green space quantity			
≤ 5%	4204	11.7	
6–10%	3292	11.9	
11–20%	5671	13.7	
21–40%	4987	12.9	
≥ 41%	2253	10.3	22.2 (< 0.001)
Parks good quality			
Do not agree	3726	16.0	
Agree	9626	12.8	
Strongly Agree	6548	9.7	
No response	507	13.4	89.2 (< 0.001)
Years since childbirth			
0-1y	1658	14.2	
2-3y	1623	8.8	
4-5y	3362	15.4	
6-7y	3440	11.0	
8-9y	3312	11.7	
10-11y	3436	12.1	
12-13y	1810	12.6	
14-15y	1766	12.9	60.4 (< 0.001)
Age group			
17 to 29	1004	16.4	
30 to 34	3198	13.8	
35 to 39	6007	12.3	
40 to 44	6084	12.0	
45 to 63	4114	11.2	26.9 (< 0.001)
Indigenous status			
No	20,108	12.3	
Yes	290	18.6	
No response	9	33.3	14.1 (0.001)
Highest educational qualification			
Postgraduate	3357	10.5	
Undergraduate	12,172	12.7	
Year 11 to 13	3172	11.4	
≤ Year 10	1693	16.1	
Other	13	23.1	38.3 (< 0.001)
Economic status			
employed	14,994	10.4	
economically inactive	4979	17.5	
unemployed	419	23.6	
no response	15	13.3	224.2 (< 0.001)

Table 1 Sample counts and percentage reporting serious mental illness, as defined by scores ≥ 13 out of 24 on the Kessler 6 Psychological Distress Scale, across sample characteristics (Continued)

	N	% K6 ≥ 13	Chi2 (p-value)
Area disadvantage			
affluent	6786	10.3	
average	6745	12.4	
deprived	6876	14.5	54.3 (< 0.001)
Geographic remoteness			
major cities	13,165	12.9	
inner regional	4331	11.1	
outer regional or remote	2911	12.2	9.9 (0.007)

began in 2004 and involved biennial follow-up of approximately 10,000 children and at least one parent each. The majority of the parents who participated were mothers [38]. Sampling for the LSAC originated with the Australian Government's provider of universal healthcare listing all permanent residents and citizens ('Medicare') in a two-stage clustered design. Representativeness of the sample across urban, regional and rural communities was obtained via sampling of postcodes stratified by state and territory and by capital city statistical division compared with the rest of the state in 2004. Recruitment and consent for participation was obtained via letters posted to parents who were randomly selected from the sample postcodes. The rate of recruitment was 50.4%, with 37.5% opting out and 15.2% being uncontactable. Data collection via face-to-face interviews had response rates > 90% at baseline and approximately 80% thereafter. Further information on the LSAC sampling and variables is available in a published data user guide [39].

This study used an accelerated cohort design [40] that made use of data on all mothers irrespective of whether their child had been classified as part of the (a) 'baby cohort', which was aged 0-1y at baseline, or the (b) 'kindergarten' cohort, aged 4-5y at baseline. Mother and child were tracked biennially for up to 4 more waves after baseline. We restricted the sample to only those mothers who did not change neighbourhood during this period, leaving 4259 (42.2%) participants in the sample from both cohorts. Further omission of participants who were not mothers and/or did not have a response on the K6 measure brought the final sample to 3897 women. By survey wave this was as follows: 2004 (*n* = 3526); 2006 (*n* = 3429); 2008 (*n* = 3191); 2010 (*n* = 3469); 2012 (*n* = 3425); and (2014 (*n* = 3367).

Mental health

Symptoms of psychological distress were measured using the Kessler 6 Psychological Distress Scale (K6) in each

Table 2 Multilevel negative binomial regression models of symptoms of psychological distress in association with green space quantity and quality among women in the postpartum period

	Green space quantity		Green space quality	
	Model 1	Model 2	Model 3	Model 4
Fixed part	Rate Ratio (95% Confidence Interval)			
Age (mean centred)	0.99 (0.98, 0.99)	0.99 (0.98, 0.99)	0.99 (0.98, 0.99)	0.99 (0.98, 0.99)
Age square (mean centred)	1.00 (1.00, 1.00)	1.00 (1.00, 1.00)	1.00 (1.00, 1.00)	1.00 (1.00, 1.00)
Indigenous status (No)				
Yes	1.30 (1.06, 1.59)	1.30 (1.06, 1.59)	1.30 (1.06, 1.59)	1.30 (1.06, 1.59)
Highest qualification (ref: Postgraduate)				
Undergraduate	1.01 (0.95, 1.07)	1.01 (0.95, 1.07)	1.01 (0.95, 1.07)	1.01 (0.95, 1.07)
Year 11 to 13	0.94 (0.87, 1.01)	0.93 (0.86, 1.01)	0.93 (0.86, 1.01)	0.93 (0.86, 1.01)
$\leq$ Year 10	1.02 (0.93, 1.12)	1.02 (0.93, 1.12)	1.02 (0.93, 1.11)	1.02 (0.93, 1.12)
Other	1.34 (0.63, 2.84)	1.34 (0.63, 2.84)	1.39 (0.65, 2.95)	1.39 (0.66, 2.96)
Economic status (ref: Employed)				
Economically inactive	1.11 (1.07, 1.14)	1.11 (1.07, 1.15)	1.11 (1.07, 1.14)	1.11 (1.07, 1.14)
Unemployed	1.10 (1.02, 1.19)	1.10 (1.02, 1.19)	1.10 (1.01, 1.19)	1.10 (1.01, 1.19)
Area disadvantage (ref: affluent)				
Average	1.04 (1.00, 1.09)	1.04 (1.00, 1.09)	1.03 (0.99, 1.08)	1.03 (0.99, 1.08)
Disadvantaged	1.08 (1.03, 1.13)	1.08 (1.03, 1.13)	1.06 (1.01, 1.11)	1.06 (1.01, 1.11)
Remoteness (ref: Major Cities)				
Inner regional	0.91 (0.85, 0.98)	0.91 (0.85, 0.98)	0.89 (0.83, 0.96)	0.89 (0.83, 0.96)
Outer regional or remote	0.94 (0.87, 1.03)	0.94 (0.87, 1.03)	0.93 (0.85, 1.01)	0.93 (0.85, 1.01)
Years since childbirth (mean centred)	1.00 (0.99, 1.01)	1.00 (0.98, 1.01)	0.99 (0.98, 1.01)	1.00 (0.98, 1.01)
Years since childbirth^2 (mean centred)	1.00 (1.00, 1.00)	1.00 (1.00, 1.01)	1.00 (1.00, 1.00)	1.00 (1.00, 1.01)
Green space quantity (ref: $\leq$ 5%)				
6–10%	0.99 (0.90, 1.09)	0.98 (0.89, 1.09)		
11–20%	1.07 (0.99, 1.16)	1.07 (0.98, 1.17)		
21–40%	1.04 (0.96, 1.13)	1.06 (0.97, 1.16)		
$\geq$ 41%	0.99 (0.89, 1.09)	1.03 (0.92, 1.15)		
Parks good quality (ref: Do not agree)				
Agree			0.95 (0.91, 0.98)	0.94 (0.90, 0.98)
Strongly Agree			0.89 (0.85, 0.93)	0.88 (0.84, 0.93)
Years since childbirth × Green space quantity				
Years × 6–10%		0.99 (0.97, 1.01)		
Years × 11–20%		1.00 (0.98, 1.01)		
Years × 21–40%		1.01 (0.99, 1.03)		
Years × $\geq$ 41%		1.00 (0.98, 1.02)		
Years since childbirth^2 × Green space quantity				
Years^2 × 6–10%		1.00 (0.99, 1.01)		
Years^2 × 11–20%		1.00 (0.99, 1.01)		
Years^2 × 21–40%		1.00 (0.99, 1.00)		
Years^2 × $\geq$ 41%		0.99 (0.98, 1.00)		
Years since childbirth ×Parks good quality				
Years × Agree				1.00 (0.99, 1.02)
Years × Strongly agree				0.99 (0.97, 1.01)

Table 2 Multilevel negative binomial regression models of symptoms of psychological distress in association with green space quantity and quality among women in the postpartum period *(Continued)*

	Green space quantity		Green space quality	
	Model 1	Model 2	Model 3	Model 4
Years since childbirth^2 × Parks good quality				
Years^2 × Agree				1.00 (0.99, 1.01)
Years^2 × Strongly agree				1.00 (0.99, 1.01)
Random part				
Level 3: Statistical Area 2	0.004 (0.006)	0.004 (0.006)	0.004 (0.006)	0.004 (0.006)
Level 2: Person	0.558 (0.016)	0.559 (0.016)	0.557 (0.016)	0.557 (0.016)

Level 1: Observation (*N* = 20,407) | Level 2: Person (*N* = 3897) | Level 3: Statistical Area 3 (*N* = 859)

wave [41, 42]. The K6 is a short form screening instrument for non-specific psychological distress based upon responses to six questions as follows: *"During the last 30 days, how often did:* (1) *you feel nervous?;* (2) *you feel hopeless?;* (3) *you feel restless or fidgety?;* (4) *you feel so depressed that nothing could cheer you up?;* (5) *you feel that everything was an effort?;* and (6) *you feel worthless?"* Responses were rated as 0 = "none of the time", 1 = "a little of the time", 2 = "some of the time", 3 = "most of the time" and 4 = "all of the time". In the current study, the sum of all six responses was used as the outcome variable, in order to examine incremental changes that may occur across the postpartum period. The score was scaled with a base value of 0, ranging up to 24. Assessment of the odds of serious mental illness was defined using scores of 13 or greater out of 24 [43].

Green space measures

Different sources of data were used to measure green space quantity and quality. The quantity of green space was measured according to the percentage of the land-use of the 'Statistical Area 2' of residence covered in 'parkland' according to the Australian Bureau of Statistics (ABS). This land-use category did not include agricultural land. Data on green space was extracted from the ABS's 2006 meshblock classification and aggregated to the Statistical Area 2 unit, which was designed by the ABS with populations of 10,000 on average (ranging from 3000 to 25,000) and to represent local communities and functional areas that contain commercial and transport hubs in areas outside of cities [44]. Mother's self-reports were used to identify the availability of good quality green space nearby. This involved reclassifying Likert scale responses to the statement: *"there are good parks, playgrounds and play spaces in this neighbourhood"* into 'did not agree', 'agreed' and 'strongly agreed'. In specifying whether a mother felt good parks and similar spaces were available nearby, this focussed on quality and avoided simply detecting whether any green space was proximal. This is an important caveat

as some previous work with a different dataset in Australia has reported lower odds of psychological distress among people living nearby higher quality green space, but no association between psychological distress and the quantity of green space per se [19].

Confounding

Socioeconomic and geographical factors play an important role in determining mental health [45] and also likely influence access to more and better quality green space [46–48]. In this study, mother's economic status and her highest educational qualification were taken into account. Economic status includes whether a mother was employed, unemployed, not working and not looking for a job ('economically inactive') or other categories, such as a student. Aboriginal and Torres Strait Islander status was also taken into account as women of these ethnic groups are known to disproportionately greater levels of socioeconomic disadvantage [49]. The geographic context where each woman lived was expressed in two different ways. First, the Accessibility/Remoteness Index of Australia was used to differentiate between mothers living in major cities, inner regional, outer regional, remote and very remote communities [50]. Second, strata of area-level socioeconomic circumstances were incorporated using the Socio Economic Index For Areas (SEIFA) relative index of social disadvantage [51], which is a composite measure of census-based indicators including local income, educational attainment and employment rates.

Statistical analysis

The percentage of the sample at high risk of psychological distress were described across the postpartum period and in relation to other sample characteristics. Multivariate analysis was then conducted using multilevel negative binomial regression models in MLwIN V3.00 [52]. Each model explicitly took into account variation in symptoms of psychological distress across three levels: (1) person-year observations (i.e. time); (2) person; (3) neighbourhood (Statistical Area 2). Negative

Table 3 Multilevel logistic regression models of the odds of serious mental illness in association with green space quantity and quality among women in the postpartum period

	Green space quantity		Green space quality	
	Model 5	Model 6	Model 7	Model 8
Fixed part	Odds Ratio (95% Confidence Interval)			
Age (mean centred)	0.98 (0.97, 0.99)	0.98 (0.97, 0.99)	0.98 (0.97, 0.99)	0.98 (0.97, 0.99)
Age square (mean centred)	1.00 (1.00, 1.00)	1.00 (1.00, 1.00)	1.00 (1.00, 1.00)	1.00 (1.00, 1.00)
Indigenous status (No)				
Yes	1.55 (0.96, 2.50)	1.55 (0.96, 2.51)	1.58 (0.98, 2.55)	1.58 (0.98, 2.56)
Highest qualification (ref: Postgraduate)				
Undergraduate	1.11 (0.93, 1.32)	1.11 (0.93, 1.32)	1.10 (0.92, 1.31)	1.10 (0.92, 1.30)
Year 11 to 13	0.92 (0.73, 1.15)	0.91 (0.73, 1.14)	0.91 (0.73, 1.14)	0.91 (0.73, 1.14)
≤ Year 10	1.26 (0.97, 1.63)	1.26 (0.97, 1.63)	1.23 (0.95, 1.59)	1.23 (0.95, 1.59)
Other	1.92 (0.28, 13.23)	1.91 (0.28, 13.06)	2.10 (0.31, 14.14)	2.10 (0.31, 14.10)
Economic status (ref: Employed)				
Economically inactive	1.47 (1.31, 1.65)	1.47 (1.31, 1.66)	1.47 (1.31, 1.66)	1.47 (1.31, 1.65)
Unemployed	1.68 (1.27, 2.22)	1.68 (1.27, 2.23)	1.68 (1.27, 2.22)	1.67 (1.26, 2.22)
Area disadvantage (ref: affluent)				
Average	1.23 (1.07, 1.42)	1.24 (1.07, 1.42)	1.19 (1.04, 1.37)	1.19 (1.03, 1.37)
Disadvantaged	1.47 (1.25, 1.72)	1.47 (1.25, 1.72)	1.37 (1.17, 1.60)	1.36 (1.16, 1.60)
Remoteness (ref: Major Cities)				
Inner regional	0.75 (0.63, 0.89)	0.75 (0.63, 0.89)	0.71 (0.59, 0.84)	0.71 (0.59, 0.84)
Outer regional or remote	0.79 (0.64, 0.97)	0.79 (0.64, 0.97)	0.76 (0.62, 0.93)	0.76 (0.62, 0.93)
Years since childbirth (mean centred)	1.03 (0.99, 1.07)	1.03 (0.97, 1.09)	1.02 (0.99, 1.06)	1.02 (0.97, 1.08)
Years since childbirth^2 (mean centred)	1.00 (0.99, 1.01)	1.01 (0.99, 1.03)	1.00 (0.99, 1.01)	1.00 (0.98, 1.02)
Green space quantity (ref: ≤ 5%)				
6–10%	1.01 (0.81, 1.27)	0.94 (0.72, 1.22)		
11–20%	1.24 (1.02, 1.51)	1.25 (1.00, 1.57)		
21–40%	1.16 (0.95, 1.42)	1.22 (0.97, 1.55)		
≥ 41%	0.89 (0.69, 1.14)	1.04 (0.78, 1.39)		
Parks good quality (ref: Do not agree)				
Agree			0.88 (0.77, 1.00)	0.86 (0.73, 1.02)
Strongly Agree			0.74 (0.64, 0.86)	0.71 (0.59, 0.87)
Years since childbirth×Green space quantity				
Years × 6–10%		0.99 (0.92, 1.07)		
Years × 11–20%		1.00 (0.93, 1.07)		
Years × 21–40%		1.03 (0.97, 1.11)		
Years × ≥ 41%		0.97 (0.88, 1.06)		
Years since childbirth^2 × Green space quantity				
Years^2 × 6–10%		1.02 (0.99, 1.05)		
Years^2 × 11–20%		1.00 (0.97, 1.03)		
Years^2 × 21–40%		0.99 (0.96, 1.02)		
Years^2 × ≥ 41%		0.96 (0.92, 1.00)		
Years since childbirth × Parks good quality				
Years × Agree				1.00 (0.95, 1.06)
Years × Strongly agree				1.00 (0.94, 1.07)

Table 3 Multilevel logistic regression models of the odds of serious mental illness in association with green space quantity and quality among women in the postpartum period *(Continued)*

	Green space quantity		Green space quality	
	Model 5	Model 6	Model 7	Model 8
Years since childbirth^2 × Parks good quality				
Years^2 × Agree				1.00 (0.98, 1.03)
Years^2 × Strongly agree				1.01 (0.98, 1.04)
Random part				
Level 3: Statistical Area 2	0.005 (0.032)	0.004 (0.032)	0.009 (0.032)	0.009 (0.032)
Level 2: Person	2.195 (0.096)	2.199 (0.096)	2.184 (0.096)	2.181 (0.096)

Level 1: Observation (*N* = 20,407) | Level 2: Person (N = 3897) | Level 3: Statistical Area 3 (*N* = 859)

binomial regressions were used to assess symptoms of psychological distress, to account for over-dispersed integer counts. Parameter estimates were expressed as rate ratios (RR). Separate models were used to examine association between symptoms of psychological distress with measures of green space quantity and quality, before and after adjusting for confounding. Mean-centred linear and square terms of age were fitted to account for potential non-linearities. A final set of models were fitted with a two-way interaction term between the number of years postpartum (also mean-centred linear and square terms to account for potential non-linearities) and each of the green space measures, to investigate whether mean associations with symptoms of psychological distress were consistent across the postpartum period. All of these analyses were repeated using multilevel logistic regression of the odds of serious mental illness, with parameters expressed as odds ratios (OR).

Results

The overall sample of 3897 included 20,407 observations nested within 859 areas and a prevalence of serious mental illness (K6 ≥ 13) at 12.4%. Table 1 reports how this prevalence was distributed by each of the sample characteristics using chi-square values. The prevalence of serious mental illness appeared to vary by only about 1.4% between mothers living in areas with ≤ 5% green space compared with those who had ≥ 41%. In contrast, compared to those who felt that there were no good quality parks nearby 16.0% K6 ≥ 13, those who agreed (12.8%) or strongly agreed (9.7%) that there were good parks nearby had a lower prevalence of serious mental illness. Some variation in the prevalence of serious mental illness was observed with respect to years since childbirth. Lower prevalence was noted with age, higher educational qualifications, among those who were employed, and living in more affluent areas. Higher prevalence was observed among mothers who identified as Aboriginal or Torres Strait Islander, economically inactive or unemployed. There appeared to be

little variation in the prevalence of serious mental illness with respect to geographic remoteness.

In adjusted multilevel negative binomial regressions there was no convincing evidence of an average effect of green space quantity on symptoms of psychological distress, nor of an interaction between green space quantity and the number of years since childbirth (Table 2, Models 1 and 2). Substituting the measure of green space quantity for that of green space quality yielded different results. Mothers who agreed (OR 0.95, 95%CI 0.91 to 0.98) or strongly agreed (OR 0.89, 95%CI 0.85 to 0.93) that local parks were of good quality had fewer symptoms of psychological distress than their counterparts who disagreed (Table 2, Model 3). There was no evidence that this association varied with respect to the number of years since childbirth (Table 2, Model 4). These patterns with respect to green space quantity and quality were also observed when switching from symptoms of psychological distress to the odds of serious mental illness as the study outcome (Table 3, Models 5 to 8). The non-significant trajectories in both outcomes for all of the final models featuring two-way interaction terms between the number of years since childbirth and each of the green space measures are illustrated in Fig. 1.

Discussion

The key finding from this longitudinal study is that green space quality, but not quantity, is associated with fewer symptoms of psychological distress and lower odds of serious mental illness among women up to 15 years postpartum. The second key finding was that the potential effect of green space quality and non-effect of green space quantity on mental health appeared to be relatively consistent across this period of time in the women's lives. To our knowledge, this is only the fourth study to have examined associations between mental health and measures of green space quantity and quality. It is the first to do so longitudinally. It is also the first study to investigate for evidence of mental health benefits of green space among women in postpartum, a period that can pose significant psychological challenges. Most of

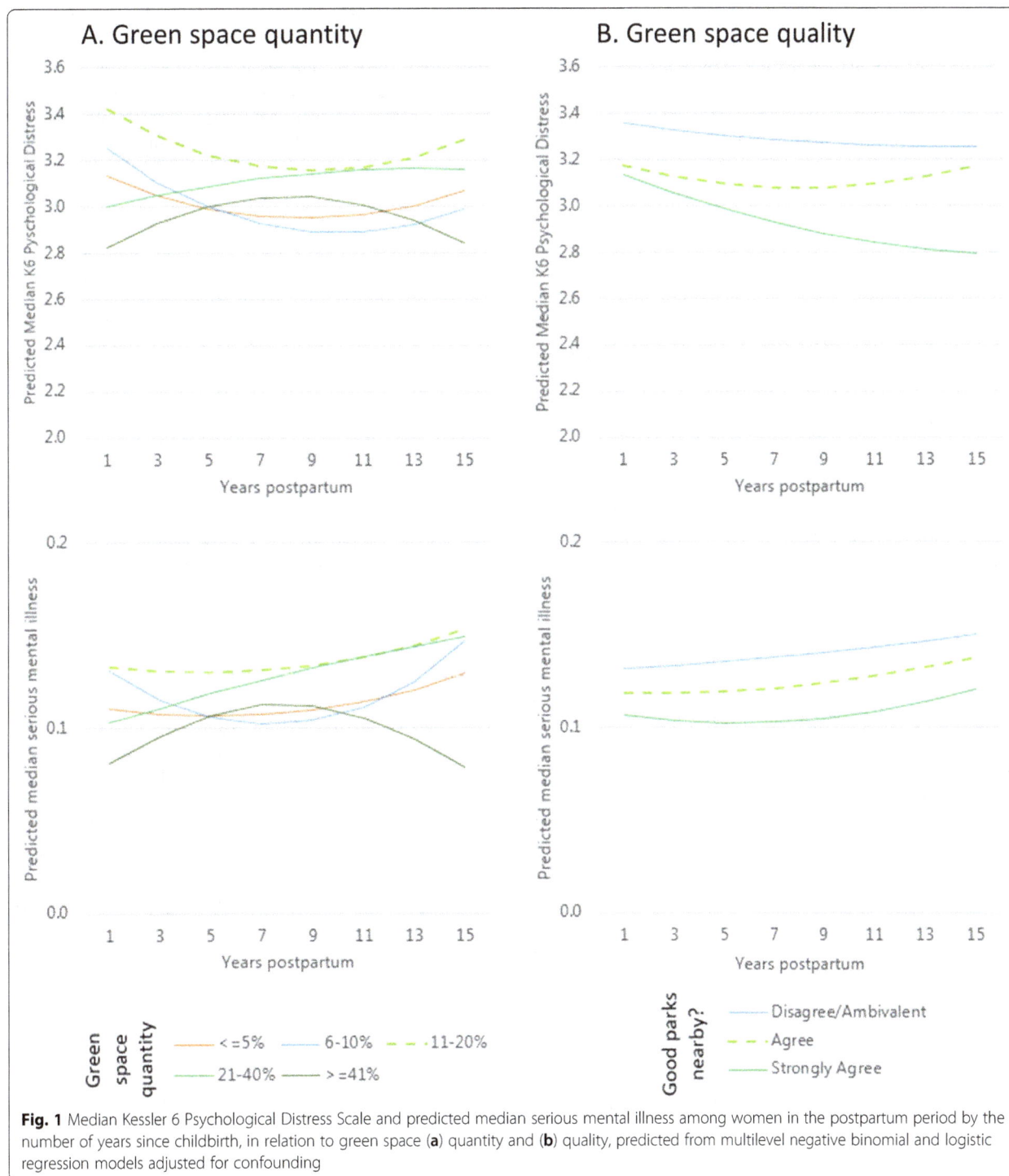

Fig. 1 Median Kessler 6 Psychological Distress Scale and predicted median serious mental illness among women in the postpartum period by the number of years since childbirth, in relation to green space (**a**) quantity and (**b**) quality, predicted from multilevel negative binomial and logistic regression models adjusted for confounding

the research on green space and health in or around this important lifecourse stage focusses upon birth outcomes such as birthweight [53]. Just two studies have been published on green space and symptoms of psychological distress in pregnant women, each focussing on quantity-based measures and finding mixed results [54, 55]. This study therefore highlights and

begins to address an important gap in understandings of green space and maternal health.

The findings from this study align relatively closely with another set in a different area of Australia on a general population sample, which also found evidence of a mental health benefit from proximity to quality green space, but not the availability of green space per se [19].

The results of both Australian studies contrast with evidence from the Netherlands where both measures of quantity and quality seemed to matter [29]. A sample size of four studies prohibits any definitive conclusions, though it may be that similarities between the Australian studies and contrasts with the Dutch findings reflect the potential for international variation in the relationship between green space quantity, quality and mental health, as well as geographical differences in how people value and interact with green spaces of varying quality. Geographical differences may be indicative of a range of aspects including cultural, socioeconomic and historical factors, variations in urban form, and climatic and topographical influences. There is also potentially important variation in the availability of green spaces within and between countries that intersect with other components of the built and natural environment (e.g. green walls, linear parks along river corridors) that may play a role, but were not specifically measured in our study. Given these possibilities, generalisations with regards to green space quality and mental health, or other health outcomes, to other countries should be only with the utmost caution. To advance the field of enquiry, there is a need for research specifically designed to examine the issue of green space quality in different countries simultaneously, not only to describe likely variations with mental health and other relevant outcomes, but also to learn about success stories in urban greening and green space restoration strategies, in order to identify what elements could be transferable across national boundaries and to promote population health in other contexts.

The results of this study with respect to green space quantity were unexpected, given the multiple pathways by which green space quantity may influence mental health. Green space quality has been found to be more important than green space quantity in another study of mental health with different data in Australia [19]. However, other studies have found green space quantity to be relevant. For example, one study used the same green space land-use data (though not the same metric) to report lower odds of psychological distress with more green space in a sample of men and women aged 45 years and older [9]. Unlike the aforementioned study, however, the geographical unit of analysis in our sample was the Statistical Area 2, which may be too large to identify associations with symptoms of psychological distress. It is plausible that the size of and distance to the nearest green space is particularly important for mothers due to well-known high levels of dependency upon parents during childhood [56]. Our measure of green space quantity may be an insufficient marker in this respect. Although all mothers in the data remained in the same location throughout the course of the study period, it is possible that in some cases the green space land-use (measured in 2006) could have changed over that time.

It is important to acknowledge potential circularity in the association between symptoms of psychological distress and self-reported green space quality. It is also plausible that in some contexts there may be good quality playgrounds and play spaces that are not set within some form of green space. Other features of the local environment not examined in this study may also play a confounding or modifying role, such as differences in walkability and places other than green spaces that mothers of young children may walk to, and potentially come into contact with green space as part of their journeys. Lastly, potentially mediating pathways linking green space quality and mental health in the postpartum period warrant dedicated investigation using longitudinal data and causal mediation models [57].

Conclusions

If the results are interpreted as reflecting potentially causal relationships, this longitudinal study has provided evidence that green space quality matters for protecting mental health among women in the postpartum period. By contrast, the amount of green space nearby was not associated with fewer symptoms of psychological distress. Although this study is not without limitations, it seems reasonably clear from the findings of this study and just a few others before it to have examined mental health in relation to measures of green space quality, that efforts to redesign and restore green spaces need to involve community consultation in order to optimise the health benefits. Further research on green space quality and mental health generally and among women in the postpartum period is warranted to better understand what aspects of green space quality matter when, where and for whom.

Acknowledgements

This paper uses unit record data from Growing Up in Australia, the Longitudinal Study of Australian Children. The study is conducted in partnership between the Department of Social Services, the Australian Institute of Family Studies and the Australian Bureau of Statistics. The findings and views reported in this paper are those of the authors and should not be attributed to Department of Social Services, Australian Institute of Family Studies, or the Australian Bureau of Statistics. We also acknowledge the Australian Bureau of Statistics for use of the 2006 mesh block data.

Funding

This project received funding from Hort Innovation Limited with co-investment from the University of Wollongong (UOW) Faculty of Social Sciences, the UOW Global Challenges initiative and the Australian Government (project number #GC15005). Xiaoqi Feng's contribution to this project was also supported by a National Health and Medical Research Council Career Development Fellowship (#1148792). Xiaoqi Feng and Thomas Astell-Burt are also supported by a

National Health and Medical Research Council project grant (#1101065). Thomas Astell-Burt is supported by a National Health and Medical Research Council Boosting Dementia Research Leader Fellowship (#1140317). The study design, analysis, interpretation of the data, writing the report, and decision to submit the report for publication are of the authors only.

Authors' contributions

XF conceptualised the study, conducted the analyses, interpreted the results and wrote the first draft of the paper. TAB helped to refine the study and analytical design, interpreted the results and supported critical editing to revised drafts of the manuscript. Both authors read and approved the final manuscript.

Consent for publication

Not applicable.

Competing interests

The authors declare that they have no competing interests.

Author details

[1]Population Wellbeing and Environment Research Lab (PowerLab), School of Health and Society, Faculty of Social Sciences, University of Wollongong, Wollongong, NSW, Australia. [2]Menzies Centre for Health Policy, University of Sydney, Sydney, NSW, Australia. [3]Illawarra Health and Medical Research Institute (IHMRI), University of Wollongong and Illawarra and Shoalhaven Local Health District, Wollongong, NSW, Australia. [4]School of Public Health, Peking Union Medical College and the Chinese Academy of Medical Sciences, Beijing, China.

References

1. Hartig T, Mitchell R, de Vries S, Frumkin H. Nature and health. Annu Rev Public Health. 2014;35:207–28.
2. Kaplan S. The restorative benefits of nature: toward an integrative framework. J Environ Psychol. 1995;15(3):169–82.
3. Bowler DE, Buyung-Ali LM, Knight TM, Pullin AS. A systematic review of evidence for the added benefits to health of exposure to natural environments. BMC Public Health. 2010;10:456.
4. Ohly H, Gentry S, Wigglesworth R, Bethel A, Lovell R, Garside R. A systematic review of the health and well-being impacts of school gardening: synthesis of quantitative and qualitative evidence. BMC Public Health. 2016;16(1):286.
5. Berto R, Baroni MR, Zainaghi A, Bettella S. An exploratory study of the effect of high and low fascination environments on attentional fatigue. J Environ Psychol. 2010;30(4):494–500.
6. Aspinall P, Mavros P, Coyne R, Roe J. The urban brain: analysing outdoor physical activity with mobile EEG. Br J Sports Med. 2015;49(4):272–6.
7. Tsunetsugu Y, Miyazaki Y. Measurement of absolute hemoglobin concentrations of prefrontal region by near-infrared time-resolved spectroscopy: examples of experiments and prospects. J Physiol Anthropol Appl Hum Sci. 2005;24(4):469–72.
8. Kim T-H, Jeong G-W, Baek H-S, Kim G-W, Sundaram T, Kang H-K, Lee S-W, Kim H-J, Song J-K. Human brain activation in response to visual stimulation with rural and urban scenery pictures: a functional magnetic resonance imaging study. Sci Total Environ. 2010;408(12):2600–7.
9. Astell-Burt T, Feng X, Kolt GS. Mental health benefits of neighbourhood green space are stronger among physically active adults in middle-to-older age: evidence from 260,061 Australians. Prev Med. 2013;57(5):601–6.
10. Mitchell R. Is physical activity in natural environments better for mental health than physical activity in other environments? Soc Sci Med. 2012;91: 130–4.
11. Cervinka R, Röderer K, Hefler E. Are nature lovers happy? On various indicators of well-being and connectedness with nature. J Health Psychol. 2012;17(3):379–88.
12. van der Wal AJ, Schade HM, Krabbendam L, van Vugt M. Do natural landscapes reduce future discounting in humans? Proc R Soc Lond B Biol Sci. 2013;280(1773):20132295.
13. Saadatmand V, Rejeh N, Heravi-Karimooi M, Tadrisi SD, Zayeri F, Vaismoradi M, Jasper M. Effect of nature-based sounds' intervention on agitation, anxiety, and stress in patients under mechanical ventilator support: a randomised controlled trial. Int J Nurs Stud. 2013;50(7):895–904.
14. Li Q, Kobayashi M, Inagaki H, Hirata Y, Li Y, Hirata K, Shimizu T, Suzuki H, Katsumata M, Wakayama Y. A day trip to a forest park increases human natural killer activity and the expression of anti-cancer proteins in male subjects. J Biol Regul Homeost Agents. 2009;24(2):157–65.
15. Wu C-F, Lai C-H, Chu H-J, Lin W-H. Evaluating and mapping of spatial air ion quality patterns in a residential garden using a geostatistic method. Int J Environ Res Public Health. 2011;8(6):2304–19.
16. Perez V, Alexander DD, Bailey WH. Air ions and mood outcomes: a review and meta-analysis. BMC Psychiatry. 2013;13(1):29.
17. Rook GA. Regulation of the immune system by biodiversity from the natural environment: an ecosystem service essential to health. Proc Natl Acad Sci. 2013;110(46):18360–7.
18. Sugiyama T, Leslie E, Giles-Corti B, Owen N. Associations of neighbourhood greenness with physical and mental health: do walking, social coherence and local social interaction explain the relationships? J Epidemiol Community Health. 2008;62(5):e9.
19. Francis J, Wood LJ, Knuiman M, Giles-Corti B. Quality or quantity? Exploring the relationship between public open space attributes and mental health in Perth, Western Australia. Soc Sci Med. 2012;74(10):1570–7.
20. Nutsford D, Pearson A, Kingham S. An ecological study investigating the association between access to urban green space and mental health. Public Health. 2013;127(11):1005–11.
21. Astell-Burt T, Mitchell R, Hartig T. The association between green space and mental health varies across the lifecourse. A longitudinal study. J Epidemiol Community Health. 2014;68:578–83.
22. Alcock I, White MP, Wheeler BW, Fleming LE, Depledge MH. Longitudinal effects on mental health of moving to greener and less green urban areas. Environ Sci Technol. 2014;48(2):1247–55.
23. Thompson CW, Roe J, Aspinall P, Mitchell R, Clow A, Miller D. More green space is linked to less stress in deprived communities: evidence from salivary cortisol patterns. Landsc Urban Plan. 2012;105(3):221–9.
24. Roe JJ, Thompson CW, Aspinall PA, Brewer MJ, Duff EI, Miller D, Mitchell R, Clow A. Green space and stress: evidence from cortisol measures in deprived urban communities. Int J Environ Res Public Health. 2013;10(9): 4086–103.
25. Vemuri AW, Morgan Grove J, Wilson MA, Burch WR Jr. A tale of two scales: evaluating the relationship among life satisfaction, social capital, income, and the natural environment at individual and neighborhood levels in metropolitan Baltimore. Environ Behav. 2011;43(1):3–25.
26. Beyer KM, Kaltenbach A, Szabo A, Bogar S, Nieto FJ, Malecki KM. Exposure to neighborhood green space and mental health: evidence from the survey of the health of Wisconsin. Int J Environ Res Public Health. 2014;11(3):3453–72.
27. Maas J, Verheij RA, de Vries S, Spreeuwenberg P, Schellevis FG, Groenewegen PP. Morbidity is related to a green living environment. J Epidemiol Community Health. 2009;63(12):967–73.
28. Van Den Berg AE, Maas J, Verheij RA, Groenewegen PP. Green space as a buffer between stressful life events and health. Soc Sci Med. 2010;70(8): 1203–10.
29. van Dillen SM, de Vries S, Groenewegen PP, Spreeuwenberg P. Greenspace in urban neighbourhoods and residents' health: adding quality to quantity. J Epidemiol Community Health. 2012;66(6):e8.
30. Stigsdotter UK, Ekholm O, Schipperijn J, Toftager M, Kamper-Jørgensen F, Randrup TB. Health promoting outdoor environments-associations between green space, and health, health-related quality of life and stress based on a Danish national representative survey. Scand J Soc Med. 2010;38(4):411–7.
31. Gascon M, Triguero-Mas M, Martínez D, Dadvand P, Forns J, Plasència A, Nieuwenhuijsen MJ. Mental health benefits of long-term exposure to

residential green and blue spaces: a systematic review. Int J Environ Res Public Health. 2015;12(4):4354–79.

32. Houlden V, Weich S, de Albuquerque JP, Jarvis S, Rees K. The relationship between greenspace and the mental wellbeing of adults: a systematic review. PLoS One. 2018;13(9):e0203000.

33. Araya R, Montgomery A, Rojas G, Fritsch R, Solis J, Signorelli A, Lewis G. Common mental disorders and the built environment in Santiago, Chile. Br J Psychiatry. 2007;190(5):394–401.

34. Seyfried LS, Marcus S. Postpartum mood disorders. Int Rev Psychiatry. 2003; 15(3):231–42.

35. Depression P. Heterogeneity of postpartum depression: a latent class analysis. Lancet Psychiatry. 2015;2(1):59–67.

36. Woolhouse H, Gartland D, Mensah F, Brown S. Maternal depression from early pregnancy to 4 years postpartum in a prospective pregnancy cohort study: implications for primary health care. BJOG. 2015;122(3):312–21.

37. Macintyre S, Macdonald L, Ellaway A. Lack of agreement between measured and self-reported distance from public green parks in Glasgow, Scotland. Int J Behav Nutr Phys Act. 2008;5(1):26.

38. Sanson A, Nicholson J, Ungerer J, Zubrick S, Wilson K. Introducing the Longitudinal Study of Australian Children-LSAC Discussion Paper No 1. 2002.

39. Australian Institute of Family Studies. The Longitudinal Study of Australian Children: An Australian Government initiative. Data User Guide. Australian Government: Canberra; 2013.

40. Raudenbush SW, Chan WS. Growth curve analysis in accelerated longitudinal designs. J Res Crime Delinq. 1992;29(4):387–411.

41. Furukawa TA, Kessler RC, Slade T, Andrews G. The performance of the K6 and K10 screening scales for psychological distress in the Australian National Survey of mental health and well-being. Psychol Med. 2003;33(2): 357–62.

42. Kessler RC, Green JG, Gruber MJ, Sampson NA, Bromet E, Cuitan M, Furukawa TA, Gureje O, Hinkov H, Hu CY. Screening for serious mental illness in the general population with the K6 screening scale: results from the WHO world mental health (WMH) survey initiative. Int J Methods Psychiatr Res. 2010;19(S1):4–22.

43. National Comorbidity Study. K10 and K6 Scales. https://www.hcp.med. harvard.edu/ncs/k6_scales.php. Accessed 22 Apr 2018.

44. Australian Statistical Geography Standard (ASGS). Volume 1 - Main Structure and Greater Capital City Statistical Areas http://www.abs.gov.au/ausstats/ abs@.nsf/mf/1270.0.55.001. Accessed 01 Feb 2017.

45. Allen J, Balfour R, Bell R, Marmot M. Social determinants of mental health. Int Rev Psychiatry. 2014;26(4):392–407.

46. Mavoa S, Koohsari MJ, Badland HM, Davern M, Feng X, Astell-Burt T, Giles-Corti B. Area-level disparities of public open space: a geographic information systems analysis in metropolitan Melbourne. Urban Policy Res. 2014:1–18. https://doi.org/10.1080/08111146.2014.974747.

47. Astell-Burt T, Feng X, Mavoa S, Badland HM, Giles-Corti B. Do low-income neighbourhoods have the least green space? A cross-sectional study of Australia's most populous cities. BMC Public Health. 2014;14:292.

48. Crawford D, Timperio A, Giles-Corti B, Ball K, Hume C, Roberts R, Andrianopoulos N, Salmon J. Do features of public open spaces vary according to neighbourhood socio-economic status? Health Place. 2008; 14(4):889–93.

49. Marmot M. Social determinants and the health of indigenous Australians. Med J Aust. 2011;194(10):512–3.

50. ARIA (Accessibility/Remoteness Index of Australia). https://www.adelaide.edu. au/hugo-centre/spatial_data/aria/.

51. Pink B. Socio-economic indexes for areas (SEIFA). Canberra: Australian Bureau of Statistics; 2011.

52. Rasbash J, Browne W, Goldstein H, Yang M, Plewis I, Healy M, Woodhouse G, Draper D, Langford I, Lewis T. A user's guide to MLwiN. 2000.

53. Banay RF, Bezold CP, James P, Hart JE, Laden F. Residential greenness: current perspectives on its impact on maternal health and pregnancy outcomes. Int J Women's Health. 2017;9:133.

54. McEachan R, Prady S, Smith G, Fairley L, Cabieses B, Gidlow C, Wright J, Dadvand P, Van Gent D, Nieuwenhuijsen M. The association between green space and depressive symptoms in pregnant women: moderating roles of socioeconomic status and physical activity. J Epidemiol Community Health. 2016;70(3):253–9. https://doi.org/10.1136/jech-2015-205954.

55. Nichani V, Dirks K, Burns B, Bird A, Grant C. Green space and depression during pregnancy: results from the growing up in New Zealand study. Int J Environ Res Public Health. 2017;14(9):1083.

56. Steinberg L, Silverberg SB. The vicissitudes of autonomy in early adolescence. Child Dev. 1986;57(4):841–51.

57. VanderWeele TJ. Marginal structural models for the estimation of direct and indirect effects. Epidemiology. 2009;20(1):18–26.

25

Is intrauterine exposure to acetaminophen associated with emotional and hyperactivity problems during childhood? Findings from the 2004 Pelotas birth cohort

Luciana Tovo-Rodrigues[1]* (ID), Bruna Celestino Schneider[1], Thais Martins-Silva[1], Bianca Del-Ponte[1], Christian Loret de Mola[2], Lavinia Schuler-Faccini[3], Fernanda Sales Luiz Vianna[4,5,6], Tiago N. Munhoz[1,7], Ludmila Entiauspe[1], Mariângela Freitas Silveira[1], Iná S. Santos[1], Alicia Matijasevich[8], Aluísio J. D. Barros[1], Luis Augusto Rohde[9,10] and Andréa Dâmaso Bertoldi[1]

Abstract

Background: Longitudinal studies have consistently reported that prenatal exposure to acetaminophen can to lead to an increased risk of attention deficit-hyperactivity disorder during childhood. This study aimed to investigate the association between intrauterine exposure to acetaminophen and the presence of emotional and behavioral problems at the ages of 6 and 11 years in a low-middle income country.

Methods: We performed a prospective longitudinal population-based study using data from the 2004 Pelotas birth cohort. From the 4231 initial cohort participants, 3722 and 3566 children were assessed at 6 and 11 years of age, respectively. The outcomes were assessed using the parent version of Strengths and Difficulties Questionnaire (SDQ). The cut-off points established for the Brazilian population were used to categorize the outcomes. Crude and adjusted odds ratio were obtained through logistic regression.

Results: Acetaminophen was used by 27.5% (95% confidence interval [CI]: 26.1–28.9) of the mothers at least once during pregnancy. The prevalence of emotional problems at 6 and 11 years was 13.6 and 19.9%, respectively. For hyperactivity problems, prevalence was 13.9 and 16.1%, respectively. Intrauterine exposure to acetaminophen increased the odds of having emotional (odds ratio [OR] = 1.47; 95% CI: 1.07–2.02) and hyperactivity/inattention (OR = 1.42; 95% CI: 1.06–1.92) problems in 6-year-old boys. At the age of 11, a small decrease in the effect was observed for both outcomes after adjustment: OR = 1.31 (95% CI: 0.99–1.73) for emotional problems and OR = 1.25 (95% CI: 0.95–1.65) for hyperactivity/inattention in boys. No association for any phenotypes at both ages was observed for girls.

Conclusion: The effect of intrauterine exposure to acetaminophen in emotional and hyperactivity symptoms was dependent on sex in a Brazilian cohort. While it seemed to be important for boys, mainly at 6 years of age, for girls, no association was observed.

Keywords: Acetaminophen (paracetamol), Prenatal exposure, Birth cohort, Behavioral symptoms

* Correspondence: luciana.tovo@gmail.com
[1]Postgraduate Program in Epidemiology, Universidade Federal de Pelotas, Rua Marechal Deodoro, 1160 - 3° andar, Pelotas, RS 96020-220, Brazil
Full list of author information is available at the end of the article

Background

Acetaminophen (or paracetamol) is one of the most commonly used analgesics worldwide [1]. It is the first choice for pain and fever medication among pregnant women [2]. In Brazil, studies reporting acetaminophen use during pregnancy are scarce [3–5]. These studies are restricted to convenience samples, and to our knowledge, there are no population-based studies that have evaluated its use.

Several birth cohort studies have reported that prenatal exposure to acetaminophen is associated with neurobehavioral and neurodevelopmental disorders during childhood [6–12]. Intrauterine exposure to acetaminophen has been associated with (i) attention-deficit/hyperactivity disorder (ADHD) [8–12]; (ii) hyperactivity/inattention and behavioral symptoms [7–11]; (iii) autism spectrum disorder (ASD) [6–10]; and (iv) impaired motor development, difficulty in communication and behavioral disorders [9–13]. In a recent meta-analysis, acetaminophen exposure during pregnancy was associated with a 20–30% increase in the risk of neurodevelopmental disorders [14]. Only one study has evaluated behavioral outcomes at two different time points during childhood [7].

Acetaminophen crosses the human placental barrier, and in vitro and in vivo findings provide additional evidence in support of observational epidemiological studies. Acetaminophen use has been shown to interfere with neurotransmitter, endocrine and immune systems, as well as with the regulation of brain-derived neurotrophic factor and cell oxidative stress, which are processes associated with brain development [15–22].

Although several variables have been included as covariates in previous studies, the results are susceptible to potential confounding effects [14], which makes it difficult to ascertain whether the use of acetaminophen is safe during pregnancy and indicates the need for more studies in the field. It is of note that current observational studies have been conducted in only European populations [23–25]. In this sense, studies in other populations, such as those from low and medium-income countries, would contribute to the knowledge in the literature and improve the current understanding of the risk of intrauterine exposure to acetaminophen.

This study aims to investigate the association between intrauterine exposure to acetaminophen and the presence of emotional and behavioral symptoms at the ages of 6 and 11 years in the 2004 Pelotas birth cohort.

Methodology
Target population

The present investigation is a prospective longitudinal study using data from the 2004 Pelotas birth cohort, a population-based study that documented hospital childbirths in the southern Brazilian city of Pelotas. Among the 4263 live births, 4231 were considered eligible and were included in the present study. So far, these children have been visited at the ages of 3, 12, 24, 48 and 72 months and 11 years, with follow-up rates of 95.7, 94.3, 93.5, 92.0, 90.2 and 86.6%, respectively [26, 27]. The present study used data from perinatal assessments and follow-ups at ages 6 and 11. At both follow-ups, the children underwent a wide-ranging health assessment with interviews [26].

Use of acetaminophen during pregnancy

A standardized questionnaire was used during the perinatal evaluation conducted after the birth of the children. The mother's use of medication during pregnancy was retrospectively framed as the following question: *"Did you use any medications during pregnancy?"* For positive answers, the mothers were asked to report the names of all medicines used during pregnancy, as well as the beginning and end of use. Our exposure variable was defined as medication composed of acetaminophen that was used at least once during pregnancy.

Outcome measurements

Behavioral symptoms were evaluated using the standardized scores from the Strengths and Difficulties Questionnaire (SDQ). The SDQ is a screening questionnaire, which measures 25 psychological attributes divided into 5 scales: inattention/hyperactive symptoms, conduct problems, emotional symptoms, peer relationship problems, and prosocial behavior. All attributes except prosocial behavior are summed to create a total difficulties score. The questionnaire was adapted and previously validated for the Brazilian population of children and teenagers aged between 4 and 16 years [28].

Trained psychologists administered the SDQ in a standardized manner to the parents or caregivers during each follow-up. The cut-off points established for the Brazilian population were used to categorize the general difficulties scale and the subscales as follows: ≥ 17 for the total difficulties score, ≥ 5 for the emotional problems score, ≥ 4 for the conduct problems score, ≥ 7 for the inattention/hyperactivity score, ≥ 4 for the peer problems score, and ≤ 4 for the prosocial score.

Confounding factors

The analyses included variables associated with psychiatric disorders and differential use of acetaminophen as follows: National Economic Index score (an economic indicator extensively used in Brazil based on information from the 2000 demographic census by the Brazilian Institute for Geography and Statistics) [29]; sex (male, female); mother's educational level (years of school attendance); mother's age (years); mother's skin color (white, black or other); mother's parity (number of children), smoking activity during pregnancy ("Did you smoke during pregnancy?"; yes or no); alcohol consumption during pregnancy ("Did you drink alcoholic beverages during pregnancy?"; yes or no); mood issues during pregnancy ("During pregnancy, did you have depression or suffer from anxiety?"; "no", "yes, not treated" or "yes, treated" and categorized into yes or no responses); infections during pregnancy (yes or no); prepregnancy body mass index (BMI); and other nonsteroidal analgesic use during pregnancy (yes or no).

Statistical analyses

Statistical analyses were performed using Stata software (version 12.1). The analyses included children who had information available regarding maternal use of acetaminophen during pregnancy and who were assessed using the SDQ at the ages of 6 and 11 years ($N = 3470$ and $N = 3447$, respectively). The crude and adjusted analyses between exposure to acetaminophen and the outcomes were performed using logistic regression. Specific effects of acetaminophen in boys and girls were also tested.

As a sensitivity analysis, to test the specificity of acetaminophen compared to other nonsteroidal analgesics, a variable regarding the use of other analgesics was created and used as a comparative exposure. All models using intrauterine acetaminophen exposure were also adjusted for this variable. Moreover, to assess the extent of the imprecision in the mood problem information (collected perinatally), we used information from the Edinburgh Postnatal Depression Scale (EPDS) [30], which has been validated for Brazilian populations [31], as a sensitivity analysis. Data were gathered when the child was 12 months old, as this time point it correlates highly with the mood problem information collected at the perinatal interview. The cut-off of 10 points, which is the recommended cut-off for screening in the Brazilian population [31], was used. The EPDS information was added as a covariable in the models, thus replacing the variable that was gathered perinatally.

Results

Acetaminophen was used during pregnancy at a frequency of 27.5% (95% confidence interval [CI]: 26.1–28.9). The prevalence of behavioral disorders assessed through the total difficulties scale of the SDQ was 10.8% (95% CI: 9.7–11.8) at the age of 6 and 13.9% (95% CI: 12.8–15.1) at the age of 11 (Table 1). The sociodemographic, behavioral, and maternal health characteristics are also shown in Table 1. The associations between the covariables and both the exposure and the main outcomes of the study are shown in Additional file 1: Table S1.

Crude and adjusted analyses for the total sample are presented in Table 2. No associations between acetaminophen exposure and total problems or SDQ subscales were

observed after adjustment. However, a significant interaction effect was observed for the emotional ($p = 0.046$) and hyperactivity/inattention ($p = 0.018$) subscales at 6 years old. Further analyses were conducted and stratified according to the sex of the children.

Table 3 presents the association between prenatal exposure to acetaminophen and the outcomes evaluated in 6-year-old boys and girls. At this age, for boys, the use of acetaminophen during pregnancy was associated with emotional (OR = 1.47; 95% CI: 1.07–2.02), as well as with hyperactivity/inattention (OR = 1.42; 95% CI: 1.06–1.92), problems in the adjusted model. The use of acetaminophen during pregnancy was not associated with other outcomes. For girls, no association was observed.

The effect sizes in the assessment at 11 years of age were slightly smaller than those of the 6 year-old assessment, and most of the associations that were observed at 6 years did not reach significance at 11 years (Table 4). Among boys, the crude analysis showed an effect for emotional problems (OR = 1.33; 95% CI: 1.03–1.71). However, this effect lost significance after adjustment (OR = 1.31; 95% CI: 0.99–1.73). Regarding the hyperactivity/inattention subscale, the estimates for crude and adjusted models did not reach statistical significance. Acetaminophen use during pregnancy was not associated with other outcomes for either boys or girls in the adjusted model.

Sensitivity analyses

To test the specificity of the effect of acetaminophen exposure during intrauterine life on the outcomes of emotional symptoms and hyperactivity, we performed another analysis to test the effect of other nonsteroidal analgesics on the same outcomes. No associations between nonsteroidal analgesics and emotional symptoms (OR$_{adjusted}$ = 1.09; 95% CI: 0.77–1.55) or hyperactivity symptoms (OR$_{adjusted}$ = 1.07; 95% CI: 0.77–1.48) were found. No association was observed for either sex for any of the other outcomes (results not shown). In addition, nonsteroidal analgesic use was not associated with any outcomes at 11 years of age.

The second sensitivity analysis aimed to test the imprecision of reported mood problems during pregnancy that were collected perinatally. We performed this analysis by replacing the mood problems variable during pregnancy with the maternal depression information assessed with EPDS in the statistical models. Adjusted analysis results are presented in Table 5. Analyses did not change substantially. The same associations as before were observed in the 6 year-old assessment. In the 11-year-old assessment, the magnitude of the effect of acetaminophen on emotional problems in boys was greater than that in the previous analysis, and the adjusted analysis became significant (OR = 1.33; 95% CI: 1.01–1.76).

Table 1 Sociodemographic characteristics, maternal health, and use of acetaminophen and other analgesics during pregnancy among mothers of boys and girls in the 2004 Pelotas birth cohort who were assessed by SDQ at the follow-ups at 6 and 11 years of age

Maternal characteristics	Follow-up at the age of 6 years		Follow-up at the age of 11 years	
	Boys (N = 1812) N (%)	Girls (N = 1658) N (%)	Boys (N = 1781) N (%)	Girls (N = 1666) N (%)
Age (years)				
≤ 24	818 (45.14)	761 (45.93)	793 (44.53)	750 (45.07)
25–29	416 (22.96)	370 (22.33)	402 (22.57)	374 (22.48)
30–34	388 (21.41)	343 (20.70)	393 (22.07)	355 (21.33)
≥ 35	190 (10.49)	183 (11.04)	193 (10.84)	185 (11.12)
Educational level (years)				
0–4	268 (14.91)	250 (15.26)	257 (14.54)	248 (15.07)
5–8	753 (41.88)	697 (42.55)	726 (41.09)	692 (42.04)
9–11	589 (32.76)	546 (33.33)	599 (33.90)	560 (34.02)
≥ 12	188 (10.46)	145 (8.85)	185 (10.47)	146 (8.87)
National Economic Index				
1 (higher)	341 (18.82)	311 (18.76)	325 (18.25)	302 (18.13)
2	362 (19.98)	366 (22.07)	355 (19.93)	363 (21.79)
3	357 (19.70)	342 (20.63)	348 (19.54)	349 (20.95)
4	389 (21.47)	329 (19.84)	386 (21.67)	337 (20.23)
5 (lower)	363 (20.03)	310 (19.70)	367 (20.61)	315 (18.91)
Skin color				
White	1125 (62.92)	1016 (61.80)	1106 (62.98)	1015 (61.52)
Black	298 (16.67)	276 (16.79)	291 (16.57)	275 (16.67)
Other[a]	365 (20.41)	352 (21.41)	359 (20.44)	360 (21.82)
Smoking during pregnancy				
No	1332 (73.51)	1202 (72.50)	1320 (74.12)	1212 (72.75)
Yes	480 (26.49)	456 (27.50)	461 (25.88)	454 (27.25)
Use of alcohol during pregnancy				
No	1750 (96.58)	1605 (96.80)	1720 (96.57)	1616 (97.00)
Yes	62 (3.42)	53 (3.20)	61 (3.43)	50 (3.00)
Parity				
1	751 (41.45)	623 (37.60)	740 (41.55)	618 (37.12)
2	477 (26.32)	443 (26.74)	472 (26.50)	454 (27.27)
3 or more	584 (32.23)	591 (35.67)	569 (31.95)	593 (35.62)
Pre-gestational BMI				
Underweight	75 (4.49)	69 (4.54)	75 (4.59)	66 (4.32)
Normal weight	1025 (61.34)	909 (59.76)	996 (60.95)	914 (59.82)
Overweight	402 (24.06)	350 (23.01)	401 (24.54)	358 (23.43)
Obese	169 (10.11)	193 (12.69)	162 (9.91)	190 (12.43)
Mood symptoms during pregnancy				
No	1362 (75.17)	1254 (75.72)	1351 (75.86)	1268 (76.20)
Yes	450 (24.83)	402 (24.28)	430 (24.14)	396 (23.80)
Infections during pregnancy				
No	1066 (58.96)	974 (58.89)	1061 (59.71)	975 (58.63)
Yes	742 (41.04)	680 (41.11)	716 (40.29)	688 (41.37)

Table 1 Sociodemographic characteristics, maternal health, and use of acetaminophen and other analgesics during pregnancy among mothers of boys and girls in the 2004 Pelotas birth cohort who were assessed by SDQ at the follow-ups at 6 and 11 years of age (Continued)

Maternal characteristics	Follow-up at the age of 6 years		Follow-up at the age of 11 years	
	Boys (N = 1812) N (%)	Girls (N = 1658) N (%)	Boys (N = 1781) N (%)	Girls (N = 1666) N (%)
Use of acetaminophen during pregnancy				
Never	1287 (71.03)	1218 (73.46)	1259 (70.69)	1229 (73.77)
At least once	525 (28.97)	440 (26.54)	522 (29.31)	437 (26.23)
Use of other analgesics during pregnancy				
Never	1430 (79.53)	1310 (79.25)	1402 (79.21)	1311 (78.83)
At least once	368 (20.47)	343 (20.75)	368 (20.79)	352 (21.17)
Outcomes				
Total SDQ (score ≥ 17 pts)	212 (11.70)	161 (9.71)	288 (16.17)	192 (11.52)
Emotional symptoms (score ≥ 5 pts)	237 (13.08)	235 (14.17)	339 (19.03)	347 (20.83)
Conduct Problems (score ≥ 4 pts)	295 (16.28)	220 (13.27)	253 (14.21)	198 (11.88)
Hyperactivity/inattention (score ≥ 7 pts)	288 (15.89)	193 (11.64)	367 (20.61)	189 (11.34)
Peer relationship problems (score pts)	277 (15.29)	213 (12.85)	269 (15.10)	190 (11.40)
Prosocial behavior (score ≤ 4 pts)	23 (1.27)	18 (1.09)	28 (1.57)	20 (1.20)

[a]Other skin color: self-classification as brown, yellow or indigenous

Table 2 Association between use of acetaminophen by the mother during pregnancy and mental health outcomes at the age of 6 years (N = 3470)

Outcomes	Frequency of outcome according to use of acetaminophen during pregnancy N (%)		Crude analysis	Adjusted analysis[a]		p-value for sex – use of acetaminophen interaction term[b]
	Exposed n (%)	Not exposed n (%)	OR (95% CI)	OR (95% CI)	p	
6 years old						
Total SDQ (score ≥ 17 pts)	102 (10.57)	271 (10.82)	0.97 (0.77–1.24)	1.15 (0.88–1.50)	0.313	0.454
Emotional symptoms (score ≥ 5 pts)	137 (14.20)	335 (13.37)	1.07 (0.87–1.33)	1.15 (0.91–1.46)	0.232	**0.046**
Conduct problems (score ≥ 4 pts)	119 (12.33)	396 (15.81)	0.75 (0.60–0.93)	0.86 (0.68–1.10)	0.222	0.572
Hyperactivity/inattention (score ≥ 7 pts)	137 (14.20)	344 (13.73)	1.04 (0.84–1.29)	1.10 (0.87–1.39)	0.427	**0.018**
Peer relationship problems (score ≥ 4 pts)	124 (12.85)	366 (14.61)	0.86 (0.69–1.07)	1.08 (0.85–1.38)	0.517	0.140
Prosocial behavior (score ≤ 4 pts)	8 (0.83)	33 (1.32)	0.63 (0.29–1.36)	0.63 (0.27–1.49)	0.376	0.967
11 years old						
Total SDQ (score ≥ 17 pts)	138 (14.39)	342 (13.75)	1.06 (0.85–1.30)	1.19 (0.94–1.50)	0.157	0.811
Emotional symptoms (score ≥ 5 pts)	213 (22.21)	473 (19.01)	1.22 (1.01–1.46)	1.20 (0.98–1.46)	0.078	0.313
Conduct problems (score ≥ 4 pts)	108 (11.26)	343 (13.79)	0.79 (0.63–1.00)	0.93 (0.72–1.20)	0.561	0.264
Hyperactivity/inattention (score ≥ 7 pts)	165 (17.21)	391 (15.72)	1.12 (0.91–1.36)	1.20 (0.96–1.49)	0.112	0.797
Peer relationship problems (score ≥ 4 pts)	131 (13.66)	328 (13.18)	1.04 (0.84–1.30)	1.21 (0.95–1.53)	0.123	0.781
Prosocial behavior (score ≤ 4 pts)	8 (0.83)	40 (1.61)	0.52 (0.24–1.10)	0.79 (0.36–1.75)	0.565	0.151

[a]Logistic regression adjusted according to sex, maternal age, parity, national economic index, maternal educational level, smoking during pregnancy, alcohol consumption during pregnancy, maternal skin color, infection during pregnancy, pre-gestational BMI, presence of maternal mood issue and use of other analgesics during pregnancy. N after adjustment: 3103. [b]p-values marked in bold denote statistically significant results

Table 3 Association between use of acetaminophen by mother during pregnancy and mental health outcomes at the age of 6 years among boys (N = 1812) and girls (N = 1658)

Outcomes	Frequency of outcome according to use of acetaminophen during pregnancy N (%)		Crude analysis	Adjusted analysis[a]	
	Exposed n (%)	Not exposed n (%)	OR (95% CI)	OR (95% CI)	p[b]
Boys					
Total SDQ (score ≥ 17 pts)	63 (12.00)	149 (11.58)	1.04 (0.76–1.43)	1.28 (0.90–1.83)	0.163
Emotional symptoms (score ≥ 5 pts)	83 (15.81)	154 (11.97)	1.38 (1.04–1.84)	1.47 (1.07–2.02)	**0.018**
Conduct problems (score ≥ 4 pts)	72 (13.71)	223 (17.33)	0.76 (0.57–1.02)	0.93 (0.68–1.27)	0.641
Hyperactivity/inattention (score ≥ 7 pts)	93 (17.71)	195 (15.15)	1.21 (0.92–1.58)	1.42 (1.06–1.92)	**0.020**
Peer relationship problems (score ≥ 4 pts)	81 (15.43)	196 (15.23)	1.02 (0.77–1.35)	1.25 (0.91–1.71)	0.167
Prosocial behavior (score ≤ 4 pts)	5 (0.95)	18 (1.40)	0.68 (0.25–1.84)	0.60 (0.19–1.88)	0.376
Girls					
Total SDQ (score ≥ 17 pts)	39 (8.86)	122 (10.02)	0.87 (0.60–1.28)	1.02 (0.67–1.54)	0.943
Emotional symptoms (score ≥ 5 pts)	54 (12.27)	181 (14.86)	0.80 (0.58–1.11)	0.90 (0.63–1.28)	0.557
Conduct problems (score ≥ 4 pts)	47 (10.68)	173 (14.20)	0.72 (0.51–1.02)	0.79 (0.54–1.16)	0.226
Hyperactivity/inattention (score ≥ 7 pts)	44 (10.00)	149 (12.23)	0.80 (0.56–1.14)	0.76 (0.51–1.12)	0.165
Peer relationship problems (score ≥ 4 pts)	43 (9.77)	170 (13.96)	0.67 (0.47–0.95)	0.88 (0.59–1.31)	0.535
Prosocial behavior (score ≤ 4 pts)	3 (0.68)	15 (1.23)	0.55 (0.16–1.91)	0.73 (0.20–2.69)	0.630

[a]Logistic regression adjusted according to maternal age, parity, national economic index, maternal educational level, smoking during pregnancy, alcohol during pregnancy, maternal skin color, infection during pregnancy, pre-gestational BMI, presence of maternal mood disorder and use of other analgesics during pregnancy. N after adjustment: 1619 for boys; 1484 for girls. [b]p-values marked in bold denote statistically significant results

Table 4 Association between use of acetaminophen by mother during pregnancy and mental health outcomes at the age of 11 years among boys (N = 1781) and girls (N = 1666)

Outcomes	Frequency of outcome according to use of acetaminophen during pregnancy N (%)		Crude analysis	Adjusted analysis[a]	
	Exposed n (%)	Not exposed n (%)	OR (95% CI)	OR (95% CI)	p
Boys					
Total SDQ (score ≥ 17 pts)	89 (17.05)	199 (15.81)	1.09 (0.83–1.44)	1.21 (0.89–1.64)	0.228
Emotional symptoms (score ≥ 5 pts)	116 (22.22)	223 (17.71)	1.33 (1.03–1.71)	1.31 (0.99–1.73)	0.052
Conduct problems (score ≥ 4 pts)	68 (13.03)	185 (14.69)	0.87 (0.64–1.17)	1.08 (0.77–1.51)	0.664
Hyperactivity/inattention (score ≥ 7 pts)	115 (22.03)	252 (20.02)	1.13 (0.88–1.45)	1.25 (0.95–1.65)	0.115
Peer relationship problems (score ≥ 4 pts)	78 (14.94)	191 (15.17)	0.98 (0.74–1.31)	1.16 (0.85–1.59)	0.339
Prosocial behavior (score ≤ 4 pts)	3 (0.57)	25 (1.99)	0.29 (0.86–0.95)	0.47 (0.14–1.63)	0.234
Girls					
Total SDQ (score ≥ 17 pts)	49 (11.21)	143 (11.64)	0.95 (0.68–1.35)	1.16 (0.80–1.69)	0.426
Emotional symptoms (score ≥ 5 pts)	97 (22.20)	250 (20.34)	1.12 (0.85–1.46)	1.08 (0.81–1.43)	0.624
Conduct problems (score ≥ 4 pts)	40 (9.15)	158 (12.86)	0.68 (0.47–0.98)	0.77 (0.52–1.14)	0.192
Hyperactivity/inattention (score ≥ 7 pts)	50 (11.44)	139 (11.31)	1.01 (0.72–1.43)	1.14 (0.79–1.64)	0.498
Peer relationship problems (score ≥ 4 pts)	53 (12.13)	137 (11.15)	1.10 (0.78–1.54)	1.30 (0.90–1.89)	0.164
Prosocial behavior (score ≤ 4 pts)	5 (1.14)	15 (1.22)	0.94 (0.34–2.59)	1.38 (0.47–4.07)	0.562

[a]Logistic regression adjusted according to maternal age, parity, national economic index, maternal educational level, smoking during pregnancy, alcohol comsumption during pregnancy, maternal skin color, infection during pregnancy, pre-gestational BMI, presence of maternal mood issue and use of other analgesics during pregnancy. N after adjustment: 1585 boys and 1494 girls

Table 5 Sensitivity analysis considering Edinburgh Postnatal Depression Scale at 12 months follow-up interview for the association between exposure to acetaminophen during pregnancy and SDQ total and subscales problems of children at 6 and 11 years of age

Outcomes	6 years		11 years	
	Adjusted analysis[a]		Adjusted analysis[a]	
	OR (95% CI)	p[b]	OR (95% CI)	p[b]
Boys				
Total SDQ (score ≥ 17 pts)	1.22 (0.85–1.75)	0.291	1.22 (0.89–1.66)	0.221
Emotional symptoms (score ≥ 5 pts)	1.42 (1.02–1.97)	**0.038**	1.33 (1.01–1.76)	**0.045**
Conduct problems (score ≥ 4 pts)	0.89 (0.64–1.24)	0.503	1.09 (0.78–1.54)	0.609
Hyperactivity/inattention (score ≥ 7 pts)	1.43 (1.05–1.94)	**0.022**	1.25 (0.94–1.65)	0.121
Peer relationship problems (score ≥ 4 pts)	1.21 (0.88–1.67)	0.251	1.14 (0.83–1.57)	0.415
Prosocial behavior (score ≤ 4 pts)	0.65 (0.21–2.03)	0.457	0.48 (0.14–1.66)	0.246
Girls				
Total SDQ (score ≥ 17 pts)	0.99 (0.65–1.51)	0.954	1.14 (0.78–1.67)	0.503
Emotional symptoms (score ≥ 5 pts)	0.90 (0.63–1.28)	0.554	1.06 (0.79–1.42)	0.694
Conduct problems (score ≥ 4 pts)	0.81 (0.55–1.19)	0.290	0.73 (0.49–1.10)	0.135
Hyperactivity/inattention (score ≥ 7 pts)	0.76 (0.51–1.13)	0.175	1.10 (0.76–1.61)	0.613
Peer relationship problems (score ≥ 4 pts)	0.89 (0.60–1.32)	0.559	1.31 (0.90–1.91)	0.155
Prosocial behavior (scor e ≤ 4 pts)	0.75 (0.20–2.80)	0.663	1.39 (0.47–4.15)	0.553

[a]Logistic regression adjusted according to maternal age, parity, national economic index, maternal educational level, smoking during pregnancy, alcohol consumption during pregnancy, maternal skin color, infection during pregnancy, pre-gestational BMI, presence of maternal depression and use of other analgesics during pregnancy. N after adjustment: 1.555 for boys and 1.137 for girls at 6 years; 1.523 for boys and 1.442 for girls at 11 years. [b]p-values marked in bold denote statistically significant results

Discussion

In this study, we examined the association between acetaminophen exposure during pregnancy and the behavioral outcomes of offspring in a Brazilian birth cohort. A differential effect for sex and exposure to acetaminophen was observed. In 6-year-old boys, intrauterine exposure to acetaminophen led to increased odds of having emotional and hyperactivity/inattention problems. At the age of 11, a slight reduction in the effect size was observed. For girls, the results were nonsignificant at both follow-up times for all the considered outcomes. These findings suggest that acetaminophen exposure in the uterus may play a role in behavioral disorders in childhood, mainly in boys.

Acetaminophen is one of the most prescribed and used medications for pregnant women in Brazil [32, 33]. Comparing our results with those of previous studies, an important difference is in exposure prevalence. Although over 50% of pregnant women report using acetaminophen in the United States and Denmark [8, 34–36], we found that 27.5% of Brazilian mothers used this substance during pregnancy. We could not find Brazilian population-based studies reporting acetaminophen use during pregnancy.

Evidence from different prospective cohort studies has shown an association between acetaminophen use during pregnancy and neurobehavioral outcomes in childhood [6–12]. Three studies evaluated behavioral symptoms using the SDQ. In 7-year-old children, Liew et al. [8]

observed an association between prenatal exposure to acetaminophen and higher total difficulties, conduct problems, and hyperactivity. The authors also observed increased risk when the medication was used over more than one trimester, especially near the end of the pregnancy. In addition, they found a correlation between increased frequency of use and increased risk. Stergiakouli et al. [11] demonstrated that children exposed to acetaminophen during the second and third trimesters were at higher risk of multiple behavioral difficulties, including hyperactivity and conduct problems at 7 years of age. Prenatal exposure to acetaminophen during a 32-week pregnancy was also associated with emotional symptoms. Using parent-reported SDQ scores, Thompson et al. [7] observed that acetaminophen was a risk factor for total difficulties, emotional symptoms, and conduct problems at 7 years. At age 11, however, only an association with the parent-reported emotional scale was observed.

Animal studies have supported epidemiological observational studies, providing biological plausibility for the findings. Acetaminophen is known to freely cross the placenta [37]. Recently, exposure to acetaminophen during intrauterine life was reported to affect the modulation of neurotransmission in rats [17]. Effects on neurodevelopment and behavior have also been observed in adult rats exposed to acetaminophen during intrauterine life [15, 16]. Defects in cognitive function and deficient levels of brain-derived neurotrophic factor (BDNF) were observed in rats that were administered acetaminophen during neonatal life [38]. Interference in the regulation of cellular oxidative stress and the endocrine and immune systems by acetaminophen has also been suggested as a mechanism that could lead to neurodevelopment disorders [18–22, 39].

Sex-related differences in symptomatology have been reported for both ADHD and emotional problems. ADHD is more commonly diagnosed in boys than in girls [40], and girls with ADHD are more likely than boys to present inattentive ADHD and separation anxiety disorder. Boys present higher rates of hyperactivity and comorbidity for disorders such as oppositional defiant disorder and conduct disorder [40, 41]. Emotional problems in early adolescence, such as anxiety and depression, are more frequent in girls than in boys [42–45]. In this study, we tested whether sex could modify the effect of acetaminophen on behavioral problems. An interaction between acetaminophen exposure and sex was observed for the hyperactivity and emotional scales, suggesting that acetaminophen may have different effects on these problems in boys and girls. Stratified analyses suggested an effect of acetaminophen on the hyperactivity and emotional scales only in boys.

A similar effect was reported for ASD symptoms in a Spanish cohort [10]. The findings in Spain revealed that exposed boys had more ASD symptoms compared to exposed girls, who showed decreased scores. Differential acetaminophen metabolization between males and females has already been reported and may play a role in this difference, as suggested by Avella-Garcia et al. [10]. Studies on animals have demonstrated that male mice show higher toxicity levels than females after acetaminophen administration [46]. Other sex differences rely on a putatively increased vulnerability to stressors [47] and to the effect of acetaminophen on testosterone regulation [39, 48], neurodevelopment, and brain masculinization [15] in male brains at the beginning of life. Thus, the hypothesis that endocrine disruption influences testicular function and the production of androgens, which further affects brain development in males, could be a plausible mechanism for the present findings.

The results presented in this study suggest that the magnitude of the effect on emotional and hyperactivity/inattention problems slightly decreased from age 6 to 11. Our sensitivity analysis using EPDS showed that the absence of an association in the adjusted analysis at the age of 11 may be due to a lack of power in the analyses for emotional problems. Our results at different ages are in line with the results reported by Thompson et al. [7], which showed differences between both ages for the parent-reported symptoms. Studies evaluating other age groups, including adolescence, are necessary to better understand the relationship between the exposure and the evaluated outcomes.

The results should be interpreted considering certain limitations. The first limitation relates to the retrospective gathering of data on medication use during pregnancy, which may have resulted in difficulty recalling acetaminophen use. Thus, the low prevalence of acetaminophen use observed in this study may be a result of underreporting. We compared our data with that collected in the same population, in 2015, by another birth cohort study (2015 Pelotas Birth Cohort). In this birth cohort, acetaminophen use information was assessed prospectively during pregnancy, as well as in the perinatal interview (retrospectively). The prevalence for use in the perinatal interview was 51% (unpublished data), which agrees with most of the data from published studies [8, 32–34]. Considering that underreporting use of acetaminophen may be a limitation for the exposure definition in our study, we expect that effect size observed in the association analyses is underestimated. Therefore, false negative results are more likely to be observed than false positives regarding this limitation. Second, both the dose-response and timing of exposure associations (higher risks for the third trimester of pregnancy exposure) had been reported previously [8–11, 13]. However, because of possible memory issues, our data did not allow for the evaluation of exposure according to the trimester of pregnancy.

Furthermore, we cannot rule out the effect of using other medications during pregnancy on behavioral outcomes. However, other types of nonsteroidal analgesics were not associated with worse outcomes. Nonsteroidal analgesic use was also included as a covariable in the models. Thus, it is unlikely that co-medication with other analgesics influenced the findings. These results are consistent with the specificity of acetaminophen observed by Thompson et al. [7] and with the results from previous studies that used the same adjustment approach with other analgesics [8]. It has also been shown that children whose mothers have externalizing disorders (e.g., conduct disorder or drug/alcohol dependence) are at an increased risk for developing behavior problems [49]. Although we do not have information regarding externalizing problems in mothers, we included smoking and drinking behavior during pregnancy, which could be considered as proxies. Other psychological variables from mothers would also improve the robustness of our findings. Fever and inflammation during pregnancy are known risk factors for the development of neurological diseases [50]. Werenberg-Dreier et al. [51] showed that exposure to fever and infection over specific timeframes during pregnancy was associated with the occurrence of ADHD. Although the women in the present study reported using the medication, their reasons for doing so were not available. This information would also be important to improve the robustness of our findings. However, this information was not collected in 2004.

Another critical limitation, which has been greatly discussed in the literature, was the presence of residual confounding due to socioeconomic variables. Additional file 1: Table S1 shows socioeconomic variables, including educational level, economic index, skin color, and parity, which are variables that behave as proxies for socioeconomic position (SEP) in Brazil. These variables were all associated with the use of acetaminophen during pregnancy and with most of the outcomes at different ages, especially hyperactivity/inattention problems. While other variables were not statistically associated with our main exposure, we included some of them in the adjusted models given recent evidence suggesting them as possible confounders of this association. However, these variables might not be as important as SEP variables in our models. It is unlikely that residual confounding due to a lack of control over other SEP measurements, such as income and work, may have biased our results. Models were adjusted for variables associated with exposure. Further, the results considered most of the effects of SEP. In addition, crude and adjusted measures of the association between acetaminophen exposure and emotional problems at 11 years of age are very similar, reinforcing the idea that the association was, probably, not confounded by these variables.

Conclusions

The use of acetaminophen in pregnant mothers was associated with subsequent emotional and hyperactivity symptoms in their 6-year-old boys. A suggestive association was observed in 11-year-old boys. Further studies that gather more precise information concerning dose and time of exposure among pregnant women are necessary to establish the long-term effects of maternal acetaminophen use during pregnancy on offspring.

Acknowledgements
Not applicable

Funding
This article is based on data from the study "Pelotas Birth Cohort, 2004" conducted by Postgraduate Program in Epidemiology at Universidade Federal de Pelotas, with the collaboration of the Brazilian Public Health Association (ABRASCO). From 2009 to 2013, the Wellcome Trust supported the 2004 birth cohort study. The World Health Organization, National Support Program for Centers of Excellence (PRONEX), Brazilian National Research Council (CNPq), Brazilian Ministry of Health, and Children's Pastorate supported previous phases of the study. The 11-year follow-up was supported by the Science and Technology Department / Brazilian Ministry of Health, with resources transferred through the Brazilian National Council for Scientific and Technological Development (CNPq), grant 400943/2013–1. This article is supported by São Paulo Reseach Foundation - FAPESP (grant number 2014/13864-6). This study was financed in part by the Coordenação de Aperfeiçoamento de Pessoal de Nível Superior - Brasil (CAPES) - Finance Code 001. Alicia Matijasevich and Iná S. Santos are supported by the CNPq (National Council for Scientific and Technological Development).

Authors' contributions
LT-R, BCS, BD-P, LE, CLdM, ADB, TM-S, FSLV, TNM conceived the work, conducted the analyses and draft the first version of the manuscript. ISS, AM, AB made substantial contributions to acquisition and interpretation of data. MFS, ISS, AM, AB, LAR, LS-F, ADB revised the manuscript critically and contributed with interpretation of the findings. All authors gave final approval of the version to be published.

Consent for publication
Not applicable

Competing interests
LAR has been a member of the speakers' bureau/advisory board and/or acted as a consultant for Eli-Lilly, Janssen-Cilag, Medice, Novartis and Shire in the last three years. He receives authorship royalties from Oxford Press and ArtMed. He has also received travel awards from Shire for his participation in the 2018 APA meetings and from Novartis to take part of the 2016 AACAP meeting. The ADHD and Juvenile Bipolar Disorder Outpatient Programs chaired by him received unrestricted educational and research support from the following pharmaceutical companies in the last three years: Janssen - Cilag, Novartis, and Shire.

Author details
[1]Postgraduate Program in Epidemiology, Universidade Federal de Pelotas, Rua Marechal Deodoro, 1160 - 3° andar, Pelotas, RS 96020-220, Brazil. [2]School of Nursing and Public Health, Universidade Federal de Pelotas, Pelotas, Brazil. [3]Hospital de Clínicas de Porto Alegre, Porto Alegre, Brazil. [4]Postgraduate Program in Genetics and Molecular Biology, Universidade Federal do Rio Grande Do Sul, Porto Alegre, Brazil. [5]Genomic Medicine Laboratory, Hospital de Clínicas de Porto Alegre, Porto Alegre, Brazil. [6]Laboratory of Research in Bioethics and Ethics in Research, Hospital de Clínicas de Porto Alegre, Porto Alegre, Brazil. [7]Department of Psychology, School of Medicine, Universidade Federal de Pelotas, Pelotas, Brazil. [8]Departamento de Medicina Preventiva, Faculdade de Medicina FMUSP, Universidade de São Paulo, São Paulo, Brazil. [9]Department of Psychiatry, Hospital de Clínicas de Porto Alegre, Universidade Federal do Rio Grande do Sul, Porto Alegre, Brazil. [10]National Institute of Developmental Psychiatry for Children and Adolescents, São Paulo, Brazil.

References
1. Brune K, Renner B, Tiegs G. Acetaminophen/paracetamol: A history of errors, failures and false decisions. Eur J Pain (London, England). 2015;19(7):953–65 Epub 2014/11/29.
2. de Fays L, Van Malderen K, De Smet K, Sawchik J, Verlinden V, Hamdani J, et al. Use of paracetamol during pregnancy and child neurological development. Dev Med Child Neurol. 2015;57(8):718–24 Epub 2015/04/09.
3. Mengue SS, Schenkel EP, Duncan BB, Schmidt MI. Drug use by pregnant women in six Brazilian cities. Rev Saude Publica. 2001;35(5):415–20 Epub 2001/11/28. Uso de medicamentos por gestantes em seis cidades brasileiras.
4. Guerra GCB, da Silva AQB, França LB, Assunção PMC, Cabral RX, Ferreira AAA. Drug use during pregnancy in Natal, Brazil. Rev Bras Ginecol Obstet. 2008;30(1):12–8.

5. Melo SCCS, Pelloso SM, Carvalho MDB, Oliveira NLB. Uso de medicamentos por gestantes usuárias do Sistema Único de Saúde. Acta Paul Enferm. 2009; 22:66–70.

6. Liew Z, Ritz B, Virk J, Olsen J. Maternal use of acetaminophen during pregnancy and risk of autism spectrum disorders in childhood: a Danish national birth cohort study. Autism Res. 2016;9(9):951–8.

7. Thompson JMD, Waldie KE, Wall CR, Murphy R, Mitchell EA, the ABCsg. Associations between Acetaminophen Use during Pregnancy and ADHD Symptoms Measured at Ages 7 and 11 Years. PLoS One. 2014;9(9):e108210 Epub 2014/09/25.

8. Liew Z, Ritz B, Rebordosa C, Lee PC, Olsen J. Acetaminophen use during pregnancy, behavioral problems, and hyperkinetic disorders. JAMA Pediatr. 2014;168(4):313–20 Epub 2014/02/26.

9. Brandlistuen RE, Ystrom E, Nulman I, Koren G, Nordeng H. Prenatal paracetamol exposure and child neurodevelopment: a sibling-controlled cohort study. Int J Epidemiol. 2013;42(6):1702–13 Epub 2013/10/29.

10. Avella-Garcia CB, Julvez J, Fortuny J, Rebordosa C, Garcia-Esteban R, Galan IR, et al. Acetaminophen use in pregnancy and neurodevelopment: attention function and autism spectrum symptoms. Int J Epidemiol. 2016; 45(6):1987–96 Epub 2016/06/30.

11. Stergiakouli E, Thapar A, Davey SG. Association of Acetaminophen use during Pregnancy with Behavioral Problems in childhood: evidence against confounding. JAMA Pediatr. 2016;170(10):964–70 Epub 2016/08/18.

12. Ystrom E, Gustavson K, Brandlistuen RE, Knudsen GP, Magnus P, Susser E, et al. Prenatal Exposure to Acetaminophen and Risk of ADHD. Pediatrics. 2017; 140(5) Epub 2017/11/01.

13. Vlenterie R, Wood ME, Brandlistuen RE, Roeleveld N, van Gelder MM, Nordeng H. Neurodevelopmental problems at 18 months among children exposed to paracetamol in utero: a propensity score matched cohort study. Int J Epidemiol. 2016;45(6):1998–2008 Epub 2016/09/03.

14. Masarwa R, Levine H, Gorelik E, Reif S, Perlman A, Matok I. Prenatal exposure to acetaminophen and risk for attention deficit hyperactivity disorder and autistic Spectrum disorder: a systematic review, meta-analysis, and meta-regression analysis of cohort studies. Am J Epidemiol. 2018; Epub 2018/04/25.

15. Hay-Schmidt A, Finkielman OTE, Jensen BAH, Hogsbro CF, Bak Holm J, Johansen KH, et al. Prenatal exposure to paracetamol/acetaminophen and precursor aniline impairs masculinisation of male brain and behaviour. Reproduction (Cambridge, England). 2017;154(2):145–52 Epub 2017/06/01.

16. Philippot G, Gordh T, Fredriksson A, Viberg H. Adult neurobehavioral alterations in male and female mice following developmental exposure to paracetamol (acetaminophen): characterization of a critical period. J Appl Toxicol. 2017;37(10):1174–81 Epub 2017/04/28.

17. Blecharz-Klin K, Joniec-Maciejak I, Jawna K, Pyrzanowska J, Piechal A, Wawer A, et al. Developmental exposure to paracetamol causes biochemical alterations in medulla oblongata. Environ Toxicol Pharmacol. 2015;40(2): 369–74 Epub 2015/08/04.

18. Shaheen SO, Newson RB, Ring SM, Rose-Zerilli MJ, Holloway JW, Henderson AJ. Prenatal and infant acetaminophen exposure, antioxidant gene polymorphisms and childhood asthma. J Allergy Clin Immunol. 2010;126(6): 1141–8.

19. Nuttall SL, Khan JN, Thorpe GH, Langford N, Kendall MJ. The impact of therapeutic doses of paracetamol on serum total antioxidant capacity. J Clin Pharm Ther. 2003;28(4):289–94 Epub 2003/08/13.

20. Thiele K, Solano ME, Huber S, Flavell RA, Kessler T, Barikbin R, et al. Prenatal acetaminophen affects maternal immune and endocrine adaptation to pregnancy, induces placental damage, and impairs fetal development in mice. Am J Pathol. 2015;185(10):2805–18 Epub 2015/08/09.

21. Kristensen DM, Lesne L, Le Fol V, Desdoits-Lethimonier C, Dejucq-Rainsford N, Leffers H, et al. Paracetamol (acetaminophen), aspirin (acetylsalicylic acid) and indomethacin are anti-androgenic in the rat foetal testis. Int J Epidemiol. 2012;35(3):377–84 Epub 2012/05/23.

22. Albert O, Desdoits-Lethimonier C, Lesne L, Legrand A, Guille F, Bensalah K, et al. Paracetamol, aspirin and indomethacin display endocrine disrupting properties in the adult human testis in vitro. Hum Reprod (Oxford, England). 2013;28(7):1890–8 Epub 2013/05/15.

23. Brion MJ, Victora C, Matijasevich A, Horta B, Anselmi L, Steer C, et al. Maternal smoking and child psychological problems: disentangling causal and noncausal effects. Pediatrics. 2010;126(1):e57–65 Epub 2010/07/01.

24. Brion MJ, Lawlor DA, Matijasevich A, Horta B, Anselmi L, Araujo CL, et al. What are the causal effects of breastfeeding on IQ, obesity and blood pressure? Evidence from comparing high-income with middle-income cohorts. Int J Epidemiol. 2011;40(3):670–80 Epub 2011/02/26.

25. Murray E, Pearson R, Fernandes M, Santos IS, Barros FC, Victora CG, et al. Are fetal growth impairment and preterm birth causally related to child attention problems and ADHD? Evidence from a comparison between high-income and middle-income cohorts. J Epidemiol Community Health. 2016;70(7):704–9 Epub 2016/01/16.

26. Santos IS, Barros AJD, Matijasevich A, Zanini R, Chrestani Cesar MA, Camargo-Figuera FA, et al. Cohort Profile Update: 2004 Pelotas (Brazil) Birth Cohort Study. Body composition, mental health and genetic assessment at the 6 years follow-up. Int J Epidemiol. 2014;43(5):1437.

27. Santos IS, Barros AJ, Matijasevich A, Domingues MR, Barros FC, Victora CG. Cohort profile: the 2004 Pelotas (Brazil) birth cohort study. Int J Epidemiol. 2011;40(6):1461–8 Epub 2010/08/13.

28. Fleitlich-Bilyk B, Goodman R. Prevalence of child and adolescent psychiatric disorders in Southeast Brazil. J Am Acad Child Adolesc Psychiatry. 2004; 43(6):727–34 Epub 2004/05/29.

29. Barros AJD, Victora CG. Indicador econômico para o Brasil baseado no censo demográfico de 2000. Rev Saude Publica. 2005;39(4):523–9.

30. Cox JL, Holden JM, Sagovsky R. Detection of postnatal depression. Development of the 10-item Edinburgh postnatal depression scale. Br J Psychiatry J Ment Sci. 1987;150:782–6 Epub 1987/06/01.

31. Santos IS, Matijasevich A, Tavares BF, Barros AJD, Botelho IP, Lapolli C, et al. Validation of the Edinburgh postnatal depression scale (EPDS) in a sample of mothers from the 2004 Pelotas birth cohort study. Cad Saude Publica. 2007;23:2577–88.

32. Costa DB, Coelho HLL, Santos DB. Utilização de medicamentos antes e durante a gestação: prevalência e fatores associados. Cad Saude Publica. 2017;33:e00126215.

33. Brum LFS, Pereira P, Felicetti LL, Silveira RD. Utilização de medicamentos por gestantes usuárias do Sistema Único de Saúde no município de Santa Rosa (RS, Brasil). Cien Saude Colet. 2011;16:2435–42.

34. Werler MM, Mitchell AA, Hernandez-Diaz S, Honein MA. Use of over-the-counter medications during pregnancy. Am J Obstet Gynecol. 2005;193(3 Pt 1):771–7 Epub 2005/09/10.

35. Rebordosa C, Kogevinas M, Bech BH, Sorensen HT, Olsen J. Use of acetaminophen during pregnancy and risk of adverse pregnancy outcomes. Int J Epidemiol. 2009;38(3):706–14 Epub 2009/04/01.

36. Jensen MS, Rebordosa C, Thulstrup AM, Toft G, Sorensen HT, Bonde JP, et al. Maternal use of acetaminophen, ibuprofen, and acetylsalicylic acid during pregnancy and risk of cryptorchidism. Epidemiology (Cambridge, Mass). 2010;21(6):779–85 Epub 2010/09/02.

37. Levy G, Garrettson LK, Soda DM. Evidence of placental transfer of acetaminophen. Pediatrics. 1975;55(6):895 Epub 1975/06/01.

38. Viberg H, Eriksson P, Gordh T, Fredriksson A. Paracetamol (acetaminophen) administration during neonatal brain development affects cognitive function and alters its analgesic and anxiolytic response in adult male mice. Toxicol Sci. 2014;138(1):139–47 Epub 2013/12/24.

39. van den Driesche S, Macdonald J, Anderson RA, Johnston ZC, Chetty T, Smith LB, et al. Prolonged exposure to acetaminophen reduces testosterone production by the human fetal testis in a xenograft model. Sci Transl Med. 2015;7(288):280–8 Epub 2015/05/23.

40. Dalsgaard S, Mortensen PB, Frydenberg M, Thomsen PH. Conduct problems, gender and adult psychiatric outcome of children with attention-deficit hyperactivity disorder. Br J Psychiatry. 2002;181(5):416–21 Epub 2018/01/02.

41. Levy F, Hay DA, Bennett KS, McStephen M. Gender differences in ADHD subtype comorbidity. J Am Acad Child Adolesc Psychiatry. 2005;44(4):368–76 Epub 2005/03/23.

42. Bakhla AK, Sinha P, Sharan R, Binay Y, Verma V, Chaudhury S. Anxiety in school students: role of parenting and gender. Ind Psychiatry J. 2013;22(2): 131–7 Epub 2014/07/12.

43. Costello EJ, Mustillo S, Erkanli A, Keeler G, Angold A. Prevalence and development of psychiatric disorders in childhood and adolescence. Arch Gen Psychiatry. 2003;60(8):837–44 Epub 2003/08/13.

44. Poulton R, Milne BJ, Craske MG, Menzies RG. A longitudinal study of the etiology of separation anxiety. Behav Res Ther. 2001;39(12):1395–410 Epub 2002/01/05.

45. Weiss DD, Last CG. The developmental psychopathology of anxiety. Developmental variations in the prevalence and manifestation of anxiety disorders; 2015.

46. McConnachie LA, Mohar I, Hudson FN, Ware CB, Ladiges WC, Fernandez C, et al. Glutamate cysteine ligase modifier subunit deficiency and gender as

Is intrauterine exposure to acetaminophen associated with emotional and hyperactivity problems...

265

determinants of acetaminophen-induced hepatotoxicity in mice. Toxicol Sci. 2007;99(2):628–36.

47. Taylor E. In: Rutter M, Bishop D, Pine D, Scott S, Stevenson JS, Thapar A, editors. Rutter's child and adolescent psychiatry. 5th ed. Oxford: WILEY-BLACKWELL; 2010.

48. Kristensen DM, Hass U, Lesne L, Lottrup G, Jacobsen PR, Desdoits-Lethimonier C, et al. Intrauterine exposure to mild analgesics is a risk factor for development of male reproductive disorders in human and rat. Hum Reprod (Oxford, England). 2011;26(1):235–44 Epub 2010/11/10.

49. Weijers D, van Steensel FJA, Bogels SM. Associations between psychopathology in mothers, fathers and their children: a structural modeling approach. J Child Fam Stud. 2018;27(6):1992–2003 Epub 2018/05/15.

50. Mann JR, McDermott S. Are maternal genitourinary infection and pre-eclampsia associated with ADHD in school-aged children? J Atten Disord. 2010;15(8):667–73.

51. Werenberg Dreier J, Nybo Andersen AM, Hvolby A, Garne E, Kragh Andersen P, Berg-Beckhoff G. Fever and infections in pregnancy and risk of attention deficit/hyperactivity disorder in the offspring. J Child Psychol Psychiatry Allied Discip. 2016;57(4):540–8 Epub 2015/11/05.

Permissions

All chapters in this book were first published in PSYCHIATRY, by BioMed Central; hereby published with permission under the Creative Commons Attribution License or equivalent. Every chapter published in this book has been scrutinized by our experts. Their significance has been extensively debated. The topics covered herein carry significant findings which will fuel the growth of the discipline. They may even be implemented as practical applications or may be referred to as a beginning point for another development.

The contributors of this book come from diverse backgrounds, making this book a truly international effort. This book will bring forth new frontiers with its revolutionizing research information and detailed analysis of the nascent developments around the world.

We would like to thank all the contributing authors for lending their expertise to make the book truly unique. They have played a crucial role in the development of this book. Without their invaluable contributions this book wouldn't have been possible. They have made vital efforts to compile up to date information on the varied aspects of this subject to make this book a valuable addition to the collection of many professionals and students.

This book was conceptualized with the vision of imparting up-to-date information and advanced data in this field. To ensure the same, a matchless editorial board was set up. Every individual on the board went through rigorous rounds of assessment to prove their worth. After which they invested a large part of their time researching and compiling the most relevant data for our readers.

The editorial board has been involved in producing this book since its inception. They have spent rigorous hours researching and exploring the diverse topics which have resulted in the successful publishing of this book. They have passed on their knowledge of decades through this book. To expedite this challenging task, the publisher supported the team at every step. A small team of assistant editors was also appointed to further simplify the editing procedure and attain best results for the readers.

Apart from the editorial board, the designing team has also invested a significant amount of their time in understanding the subject and creating the most relevant covers. They scrutinized every image to scout for the most suitable representation of the subject and create an appropriate cover for the book.

The publishing team has been an ardent support to the editorial, designing and production team. Their endless efforts to recruit the best for this project, has resulted in the accomplishment of this book. They are a veteran in the field of academics and their pool of knowledge is as vast as their experience in printing. Their expertise and guidance has proved useful at every step. Their uncompromising quality standards have made this book an exceptional effort. Their encouragement from time to time has been an inspiration for everyone.

The publisher and the editorial board hope that this book will prove to be a valuable piece of knowledge for researchers, students, practitioners and scholars across the globe.

List of Contributors

Masanori Nagamine and Kunio Shimizu
Division of Behavioral Science, National Defense Medical College Research Institute, 3-2 Namiki, Tokorozawa, Saitama 359-8513, Japan

Jun Shigemura, Masaaki Tanichi, Taku Saito, Hiroyuki Toda and Aihide Yoshino
Department of Psychiatry, School of Medicine, National Defense Medical College, 3-2 Namiki, Tokorozawa, Saitama, Japan

Toshimichi Fujiwara and Fumiko Waki
Japan Ground Self-Defense Force Medical School, 1-2-24, Ikejiri, Setagaya-ku, Tokyo, Japan

Stanley N. Caroff
Department of Psychiatry, Corporal Michael J. Crescenz VA Medical Center and the Perelman School of Medicine at the University of Pennsylvania, 3900 Woodland Avenue, Philadelphia, PA 19104, USA

Fan Mu and Rajeev Ayyagari
Analysis Group, 111 Huntington Ave, Boston, MA 02199, USA

Traci Schilling, Victor Abler and Benjamin Carroll
Teva Pharmaceutical Industries, 41 Moores Rd, Frazer, Malvern, PA 19355, USA

Lian Tong and Qiong Yan
Department of Maternal, China and Adolescent Health, School of Public Health, Fudan University/ Key laboratory Public Health Safety, Chinese Ministry of Education, 138 Yixueyuan Road, Shanghai 200032, China

Yan Ye
Department of Behavior and Psychology Science, Zhejiang University, Hangzhou, China

Suzanne McCarthy
School of Pharmacy, University College Cork, Cork, Ireland

Antje Neubert
Department of Paediatrics and Adolescents Medicine, University Hospital Erlangen, Erlangen, Germany

Ian C. K. Wong
Centre for Paediatric Pharmacy Research, Research Department of Practice and Policy, UCL School of Pharmacy, London, UK
Centre for Safe Medication Practice and Research, Department of Pharmacology and Pharmacy, Li Ka Shing Faculty of Medicine, The University of Hong Kong, Hong Kong, Hong Kong

Kenneth K. C. Man
Centre for Paediatric Pharmacy Research, Research Department of Practice and Policy, UCL School of Pharmacy, London, UK
Department of Paediatrics and Adolescent Medicine, Li Ka Shing Faculty of Medicine, The University of Hong Kong, Hong Kong, Hong Kong
Department of Medical Informatics, Erasmus University Medical Center, Rotterdam, Netherlands

Tobias Banaschewski, Alexander Häge and Konstantin Mechler
Department of Child and Adolescent Psychiatry and Psychotherapy, Medical Faculty Mannheim, Central Institute of Mental Health, University of Heidelberg, Mannheim, Germany

Jan Buitelaar
Department of Cognitive Neuroscience, Donders Institute for Brain, Cognition and Behavior, Radboud University Medical Centre, and Karakter Child and Adolescent Psychiatry University Centre, Nijmegen, The Netherlands

Sara Carucci and Alessandro Zuddas
Child and Adolescent Neuropsychiatry Unit, Department of Biomedical Science, University of Cagliari and "A. Cao" Pediatric Hospital, Brotzu Hospital Trust, Cagliari, Italy

David Coghill
Departments of Paediatrics and Psychiatry, Faculty of Medicine, Dentistry and Health Sciences, University of Melbourne, Melbourne, Australia
Murdoch Children's Research Institute, Melbourne, Australia
Division of Neuroscience, School of Medicine, University of Dundee, Dundee, UK

Marina Danckaerts
Department of Child and Adolescent Psychiatry, University Psychiatric Center, Leuven, KU, Belgium
Department of Neurosciences, University Psychiatric Center, Leuven, KU, Belgium

Bruno Falissard
University Paris-Sud, Univ. Paris-Descartes, AP-HP, INSERM U1178, Paris, France

Peter Garas and Peter Nagy
Vadaskert Child and Adolescent Psychiatric Hospital, Budapest, Hungary

Chris Hollis
Division of Psychiatry and Applied Psychology, Institute of Mental Health, School of Medicine, University of Nottingham, Nottingham, UK

Elizabeth Liddle
Division of Psychiatry and Applied Psychology, Institute of Mental Health, School of Medicine, University of Nottingham, Nottingham, UK
Institute of Mental Health, Nottingham, UK

Sarah Inglis
Tayside Clinical Trials Unit, University of Dundee, Dundee, UK

Hanna Kovshoff
Department of Psychology, University of Southampton, Southampton, UK

Eric Rosenthal
Department of Paediatric Cardiology, Evelina Children's Hospital, St Thomas' Hospital, London, UK

Robert Schlack
Unit of Mental Health Department of Epidemiology and Health Reporting, Robert Koch Institute, Berlin, Germany

Edmund Sonuga-Barke
Department of Child and Adolescent Psychiatry, Institute of Psychiatry, King's College London, London, UK
Department of Experimental Clinical and Health Psychology, Ghent University, Ghent, Belgium

Stephanie Book, Katharina Luttenberger and Elmar Graessel
Center for Health Services Research in Medicine, Department of Psychiatry and Psychotherapy, Friedrich-Alexander Universität Erlangen-Nürnberg, Schwabachanlage 6, 91054 Erlangen, Germany

Mark Stemmler
Institute of Psychology, Friedrich-Alexander-Universität Erlangen-Nürnberg, Nägelsbachstr. 49c, 91052 Erlangen, Germany

Sebastian Meyer
Institute of Medical Informatics, Biometry, and Epidemiology, Friedrich-Alexander-Universität Erlangen-Nürnberg, Waldstraße 6, 91054 Erlangen, Germany

Eric Achtyes
Cherry Health and Michigan State University College of Human Medicine, Grand Rapids, MI, USA

Adam Simmons, Anna Skabeev, Nikki Levy, Ying Jiang and Peter J. Weiden
Alkermes, Inc., Waltham, MA, USA

Patricia Marcy
Vanguard Research Group, Northwell Health System, Manhasset, NY, USA

Tarek Rajji
Division of Geriatric Psychiatry, Centre for Addiction and Mental Health, Toronto, Canada
Department of Psychiatry, University of Toronto, Toronto, Canada

Pallavi Dham
Division of Geriatric Psychiatry, Centre for Addiction and Mental Health, Toronto, Canada
Department of Psychiatry, University of Toronto, Toronto, Canada
Centre for Addiction and Mental Health, 80 Workman Way, 6th floor, Room 6312, Toronto, ON M6J1H4, Canada

Neeraj Gupta, Jacob Alexander, Warwick Black and Elaine Skinner
Departments of Psychiatry, Rural and Remote Mental Health Services, Adelaide, South Australia

Johan Bjureberg, Hanna Sahlin and Clara Hellner
Centre for Psychiatry Research, Department of Clinical Neuroscience, Karolinska Institutet, and Stockholm Health Care Services, Stockholm County Council, Norra stationsgatan 69, SE-11364 Stockholm, Sweden

Brjánn Ljótsson
Centre for Psychiatry Research, Department of Clinical Neuroscience, Karolinska Institutet, and Stockholm Health Care Services, Stockholm County Council, Norra stationsgatan 69, SE-11364 Stockholm, Sweden
Division of Psychology, Department of Clinical Neuroscience, Karolinska Institutet, Nobels väg 9, SE-171 65 Stockholm, Sweden

Jussi Jokinen
Centre for Psychiatry Research, Department of Clinical Neuroscience, Karolinska Institutet, and Stockholm Health Care Services, Stockholm County Council, Norra stationsgatan 69, SE-11364 Stockholm, Sweden
Department of Clinical Sciences/Psychiatry, Umeå University, By 23, Enheten för psykiatri, 901 85 Umeå, Sweden

Erik Hedman-Lagerlöf
Division of Psychology, Department of Clinical Neuroscience, Karolinska Institutet, Nobels väg 9, SE-171 65 Stockholm, Sweden

Kim L. Gratz and Matthew T. Tull
Department of Psychology, University of Toledo, 2801 W. Bancroft Street, Toledo, OH 43606, USA

Erlend Bugge and Ole Kristian Grønli
Division of Mental Health and Addictions, University Hospital of North Norway, N-9037 Tromsø, Norway

Rolf Wynn
Department of Clinical Medicine, UiT The Arctic University of Norway, N-9038 Tromsø, Norway

Tom Eirik Mollnes
UiT The Arctic University of Norway, K.G. Jebsen TREC, N-9038 Tromsø, Norway
Research Laboratory, Nordland Hospital, Bodø, Norway
Faculty of Health Sciences, K.G. Jebsen TREC, University of Tromsø, Tromsø, Norway
Department of Immunology, Oslo University Hospital, and University of Oslo, Oslo, Norway
Centre of Molecular Inflammation Research, Norwegian University of Science and Technology, Trondheim, Norway

Solveig Klæbo Reitan
Norwegian University of Science and Technology, Faculty of Medicine and Health Sciences, N-7491 Trondheim, Norway

Junling Li
School of Traditional Chinese Medicine, Capital Medical University, Beijing 100069, China
Beijing University of Chinese Medicine, Beijing 100029, China

Kai Xia, Tian Wang, Kuo Gao, Jianxin Chen, Huihui Zhao and Wei Wang
Beijing University of Chinese Medicine, Beijing 100029, China

Ran Yang
Cardiovascular department of Guang'anmen Hospital, China Academy of Chinese Medical Sciences, Beijing 100053, China

Binbin Nie
Key Laboratory of Nuclear Analytical Techniques, Institute of High Energy Physics, Chinese Academy of Sciences, Beijing 100049, China

Yubo Li
Institute of Basic Theory for Chinese Medicine, China Academy of Chinese Medical Sciences, Beijing 100700, China

Robbin H. Ophuis, Branko F. Olij, Suzanne Polinder and Juanita A. Haagsma
Department of Public Health, Erasmus University Medical Center, 3000, CA, Rotterdam, The Netherlands

Yimenu Yitayih, Mubarek Abera, Eliais Tesfaye, Almaz Mamaru and Matiwos Soboka
Department of Psychiatry, College of Health Sciences, Jimma University, Jimma, Ethiopia

Kristina Adorjan
Center for International Health, Ludwig-Maximilians-Universität, Munich, Germany
Department of Psychiatry and Psychotherapy, Medical Center of the University of Munich, Munich, Germany
Institute of Psychiatric Phenomics and Genomics (IPPG), Medical Center of the University of Munich, Munich, Germany

Åsa U. Lindh, Karin Beckman Marie Dahlin and Bo Runeson
Centre for Psychiatry Research, Department of Clinical Neuroscience, Karolinska Institutet, and Stockholm Health Care Services, Stockholm County Council, S:t Görans Hospital, Vårdvägen 1, SE-112 81 Stockholm, Sweden

Margda Waern
Department of Psychiatry and Neurochemistry, University of Göteborg, Gothenburg, Sweden

Ellinor Salander Renberg
Department of Clinical Sciences, Division of Psychiatry, University of Umeå, Umeå, Sweden

Tarran Prangley
School of Medicine, University of Wollongong, Wollongong, Australia

Sabrina Winona Pit
School of Medicine, University Centre for Rural Health, Western Sydney University, 61 Uralba Street, Lismore, NSW 2480, Australia
Sydney Medical School, University of Sydney, 61 Uralba Street, Lismore, NSW 2480, Australia

Trent Rees
The Buttery, Bangalow, Australia

Jessica Nealon
Faculty of Science, Medicine and Health, School of Medicine, University of Wollongong, Wollongong, Australia

Nicola J. Reavley, Amy J. Morgan, Julie-Anne Fischer and Anthony F. Jorm
Centre for Mental Health, Melbourne School of Population and Global Health, University of Melbourne, 207 Bouverie Street, Carlton, VIC 3010, Australia

Betty Kitchener and Nataly Bovopoulos
Mental Health First Aid Australia, 369 Royal Parade, Parkville, VIC 3052, Australia

Joanne C. King and Christopher W. N. Saville
School of Psychology, Bangor University, Bangor, Gwynedd, UK

Michaela A. Swales
School of Psychology, Bangor University, Bangor, Gwynedd, UK
Besti Cadwaladr University Health Board, Bangor, Gwynedd, UK

Richard Hibbs
Integral Business Support Ltd, Wrexham, UK

Ian D Maidment, Niyah Campbell and Rachel Shaw
School of Life and Health Sciences, Aston University, Birmingham B4 7ET, UK

Sarah Damery
Institute of Applied Health Research, College of Medical and Dental Sciences, University of Birmingham, Edgbaston, Birmingham B15 2TT, UK

Nichola Seare
Aston Health Research Innovation Cluster, Aston University, Birmingham B4 7ET, UK

Chris Fox
Norwich Medical School, University of East Anglia, Earlham Road, Norwich, Norfolk NR4 7TJ, UK

Steve Iliffe and Jane Wilcock
Research Department of Primary Care and Population Health, University College London, Royal Free Campus, Rowland Hill St, London NW3 2PF, UK

Andrea Hilton
Faculty of Health Science, University of Hull, Hull HU6 7RX, UK

Graeme Brown and Nigel Barnes
Birmingham and Solihull Mental Health NHS Foundation Trust, Unit 1, B1, 50 Summer Hill Road, Birmingham B1 3RB, UK

Emma Randle
National Centre for Mental Health, Research and Innovation Department, The Barberry, 25 Vincent Drive, Birmingham B15 2FG, UK

Sarah Gillespie
Department of Clinical Healthcare, Faculty of Health and Life Sciences, Oxford Brookes University, Gipsy Lane Campus, Headington, Oxford OX3 0FL, UK

Garry Barton
Norwich Clinical Trials Unit, University of East Anglia, Earlham Road, Norwich, Norfolk NR4 7TJ, UK

Katharina Piontek
Institute for Medical Psychology, University Medicine Greifswald, Greifswald, Germany
Department of Psychosomatic Medicine and Psychotherapy, University Medical Center Hamburg-Eppendorf, Hamburg, Germany

Meike C. Shedden-Mora, Maria Gladigau, Amina Kuby and Bernd Löwe
Department of Psychosomatic Medicine and Psychotherapy, University Medical Center Hamburg-Eppendorf, Hamburg, Germany

Allitia DiBernardo, Xiwu Lin, Qiaoyi Zhang, Jim Xiang, Lang Lu, Carol Jamieson and Kwan Lee
Janssen Research and Development, LLC, Titusville, NJ, USA

Gang Li
Janssen Research and Development, LLC, Titusville, NJ, USA
Real World Evidence, Statistics and Decision Sciences, Janssen R&D US, 920 US Highway 202 S, Raritan, NJ 08869, USA

Carmela Benson
Janssen Scientific Affairs, LLC, Titusville, NJ, USA

Robert Bodén
Department of Neuroscience, Psychiatry, Uppsala University, Uppsala, Sweden
Centre for Pharmacoepidemiology, Clinical Epidemiology, Department of Medicine Solna, Karolinska Institutet, Karolinska University Hospital, Stockholm, Sweden

Lena Brandt, Philip Brenner and Johan Reutfors
Centre for Pharmacoepidemiology, Clinical Epidemiology, Department of Medicine Solna, Karolinska Institutet, Karolinska University Hospital, Stockholm, Sweden

Kamelia Harris
Division of Psychology and Mental Health, School of Health Sciences, University of Manchester, Zochonis Building, Brunswick St, Manchester M13 9PL, UK

Emma Shaw-Núñez
Division of Psychology and Mental Health, School of Health Sciences, University of Manchester, Zochonis Building, Brunswick St, Manchester M13 9PL, UK
Greater Manchester Mental Health NHS Trust, Manchester, UK

Sarah Peters and Patricia A Gooding
Division of Psychology and Mental Health, School of Health Sciences, University of Manchester, Zochonis Building, Brunswick St, Manchester M13 9PL, UK
Manchester Academic Health Science Centre, MAHSC, Manchester, UK
Manchester Centre for Health Psychology, University of Manchester, Manchester, UK

Yvonne F Awenat, Daniel Pratt and Gillian Haddock
Division of Psychology and Mental Health, School of Health Sciences, University of Manchester, Zochonis Building, Brunswick St, Manchester M13 9PL, UK
Manchester Academic Health Science Centre, MAHSC, Manchester, UK
Greater Manchester Mental Health NHS Trust, Manchester, UK

Maria Basta, Alexandros Vgontzas, Maria Anastasaki and Panagiotis Simos
Department of Psychiatry, University Hospital of Heraklion, Voutes, Heraklion, 71110 Crete, Greece

Anastasia Kastanaki, Manolis Michalodimitrakis and Katerina Kanaki
Department of Forensic Science, School of Medicine, University of Crete, Voutes, Heraklion, 71003 Crete, Greece

Katerina Koutra
Department of Psychology, School of Social Sciences, University of Crete, Gallos, Rethymnon, 74100 Crete, Greece

Christian Dalton-Locke, Rosie Attard and Helen Killaspy
Division of Psychiatry, University College London, Maple House, 149 Tottenham Court Road, London W1T 7NF, UK

Sarah White
Population Health Research Institute, St George's, University of London, Cranmer Terrace, London SW17 0RE, UK

Aslak Steinsbekk
Department of Public Health and Nursing, Norwegian University of Science and Technology, 7491 Trondheim, Norway

Eirik Roos
Department of Public Health and Nursing, Norwegian University of Science and Technology, 7491 Trondheim, Norway
Health and Welfare, Trondheim, Norway

Ottar Bjerkeset
Faculty of Nursing and Health Sciences, Nord University, Levanger, Norway
Department of Mental Health, Norwegian University of Science and Technology, Trondheim, Norway

Xiaoqi Feng
Population Wellbeing and Environment Research Lab (PowerLab), School of Health and Society, Faculty of Social Sciences, University of Wollongong, Wollongong, NSW, Australia
Menzies Centre for Health Policy, University of Sydney, Sydney, NSW, Australia
Illawarra Health and Medical Research Institute (IHMRI), University of Wollongong and Illawarra and Shoalhaven Local Health District, Wollongong, NSW, Australia

Thomas Astell-Burt
Population Wellbeing and Environment Research Lab (PowerLab), School of Health and Society, Faculty of Social Sciences, University of Wollongong, Wollongong, NSW, Australia
Menzies Centre for Health Policy, University of Sydney, Sydney, NSW, Australia
Illawarra Health and Medical Research Institute (IHMRI), University of Wollongong and Illawarra and Shoalhaven Local Health District, Wollongong, NSW, Australia
School of Public Health, Peking Union Medical College and the Chinese Academy of Medical Sciences, Beijing, China

Luciana Tovo-Rodrigues, Bruna Celestino Schneider, Thais Martins-Silva, Bianca Del-Ponte, Ludmila Entiauspe, Mariângela Freitas Silveira, Iná S. Santos, Aluísio J. D. Barros and Andréa Dâmaso Bertoldi
Postgraduate Program in Epidemiology, Universidade Federal de Pelotas, Rua Marechal Deodoro, 1160 - 3° andar, Pelotas, RS 96020-220, Brazil

Tiago N. Munhoz
Postgraduate Program in Epidemiology, Universidade Federal de Pelotas, Rua Marechal Deodoro, 1160 - 3° andar, Pelotas, RS 96020-220, Brazil
Department of Psychology, School of Medicine, Universidade Federal de Pelotas, Pelotas, Brazil

Christian Loret de Mola
School of Nursing and Public Health, Universidade Federal de Pelotas, Pelotas, Brazil

Lavinia Schuler-Faccini
Hospital de Clínicas de Porto Alegre, Porto Alegre, Brazil

Fernanda Sales Luiz Vianna
Postgraduate Program in Genetics and Molecular Biology, Universidade Federal do Rio Grande Do Sul, Porto Alegre, Brazil
Genomic Medicine Laboratory, Hospital de Clínicas de Porto Alegre, Porto Alegre, Brazil

Laboratory of Research in Bioethics and Ethics in Research, Hospital de Clínicas de Porto Alegre, Porto Alegre, Brazil

Alicia Matijasevich
Departamento de Medicina Preventiva, Faculdade de Medicina FMUSP, Universidade de São Paulo, São Paulo, Brazil

Luis Augusto Rohde
Department of Psychiatry, Hospital de Clínicas de Porto Alegre, Universidade Federal do Rio Grande do Sul, Porto Alegre, Brazil
National Institute of Developmental Psychiatry for Children and Adolescents, São Paulo, Brazil

Index